For Those Who <u>Only Want the Best</u>, We Offer...

The World's Most Premium Herbal Based Gut Cleansing Formula For Candida & Gut Disorders

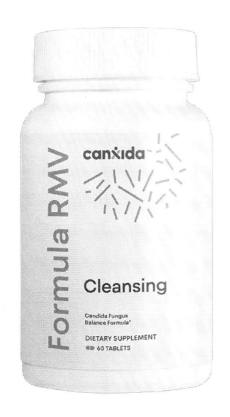

CanXida Remove (RMV) is:

- Clinician formulated based on +30 years of experience treating Candida, IBS, SIBO, Leaky Gut, IBD & more.

- Uses standardized ingredients in a sustain release form (targets all parts of GI tract).

- Gentle on the digestive sytem. Suitable for seniors & people with poor gut function.

- Designed to work even for severe cases where the patient has been sick for YEARS.

- Comes with 28 page User Guide booklet & YouTube channel with +2,000 gut health related videos to help patients get well.

Click Here or Visit <u>www.canxida.com</u> Today to Learn More

TABLE OF CONTENTS

ADDITIONAL RESOURCES

To further support your journey, we are delighted to offer you an array of complimentary resources designed to complement the insights and strategies shared within this book.

As a valued reader, you have exclusive access to a suite of helpful tools, including:

- **Comprehensive Handouts:** A detailed list of foods to eat and avoid to maintain a balanced diet.

- **Candida Diet and Cleanse Progress Tracker:** Monitor your progress with a tailored tracker that keeps you motivated and on course.

- **Curated List of Candida Diet-Friendly Recipes:** Discover delicious, healthy recipes that align with your dietary goals.

- **Candida Health Planner:** A personalized planner to help organize your health journey and optimize your daily regimen.

- **Additional Informative Handouts:** Gain further insights and tips to make your treatment journey smoother and more effective.

- **Significant Discounts on CanXida Supplements:** Readers of this book get special introductory discount on all CanXida products.

These resources are designed to make your treatment journey as straightforward and effective as possible. To access your free resources, please visit **CanXida.com**, or reach out to us directly via email at **support@canxida.com** or by phone at **+1 (888) 508-3171**. When contacting our customer care team, simply mention that you have read our book and are calling or writing to request the resources included with the **Candida Crusher** book.

We are here to support you every step of the way. Don't hesitate to get in touch for any further assistance or information.

CHAPTER 1

Introduction

Welcome To Candida Crusher

By Eric Bakker B.A.Sc. (Comp.Med). N.D.

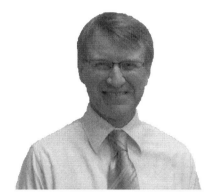

Candida albicans, candidiasis or a yeast infection has become a hidden epidemic in many parts of the world. It has been and is increasingly becoming a major illness in its own right, as well as a contributing and underlying causative factor in many other chronic illnesses. Health problems involving yeast infections are one of the primary reasons patients come to see us as natural healthcare professionals, and for over twenty years, people have come seeking my assistance with many different yeast infection related health issues.

If you suspect or know that you may be suffering from a yeast infection, Candida Crusher provides you with right guidelines for understanding the causes of candidiasis, as well as diagnosing and treating this common condition with nutrition and natural medicine in addition to incorporating the appropriate lifestyle changes.

There are several reasons why candida is such a major issue today; just as big a problem if not bigger than it was in the eighties when everybody talked about it. It is easy to think that this condition only affects a few people when in fact yeast overgrowth and dysbiosis are rampant conditions affecting countless people we see today. It has been estimated that more than 60 million people in America alone are affected by yeast infection and the number is increasing.

In the eighties it was called a yeast infection or candidiasis, but many people today who have a yeast infection believe they have (or may mistakenly been diagnosed as having) irritable bowel syndrome, a food allergy, gluten intolerance, inflammatory bowel disease, psoriasis or many other different conditions which may appear at first to be an illness in their own right, but in fact have a yeast infection as one of their underlying and primary causes. Yeast infections today are more prevalent than they have ever been since not only the discovery and rampant prescribing of antibiotics and steroidal drugs, but other drugs such as immune modulating drugs and non-steroidal anti-inflammatory drugs, aka NSAIDS. Sugar-laden foods have never been so cheap and widely available in history previously, and our ever-increasing consumption of sugars in our diets (like high fructose corn syrup) along with an increasing reliance of packaged, processed and take-out foods, we can expect yeast infections to only get worse in the future.

Today, our high level of technological advances coupled with sedentary lifestyles mean that many people do not exercise adequately nor pay sufficient attention to maintaining healthy (home-cooked) diets and balanced (low-stress) lifestyles. Yeast infections therefore play an even greater role today than they ever have at any time in our history, and they seem especially common in the hurried, worried and stressed kinds of people. The people who most commonly seem to get yeast infections are the same kinds of people who tend to get adrenal fatigue, they tend to be the busy people, the workers, the doers, the A-type people, carers or over-achievers.

I have commonly found that people who have imbalanced lifestyles are especially prone to a yeast infection, and the 21st century with all its technological advances has spawned a whole new generation of hurried, worried and stressed individuals showing signs of candidiasis. Candida, just like heart disease, diabetes and cancer, is a disease of modern civilization and if left unchecked and allowed to take its course can lead to a more widespread chronic and degenerative illness. It is the small yet continuous dietary and lifestyle indiscretions that need adjustment in a person's life before they become major health crises, and any health-care professional is all too well aware that every dollar spent today on preventive health will save four dollars tomorrow. Candida Crusher is all about revealing these indiscretions and what you can do about them right now, today.

I am going to tell you what most books on this topic won't, that it is not easy to get really well and to remain really well, it will require plenty of commitment and will power to stay on track the first month or two, especially if you have been suffering with a chronic yeast infection several years duration! Have you been lured into believing the sales pitch "Yeast Infection Cured In Two Weeks" for example? Or what about "The 12 hour Cure", what a bunch of baloney, you simply cannot "cure candida in 12 hours"; it needs a clear plan of action, consistent effort, application, and plenty of self-discipline and perseverance. I have tried to write Candida Crusher as informative and "baloney-free" as possible yet tried to maintain a degree of simplicity and a minimum of technical jargon, and trust that it is light, easy to read, humorous in parts yet informative and comprehensive enough to use as a self-help guide for those who present with the many and varied manifestations of a yeast infection.

When I first started treating yeast infections in the late 80's, my knowledge and treatment protocols were largely based on the work of American pioneers in this field such as Doctors William Crook, Orian Truss, Sidney Baker, and John Trowbridge, but in addition, my treatments were also based on lesser-known naturopathic pioneers from Australia from the 1970's and 1980's such as William Vayda, Denis Stewart, Walter Last and Dorothy Hall. These early candida pioneers employed techniques that have served me well initially, and some of them I still use today because they have proven to work so consistently and reliably. Why make changes when you get results? "If it ain't broke then don't fix it" a mechanic friend told me once.

My teachers and mentors used their collective experiences and empirical observations along with a good deal of common sense yet employed no fancy technology or the internet to work out the best treatment outcomes for their patients. My belief is that some of the best health practitioners lived many years ago when limitations were at there greatest, and a sharp and observant mind, minimal tools and a keen sense of learning were some of the best tools they had. Their very reputations were based on gaining the best outcomes for their patients.

In the early 90's I completed post graduation education with Dr. Subrata Banerjea, who taught me the finer art of classical homeopathy. I practiced as a homeopath for the first several years in my natural medicine career, and then went on to study nutrition, naturopathic medicine and herbal medicine that culminated in my Bachelor Degree of Science majoring in Complementary Medicine. In my later years of practice, Dr. Alan Gaby from America inspired me to take up nutritional medicine to a greater degree and I completed his Nutritional Therapy in Medical Practice training in Seattle.

Dr. Gaby made me aware of the critical role of nutritional medicine in clinical practice, and you will find a strong emphasis on many aspects of diet and nutrition in the Candida Crusher. Other diet and nutrition authors who have influenced my work over the years include authors such as Sally Fallon, David Wolfe, Pierre Dukan, Michael Barbee, Michael Pollan, Donna Gates and many others.

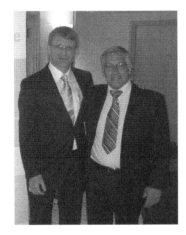

More recently, my current mentor and good friend is Dr. James Wilson from Arizona, USA. Dr. Wilson is the world's authority in adrenal fatigue. After having studied adrenal fatigue since 2007 and having treated several thousand patients using Dr. Wilson's unique protocols, I have come to see adrenal fatigue as one of the missing links in chronic yeast infection treatment, particularly in the deep recovery phase of those with severe yeast infections of long duration. There is a considerable emphasis on stress and adrenal fatigue in the Candida Crusher, and it is one of the main reasons my chronic cases have responded so well and have had the ability to recover deeper and faster than by any other methods I have tried.

Patients however have always been my best teachers, and no matter how many years I have been in clinical practice, there will always be something more to learn and for that reason I am always on the lookout for better tools and clinical protocols that will enable my patients to improve and recover more rapidly with the least amount of aggravation.

Candida Crusher is the culmination of knowledge regarding yeast infection I have distilled from my association with various mentors as well as with countless patients. I would like to personally thank every patient for trusting me enough by placing the treatment of his or her yeast infection in my care.

The book you now hold in your hands is the end result of many thousands of hours spent in the clinic with patients with all manner of acute and chronic yeast related complaints; time spent researching countless books, online resources as well as trial and error and plain old common sense. But in addition to my clinic there has been much time I've invested with many health-care professionals in many different healing disciplines spanning more than two decades, taking into account their ideas on the most effective ways of treating yeast infections, digestive problems, stress-related issues, and many other health concerns. Every practitioner has his or her own professional experience to share and it is the combination of these many shared and accumulated experiences from both patient treatments and practitioner relationships that I have distilled into Candida

Crusher, hard earned knowledge from which I hope you will gain an insight into your yeast-related health concerns.

Writing a non-fiction book is no easy task, it takes plenty of time and has to be factually correct. Candida Crusher took three years to complete after constant requests from many patients who have been waiting for my book on yeast infections for a long time. The completion of this book has also been very much to the relief of my wife!

Candida Crusher contains a simple step-by-step approach that will guide you through the program clearly and logically. Chapter 7 is the main treatment chapter in this book and contains five sections, it will show you in many highly effective ways that it is all about creating a healthy balance inside and outside your body, and how you can restore your body back to a healthy balance by adopting a holistic approach to your candida program.

You may find the Table Of Contents (TOC) of the Candida Crusher to be a bit extreme being literally dozens of pages, but I did this for a very valid reason. The great thing about an e-book is that all the links in the TOC are clickable, all you need to do is to scroll away until you find what you want to read, then click on the section and you will be instantly transported to that section of the book. Hit the back button and you are back to the TOC. Who needs an index when you can use the Table Of Contents much quicker instead? You may also find the sheer size of the Candida Crusher book a bit extreme, but by using the clickable TOC navigation will be a snap, and I'm sure many will appreciate having the extra information. Did you print it out? That's fine too; just use the page numbers to navigate. I use slips of paper to bookmark the important places in my books.

Many books I have seen on candida are extensions of recipe or cookbooks, and I didn't want to create just another yeast infection book three quarters full of re-hashed recipes. If you are interested in yeast infection recipes, you will find countless recipes online, and will be able to key-word search for the exact recipe you are looking for. The diet and nutrition section of Candida Crusher however is very comprehensive and contains a great deal of useful information along with plenty of unique hints and tips on treating and overcoming your yeast infection by dietary means you simply won't find anywhere else in any book, blog, forum or web page on the topic.

One of the most important points of the Candida Crusher, and hence its size, is to not only help you overcome your yeast infection, but to teach you how to maintain a healthy body and thereby reduce your chances of prematurely developing many different chronic illnesses. Candida Crusher is about holistic treatment, and the term holistic implies treating the entire person, taking into account their physical, nutritional, environmental, emotional, social, spiritual and lifestyle values, and avails itself all modes of diagnosis and treatment. And because holistic treatment is the best way to permanently rid your body of a yeast infection, Candida Crusher involves a holistic program that includes a comprehensive dietary; cleansing, lifestyle and nutritional supplementation program that can help you remain candida free for life. That's why the by-line of this book is called "Permanent Yeast Infection Solution".

Like many health-care professionals, I have spent many years helping others overcome their health care challenges and will try any protocol or product I know or have learned to help patients attain a higher state of health in the minimal amount of time, yet always try to remain realistic about the advice I recommend and do try to keep costs down. I have no bias towards any treatment or product, and the products I recommend in the Candida Crusher are purely based on my own personal experiences with regard to offering you the best value for money and therapeutic results. They are recommended because I have found them to work very well and consistently, after trying many other products.

If a better tool or treatment protocol to treat and eradicate yeast infections comes along I will use it, and no doubt in time you will find that I will have updated the Candida Crusher to include these updated tools and protocols.

You may like to visit our blog and any comments can be left, this will give you the opportunity to ask questions about candida yeast infections, and I will reply, time permitting, perhaps giving others answers to similar questions they may have as well.

We have comprehensive male and female candida yeast infection quiz that you can check by visiting https://quiz.yeastinfection.org/. The specialized candida crusher products can be ordered at CanXida.com.

Our YouTube channel can be found at https://www.youtube.com/@canxida.

So, are you ready to join me, and allow me to explain to you in detail what I believe to be one of the best yeast infection methods currently available, to help you finally rid your body of that annoying yeast infection which has plagued you possibly for many years? Please understand that by only following one chapter The Candida Crusher Program without really understanding the significance of using all the information provided, will give you a very average and limited result. By following all the advice, particularly the advice contained in chapter 7, and actually adopting all the recommendations, you will notice some truly amazing changes to your health in general. And by watching my educational You Tube videos and participating in our blog and forum you will gain even more useful information.

After having been in naturopathic practice for twenty-five years and having helped countless thousands of yeast infected patients back on their feet, it gives me great satisfaction that the Candida Crusher is now finally in your hands.
I sincerely encourage you to take full control of your health through a balanced and intelligent approach with your health-care choices, and by adopting the principles I have outlined in the Candida Crusher you will be ensuring that your body is nourished in the most optimal holistic way leading to a long, healthy and happy life. The best news of all is that you yourself can do most of what is necessary to fully recover!

Now let's get started and Crush that Candida!

Eric

Eric Bakker ND
Havelock North   New Zealand   January 2013

For more information along with updates, be sure to visit CanXida.com.

About the Author

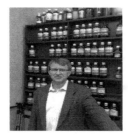 Eric Bakker N.D. is the clinical director of a New Zealand naturopathic clinic called The Naturopaths. Eric has a Bachelor Degree of Science majoring in Complementary Health Care, as well as separate diploma and degree qualifications in Naturopathy, Herbal Medicine and Homeopathy.

Eric has completed ten years of natural medicine study, has 25 years of clinical experience in natural and integrative forms of medicine and has pursued continuous post-graduate education in Australia, America, India as well as in New Zealand.

Eric has been a respected consultant to the natural medicine industry in both New Zealand and Australia for over 20 years. He is the past Vice President of the NZ Natural Medicine Association and is on their editorial advisory board. He is a feature article writer for the New Zealand Journal of Natural Medicine. Ericis a professional member of the New Zealand Natural Medicine Association.

Eric has worked as a technical and clinical services consultant in natural medicine representing several of the world's leading nutritional supplement brands for more than 20 years. In 2006, Eric became the Technical and Clinical Services President of his own New Zealand Company, Nutrisearch, offering a small yet highly researched range produced to his exacting standards. Eric has been researching the best ways to treat yeast infections with diet, lifestyle, dietary supplements and herbal medicines for many years and will release his Candida Crusher formulations later in 2013.

International Lecturer

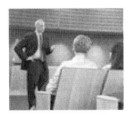

Eric attends the latest national and international natural and integrative medicine conferences in New Zealand, Australia, Europe and in America annually to keep up with the latest science and trends, and follows the cutting edge in natural medicine. He lectures regularly to the public as well as to various medical associations such as the Australasian Integrated Medical Association, his popular seminars series including topics such as "Are You Heart Smart", "The Art Of Stress Management and Adrenal Fatigue", and "Detox To Thrive" and "Hard To Stomach".

In addition, he presents highly focused and well-researched health presentations at natural medicine colleges throughout Australia and New Zealand, as well as researching and writing for several journals, websites and health publications.

Experienced Clinician

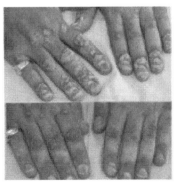

Eric has been treating and specializing in many different types of yeast infections for over twenty years. He has developed an incredibly successful treatment program called the Candida Crusher, based on several thousand successfully treated cases of vaginal thrush, endometriosis, jock itch, toenail fungus, athlete's foot, psoriasis and the many other manifestations of a yeast infection. Patients regularly consult with Dr. Bakker from over 30 countries around the world online through Skype, seeking assistance with their difficult to manage cases of yeast infection.

COPYRIGHT NOTICE

Please do not forward this electronic document

The License and Conditions

Terms of Use

Copyright

The entire contents of the Licenced eBook Candida Crusher and other material available through your registration are protected by copyright, unless otherwise indicated. Full-scale copying of Licenced eBook Candida Crusher contents is expressly prohibited. You may not remove, delete, transmit or create derivative works from any of the Licenced eBook Candida Crusher content. No part of any chapter of any book may be transmitted in any form by any means or reproduced for any other purpose, without the prior written permission from Eric Bakker N.D. except as permitted under relevant fair dealing provisions. Any other use violates this Agreement and is strictly prohibited by law.

Eric Bakker N.D. is the exclusive owner and or licensee of the content, products and services ("Content") offered in the e-book Candida Crusher and retains all proprietary rights in and to such Content, including all copyrighted material, trademarks, and other proprietary information of Candida Crusher.

Except for that information for which you have been given written permission, you may not copy, modify, publish, transmit, distribute, perform, display, or sell any such proprietary information.

All interfaces, look and feel, navigation schemes, designs and program features and functional of the Licensed eBook Candida Crusher are the property of Eric Bakker and may not be copied or reproduced or used in derivative works.

Legal Disclaimer

THE LICENCED E-BOOK CANDIDA CRUSHER IS PROVIDED "AS IS", WITHOUT WARRANTY OF ANY KIND, EXPRESSED OR IMPLIED INCLUDING WIHTOUT LIMITATIONS ACCURACY, OMISSIONS, COMPLETENESS OR IMPLIED WARRANTIES OR MERCHANTABILITY OR FITNESS FOR A PARTICULAR PURPOSE OR OTHER INCIDENTAL DAMAGES ARISING OUT OF THE USE OR THE INABILITY TO USE THE LICENCED E-BOOK. YOU ACKNOWLEDGE THAT THE USE OF THIS SERVICE IS ENTIRLY AT YOUR OWN RISK.

New Zealand law governs this Agreement. You acknowledge that you have read this Agreement, and agree to be bound by its terms and conditions.

Candida Crusher Disclaimer

The author does not assume any liability for the misuse of information contained herein. The content in this guide is provided for educational and informational purposes only, and is not intended, nor should it be, a substitute for professional medical advice, diagnosis, or treatment. The author is not a medical doctor, nor does he claim to be. Never disregard professional medical advice or delay in seeking it because of something you have read in Candida Crusher or on the websites candidacrusher.com or yeastinfection.org. Always consult your primary health care provider about the applicability of any opinions or recommendations with respect to your own symptoms or medical conditions.

The publishing company Bak to Health Ltd., the websites ericbakker.com, candidacrusher.com or yeastinfection.org and author Eric Bakker N.D. shall have neither liability nor responsibility to any person or entity with respect to any loss, damage, or injury caused or alleged to be caused directly or indirectly by the information contained in this e-Book Candida Crusher.

While every attempt has been made to provide information that is both accurate and proven effective, the author and, by extension, this guide, Candida Crusher, make no guarantees that any remedies, suggestions, treatments or protocols presented herein will help everyone in every situation. As the symptoms and conditions for each person are unique to individual histories, physical conditioning and body type, and the specifics of the actual yeast infection presentation, successes will vary. If you are taking any medications, you should consult with your physician, health care professional or health care provider before making any changes in your health maintenance program or profile before, during or after reading any information contained in the Candida Crusher.

By buying the e-book Candida Crusher and adhering to these terms and conditions, you hereby agree to indemnify and hold harmless Bak to Health Ltd., its subsidiaries, affiliates, officers, agents, licensors, partners and employees, from any loss, liability, claim, or demand, including legal fees, made by any third party due to or arising out of your use of the information contained herein, products and services, in violation of this agreement and/or arising from a breach of this agreement.

All links are for information purposes only and are not warranted for content, accuracy or any other implied or explicit purpose.

CHAPTER 2 The Yeast Connetion

What is Yeast Infection?

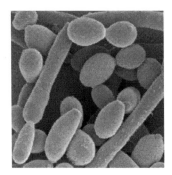

Candida albicans is a type of yeast like fungus that inhabits the intestines of over 90% of people as well as the genital tract and mouth of the host. In women the condition migrates readily from the large intestine to the vagina.

Candida is microscopic yeast in a sub-group of fungi or moulds. And moulds are truly everywhere; these bugs live in and on the soil, on all plants, in the air and in fact thrive on all living creatures' great and small. You may be familiar to fungi as the green "fur" which you occasionally see on a piece of mouldy cheese, bread or fruit. Moulds and yeasts spread and reproduce by releasing many millions of microscopic spores into the atmosphere, they literally float on air and eventually settle on a surface and if the conditions are favourable enough, the spore will grow into another mold plant.

Many people think of candida yeast infections as a woman's problem, affecting only the vagina. This is incorrect, in fact candida can affect women, men and children equally, and the main area this little yeast will inhabit is the digestive tract. A yeast infection can manifest in many different ways in or on a person's body and can result in jock itch, athlete's foot, dandruff, vaginal discharge, irritable bowel syndrome, a heavily coated tongue, and colic and thrush in infants. Chapter 3 will expand on the long list of potential signs and symptoms associated with a yeast infection.

Case History # 1

Kirsty, 19 years

Kirsty is a young female student who came to our clinic about two years ago complaining of chronic fatigue. She was absolutely exhausted and found it hard to concentrate at university. Kirsty was falling asleep during her afternoon lectures and was becoming increasing anxious at her inability to concentrate. Her main complaints were foggy thinking, anxiety and depression, occasional thrush, intermittent pains in her tummy, nausea and small whitish spots on her body. Her mother had been a patient of our practice for some time and referred Kirsty to me. When I questioned her about her daughter's diet and lifestyle, she said that she was tired of receiving phone calls from her daughter several times a week complaining about her health and that Kirsty liked to have a drink on Friday and Saturday nights, which was of concern to her. I have occasionally found it invaluable before the consultation to (discretely) make enquiries about a patient through their relatives, especially regarding younger patients and alcohol. You can learn a lot about the patient's case history this way, and may miss something the patient may be not willing to tell you - the practitioner.

Kirsty showed me her arms and I immediately identified a fungal skin complaint I have commonly seen on the arms, legs and torso of many chronic candida patients over the years.

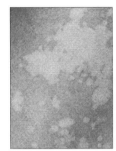 (See picture) I knew this was another chronic candida sufferer. Her doctor ran all the tests and found nothing wrong; a skin scraping which was sent to the pathology lab was "inconclusive". I have even seen similar skin rashes diagnosed by some doctors as psoriasis, eczema and even vitiligo, when in fact it was a fungal skin rash. How can I be so sure? Because careful case taking and after treating many patients with similar skin rashes I've discovered that most go away with the Candida Crusher Program. Skin conditions such as psoriasis, eczema and vitiligo may temporarily improve but do not disappear when you don't treat for candida. Kirsty loved white wine, but also bread and two-minute noodles.

We had several consultations, and I had to really convince her that alcohol just had to go. She was so sick and tired of feeling sick and tired that in the end she complied. This was Kirsty's tipping point, but Kirsty's case proved to be quite difficult indeed and took almost one year to come right. The problem here was that Kirsty is an extreme person, and after I told her to go "real easy" with treatment initially, she disregarded my advice and tripled the dosage of all the supplements as well as going rather extreme with the diet. She avoided just about everything except for meat proteins, green leafy vegetables and brown rice. The result? She felt totally awesome for the first seven days, but then felt absolutely terrible. This is due to the Herxheimer reaction, and you can read all about this later on in the book. You want to avoid this at all costs, and you can if you just follow the program carefully.

Yeast Infections Are Common Place

You and I have candida living on our skin and they thrive on all the mucous membrane surfaces lining all body cavities. While we all have bugs like bacteria and yeasts growing in and on our bodies, we all have our own particular blend of bacteria and yeasts which live in harmony with each other without causing the least discomfort or disease. But like any eco system, when the natural balance becomes disturbed the resulting effects may range from being minor and trivial to widespread and catastrophic.

Until not all that long ago, only a very few doctors would even find it conceivable to consider candidiasis (candida albicans) as a possible diagnosis when they were confronted with a patient complaining of many and varied signs and symptoms. This is certainly no longer true today, and there have been countless books written on candida since the 1980's by both medical and non-medical health care professionals.

Until fairly recently, Candida's most common manifestation, vaginal thrush, discharge or irritation which plagues so many women, was brushed off by many doctors as a purely "trivial women's ailment" and treated locally with a cream and an applicator, often unsuccessfully. I have given up counting how many women I have seen in exactly this situation, they have just been offered local treatment only to find that the condition resurfaces down the track, time and again, and again, and yet again.

Similarly, we see men in the clinic who presented to their doctor with jock itch; a groin rash or athlete's foot only to be offered local treatment once again. And yes, the recurrence rate for these male complaints is as high as it is for the women's manifestations of candida. And after awhile, many simply give up on treatment.

When you visit your health-care professional with a yeast-related health problem, be sure to ask that if they interested primarily in treating your symptoms or are also interested in looking deeper into the case for the cause. Is the treatment going to make your healthy and strong and prevent further problems, or is the treatment primarily about reducing the symptoms, and keeping you reliant on medications?

Is the antibiotic, antifungal drug or cream going to fix your problem and prevent further problems and recurrences, or is it a medication you will require on/off for years? Secondly, ask the physician to actually treat you and *not the disease.* It's your choice, you decide what is right for you, and if you are smart you will want to treat the cause.

The Cause Is Never Deemed As Important As The Treatment

If I could live my life over again, I would devote it to proving that germs seek their natural habitat, diseased tissues, rather than being the cause of disease.
Dr. Rudolph Virchow (the germ theory)

In 1965, a pioneering doctor named Jack Geiger helped to start America's first health centers in the Mississippi Delta and in Boston for the lower income population. Dr. Geiger treated many children who were ill and so malnourished that his prescriptions were not for pharmaceutical drugs, but "prescriptions" for basic healthy foods like meat, fruit and vegetables. These prescriptions were funded by his community center pharmacy budget, and once word got out to Washington, a government official was sent to reprimand Geiger for his "reckless spending". The point was made to Geiger that his pharmacy's budget was for "medical purposes" only and was not intended to cover foods. Geiger's reply was simple: " The last time I checked my textbooks the specific therapy for malnutrition was in fact … food."

The point here is that even in 1965, American government health officials did not recognize nutrition as having much bearing on human health. Having a poor and impoverished diet was not seen to be a contributing or causative factor in poor health and disease, and the sad fact is that even today there are doctors and governments who still believe that nutrition plays little role in human health, and that ill health in people can be attributed to some kind of "deficiency of a pharmaceutical drug".

The interesting thing I find with conventional medicine is that it has developed an elaborate system cloaked in science aimed at treating the patient over a prolonged period of time, for the same complaint, and in cases like yeast infection - without much expectation of any complete resolution, for years on end, even decades. It reeks of profits for big pharma to me; there is no profit in health, only in ill health.

There is no doubt about it, Western medicine has given us many fantastic advances, but are medical doctors really looking for the actual causes of our illness or merely addressing the symptoms with potentially toxic drugs?

Like many different types of infections, yeast infections can lead to a host of chronic diseases. If you think about it for one minute, did you wake up one morning and have irritable bowel disease, ulcerative colitis, arthritis, psoriasis, heart disease, fibromyalgia, chronic fatigue syndrome or any one of a number of other chronic health issues? Chronic problems most always have their origin in small beginnings, like a small infection. A house that needs demolition from rot starts with the tiniest amount of rot, but it remains hidden and undetected for years, sometimes decades until one day it was exposed and then it was too late, demolition was called for. This is just like cancer, no symptoms or pain for years, yet the same contributing underlying factors which are often hidden and then one day "OMG, I've got cancer".

Conditions like vaginal thrush and athlete's foot are generally seen as local and "trivial", and if the patient returns with the same problem, the cause is not generally sought for and medications are prescribed time and again.

What other professional person would you consult, and be expected to pay a fee to, who just shrugs his or her shoulders when you enquire as to the actual cause of your complaints? That's right – nobody. If a plumber or mechanic kept repeatedly giving you lame excuses, would you pay them and take them seriously? Of course you wouldn't, you would take your problem and your wallet somewhere else. Well, that's exactly what happens to thousands of people who consult their doctors with a yeast related problem every day; they are treated symptomatically because all the emphasis is on the symptoms and not the actual cause. In my opinion, *the treatment is never as important as discovering the actual cause*, and any intelligent person would be quick to add that if you get the cause sorted you wouldn't end up with any crippling symptoms and their long-term consequences. Same with heart disease, same with cancer, same with candida, in fact, the same with any chronic illness.

Candida problems have become so widespread today, that if a random sample of patients, those unsuspecting candida infections, yet complaining of miscellaneous symptoms is given anti-candida therapy, many of them will exhibit a marked reduction in symptoms over the next few months and some will even exhibit a dramatic return to good health. I have found this to be the case in many situations in my clinic. Candida problems can present themselves in all shapes and sizes and have many disguises, so don't be fooled into thinking that candida is purely a "digestive problem" or a "vaginal problem", or "toe nail fungus" by any means, and this will be amply illustrated with the many case-studies you will encounter in the Candida Crusher book. Candida is a widespread digestive and systemic problem, but more often begins in the digestive system and then trans-locates to other parts of the body by way of the blood stream. If you have a local occurrence of candida, you will almost certainly have it in the digestive system and/or vagina, and it may be under control or ready to ramp up and go out of control.

Candida yeast infection was dubbed as the twentieth-century disease, but now into the twenty-first century nothing has changed, in fact I believe that you will probably see more cases of candida yeast infection than you will ever have seen before in history. In the Candida Crusher I would like to talk about my experiences treating people with yeast infections and show you many case studies along the way and in addition give my take on what I consider to be the most clinically effective solution to this scourge which we see so regularly in any natural or medical practice. I'll address the many and varied causes throughout the book, especially in chapter 7. Be sure to underline anything that stands out or use a high lighter, this is your personal copy!

The Primary Cause And
The Maintaining Causes Of Yeast Infections

If there is but one thing I have discovered over the years working with many yeast-infected patients is that there is always a cause, and generally there are two distinct types of causes, the primary cause (what actually started or helped to start the yeast infection) and the maintaining causes (what keeps it going on, and on, and on).

The Primary Cause

Do you know what your primary (exciting) cause or causes were in the past; could you remember what possibly triggered it? Was it that course of antibiotics you had after you had a cough, cold or an infection? Perhaps like many people, you have had several courses of antibiotics and have never been well since. If you are likely to tell me this in my room, I will write "NBWS" behind such an event and mark it out as a primary cause. Was it after you came out of hospital, or when you came back from that holiday? Think of an event (*any*) that took place just before it started. Think of a drug or treatment that coincided with the onset of candida.

It is pretty foolish to believe that your yeast infection came out of nowhere and just "happened", there *IS* always a cause for your yeast overgrowth, and with a bit of detective work you should be able to figure out how long ago this whole mess started.

Primary causes are more dramatic and there is almost always a strong relationship between cause and effect, and most patients can remember the one or several primary causes. As people get older and they have had their yeast infection for many years, the memory may not be that good anymore and it may be harder to track the primary cause.

The Maintaining Cause

These are generally a lot easier to discover, they will be happening right now and a bit of detective work will soon uncover these, there will often be several maintaining causes or one big one, like eating chocolate several times a week or drinking alcohol daily. What are you doing to keep your yeast infection going? Is it something specific in your diet or is it something to do with your lifestyle or is it both? Do you eat commercial chicken every week that may contain antibiotics? You may be suffering from stress or adrenal fatigue, but more about this later. Maintaining causes can be dietary or lifestyle or generally a combination of both, as you go through chapter 7 more will be explained.

The 11 Main Yeast Infection Causes

There are a number of factors that allow a yeast infection to go wildly out of control, but there is seldom just one factor responsible for preventing people gaining control of their yeast infection and turning the corner.

I have listed the main risk factors for a yeast infection below, but suffice to say, candida overgrowth is most often due to chronic antibiotic use, particularly the broad-spectrum variety. Antibiotics kill the gastrointestinal bacteria that normally help to keep a yeast overgrowth at bay, and of no surprise, when antibiotic use first became widespread it was soon noticed that yeast infections were on the rise.

What are the key reasons why a yeast infection is so prevalent in the digestive tracts of people living in the Western industrialized countries? I believe that we principally have our hectic 21st century lifestyles and nutritionally depleted, highly refined & processed and sugar laden diets to blame, but technology is also to blame to a degree and the way we use and abuse science and technology. Here are the major factors that allow candida to get out of hand; there are potentially many more, but these represent the core:

Antibiotic drugs. Most probably the number one cause in my opinion of chronic yeast infection is the prolonged, inappropriate, and excessive use of certain types of pharmaceutical drugs like broad-spectrum antibiotics. Antibiotics are used to kill disease-causing bacteria, but unfortunately they also kill normal, protective bacterial flora throughout your body and actually encourage yeast infections. Did you know that most antibiotics are actually made from chemicals found in some fungi species? The fungi themselves make certain types of chemicals that protect them from many different types of bacteria, and this is one of the major reasons why antibiotics work so well against bacteria, but unfortunately also one of the main reasons why they support the growth of fungi.

Antibiotics in meat. Many different kinds of antibiotics are also found in commercial poultry, pork, beef and other meats. Be particularly careful to avoid commercial poultry, as thousands of chickens are crammed into cages and routinely fed high protein foods full of antibiotics. Buy free range and certified organic chicken just to be sure.

An underlying inherited or acquired immune system deficiency. There are several reasons why your immune system may be impaired and an investigation may well reveal the cause. Be sure to have the appropriate blood tests to uncover any potential causes like neutropenia, which means poor levels of neutrophils

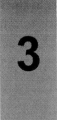

3 or white blood cells (get a full blood count), vitamin B12 or folate deficiencies. Nutrient deficiencies are one common source of an immune deficiency. See your health-care professional and get the appropriate medical or functional medicine testing, especially if you have had a chronic yeast infection for some time. If your doctor is resistant and "does not believe" in your self-observations of candida, find yourself another doctor who hasn't got a hearing problem.

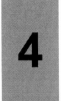

4 The liberal use of steroidal or other drugs. Particularly steroids whether they be hydrocortisone or prednisolone. These steroidal drugs can be inhaled, in a tablet, capsule or cream form. Inhaled steroids (asthma) also feature high on this list. The oral contraceptive pill is in this category too, and so are heartburn or anti-ulcer preparations.

5 Alcohol. In my experience, not many avoid alcohol. While I do occasionally see some people with a yeast infection who don't drink, they tend to be uncommon. Most all folks I've seen with a chronic yeast infection drink alcohol regularly. And the types of alcohol I associate the most with a yeast infection are beer, white wine and spirits like whisky, rum and bourbon. Any alcohol can be implicated, but these are the big ones. Why these spirits? Any spirits that a person will routinely mix Coke (or a high sugar soda drink) with is more likely to get a yeast infection because they are consuming plenty of sugar. Those with yeast infections are drawn to alcohol, like moths are to a flame. Is there any "safe" alcohol? Not really, all alcohol can promote candida, whether it is gin, vodka, whiskey or wine. Most yeast infection sufferers have poor digestive health leading to nutritional deficiencies, and alcohol is often implicated here too.

6 Candida friendly diets. (Sugar, alcohol, refined flour, etc). Just like alcohol, this group of foods encourages the growth and proliferation of a yeast infection. Typically craved foods are breads, chocolate, moldy cheeses (brie, camembert, etc.), pickles, sweet sauces, and the sweet fruits like oranges, bananas, grapes, and dried fruits. I won't elaborate on foods too much here, you can read a lot more about foods and drinks and yeast infections in section 1 (Chapter 7) of The Candida Crusher Program.

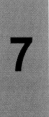

7 Stress, which eventually depletes our body's ability (adrenal glands) to produce sufficient cortisol that in turn reduces the immune system's functionality. Fluctuating cortisol levels also cause blood-sugar dysregulation (hypoglycemia) that is a further risk factor for candida. Those with prolonged stress often end up developing adrenal fatigue (see Section 2 – Understanding Stress and Immunity). In my experience, most all chronic yeast infection patients have some degree of adrenal fatigue, which is best treated at the same time as their yeast infection.

8 Exposure to pesticides, herbicides, chemicals, toxic metals (lead, mercury). Many people with chronic yeast infections are toxic people, and hair or urine testing may reveal a heavy metal problem. Mercury has been implicated with chronic candida, be sure to read the section 3 in chapter 7 that explains all about the most effective ways to detoxify.

9 Diabetes. Diabetics are more prone to candida yeast infections for several reasons, but the main connection is that diabetics have problems regulating their blood sugar levels. There are two main types of diabetes, however, all forms of diabetes have one thing in common, which is insulin production problems or insulin resistance. The pancreas in a healthy person produces insulin. Type 2 diabetics (diabetes mellitus) have generally a problem with insulin resistance in that the cells of their body have a problem accepting insulin's ability to regulate blood sugar. The purpose of insulin is to process blood sugar (glucose) into energy. And sugar, as you are aware, is the primary agent that feeds a yeast infection. Since people with diabetes have higher concentrations of glucose in their body, they are therefore also at a higher risk of developing recurrent and chronic candida yeast infections.

10 Chlorinated water. Chlorinated water is a big but commonly overlooked problem in the development of a yeast infection. By swimming in a chlorinated pool or a Jacuzzi (spa pool) you are allowing your body to absorb plenty of chlorine, an antibiotic. Why is this so? Why do you think they throw that stuff into the water? They throw it in to kill any bacteria and algae, and not unlike an antibiotic you swallow, you are allowing the yeasts to thrive by reducing the beneficial bacteria levels in your body. Just as chlorine kills bacteria in the water, it also kills the body's normal bacterial flora.

11 Mold exposure. Just like chlorine, mold is a frequently overlooked problem when it comes to candida. Mold will hurt the immune system by suppressing it. I have seen many patients who improved once they moved out of their house. Think about carpets, rugs and walls in bedrooms, kitchens and bathrooms. Sometimes mold is obvious on walls or ceilings and sometimes it is not. If you have a mold problem it will continually send out microscopic spores into the air that you inhale. Read more about mold in section 5 of chapter 7.

Thumbtack Disease

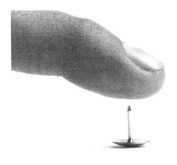

Here is a recent scenario that happened to me and perfectly illustrates cause and effect. I have been busy renovating my house for the past several months and recently have been painting the outside of my old home. I developed a sore right foot and when I had a bath later that evening I noticed a painful red sore on the sole of my right foot. I treated this promptly with tea tree oil and a plaster. I checked the shoe for a rose thorn or nail but found nothing.

But after a few days, the pain would not go away and each time I climbed up the ladder and placed my right foot on a rung, I felt a sharp pain in my foot.

That's when I decided to take a much closer look at the bottom of my shoe and found a tiny panel pin that had worked its way into the sole of my shoe, it was the primary cause and it was partially hidden. I could only feel a sharp prick when I placed my hand in the shoe and applied pressure. Once I removed the tiny pin I no longer had any pain and my foot healed fine. You are probably thinking why didn't he look carefully right away? Well I did, but when I looked much more carefully I saw the tiny head on the panel pin (a very small nail), but it was barely visible on first inspection and could only feel the pain under pressure. Leaving the panel pin in my shoe was the maintaining cause of the pain, unbeknown to me.

The moral of this story is that if you don't find a cause then look very carefully for the hidden cause, because you may well initially glance right over the cause when you first look at a problem, just like I did. There is always a cause, but sometimes it is not that obvious and staring you right in the face, and that's why most people miss the cause and just end up treating the effect.

On other occasions, things are right there in front of us but we don't see them! Have you ever been in your kitchen and looked for the can opener or a particular knife and couldn't find it, but it was right there in front of you, staring right at you?

Sometimes the solution to our problem is staring us right in the face but we have become blind due to familiarity. And at other times we know what the cause is but just ignore it for some reason, like the person who keeps on drinking and is in denial. Like a pharmacist's wife I once saw who brought me her 11-year-old son with a major yeast infection who had been on an antibiotic almost continually for eighteen months due to an unresolved cough and cold.

Your Body is Like a Car

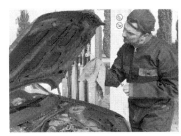

Your body is much like your motor vehicle. It is reliable and with a little care and maintenance can last for many years. When things go wrong, it will give you the appropriate warning signals; even in the very earliest stages of a big mechanical problem it will tell you that something is wrong. But cars are like humans too in the sense that something unpredictable may happen, although the odds are quite rare, they do increase with age. For example, your risk of a heart attack may increase with age just like your car may experience major mechanical failure with age, but with routine and regular maintenance checks the likelihood will be considerably more slim.

Signs and symptoms of an impending yeast infection like increasing gas and bloating, bowel motions that are changeable and digestive pain that is occurring much more regularly are all signs that something is amiss. All of those digestive problems are telling us our digestive system isn't functioning properly. This can lead to poor absorption of nutrients and even deficiencies causing fatigue, irritability, poor moods, etc. How can you expect your body to overcome any ailment or re-build itself if the food and nutrients aren't absorbed? And in addition, you become a sitting duck for a yeast infection, and some cancer researchers even go as far as saying that a yeast infection of many decades of neglect may even turn into some forms of cancer.

Many women will experience occasional vaginal discomfort or a discharge but the cause should be addressed before the problem becomes chronic and most uncomfortable, when most women seek help. Sometimes a simple treatment and diet change is all that is needed in the earliest stages of a health problem, and the best time to treat any illness is right at the beginning, before any real disease or pathology has taken place. The longer you wait, the more difficult and expensive the treatment will be. This is what I think "drives" a person in to see their mechanic at the first sound of a noise in their car, a costly repair job!

It is our job to address these signs and symptoms as soon as we feel something isn't right, we need to establish the root cause and establish it as soon as possible to get our health back on track. But, if you are the kind of person who ignores the red light flashing on the dashboard of your car then your problems could grow and escalate into a major health problem. Have you learned anything from your ill health? Was it something you could have prevented? Maybe you could learn something from it and prevent any such further episodes.

 A wise man should consider that health is the greatest of human blessings, and learn how by his own thought to derive benefit from his illnesses.

Hippocrates

Dr. William Crook and Dr. Orion Truss

These two doctors were the first true pioneers in the discovery of the true extent of candida infections in the population. I can remember reading a book written by Dr. William Crook called *The Yeast Connection* in 1983 when my father bought a copy to try and sort his own digestive problems out. To understand more about the background, you have to understand Dr. William Crook. In 1979, Dr. Crook learned from Dr. Orian Truss about the relationship of common yeast called *Candida albicans* with many illnesses.

Dr. Truss wrote a book in 1983 entitled "The Missing Diagnosis" and made the suggestion that since the 1950's, the widespread use of antibiotics, combined with the universal use of the oral contraceptive pill and immune suppressing drugs like steroids (hydrocortisone, prednisone, cortisol and asthma preventative steroidal inhalers) coupled with a high carbohydrate type diet (such as bread, alcohol processed and take-out foods) has caused a dramatic increase in yeast like overgrowths in the human population.

William G. Crook, MD, passed away in October 2003, at the age of 85. To many involved in natural medicine, Dr. Crook was a mentor and a true role model. He was a passionate man who worked tirelessly to improve the public health, primarily by helping publicise the importance of food allergy and of candida yeast infection as causes of illness. As a pediatrician, Dr. Crook became interested in the idea that hidden food allergies were a triggering factor for conditions such as hyperactivity, learning disabilities, fatigue, bedwetting, migraine, colic and other common pediatric problems. After helping thousands of children overcome chronic conditions by means of an elimination diet, Dr. Crook then began to spread the word by writing books and articles on the subject. Many medical and natural medicine practitioners used his book "Tracking Down Hidden Food Allergies" as a blueprint for identifying food allergies in both children and adults.

Dr. William Crook is best known for his role in increasing public awareness of candida albicans yeast infections as a cause of chronic physical and emotional problems. Although Orion Truss MD, is credited with alerting the medical profession to the yeast-illness connection, it was Dr. Crook's landmark bestselling book "The Yeast Connection" that gave recognition to a condition which is as big today as it has ever been.

To this day, the candida yeast infection syndrome remains a controversial diagnosis, ignored or ridiculed by the majority in the medical profession. However, thousands of open-minded practitioners have been able to help countless numbers of patients, largely because of Dr. Crook's books and lectures on the subject. Thanks to the pioneering work by doctors such as Truss and Crook, chronic candida infection has been known for over thirty years in medicine now. Before the early seventies however, neither the public nor the health care professional had much of idea of the magnitude of this problem or in fact had ever really heard of a patient with a candida infection.

Like many conditions that people present with, it is once again not the condition they present with so much that is the real issue – it is the continuation of a dietary and lifestyle habit underpinning candida that needs the attention.

Are Your Health Problems Yeast Related?

One of the best ways to discover if a candida yeast infection is a factor in your health complaints is to complete one of the several surveys we have placed online for your convenience, just go to www.yeastinfection.org

Some of the key things to look out for are the following:

- Do you crave sweets or sweet foods?

- Do you feel sick all over?

- Do you have vaginal thrush?

- Do you have jock itch or toenail fungus?

- Are you itchy anywhere?

- Have you taken any antibiotics?

- Have you been on the oral contraceptive pill for some time?

- Do you have any unresolved digestive issues?

- Have you seen many doctors and have not found help?

- Have you been developing an increasing amount of food allergies?

Here is a typical case history of a chronic candida patient, you may be able to relate with this patient, because she has multiple systems affected by candida and is typical of a chronic case I would tend to see in my clinic. Chronic cases such as these may give you an insight as to whether your case is related to a chronic low-grade yeast infection.

Case History # 2

Susan, 39 years

Susan is an Australian lady who visited our practice several years ago complaining of a number of chronic health problems that had plagued her for over twenty years. Many of Susan's health issues are typical of some of the clinical complaints people have when they endure a chronic generalized yeast infection.

Susan suffered from sinus and hay fever all her life and has taken many different drugs for her allergies but had to keep changing them because they were only of temporary relief. She had learned to live with a stuffy or perpetually blocked nostril, post nasal drip, sneezing, itchy upper palate, sore throats and had dark circles under her eyes. She also suffered from the worst headaches imaginable since she was sixteen, at times like a nail piercing her skull as she described them. These headaches were typically much worse about four days before her menstrual cycle.

Susan went to her doctor about five years ago complaining of the headaches and he referred her to a neurologist who concluded after an ECG (brain wave scan) that all was well and that the headaches were caused by stress and tension and to take analgesics as required. Several hundred dollars later, and none the wiser, Susan started to take paracetamol (Acetaminophen) several times a day with only a temporary relief.

When Susan was in her late twenties she started to become more aware of the fluid retention she was suffering from, including a huge weight gain since her teens (over 150 pounds). After she ate a carbohydrate rich meal she would bloat considerably and retain as much as eight pounds of fluid or more at times (four kilograms). Her doctor told her it was because of salt, so Susan excluded all salt from her diet as much as possible, only to find out that salt reduction made absolutely no difference to her fluid retention.

What she did notice was how much worse her fluid retention was before her period, and it co-incided with feeling very emotional and depressed. Maybe there was a link, Susan thought? Susan was placed on the Candida Crusher Program and after five months the results were staggering, it was the first time that this lady started to feel normal as she put it.

 Here is a quote from Dr. Leo Galland, MD, of New York, is one of America's leading natural medicine specialists who has specialised on treating many difficult cases of candida-related health problems:

 The intestinal tract is one of the most important parts of the body as far as whether one is sick or well. I'm not talking just about food allergies, but the reason we're seeing an increasing prevalence of food intolerance is because of an unhealthy and imbalanced gut flora. The problem may be with the diet itself, or it may be from antibiotics or parasitic infestation such as a yeast infection. "

I'll talk more about Dr. Galland's dietary recommendations for the candida patient in Section 1 of Chapter 7.

Yeasts And How Acetaldehyde Can Make You Sick

Yeasts like to grow in a warm, dark and moist environment and like all plants have a stem, leaf and root system.

Normally many plants will take root in water, they will take up nutrients and carbon dioxide through its roots, stem and leaves and take in and release oxygen as a waste product into the atmosphere. Candida however, works the other way around as its nutrients are taken in through the top and waste products are released through its roots. The root system of Candida sinks into the mucous membranes of the body, which to Candida are like a fertile soil. This little parasitic plant likes to feed on sugars and refined products like white flour, candy, soda drinks and then will go about depositing its wastes deep into the mucous membranes into which it is anchored.

And when this little plant comes into contact with its food source, enzymes in its leaves then convert food into chemicals that the yeast needs to sustain its life.

The waste product deposited which is a by-product of this enzymatic conversion, and is a toxic chemical called acetaldehyde, otherwise known as acetic aldehyde ethanol, a relation of the alcohol family.

As the yeast proliferates throughout the mucous membranes it begins to secrete more and more acetaldehyde. It is important to bear in mind that acetaldehyde is in fact a chemical even more potentially toxic to the human brain than ethanol itself, which insidiously undermines brain functions and damages neurological structures.

We will talk a little later on about another chemical called gliotoxin produced by candida, which also has neurotoxic effects and can even secrete a chemical that kills various kinds of white blood cells around it, making it immune suppressive.

Apart from its toxic neurological effects, acetaldehyde in turn produces an allergic reaction in a person's mucous membranes lining the mouth and whole digestive tract, as well as sinuses and respiratory tract causing the mucous membranes to stimulate the production of mucous. Does this sound familiar to you? How many people do you know with digestive problems for example that have a sniffle or need to clear their throat on a regular occasion? I have always associated increased phlegm and mucus with a yeast infection, and that once the digestive system is finally cleared of the yeast overgrowth that this phlegm or mucus slowly clears up.

As candida is increasingly produced, more mucus is produced which is a perfect breeding ground for bacteria, requiring yet more antibiotics, and so the cycle continues. Those on a regular antibiotic should always be treated as a candida case, regardless of their presenting symptoms.

It is interesting to hear those who are chronically infected with candida yet who don't drink alcohol, say that they may even feel "drunk", spaced out or a bit inebriated or stoned. I've heard many patients over the years tell me that they feel "unreal" or "not quite with it", and now you know why. Can you remember the last time you drank a little too much alcohol? Remember how it felt? Then you will understand how some patients feel with candida infections.

If you have a history of phlegm or mucus, and especially if you notice an increase in the production of this phlegm or mucus after eating or drinking anything, see if you can work out what food or drink is causing this increased production. In many instances, that food or drink contained some form of sugar. Sugar is the perfect food for this little fungus, and what you will find is that even foods like milk (containing lactose, or milk sugar) can very easily stimulate the production of phlegm. It is further important to remember that a candida yeast infection is often found in combination with food allergies, and once the candida is dealt with then the person in most cases will again be able to tolerate that food once again.

Acetaldehyde Is A Chemical
That Enters Your Body In Various Ways

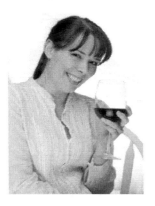

- Drinking alcohol

- Inhaling exhaust fumes or cigarette smoke (active or passive)

- Having an overgrowth of candida in your body

When we drink alcohol, an enzyme found in the liver called *alcohol dehydrogenase* converts it into acetaldehyde, after this process, another enzyme breaks it down further into acetate, which gives our cells energy.

The problem is that in alcoholics or people with a high level of toxicity, the body's ability to convert acetaldehyde is undermined, and high levels of acetaldehyde remain in the body and can cause a kind of poisoning which not only does physical damage but also can very much distort mental perceptions.

This is one of the reasons why some people with chronic and systemic candida, especially those who drink plenty of alcohol, can have depression, anxiety, mood swings and irritability.

It is important for you to understand that if you like a drink and have candida you simply must stop drinking for some time and restore your digestive system, repair the leaky bowel and work on building a healthy bacterial population and then in time re-introduce alcohol.

It may take six to twelve months though, so be patient. This is by far the most important component of your dietary regime for you to adhere to if you truly want to recover; you have to ease up on the drink. If you bought the Candida Crusher because you want to beat your yeast infection but you can't be bothered or enjoy alcohol more than your yeast infection, then I'm afraid you have just wasted your money on this book. In that case, you may want to give it to somebody who can use this information more effectively and put it to good use, a person like this may take his or her health more seriously.

 Take your health seriously, or take it somewhere else.
James L. Wilson DC, ND, PhD.

Why Is Candida Albicans Yeast Overgrowth So Prevalent?

This question is not that hard to answer, we have so many bacteria, microbes and fungi living in and on our body's surface, it is all a matter of balance. From the day of your birth your body lives in a sea of bacteria. Infectious germs known as microbes swim throughout your body at all times. These microbes can live in your throat, mouth, nose, gums, gastrointestinal tract, blood, bladder, vagina, and numerous other body tissues.

These microorganisms that may be bacteria, viruses, fungi, or parasites, are as much a part of every human being as foods and chemicals. Figuratively speaking, they are constantly trying to 'eat us alive'. In some people these bugs actually succeed and death follows. An example of this is deaths we have had in many other parts of the world due to the HN1 swine flu virus. The influenza virus is so small is impossible to see without amazingly powerful magnification, yet is capable of causing perfectly healthy people to die.

And, even if when we do die of natural causes the bugs eventually eat our physical remains. Only healthy cells and tissues within our living bodies can effectively defend us against infectious microbes.

Immunologists, gynecologists and other health-care professionals generally tend to see the candida syndrome as a fictional one, probably because the manifestations are seen too often, the need for treatment too frequent, and the conventional testing for its presence and effect too inadequate, and because almost everyone suddenly has become an expert in its presence or absence.

Many naturopaths and natural health-care professionals see candida as a scourge, affecting patients so widespread that some like myself actually specialize in this condition. Some do a great job, but many do an average job because they have their patient follow a "candida program" which can last anywhere generally from one to six weeks and that's it. Many pay lip service to the importance of the correct diet and lifestyle ongoing, and whilst the patient may initially feel OK, the candida comes back with vengeance and the patient is disillusioned and begins over the years to hop from one practitioner to another.

We call this in our business "doctor-hopping", and such patients generally end up on my doorstep with bags or boxes of dietary supplements as well as medical prescriptions for all manner of creams, pills and lotions with the condition remaining unresolved.

Candida can be a real trap for most medical natural health care professionals; this is another prime reason why candida is just so prevalent today. Most shocking, since many medical doctors do not recognise systemic candida as a problem, they often misdiagnose the condition and mistreat accordingly. And the patients are the ones I find who suffer, and suffer and continue to… suffer. But don't be alarmed, with an ounce of proper treatment and the correction of the underlying dietary and lifestyle patterns today, you can overcome candida and save yourself a ton of health misery down the track tomorrow. The connection between your digestive system and the rest of your health, in particular your mental and emotional health is only just starting to become apparent to the many enlightened medical health professionals.

Let's take a look at drug treatments today. We have such powerful drugs like the broad spectrum antibiotics which kill the friendly bugs in your digestive system, chemotherapy (immuno-suppressive) drugs, and steroidal drugs like asthma puffers, hydrocortisone creams for all manner of skin afflictions and prednisone whenever a patient has an incontrollable immune condition which again needs suppression. We will go more into these causes a little later. Pharmaceutical drugs such as these along with a diet laden with sugar, alcohol, breads, convenience foods, etc, are hugely responsible for the candida problem. Most all cancer patients have candidiasis. The candidiasis was not the cause of their cancer; rather it was part of the lowered resistance that had likely contributed to the cancer itself due to the chemotherapy treatment.

Many sick people in my observation have yeast overgrowth to some degree, but yeast overgrowth is not what makes so many people sick, rather it is their lowered resistance and their increasing susceptibility. So, as our population continues to develop more and more degenerative ailments, what do we do? As a Western culture, ultimately, in addition to treating the effects of our lifestyles, e.g. the yeast, at some point the way of life in this country led by so many people has got to be changed in some very fundamental ways. In chapter 7, I will explain the many ways in which we can change, thereby making our bodies much stronger and more capable of fighting a yeast infection.

Systemic Candidiasis Is A Scientifically Proven Fact

While gastrointestinal candidiasis has long been acknowledged as a fact, systemic candidiasis has been a subject of controversy for more than thirty years, particularly since most of the books on candida have been launched in the early to mid eighties.

Candida albicans has only been considered a serious organism by the medical profession in those who are severely immune compromised, such as leukemia patients, those with AIDS, people undergoing chemotherapy, radiation or those being treated with immune-suppressive drugs.

In particular, ever since Dr. Orion Truss published his book "The Missing Diagnosis" in 1983, followed by Dr. William Crook's book "The Yeast Connection" in 1984, a controversy has raged in both the scientific circles and the media regarding the ability of gastrointestinal candidiasis to cause systemic yeast infection.

Interestingly, a *study was published in 1969 in *Lancet,* the prestigious medical journal, which demonstrated that candida albicans is perfectly capable of escaping from a human being's gastrointestinal tract and trans-locating into the person's bloodstream within literally hours.

The researcher, W. Krause, was first tested and examined to the satisfaction of his medical peers to exclude any digestive, immune, and respiratory or kidney diseases and had not used any antibiotics in the previous ten years. He was thoroughly tested to eliminate any possibility that had any pre-existing yeast infection. He then ingested a significantly large dose of candida albicans orally (10^{12}). That is an incredible 10,000,000,000,000 candida albicans organisms!

Within two hours of swallowing candida albicans, he developed a fever, a headache and was shivering. Incredibly, candida albicans was cultured from a blood sample taken at 3 and 6 hours after ingestion. Candida was also cultured from urine samples taken from the same person at 2 ¾ and 3 ¼ hours after the ingestion of candida.

This study, although performed in 1969, clearly demonstrates that gastrointestinal candidiasis can shift from the digestive system into the bloodstream in a non immune-compromised host.

Krause W, Matheis H, Wulf K, Fungaemia and funguria after oral administration of Candida albicans, Lancet 1969; 1:598 -599.

These and many more underlying factors can transform candida, which is commonly found but kept under control by beneficial bacteria, from its docile state into that of a predator.

Most Common Western Medicine Risk Factors Involved In Yeast Overgrowth

- Anti-ulcer drugs

- Broad-spectrum antibiotics

- Corticosteroids

- Diabetes

- Immune-suppressive drugs

- Intravascular catheter usage

- Intravenous drug usage

- Oral contraceptive pill

- Prolonged hospital stay

Poor Yeast Infection Recovery Is Most Common

Are people not getting and staying well because of changing yeast forms, or is it perhaps that the person is not strict enough with their diet or lifestyle, or maybe not enough time given to allow the treatment to be fully effective? Perhaps there is some self-responsibility lacking? I believe that there are as many reasons for a poor recovery as there are people.

I think it is also because most patients never really give their body the chance to maximize its healing capacity by way of rest, sleep, sunshine, peace of mind, thereby providing a conducive healing environment. These health-promoting factors are generally encouraged by the medical professional, and sadly to say not even by many natural health-care professionals these days. So, armed with pharmaceutical drugs, all manner of self-prescribed supplements, a magazine or internet diet and a bit of will power thrown in, a few recover partially here or there, the lucky few fully recover, but the vast majority will tend to stay with a yeast infection and rarely fully and permanently recover. These are the walking wounded that tend to fill up our waiting rooms as naturopaths.

I truely hope that the information I have provided for you in the form of The Candida Crusher can change all that, because you can get rid of candida by changing the way you think, by changing the way you eat and changing the way you live.

And, I will tell you repeatedly in this book, it takes time to improve and finally beat a chronic yeast infection, it is not going to happen overnight. If you think you will shake it in a few weeks by taking this or that magic brew or potion then the Candida Crusher is not for you and you have wasted you money buying it, sorry.

You will hear the same from me in the Candida Crusher as you would if you consulted me, *but with one exception*. I can have a tendency to be a little tough on patients who keep coming back to me complaining of no or very little results in terms of the candida problem over several months of treatment duration. I just don't buy it it, because if you follow the rules, you will get results. If you play the game with a view of winning the game, chances are you will win, especially if you put your heart and soul into it.

It may take three to four months on average, but it may take one year if you have been chronically unwell for a long time, but you will start feeling better and increasingly better over a reasonable time. And if we just aren't getting there in terms of results, then there will be a hidden cause which we will talk about at the end of section 5 in chapter 7 entitled: "What to do if you don't seem to come right".

Case History # **3**
Trudy, 62 years

Yeast infections are so prevalent because they are oven just plain over looked. Here is a typical case study I see, if you are a health professional, you will most probably think of a few cases you may have right now which resemble Trudy. Trudy came to see me several years ago complaining of irritable bowel syndrome (IBS). She had ongoing constipation and diarrhea for over ten years, "too many years to remember" she told me.

Trudy has been treated as an IBS patient by every practitioner she has seen, and was never considered to be a person who may have a serious yeast infection. Because she told them all that is what a medical doctor had diagnosed her with several years ago. There were the natural medicine practitioners who had placed her on strict exclusion diets and the allergy diets; her doctor had treated her several times with antibiotics before he washed his hands of her and placed her in the too hard basket.

The bowel specialist concluded that there was nothing the matter with Trudy after all the standard investigations like a colonoscopy, endoscopy, abdominal x-rays, and the many blood tests. I have heard this one hundred times before. Whenever I teach students about digestive problems, I say: "If the health professionals diagnose IBS or can't find a reason for the patient's digestive dysfunction, suspect a yeast infection".

Trudy mentioned that she had an itchy scalp and on close inspection I noticed that both her big toenails were thickened and discoloured. We completed a stool analysis and there it was – yeast in all three stool samples. But not only yeast, she also had several other bad bacteria and parasites present which is typical of a chronic ongoing digestive case like this. The opportunity exists for such a proliferation of dysbiosis; hence the term opportunistic infection is generally used. Trudy had a stool test completed years ago but was only tested for the basic pathogens like giardia, campylobacter, cryptosporidium and rotavirus, because she used to work at a children's day care centre on occasion. All results were negative as usual, and Trudy was left with no answers. It took almost six months to get Trudy in fine form.

One of my biggest disgusts with conventional treatment of digestive complaints is the routine and overzealous prescribing of anti-biotics by the doctors. And I have seen many hundreds of candida patients over the years that have never been well since a round of anti-biotics that was prescribed to them many years ago. Trudy was just another case. She had developed sore throats and chesty coughs in her late forties and was prescribed penicillin at least three to four times a year for a few years and then developed the digestive problems that were again treated with yet more antibiotics. As long as the doctors keep on prescribing these antibiotics, it will keep the naturopath in business trying to help the patient recover from a yeast infection.

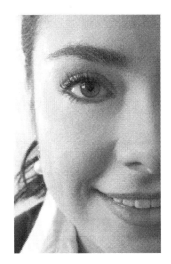

A Typical Chronic Candida Patient Profile

Here is a case illustration of the type of person I typically see in my consultation room with a chronic yeast infection. She will be female, middle income earner and will have been to one or several practitioners seeking help. She may have a history of the oral contraceptive pill, may have taken a steroid medication or an antibiotic in the past. She may well be under stress with children, her marriage, business, etc. Be sure to read Chapter 3 - Diagnosing, Identifying and Testing for Candida Yeast Infections for a most complete description of all the likely signs and symptoms you are likely to discover in those with yeast infections.

Gender: Female

Age: 18 to 55 years of age

General Symptoms: Chronic tiredness & fatigue, loss of energy, general unwellness and malaise, poor or no libido.

Gastrointestinal Symptoms: bloating, gas, constipation or diarrhea, irritable bowel syndrome, intestinal cramps or spasms, rectal itching, sweet cravings.

Genital and Urinary Symptoms: vaginal yeast infections and thrush, regular (itchy) discharge worse before the period, recurrent bladder or urinary tract infections, and premenstrual complaints.

Nervous System Symptoms: Depression, anxiety, irritability, poor memory and concentration and sleeping disturbances.

Immune System Symptoms: food allergies, environmental allergies and sensitivities, recurrent acute infections (coughs, colds, sinus, etc.), psoriasis.

Conditions Commonly Associated With Yeast Infections

- Premenstrual syndrome
- Low-blood sugar (hypoglycemia)
- Constipation, diarrhea, gas, bloating
- Food allergies and chemical sensitivities
- Leaky gut syndrome
- Psoriasis
- Irritable bowel syndrome
- Ulcerative colitis and Crohn's disease

Candida Predisposing Risk Factors

Here are some of the main predisposing factors when it comes to getting a yeast infection. A chronic yeast infection is not a condition acquired by some external source, it almost always the result of improper living habits, as well as dietary factors and even environmental and emotional influences that all can potentially lead to a reduced level of proper functioning of the entire body. But what are the main pre-disposing factors an individual will face when it comes to a yeast infection, what are some of the key drivers behind a person developing this condition?

Yeasts and other microorganisms like parasites and bacteria have no real place in your body to multiply and grow out of control into mutated forms unless the right conditions for them to do so exist. These conditions are created by a person's mode of living and diet. Always remember that the candida yeast organism has a place in the normal ecology of your healthy digestive system when these hostile conditions are not present, as they are kept in balance by the friendly organisms.

The factors you see below are the main ones I find which contribute to disturbing the intestinal tract's ecology, and once the balance is disturbed the concentration of healthy species will become diminished and it is at this point that candida can begin to get the upper hand and mutate into their more harmful fungal forms.

Once in this mutated form, the fungal rhizoids have the ability to penetrate the delicate intestinal lining with their elongated root-like structures. It is at this stage that they have successfully migrated from the intestinal tract into the systemic circulation, and at this point they have the ability to colonize different parts of your body because wherever the circulation (bloodstream) takes them the potential is there for harm. The rhizoid form more so than the candida yeast form has the ability to produce powerful toxins which have the potential to cause a great deal of suffering to their host, and in some cases can completely overwhelm the body's detoxification system. I'll talk a lot more about these forms and how they can affect your body later on.

- **Inappropriate Diet.** I expand greatly on diet in section 1 of chapter 7 (Understanding Digestion and Nutrition) but suffice to say this is a big problem with many people living with a yeast infection. It probably won't be when they see me in my clinic, I have noticed that by the time they come to see me that most will have cleaned up their diet as they have learned over time that many foods have the potential to make them feel terrible and must be avoided. These foods often include such items as alcohol, chocolate, rich and creamy foods like ice cream and cakes, but may even include commercial bread and milk. But for years these foods and drinks were not avoided and along with other factors may have contributed to the yeast infection. A number of dietary factors certainly promote the overgrowth of a yeast infection, and the recovery diet needs to be free of sugars, fruit juices, refined foods and any foods or drinks with a high content of sugar. Foods with a potential to mold or yeast must be avoided as well, and these include alcoholic drinks, peanuts, melons, cheeses and dried fruits. Cow's milk contains lactose (sugar) and is potentially one of the most allergy-forming foods and should be avoided for some time, especially until the digestive system has much improved. I'm big on removing all potentially allergenic foods from the diet as well, because most with a chronic yeast infection have developed a "leaky gut" (gastro-intestinal permeability) and have an increased risk of food allergies because of it. Please read section 1 if chapter 7 for much more detailed information about this most important predisposing factor – diet.

- **Alcohol.** Candidiasis patients should also stay away from all alcohol since it is composed of fermented and refined sugar. It is more toxic than sugar in candida problems and really feeds the yeast. Alcohol suppresses the immune system, disturbs the whole adrenal – stress axis, and there in no doubt that it makes anyone with candida feel much worse in the long run.

  I have seen several patients in particular who find it almost impossible to stay away from alcohol yet who have digestive issues, skin complaints and fatigue. This to me is saying that you have a money problem yet you keep taking on more credit with the bank and continue a gambling habit. Of course you have a problem, and the cause is right under your nose but you are either in denial or you just can't be bothered. With women it is usually the wine and chocolate, with guys it will be beer or wine. I can't think of any food or beverage more destructive for the candida patient than alcohol. The more resistant the patient is in wanting to give up all alcohol entirely for at least 6 months (to allow the digestive system to recover), the more likely it is that alcohol is underpinning the candida condition.

Many candida patients also have anxiety, mood swings, impatience, irritability and even depression. These conditions appear to go hand in hand with chronic candida sufferers, especially if regular alcohol intake is apparent. Some candidiasis sufferers will feel, and appear to be, intoxicated. An unusual symptom of certain people with severe candidiasis is the presence of alcohol in the blood stream even when none has been consumed. First discovered in Japan, and called "drunk disease," this condition creates strains of candida albicans which turn acetaldehyde (which is the chemical created by sugar and yeast fermentation and as a waste by-product of candida) into ethanol. This is a process well understood by distillers of homemade brew.

A medical test has been developed in which, after an overnight fast, the individual is given 100 grams of pure sugar. Blood samples taken both before the sugar loading, and an hour after, are measured for alcohol. An increase of alcohol indicates yeast "auto-brewery" intoxication. Another connection between alcohol and candidiasis has been found in a study of 213 alcoholics at a recovery center in Minneapolis, USA. Test and questionnaire results indicated that candidiasis is a common complication of moderately heavy drinkers and alcoholics due to the combination of high sugar content in alcohol and the inability of drinker to assimilate nutrients. Additionally, female heavy drinkers with candidiasis were significantly sicker than non-drinking women with candidiasis.

Many of the symptoms exhibited in drinkers such as insomnia, depression, loss of libido, headaches, sinusitis/post-nasal drip, digestion and intestinal complaints, overlap with those in candida overgrowth.

- **Reduced Digestive Function.** A common theme with many patients with yeast infections is an impaired ability of the upper digestive system to function adequately. It's amazing how common those drug advertisements are on the TV at night, aimed at putting out the fire of an over-acid stomach. A condition we commonly see in the clinic is hypochlorhydria, or an under acidity of the stomach. Unfortunately, the symptoms of this condition can include reflux, heartburn or a low-grade feeling of nausea. The doctor may be quick to prescribe an acid blocker (believing the patient has a stomach over-acidity) that relieves the symptom but keeps the patient reliant on a drug continuously. Digestive secretions like hydrochloric acid (stomach) and pancreatic enzymes as well as bile all play a very important role in the inhibition of candida and prevent its infiltration from the small intestine into the bloodstream because they create an environment hostile to yeasts.

A very much over-looked area in natural medicine, and completely over-looked in conventional medicine, is the recommendation of digestive enzymes. A reduced or poor output of enzymes like amylase due to stress, alcohol, soda drinks, sugars, etc., will create incomplete digestion of proteins and carbohydrates and predispose the person to the development of intestinal toxemia and food allergies, as well as yeast infections. Bowel toxins are more easily formed creating a problem for the intestinal tract, leading the unsuspecting patient and practitioner on a progressively downward spiral of chronic fatigue, increasing allergies, mental and emotional irritability and "unexplained" digestive problems, sometimes for many, many years. A little known fact is that an important role of the pancreatic enzymes is to prevent any unwanted bacteria, yeasts or parasites form entering into the small intestine, preventing their overgrowth. This is one of the main reasons I recommend most all patients with yeast infection to take a top-quality digestive enzyme to help the digestive secretions along.

Pancreatic insufficiency. Some of my best success stories in the clinic come from treating pancreatic problems in patients who were passed-off by their practitioner as being in the too hard basket or just plain unresponsive to their regular treatments. Some of the most difficult of all candida cases I've seen have at times proven to be the pancreatic insufficiency patients, and this is a good tip if you are a practitioner reading this right now. Take a digestive enzyme product (containing amylase in particular) if you suspect problems here. Your patient will be glad she did.

Liver/gallbladder cases. The second category of difficult digestive cases I tend to see with regards to the unresolved candida cases are those women with obstructed livers and congested gallbladder function. Liver and gallbladder stones and gravel are very common indeed, and most people will have some degree of stones. As the stones grow in size and become more numerous, the liver and gallbladder become increasingly compromised in their ability to make and expel bile. This prevents the liver from eliminating harmful substances like parasites, bacteria, yeasts and many different chemicals. Cholesterol levels may rise and frequently drop down after a liver/gallbladder cleanse.

In addition, stones are porous and contain bacteria, yeasts, parasites, viruses and various other pathogens and chemicals. This way, nests of potential infection and re-infection form that can repeatedly seed the body, often causing "unexplained" infections. A healthy liver will normally filter candida toxins from the blood, and many expert practitioners believe that conditions especially like psoriasis come about due to the liver's impaired ability to filter the candida toxins.

Case History # 4
Alan, 58 years

Alan and Susan are patients well known to our practice. Together they own and run a large and highly successful national franchise chain, and have worked hard all their lives to achieve the amazing level of success they now enjoy. Alan is a diabetic (Type 2 diabetes) who has a major case of psoriasis that occasionally used to spiral out of control. The scaly patches of skin up his arms and legs are quite an embarrassment to him and he once mentioned to me that would dearly love to have a clear skin for the summertime when he enjoys golf and the beach. The problem is that Alan also really enjoys red wine and chocolate, and these only helped to promote his psoriasis.

After a successful bowel and liver detoxification program outlined in section 3, chapter 7 – Understanding Cleansing and Detoxification, Alan experienced an almost total and complete remission of his psoriasis. Presently, when Alan does decide to adhere to the principles of the Candida Crusher Program, he does not have any flare-up of his psoriasis, but when he wanders off track for too long with his beloved red wine and chocolate, it returns with a vengeance. Psoriasis and yeast infections are very commonly found together, and if you follow the principles of eating without sugar-laden foods and engage in a good detox you will find to your surprise that your psoriasis will most certainly clear up and stay that way, only to return if you go back to your old ways and maintain these ways for weeks on end. You will need to work out for yourself whether you want a skin free from psoriatic lesions, and more importantly, to what extent you are willing to put up with psoriasis based on your level of "offending". Some can only offend a little, whereas others can offend a lot and are willing to put up with a lot. The ball is in your court. I have witnessed this with several hundred psoriasis cases in my clinic, and one of these days I may just write a booklet on this topic because there is too much bull manure written about psoriasis, even more so than about candida.

- **Nutritional Deficiencies.** Optimal immune function relies on optimal nutritional levels, and virtually any nutritional deficiency can lead to a compromised immune system. Possibly the most important nutrients in this respect are iron, folic acid, magnesium, essential fatty acids, zinc, selenium, vitamins A, C, D and E and B_6. There are ample studies that document that deficiencies of these key nutrients in particular contribute to chronic yeast infections.

Case History # 5
Gerry, 36 years

Gerry is single man who never married and works as a factory security guard at night. He came to see me some time ago complaining of jock itch, athlete's foot, heartburn and fatigue and was sent in by a lady friend who I helped to get rid of her yeast infection. Gerry's hobby is stock-car racing which takes up much of his spare time, and he spends many hours in his garage tinkering with his cars which includes a lot of welding and grinding as well as general mechanical work most afternoons during the week as well as almost every weekend.

He mentioned that he wears coveralls for several hours a day and when I questioned him about his diet it was what I expected – fast foods that are nutritionally depleted and over-processed.

Gerry would routinely skip breakfast, (having a cigarette and a coffee instead) for lunch he would usually go through to the drive-through of a fast food restaurant (deep fried chicken, pizza or burgers) and his evening meal always consisted of a TV dinner, an ice cream and a few cans of beer. Is it any wonder he had a major yeast infection? His coveralls provided the perfect warm and moist environment for a yeast infection and his diet contained sufficient sugar to maintain it.

The first change I recommended was to get rid of the coveralls and to wear 100% cotton loose fitting clothing, especially around the groin region. He was to wear 100% cotton socks and to remove them and go barefoot as soon as he was finished for the day. Gerry had developed the habit of keeping his socks on from early morning until almost bedtime when he would have his bath. I have noticed that those with tinea (athlete's foot) tend to wear shoes or boots and socks for many hours a day and rarely have their feet exposed to air, light and sun.

I asked Gerry if he could have a shower twice daily at the very least, but preferably three times daily. He is the shower once on rising and then again after work and once before bed, and if hot and sweaty also before he begins his night shift as a security guard. I recommended the use of Tea Tree oil soap and shampoo as they are very anti-fungal personal care products and have an excellent effect in many people with candida.

The biggest challenge for Gerry was to change his diet to a fresh, wholefoods diet and to take a top-quality multivitamin and mineral supplement along with an omega 3 supplement, probiotic and digestive enzyme tablet. After six months the improvements were staggering to say the least, his athlete's food and jock itch were entirely gone and he was delighted.

- **Reduced immune function.** Once a person's immune system becomes compromised, a yeast infection can get the upper hand and it stands to reason that a healthy and vibrant immune system is an important prerequisite in overcoming and successfully crushing a yeast infection. This is also one of the main reasons why a yeast infection can become a recurrent problem spanning many years, there could be an underlying and unresolved chronic low-grade problem preventing the immune system from working at its full capacity. Your immune system can become weakened by many different factors, including drug use, nutritional deficiencies, stress, various chronic diseases like cancer, diabetes, hepatitis, diseased teeth, heavy metal toxicity, being HIV positive, etc.

Remember we spoke just before about the liver gallbladder containing and stones and gravel potentially harboring bacteria and viruses? The tonsils, appendix, and ileocecal valve (the connection between your small and large bowel) and especially suspect, diseased teeth (and their roots) are all common places for bugs to hide-out and become potential hot-spots for viruses, yeasts and bacteria. This is an extremely commonly over-looked area in medical but also in natural medical practice.

Your body is clever in that your immune system will produce antibodies to respond to a particular antigen, and an antigen is something your body senses as foreign which stimulates a response by the immune system.

Candida itself has many antigens, and there can be an inborn inherent defect of your immune system that stimulates a strong response against one or more particular antigens. There are great variations also in the response to these antigens, because we are all biochemically individual.

Our ability to handle a yeast infection varies greatly from one individual to another, and some people will be more able than others to keep candida under control and limit its spread. The most common areas for candida to spread in your body, the hot spots, are into the throat, the mouth/tongue and into the vaginal area (thrush), the feet (athlete's foot), the groin and armpits. These areas will then flare-up as the body's resistance drops, and every person with a yeast infection will tend to have his or her "weak spot". These weak spots will then typically flare up from time to time due to factors such as stress, poor nutrition, lack of sufficient sleep, pollution/toxicity as well as the use of pharmaceutical drugs which all serve to weaken the immune system even further.

Eventually, over a longer period of time as your immune system becomes increasingly weaker, the yeast infection will be less inclined to invoke acute flare-ups, but will tend to remain symptomatic in a semi-permanent or a chronic state.

All patients who see me can remember those initial flare-ups of their yeast infection, and can then recount over time how the symptoms became more regular and then daily. Eventually their life becomes so compromised that all they do is try to counter the increasing severity of their yeast infection with a larger and larger array of pills and potions, different therapies, different practitioners, until the whole thing starts to spiral out of control.

As you can see, one of the primary objectives of the Candida Crusher Program is to help identify and remove these weak spots, to boost immunity and keep it operating at its maximum level. Be sure to read section 2 (Chapter 7) entitled Understanding Stress and Immunity for more comprehensive information on how you can achieve this objective.

Infections – a major cause One of the commonly overlooked causes of a yeast infection was an infection in the past, and the person was prescribed an antibiotic. Candida yeast infections are often precipitated by recurring infections such as bronchitis, sinusitis, or other respiratory infections, urinary tract infections, acne skin infections. The more severe the infection, the more likely that antibiotics will be repeatedly prescribed and the more likely that increasingly stronger dosages or prescriptions are used. Some doctors seem to think "the bigger the problem the bigger the hammer" and will continually prescribe, sometimes for years.

Case History # 6
Aaron, 18 years

Aaron's case is not uncommon, but most distressing for me to see this young man who has developed a chronic illness as a result of antibiotics prescribed for three years continually for facial acne. His mother took him to a doctor when he had just turned 15 years of age, because he had a rather severe case of acne vulgaris. The doctor recommended low-dose Tetracycline (antibiotic), and initially Aaron noticed an improvement and his mother was happy, but after twelve months the acne did not clear up, so his doctor just increased the dose. Not once was Aaron instructed in any facial hygiene protocols, lifestyle or dietary changes, he was just recommended to take the antibiotics. After having been on the antibiotic for three years, his father brought him to me (his mother does not believe in natural medicine) because Aaron was feeling terrible. After we ran some blood tests we discovered that his liver enzymes were significantly elevated as a result of the antibiotics, the drugs were poisoning his liver.

Besides, Aaron had developed a rather severe case of jock itch and athlete's food. The doctor has prescribed an antifungal cream for the jock itch and ignored the athlete's foot, but most incredibly – he maintained Aaron on the antibiotics, stating that the jock itch and athlete's foot were unlikely to be related to the antibiotic.

My first initial recommendation was for Aaron to thrown the drugs in the garbage can and began by instructing him to stop all those soda drinks he was consuming and to concentrate on a fresh food diet, we began him on a regime of antioxidants and an intensive facial cleansing regime. It took over 6 months before we got rid of his chronic yeast infection, but we eventually beat it. In Aaron's case, the exciting cause was the antibiotics, and the maintaining cause was the soda drinks and poor diet.

- Drug Use. One of the devastating effects I have seen in many women over the years that have complained of thrush and endometriosis is the long-term use of the oral contraceptive pill. I have certainly seen a strong correlation with women who have had a history of thrush and who used suppressive drug treatments to "cure" the complaint and who then went on to develop endometriosis. The most widespread use of pharmaceutical steroids is not in inhalers for asthma, nor in steroid creams for bothersome skin – but in the use of the contraceptive pill. This type of medication has a subtle but powerfully suppressive effect on the immune system as well.

Antibiotics and Yeast Infections. According to many authorities in natural medicine, antibiotics may be the single greatest cause of candidiasis, because antibiotic treatment for infections is non-discriminatory, killing the good intestinal chemistry-balancing bacteria, as well as the bad infection-causing bacteria. Since antibiotics were discovered in the late 1940's, the incidence of diseases related to the digestive system has increased dramatically. And candida is no exception; we have seen an alarming increase in candida overgrowth since antibiotics were first used in medical practice. A tremendous amount of research articles have been published since the 1950's with regard to candida and antibiotic use. Since then, more than 27,000 articles have been published on this association alone. That's enough research to enable you to study one paper every single day for the next 73 years. The common thread I have noticed in many of these articles is that the regular use of antibiotic drugs leads to the development of a yeast infection.

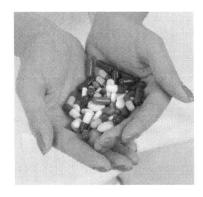

Let me enlighten you a little about how candida infections and their link with antibiotics, a link initially discovered by an American doctor not long after antibiotics were first introduced into general practice. When antibiotics were first developed, they contained an antifungal medicine built in to discourage the re-growth of fungal conditions that commonly occurs after a course of antibiotics. Not long after, the antifungal component was taken away, splitting these drugs into two different drugs, an anti fungal and an antibiotic drug.

Further down the track when antibiotics were introduced into the food chain the problem became even worse, and today there are many animal types of meat that contain traces of antibiotics, for example commercial poultry.

Not long after, also in the early 1950's, Dr. Orian Truss discovered the devastating effects of these antibiotics in an American hospital. During a hospital round, an elderly looking man who appeared to look as if he was dying intrigued Dr. Truss.

But this was no elderly man; this man was in his forties and in hospital for several months. No medical expert was able to make a diagnosis, they simply couldn't figure out why he wasn't getting better. Out of curiosity, Dr. Truss asked the patient when he was last completely well.

The man answered that he was well until six months before when he had cut his finger He had then received antibiotics and shortly afterwards developed diarrhea and his health has deteriorated ever since. Truss had plenty of experience and had seen a few years before how antibiotics caused diarrhea and he learned that fungal conditions such as candida were opportunistic and thrived in debilitated patients. Dr. Truss treated the man's candida infection which not only cleared rapidly, but the health improved remarkably overall.

Like many practitioners, I have seen countless cases of patients who have never been well since one or several rounds of antibiotics. Antibiotics are almost not necessary in most instances, in fact, and I have never used them with my family for more over twenty years. My four children have had the usual coughs, colds, cuts and broken bones, yet we have never once had to resort to antibiotics, not one single time. I have seen patients who have been unsuccessful on long-term antibiotic treatment recover within weeks with natural medicines when correctly administered. Quality natural medicines *do work* with infections and I am emphatic in the belief that antibiotics ("anti-life") may only really be necessary in bacterial pneumonia.

You may have different views, but I believe that conventional medicine is still based largely on the fear factor, and if you make somebody scared enough you can have them submit more easily to your way of treatment. Your patient may do something that he or she may later regret like an unnecessary operation, taking a drug long-term or undergo an unnecessary invasive medical procedure.

In the half percent of the cases in which antibiotics are absolutely necessary, the serious after-effects of antibiotic drugs could easily have be avoided using a probiotic. It never ceases to amaze me how readily many doctors still prescribe antibiotics for a simple cut to the finger as a "precautionary" measure. Yeast infected patients are at a particularly high risk of such prescribing when visiting their doctor with various ear, nose, throat or skin infections.

When beneficial bacterium were recommended in the 1960's in therapy they were not taken seriously by the majority of those in medicine, but today things are different and there has been a big shift towards recommending them after antibiotics, lactobacillus acidophilus is one such bacterium killed by antibiotics and highly recommended. A few years ago you didn't hear much about probiotics; today they are big news on TV and in the chemist shop (drug store) and health-food shop. Lactobacillus species happily reside in your intestines where they assist in the breakdown of foods like proteins and carbohydrates in lactic acid that allows your digestive system to maintain a balance between the good and not so good bacteria and yeasts.

Candida and other pathogenic yeasts start to grow and overtake the friendly bacteria once the friendly bacteria are in decline.

But what happens as the bad bugs grow and multiply, and multiple courses of antibiotics are given, is that each successive generation becomes a little more antibiotic-resistant than the last.

And the consequence of this is that increasingly higher dosages and stronger antibiotics are required. And so the yeast infection grows.

It is most unfortunate that many in general doubt the effectiveness of natural medicines against apparently serious infections, but experience leads me to believe that natural therapies are just as effective if not even more so, yet without causing the chronic and recurring fungal or other opportunistic infections usually seen after antibiotics.

Dr. Orion Truss who himself had completed much research into antibiotics and their side-effects, was a firm believer that antibiotics cause more harm than good in most instances. He frequently used to say that antibiotics were often used "inadvisably", and in many cases were they had no role to play in healing. For example, in situations of incorrectly diagnosed viral or fungal infections, in which case there is the strong likelihood of an actual worsening of the case. Truss was very much against the routine prescribing of tetracycline for acne, and believed that there was no way of controlling resulting yeast infections with routine prescriptions of antibiotics or the Pill. Truss discovered in fact that in many cases acne was as a direct result of a yeast infection, which worsened rather than improved on treatment.

Antibiotics in the Food Chain. At this point it is worth mentioning that there is another often totally ignored source of antibiotics and hormonal residues coming into your diet, this is of course the commercially raised meat and especially poultry you may well be consuming. Antibiotics and hormones are fed to commercially raised animals to control their heightened susceptibility towards diseases in addition to speed up their rate or growth. I can remember reading about this in the early 1980's in many candida books, that authors showed concerns about these chemicals in our daily food supply and that back then, just like today, that little research if any, has ever been conducted on the link between yeast infection and commercially raised meat. It is the ongoing and low levels of these chemicals in our diets that are a part of the problem, and my advice for you is to avoid commercially raised poultry in particular, and go for free range instead. These companies will be quick to mention that they use "no growth hormones", but there is no mention of the antibiotics that they nearly always use because of the way they house their chickens.

Steroidal Drugs. Needless to say, I am not a big fan of steroidal drugs with patients for too many reasons to mention in this book. Steroidal drugs produce side effects in almost every system of the body. They disturb the delicate hormonal system and by doing so disturb a person's entire body chemistry. In particular, they cause strong suppression of the adrenal gland that produces the body's own natural steroidal drugs such as cortisone.

A short course of prednisone for a few days to one week will not produce a great deal of side effects, but repeated courses can result in significant side effects and some patients we see have been on steroids for more than twenty years. Steroids are implicated in causing fermentation dysbiosis with yeast infections.

For many years, fungal infections in those who were taking steroidal medications were considered as "nuisance diseases" such as athlete's foot or vaginal yeast infections. However, advances in medical technology, including organ and bone marrow transplants, chemotherapy, and the increased use of antibiotics have only added to the increase in fungal infections.

Are you taking a steroidal inhaler for your asthma, a sinus steroid spray for your sinusitis, or maybe a steroidal tablet to suppress your immune system due to an inflammatory illness like rheumatoid arthritis? You may want to be particularly vigilant because you will be at a particularly high risk of developing a yeast infection due to the immune-suppressing effects of the steroid drugs. I highly recommend that you speak to your health-care professional about your concerns and to see if you can either reduce the dosage or switch to a different class of drug with less side effects.

Non Steroidal Anti-Inflammatory Drugs (NSAIDS). This group of drugs comprises any drug which has an anti-inflammatory action yet is not steroidal in nature, such as Ibuprofen (Advil, Motrin), Aspirin (Ecotrin), Naproxen (Naprosyn and Midol), Diclofenac (Voltaren) and Acetaminophen (Panadol or Tylenol). Are you taking one of these drugs long-term? WHY? Do you know the damage they are causing to your digestive system? There is no question that the risks of NSAIDs can be serious, even life-threatening. According to the American Gastroenterological Association (AGA), each year the side effects of NSAIDs hospitalize over 100,000 people and kill 16,500 in the U.S alone., mostly due to bleeding stomach ulcers.

I'll be writing and talking a lot more in the future about the horrific affects I see daily in my clinic with these terrible "medicines" which are so widely and freely recommended and taken by so many people yet are so incredibly damaging to the liver, stomach and digestive system in general. I am worried about the many different chronic digestive problems I've been seeing in patients who take these drugs, sometimes for years on end with serious health issues. Huge pharmaceutical drug company spending is thrown at these poisons, as they are a big cash cow for the drug companies. Once a person is hooked on the belief that a pill will take away all their pain, there is no reason to look at the underlying cause of this pain. And in many cases it will be found to be some kind of stress related to muscular tension.

Remember I said previously that there is no profit in prevention, only treatment? Time to wake up, the only way to get you health back on track is to address the cause, regardless of whether you are suffering from a headache, backache, period pain or a yeast infection.

Gastric bleeding and all manner of blood and immune based problems occur in those who take NSAIDS long-term, and I've seen in my clinic many patients with ulcerative colitis and Crohn's disease who took NSAIDS regularly. Many patients with chronic candida have a past and present history of taking some kind NSAID drug. Are you a routine pill-popper whenever you have a backache, headache or menstrual pain? You may be causing a lot more harm than good. I'll stick with my daily pill, a chill pill called relaxation; it seems to work wonders at preventing my stress-related aches and pains.

Case History # 7
Val, 73 years

Val came to my rooms complaining of severe fatigue, burning and itchy ears, eyes burning and watery, an irritable burning throat and many digestive problems on top of her chronic and debilitating fatigue. Val had childhood asthma and was placed on steroid medications just over 60 years ago, and remained on them for almost 50 years. She has spent countless hours over the years in various hospitals and finally (after a total of consulting with more than 30 doctors) after two epileptic fits it was decided that she should have "no more steroids" after almost 50 years of continuous use. Ventolin (Salbutamol) was taken for 25 years and other drugs like antibiotics were routinely prescribed on and off. Over the past 30 years her sinus, nose, eyes and ears were getting worse by the day, but still the doctors persisted with the steroidal drug recommendations. It is early days for Val, but things are already starting to look great. I first recommended that all drugs be neatly flushed down the lavatory from this point forward, and we started Val on an adrenal fatigue treatment program. The results have been incredible to say the least, and it just goes to show that no matter how old a person is, how debilitated they are or how screwed up they have become due to chronic over-prescribing of drugs, the body keeps on maintaining the ability to restore its vital function. After just 6 months of adrenal treatment we have had a staggering 40% improvement already, but I suspect that Val will need adrenal support for up to two years or even more before we get a full-recovery which I now believe is on the cards.

Are you a victim of a lifetime of steroids like Val? Then please visit a doctor who understands adrenal fatigue and its proper management. You are worth it!

> **The Oral Contraceptive Pill and Yeast Infections.** Dr. Truss also learned that about 35% of women who take the oral contraceptive pill have acute vaginal candidiasis associated with it. Truss mentioned "Chronic yeast vaginitis tends to be at its worst when progesterone levels are at their highest, as in pregnancy, or during the luteal phase of the menstrual cycle". Truss felt that the progesterone component of the Pill might well be responsible for the increased incidence of vaginal thrush whilst on the Pill.

Taking into account the 35% of women who develop thrush while on the Pill, we must also understand then that about 65% of women don't. This again highlights the fact that genetic weaknesses are possible that one third of women have a heightened susceptibility.

And in these cases it is important to control the factors which are under our control and which may make a difference, such as taking antibiotics, the Pill, as well as other factors like stress and nutritional requirements.

Any intelligent approach to eradicating a yeast infection permanently surely must take into account these factors, and these include building up our immune system and reducing the aggravating factors that help sustain the yeast infection in advance. The most important point here is eliminating the use of antibiotics (unless in serious situations like blood poisoning, bacterial pneumonia, etc.) and the avoidance of hormones and steroids.

Diabetics are particularly prone to candida yeast infections as their alterations in blood sugar levels can make them more prone to sugar cravings.

For this reason, those with diabetes must be even more rigorous in their efforts to control candida. Here is a true case history of a patient I am seeing who started early on antibiotics, and was prescribed them regularly throughout her life. Is it any wonder that Nikki eventually developed endometriosis?

Case History # 8
Nikki, 32 years

Nikki had her first antibiotics prescribed to her when she was 5 years of age for minor health concerns, tonsillitis and repeated ear infections. As she grew up she started to develop bladder infections (cystitis) during her years at boarding school. Her doctor prescribed a broad-spectrum antibiotic for this, and Nikki was given penicillin at least twice annually for over four years until she was about 16 years of age. Her skin started to develop a good deal of acne at this stage and the doctor once again prescribed an antibiotic long term. At 17, Nikki developed a bad case of bronchitis that left her with a wheeze, and the doctor then prescribed her with an asthma inhaler (salbutamol, a bronchodilator) and a preventive steroid inhaler. She also started to develop vaginal thrush when she was about 17 and her doctor prescribed fluconazole and she also had regular prescriptions of creams that she applied regularly. At 18 Nikki was prescribed the oral contraceptive pill and remained on the Pill for ten years, until she decided to have a baby when she was 28. It took almost one and a half years for Nikki to conceive after she went off the Pill, and she has been unable to have her second child due to a diagnosis of endometriosis. I have been working with Nikki for the past year to help her overcome her candida yeast infection. She has gained a considerable amount of weight and was also prescribed Prozac for depression last year. This is a typical case I see and you can see the progression of illness as the pharmaceutical drugs have been prescribed for almost twenty years in this case. It will take two years for Nikki's health to return to normal, and my strict instructions to her are to avoid all forms of steroids and antibiotics in the future if she is to remain well. It is also interesting to note that Nikki's child was born with oral thrush, and it didn't surprise me. Her child was exposed to many candida antigens in Nikki's womb from all the candida activity in her body, all the while inheriting the strong possibility of a weakened immune system, and so the cycle may likely repeat itself. Can you see any similarities here with your child or your upbringing with antibiotics? You may want to break the cycle and say "no" to continual and repeated antibiotic prescriptions like in Nikki's case.

- **Stress.** Stress is a frequently overlooked exciting cause in yeast infection is stress, which can be of psychological, emotional, environmental, or infectious in origin or a combination of many of these causes. My stress-mentor Dr. James Wilson, author of the book "Adrenal Fatigue, The 21st Century Stress Syndrome" has taught me a considerable amount about stress over the past 5 years. You can read a lot more about stress and yeast infections in Chapter 7, Section 2 (Candida Crusher Lifestyle – Understanding Stress and Immunity)

Common Candida Yeast Infection Myths

I would like to dispel some commonly held beliefs about candida yeast infections. There are so many myths relating to yeast infections, I think I have heard them all. Many people have accepted a lot of these beliefs as facts.

" All Yeast Infections Are Due To Candida Albicans "

After having completed over several thousand comprehensive stool tests on patients with yeast infections over the years I have noticed that approximately 70% of the yeast found was candida albicans, the remainder being candida tropicalis, candida glabrata and candida parapsilosis. Occasionally I see more rare strains like candida krusei, but not very often. Did you know there are about 250 different candida strains, and that some are easier to eradicate than others? In my experience, candida tropicalis is much more difficult to shift than candida albicans.

While about 80-90% of yeast infections are caused by candida species, there are more than 200 different strains of yeast that can affect you. Sometimes, if you have been using drugs to wipe out the most common yeast strain, other non-candida strains can increase and cause a yeast infection. If you have recurrent issues with yeast it would be best not to self-medicate yourself but to get checked by your health provider who can send your culture to a lab for more detailed analysis.

" Strict Diets Cure Candida "

Following a strict candida diet, which some call the impossible diet will most certainly provide symptomatic relief of your yeast infection but will not "cure" you. It is virtually impossible to eliminate the yeast in your body, but it certainly is possible to bring it under control. What you want to achieve is balance and awareness of the fact that your yeast population is carefully kept in balance with the many species of bacteria that inhabit your digestive system in particular. Whilst some experts believe that high yeast, high starch, or a high sugar diets do not "feed" a person's yeast infection, I would tend to disagree here. Reducing the key trigger foods (which can vary greatly from person to person as I have discovered) allows the body to better handle the candida problem and helps to prevent an accelerated candida overgrowth, but in order to help accelerate the eliminate of the yeast problem on a long-term and even permanent basis we need to look elsewhere – the immune system and in particular the immune system residing in the digestive system.

" Only Supplements Are Required, Your Diet Is Not That Important "

Again, I have read this statement in countless blog posts, paper and e-books. This is simply not true, in fact in some cases nutritional supplements are not even required nor desired to affect a complete cure. I have seen this but it is the exception rather than the rule.

Best results will always be obtained by adopting the right diet, taking a few carefully chosen herbal or nutritional supplements and adopting the right lifestyle principles I outline as part of my Candida Crusher Program. (See chapter 7)

" My Treatment Plan Is The Only One That Works "

Bear in mind that there will be as many candida protocols as there will be religious belief systems, and there are literally thousands of them. Do yourself a favor and side step any fanatical belief systems, whether they be medical, religious or political! Have you noticed that some practitioners have extremely rigid treatment protocols and believe that their treatment plan is the only way to go? I'd suggest that you avoid any such doctor or practitioner who believes that his or her yeast infection protocol is the only way to cure your yeast infection. The Candida Crusher Program is certainly very effective, and several thousand patients have shown me that my system certainly does work, but I'm also sure that there will be other effective yeast infection eradication programs out there as well. Some believe in Jesus, some in Buddha and some simply don't want to believe at all, and I'm happy with that. If you are open minded and mature enough then you will discover that there is plenty of room for many different belief systems, in medicine, in religion and in politics.

" Probiotics Can Cure Candida "

Although a good probiotic can be very effective in preventing a candida overgrowth in the first place, there is certainly no evidence to suggest that any probiotic can actually cure candida. A top quality probiotic can be most effective, but you will need to be cautious of many retail purchased products, many of which I have found to be therapeutically of little value.

Once the candida becomes more widespread in the body you will find that probiotics have little effect unless you use a good eradication product and work hard out on diet modification. It is the combined and consistent effort placed on diet, supplements and lifestyle that will win the day in more than 90% of the most difficult cases I have seen. And of course, it pays to get in early before candida becomes too widespread.

" Candida Yeast Infections Are Caused By Heavy Metals "

This is another popular myth that has done the rounds, that mercury toxicity "causes" a candida yeast infection. I have read many blog posts and several e-books proclaiming that the only sure fire way to completely eliminate a yeast infection from the body is to get rid of all of one's amalgam mercury fillings. Whilst eliminating heavy metals from the body is a good idea, there is no scientific evidence to suggest that all cases of yeast infection are improved by removing one's mercury fillings. Heavy metals can certainly depress the immune system and thereby exacerbate a yeast infection, but I am not convinced that they actually cause candida directly.

Detoxification does make sense to me though, and as a candida patient improves and regains more strength and vitality then I do recommend a detox. You can read about more of detoxification in chapter 9.

" If I Feel Itchy, It Must Be A Yeast Infection "

I know of too many women who run down to the drug store to get Monistat, Fluconazole or another yeast medication as soon as they develop vaginal itchiness, believing that it must be a case of vaginal thrush (yeast) infection. The fact of the matter is the most common condition causing itchiness in women is BV, or bacterial vaginosis, and NOT thrush. There are potentially many other conditions that may be the cause of itchiness, and this is why it is important to get checked out at your doctor's office before you decide on the correct line of treatment.

A swab will quickly and accurately tell you what kind of vaginal irritation you have, and whether it is itchiness due to an allergy, a case of BV, chlamydia of vulvodynia.

" A Yeast Infection Can Make Me Infertile "

False, there is zero evidence to suggest that a yeast infection can or will make you infertile. One of the most common reasons today affecting women and fertility is the stressful and very hectic lives they lead, and many are now leaving it until their late thirties or early forties until they have their first child. There are of course many other reasons for infertility, such as low sperm counts, but a yeast infection is not one of them, but there is some evidence that a case of vaginal yeast infection when routinely treated and suppressed with vaginal applicator creams can lead to driving the condition further into the endometrium (womb) and being implicated in endometriosis. If you do have vaginal thrush, make sure you treat it locally as well as by way of a healthy diet and lifestyle.

" Douching Can Cure My Yeast Infection "

There is the false belief that just by regular douching you can get rid of a yeast infection permanently. What many women don't know is that an acidic douche like vinegar does not necessarily kill a yeast infection, because candida can live in an alkaline environment as well as an acid environment. Douching does not generally have an effect on the entire vaginal environment either, as candida can thrive around the cervix, and area notoriously difficult to access by way of douching. This way of vaginal cleansing will often have a temporary effect and can in some instances even shift bacteria and yeast further up the vagina or into the urethra, causing a urinary tract infection.

" I Don't Have A Yeast Infection Because I Have Never Had A Vaginal Discharge "

It is not true that all yeast infections include a vaginal discharge; indeed, many women suffer with candida overgrowths that have never had a discharge. Many female patients I have seen over the years have complained of intense itchiness and soreness yet with no discharge at all.

" Yogurt Will Cure My Yeast Infection "

I have not found this to be the case al all, yogurt can relieve the symptoms of burning and itching in particular, but I've never seen it actually cure any vaginal yeast infection. It certainly does make a lot of sense to continue eating a small amount of good quality yogurt each day to help repopulate the digestive system with plenty of beneficial bacteria, and in addition to continue to use yogurt as part of your treatment plan to help relieve any local symptoms.

" Yeast Infections Are Not Sexually Transmitted Diseases (STDs) "

Yeast infections are not true STDs, but yeast infections can certainly be transmitted between partners during sexual relations.

It is therefore important that both partners are treated for a yeast infection at the same time and in addition observe cleanliness before and after intercourse to prevent transmission.

" Cancer Is Caused By Candida, And Taking Sodium Bicarbonate Will Prevent Or Cure Cancer "

Some alternative practitioners, especially Dr. Tullio Simoncini from Italy, promote sodium bicarbonate as a cure for candida and for cancer. This claim is made on several Web sites, and in You Tube videos that Dr. Simoncini has posted on the Internet, and in a book he has written as well. Scientists require evidence and studies before they can recommend certain treatments. No peer-reviewed articles in medical journals are to be found supporting the theory that cancer can be cured or prevented using sodium bicarbonate. And any available peer-reviewed medical journals do not support claims that sodium bicarbonate has worked as a cancer treatment.

While I do subscribe to the theory that alkaline diets have their place in preventing many chronic diseases and helping to reduce the chances of developing a yeast infection, I don't subscribe to the fact that giving somebody continual doses of sodium bicarbonate will cure their yeast infection or prevent cancer.

CHAPTER 3 — Diagnosing, Identifying & Testing for Candida Yeast Infections

Signs and Symptoms – The Common and Not so Common

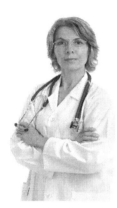

It has been stated by many health-care professionals that virtually everyone exhibits minor symptoms of candidiasis, while about one third of the population, at least in the West, is affected, and some severely. Based on my experiences in the clinic over many years I certainly support this remarkable assertion. In many cases, a definite diagnosis is quite difficult, if not impossible, but according to Western medicine in order to effectively treat something you first have to accurately diagnose it. In most cases of yeast infection with a bit of help from a practitioner and by completing various home tests yourself, you will be able to diagnose candida yourself.

This chapter is extensive and contains an exhaustive list of all the major and minor symptoms of a yeast infection. I'll explain how you can spot yeast infections in women, men and children and show you the home tests I have developed and been using in my clinic for several years with great success. You will also find my Candida Test Tracker © and Candida Symptom Tracker ©, two tools which will enable you to successfully track your Candida Crusher Program progress over a four-month period. I have found these tools invaluable and use them routinely in my clinic.

Just look further ahead in this book at the several home tests for a yeast infection and try some of these yourself, most you can track weekly, others monthly or bi-monthly.

Sometimes only a series of vague symptoms will show the patient that everything is right, and at times no end of medical tests, examinations or pathology (lab) tests will confirm a definite "disease".

Sometimes an inexperienced practitioner will overlook these vague symptoms and treat the patient for something other than candida. I know this all too well, after having helped many patients with candida for years that had visited other practitioners and were diagnosed with irritable bowel syndrome, constipation, diarrhea, parasites, food allergies, constipation, gallstones, inflammatory bowel disease, and a whole host of other complaints.

Some of these patients were desperate to get help and had become disillusioned about treatment and wondered if they would ever get well. Some of these cases have proven to be quite difficult to deal with, and is it any wonder? If you were told that you have no diagnosable health problems but you knew yourself for certain that you did, if you had been to several practitioners with little success and in addition tried self-help but improved little as a result, then you probably would be disillusioned yourself.

I can still remember how I felt when I had chronic candidiasis in the 1980's, no one to turn to and not being taken seriously by practitioners, family or friends, and mainly because there was no clear cut diagnosis. That is why chapter 3 is an important chapter and I therefore do hope you get a good understanding of testing and candida.

When you specialize in candida, you come to understand the mindset of the chronic candida patient over time, and if you put yourself in the shoes of somebody who has a chronic yeast infection, a person who has had this condition for several years without much help or relief, then you will know precisely what I mean.

Spot the Candida Patient

When a patient comes into my clinic with a very restricted or limited diet and multiple digestive complaints, complaining of many food allergies and sensitivities that there is a big chance they will have a major problem with intestinal dysbiosis, including various strains of bad bacteria, yeasts and possibly parasites. Some of these patients will have visited many practitioners, others will have spent many an hour online and can often tell you exactly what is wrong with them, and all you need to do is listen. Why am I confident in assuming they have these digestive kinds of issues? Because of comprehensive stool testing, and if you look in the right places you will generally find what you are looking for.

These patients may have a bag or two full of dietary supplements including products such as digestive enzymes, parasite cleansers, immune boosters, bowel products such as probiotics, psyllium, constipation or diarrhea aids, glutamine, aloe vera and more. Is this you? Then you are in the right place at the right time. Perhaps you are a practitioner who is reading this? Then suspect candida and dysbiosis in your patient and try the several tests I have outlined ahead. In today's Internet age, the patient will tell you that he or she has been doing some reading online with the help of Dr. Google and can maybe relate to having yeast infection issues. By analyzing the many potential signs and symptoms of a yeast infection in this chapter, a yeast infection sufferer will soon be able to confirm or deny the presence of candida. And the way to clinch the diagnosis is by going online to complete my comprehensive online candida questionnaires for females, males and children.
Just go to www.yeastinfection.org

A candida overgrowth can potentially cause so many symptoms, the most common of which in my experience are fatigue, bloating, gas, food allergies, carbohydrate craving, vaginal thrush, anxiety and/or depression, impaired memory, poor concentration, brain fog with feelings of unreality, and general weakness, tiredness or malaise. Additionally, numerous other symptoms may also be exhibited and of these, those I see most frequently in the clinic include cystitis/urethritis (urinary tract infection – painful, burning or stinging sensations when trying to urinate), menstrual irregularities, loss of libido, stiff, creaking and painful joints, muscle pain, indigestion, diarrhea/constipation (very common), inhalant allergies, multiple chemical sensitivities, mucus or catarrh (very common), hay fever, sinusitis, persistent cough (common), heart arrhythmias, discolored nails (common, especially the big toe nails), acne and other skin eruptions (nail and skin issues are classic telltale symptoms of candida), earaches, headaches, and dizziness.

Candida – The Great Contributor

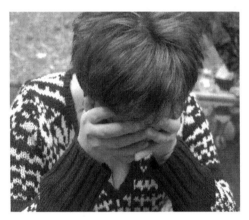

Candida may also contribute significantly to the underlying cause of a number of medical conditions as diverse as premenstrual tension, irritable bowel syndrome, asthma, eczema, psoriasis, urticaria (itchy skin/hives), epilepsy, schizophrenia, multiple sclerosis, adrenal fatigue, hypothyroidism, hypoglycemia (low-blood sugar levels), ileocecal valve dysfunction (pain in the lower gut on the right side), and childhood hyperactivity (common). The role and specificity of candida in some of these conditions is discussed below under the headings male, women and children.

Now let's look at these symptoms in a little more detail. The symptoms listed occur with digestive and systemic candidiasis, they are not all found at the same time in each and every person, but candida patients may have experienced one or several. Many of these signs and symptoms have been relieved and even completely eradicated by the Candida Crusher Program.

In medicine, symptoms and illnesses are grouped together according to the organ or system affected. This suits medicine, because then the patient can be sent to the appropriate specialist to solve the presenting problem associated with his or her specialty. This is not how we work as natural therapists however, we prefer to treat the cause and treat the whole person, not just their affected part.

The candida toxins you will read about ahead can affect just about all cells of all organs and systems of a person's body thereby causing any or all the symptoms listed below. I have grouped them together in categories simply for your convenience:

Mental, Emotional and Visual Symptoms (Central Nervous System)

- Alterations or disturbances of smell, taste, sight or hearing.

- Blurry vision, spots before the eyes.

- Eyes: erratic vision, spots in front of eyes (eye floaters) and flashing lights off to the side of vision, redness, dryness, itching, excessive tearing, inability to tear, etc. Many and varied eye/visual symptoms can be present.

- Feeling of swelling and tingling in the head, brain fog.

- Loss of self-confidence or self-esteem.

- Irritable person who can have a very short fuse, impatient.

- Nervousness, jitteriness and panic attacks.

- Poor concentration

- Headaches – dull, background headaches

- Earaches and especially the sensation of having itchy ears.

- Confusion

- Mood swings

- Dizziness and feelings of being light-headed.

- Drowsiness, especially when inappropriate.

- Numbness, tingling or weakness. This can be the tongue, hands or feet.

- Poor memory – especially short term.

- Hyperactivity – especially with children.

- Agitated, feelings of mania.

- Crying or emotional spells.

- Depression, especially the week before a period in women.

- Feeling of "cotton wool" in the head.

- Feelings of "unreal" or spaced out.

- Feeling of being drunk or inebriated.

- Feeling stoned or "out of it".

Gastro-Intestinal Symptoms

- Bloating or abdominal distention, needs to loosen the waistband regularly.

- Flatus and lots of gas. This is a KEY symptom, especially with bloating.

- Indigestion, easy after meals. Foods can upset the digestion easily.

- Heartburn, some foods can be real triggers, and you may know them well.

- Abdominal pain. You may have one particular spot that raises concern.

- Persistent diarrhea or constipation or alternating bouts of each.

- Mucus in stools.

- Hemorrhoids with rectal itching.

- Peri-anal itching, around or in the anus.

- Burning tongue, tongue symptoms are common with many.

- Appetite can be affected; a person may feel a low-grade nausea.

- Cravings or addictions for sugar, bread, pasta and other high carb foods, and also particularly alcohol in the forms of wine and beer or fruits.

- Mouth sores or blisters, canker sores, dryness, bad breath, a white or yellow coating on the tongue in the middle or back. Oral thrush.

- Blocked salivary glands and even recurring stones in the submandibular or parotid glands I have seen associated with a few chronic candida cases.

- Stomach complaints: helicobacter pylori bacteria (causes 90%+ of stomach ulcers), heartburn, indigestion, hiatus hernia, acid reflux, belching, vomiting, burning, stomach pains, needle-like or sharp, darting pains, food that seems to sit in the stomach like a lump. Any fullness after meals that is not related to hypochlorhydria (an underactive stomach).

- Person is suffering from recurring bacteria gut infections, i.e. salmonella, E. coli, h. pylori, etc.

Genito - Urinary Symptoms

- **Kidney & Bladder:** infections, especially when recurring, cystitis (inflammation of the bladder with possible infection), urinary frequency or urgency, low urine output, smelly or consistently strange colored urine, difficulty urinating, and burning pain when urinating.

- **Male associated urinary/sexual problems:** jock itch, loss of sex drive, impotence, prostatitis, penis infections, difficulty urinating,

- urinary frequency or urgency, painful intercourse, swollen scrotum, etc. Is the male a beer drinker? Suspect candida if he is and drinks beer regularly and complains of prostatitis, itchy skin, burping, bloating, and other symptoms listed here.

- **Female associated** urinary/sexual problems: infertility, vaginitis, vaginal thrush or irritations, unusual odors, napkin staining, endo-metriosis (irregular or painful menstruation), cramps, menstrual bleeding or irregularities, pre-menstrual syndrome (PMS – especial-ly cravings for sweet, hydration and depression two to three days before period), discharge, painful intercourse, loss of sexual drive, redness or swelling of the vulva and surrounding area, vulvodynia (pain), vaginal itching, burning or redness, or any persistent infec-tions.

- Fluid retention, puffiness around the body.

- Cystitis – burning on urination is a very common symptom, especially if recurring in male, female or child.

- Bed-wetting

Skin and Nail Symptoms

I have seen many and varied skin rashes, itches and strange, unexplained patches clear up on people's bodies after a successful course of the Candida Crusher Program. Many of these patients were diagnosed with skin conditions with weird names by a dermatologist and were prescribed a cream to cure the complaint. I've often wondered how applying a cream or lotion can supposedly "cure" a chronic skin complaint. In homeopathy you learn that these types of topical treatments lead to disease suppression, i.e.; they drive the illness deeper into the body. With effective treatment down the track, this condition is pushed to the surface, and it is not uncommon for me to see the return of old symptoms with successful treatment. To the enlightened person it is obvious that you won't cure a skin complaint without treating the underlying cause. Here are some of the more common manifestations of skin and nail related symptoms:

- Jock itch, groin infection in men.

- Oral candidiasis, oral thrush.

- Dryness, red or white skin patches.

- Chronic or recurring mouth ulcers.

- Intertrigo - skin fold problems (under breasts for example) and related skin irritations.

- Athletes foot, or tinea pedis (red, itchy feet and toes).

- Nail problems - discoloration / brittle, thickening nails.

- Itchy scalp and dandruff.

- Red, scaly eyelids

- Psoriasis, I treat all psoriasis cases for candida first.

- Seborrhea

- Contact dermatitis, I treat ALL dermatitis cases for candida first.

- Acne rosacea and vulgaris. Many acne cases respond well to dysbiosis control.

- Babies: colic, diaper rash, thrush (coated white tongue), and cradle cap.

- ANY fungal infections of the skin or nails, i.e. ringworm, seborrheic dermatitis, dark and light patches on the skin (tinea versicolor), etc.

- Odors: of the feet, hair or body that are not relieved by washing or deodorants. Several patients over the years have come back 12 – 18 months after the Candida Crusher Program and commented on how they "don't smell that bad anymore" from the armpits and body in general. Do you have a strange odor you can't seem to wash away? Then suspect a candida overgrowth.

Musculo-Skeletal Symptoms

This category is more difficult to determine and also very commonly overlooked. Most health-care professionals will never think about candida when it comes to aches and pains involving their muscles, nerves, bones, and connective tissue. I have found that the key areas affected in people include the upper back, the sides of the neck and also the shoulders. Many people may mistakenly believe that they are suffering from stress or overwork, when in fact candida toxins could be implicated.

Just exactly how candida affects the muscles and connective tissues is uncertain, but both Dr. Crook and Dr. Truss believed it is due to the buildup of aldehyde toxins and their metabolites causing both depletion as well as interfering with the uptake of minerals such as potassium, magnesium and possibly sodium. This could account for both muscle and nerve problems as these minerals are crucial for the proper functioning on the musculoskeletal system.

Truss was of the opinion that those with high levels of aldehyde could potentially develop problems with red blood cell membrane integrity. This can cause many issues, especially with blood flow to the extremities and through the muscles and may explain in part why some patients I see complain of cold hands and feet, numbness and tingling and cramps. If the body's microcirculation is affected and blood cannot travel freely through the body's smallest blood vessels, the capillaries, then many different symptoms may occur. The other issue is that nutrients and oxygen won't be sufficiently delivered to the muscles and waste products won't be carried away either, causing more problems. Metabolic by-products like gliotoxin and mannan remain trapped as well and can cause further havoc. You can read a lot more about acetaldehyde, gliotoxin and mannan in chapter 7, section 2.

You would be surprised how common musculo-skeletal problems occur in those with candida, I have seen many over the years who have even been diagnosed with conditions named as arthritis which resolved once the yeast infection was cleared up. Most patients with autoimmune musculo-skeletal problem have an unresolved yeast infection, along with other parasites. People who have conditions like ankylosing spondylitis and mixed connective tissue diseases like scleroderma, myositis, systemic lupus erythematosus (SLE), rheumatoid arthritis, polymyositis, and dermatomyositis generally have a yeast infection. But why would this be so you ask? Because most will have been on a steroidal or NSAID drug for years and all too often end up with a dysfunctional digestive system as a consequence. These patients may have also been on an antibiotic over the years, and the antibiotic was prescribed after the person developed an infection because of the immune-suppression that occurred after having been on a steroid (immune suppressing drug) for many years. Talk about a can of worms being opened, it sounds more like the entire worm farm got knocked over to me. Isn't it amazing how a small problem can escalate into a major problem over the years?

Arthritis like pains which improve significantly with yeast infection treatment are common, and if you have been diagnosed with one of these diseases then I highly recommend you get tested for candida, and a stool test is one of the best ways.

- Muscle aches and pains, especially if unresponsive to other treatments.
- Painful sides of neck, upper back and shoulders.
- Heart problems, rapid pulse, pounding or irregular heart or palpitations.
- Joint pain, stiffness and swellings – both the small and large joints.
- Rheumatoid arthritis diagnosis, get tested for candida or dysbiosis first..
- Creaking of joints.
- Numbness, burning or tingling sensations in muscles.
- Lack of strength and co-ordination.
- Bruising easily.
- Cheekbone or forehead tenderness or pains.
- Cold hands or feet, low body temperature.

Ear, Nose, Throat and Respiratory Symptoms

- Persistent nasal congestion or stuffiness is a KEY symptom.
- Sinus inflammation, swelling and excessive mucus or infection.
- Flu-like symptoms, coughs (low-grade the will not go away, can be worse in warm, cold or stuffy environments) and recurring colds.

- Excessive mucus in the throat, nose and ear canals (ears "popping"), sinuses, bronchial tubes or lungs. This can be particularly worse after meals or on rising.

- Joint pain and swellings – both the small and large joints.

- Cheekbone or forehead tenderness or pains.

- Ringing in the ears, tinnitus, funny "fluttering" sounds in the ears, ear infections, swimmer's ear, dryness, itchiness, ear pain, earaches, ear discharges, fluid in ears, deafness, abnormal and/or a continual wax build-up. I have discovered that there are many different ear and hearing problems associated with a candida infection.

- Sore throat, hoarse voice, constant tickle in the throat, laryngitis (loss of voice).

Other Signs and Symptoms of a Yeast Infection

- Hypoglycemia (low blood sugar), and diabetes. I always treat the diabetic for candida at some stage.

- Hypothyroidism, Wilson's Thyroid Syndrome, Hashimoto's disease, hyperthyroidism, erratic thyroid function, etc. The thyroid is very sensitive to the toxic by-products of systemic candida.

- Cysts and polyps, abnormal formation of, in different parts of the body, especially around the ears, neck, throat, and ovaries, and in the bladder, groin or scrotal region.

- Glands: swollen lymph nodes.

- Sleep: insomnia, waking up frequently, nightmares, restless sleep, etc.

- Sick all over feeling.

- Can feel like nobody understands you and why you feel so terrible in spite of all the doctor's tests coming back as normal.

- Fatigue (chronic fatigue syndrome or Epstein Barr) or a feeling of being drained of energy, lethargy, drowsiness.

Recognizing Women, Men And Children With Yeast Infections

You will find many of the following points quite relevant in recognizing yeast infections in people. Some of these indications you will know, others you may not, but they can all greatly aid in the recognition of a yeast overgrowth whether you are a yeast infection patient yourself or a practitioner who treats people with candida related problems.

How to Recognize the Female Candida Patient

- The case history will tell you if you are dealing with a female who has candida or not. Has she had a history of taking the oral contraceptive pill?

- A mature woman with a history of hormone replacement therapy (estrogen therapy).

- Look for the woman with persistent vaginal thrush, especially if she has had her vaginal yeast infection treated with fluconazole or Monistat.

- If there has been a history of re-current antibiotic use before the onset of the digestive health problem, you can almost guarantee that this lady will have a yeast infection to some degree.

- Any woman with an annoying, irritating whitish discharge.

- A female who experiences painful sex or who avoids sex.

- Suspect any woman with chronic polycystic ovarian syndrome or endometriosis.

- Look for the female who has a strong sweet or sugar craving, careful questioning during the case taking will elicit this crucial information. Does she crave chocolate, sweets or breads?

- Don't just look for a craving or strong desire for chocolate, bread, candy or sweets, look for the desire to consume orange juice, soda or fizzy drinks, dried fruits like dates, figs, sultanas or chewing gum, biscuits and a host of other foods high in sugars.

- Look for the woman who eats many pieces (3 or more) of fruit each day. Fruit has plenty of sugar in it, especially oranges, grapes and dried fruits.

- Women who love to drink wine, especially if there has been a history of the oral contraceptive pill or antibiotics.

- Women who love moldy foods like soft cheeses and sweet foods or drinks.

- Look for a woman who takes many kinds of dietary supplements including probiotics, digestive enzymes and bowel products.

- Look for a history of unresolved digestive problems, particularly if this has been of long duration involving many visits to doctors or naturopaths.

- Women whose partners suffer from yeast infections like jock-itch, the problem gets passed from one to the other.

- Ladies with toenail fungus, suspect digestive yeast related problems as well, especially if the localized toenail problem is of long duration.

- Poor motivation, depression and anxiety or any one of many different disorders may develop in women who remain without a firm diagnosis for candida.

Men's Problems and Yeast Infections

In my clinical practice, about seventy five percent of patients presenting with yeast-infection related problems are women, yet guys develop yeast related problem as well. If fact, I suspect that there are a lot of men out there who have yeast infections yet do little about getting well.

I saw my father try to conquer his yeast problems for many years, and it was only after many years that he went to a doctor who prescribed him an antibiotic after finding nothing wrong with him. And this was in spite of several trips to the gastroenterologist where he was examined by way of an endoscopy and had a barium enema performed in addition to having every other test thrown at him. The diagnosis was that there was "no abnormal disease" and dad was prescribed yet more antibiotics. This was in 1982, and unfortunately today almost thirty years on nothing much has changed, candida yeast infected patients are still diagnosed today by the mainstream doctors as having no abnormal disease if they present to their medical doctor with several yeast related signs and symptoms. So take heed, if you have done the rounds, consulted many different practitioners then I strongly urge you to consider candida treatment.

How To Recognize The Male Candida Patient:

- I carefully check the toenails and see if there is any athlete's foot, I find that men for some reason unknown more commonly complain of athlete's foot than women do. I will often check the hands and scalp carefully too, particularly if they are manual workers. Guys in general have a tendency to be less interested in hand and foot care and every male patient who I suspect of having a yeast infection will be asked to take his shoes and socks off – and what do I find? Athlete's foot.

- Guys who adjust their groin region regularly, just go to a bar and look around, especially where alcohol is served. Many men subconsciously touch their groin area and I'll bet that they are either oblivious to the fact that they have a yeast infection or are too embarrassed to seek any treatment.

- Many of the typical male candida patients I see are the blue-collar workers, or working class men. They typically enjoy a beer, rum and coke, bourbon, wine, etc, after work, a social drink at weekend and snack on sweet foods. They may not have the best of diets and when questioned carefully you will find that they bloat, burp and have plenty of gas.

- White-collar (office) workers also get yeast infections; many are under stress and work long hours at the office. They may drink alcohol as well and may not have the healthiest of diets with take-out meals occurring regularly.

- Some spend time with clients and conduct business over lunch, dinner or at conventions where alcohol is often served as well.

- Men with yeast infections are typically the ones who consume lots of beer, bread and sweet foods. Guys who crave alcohol in general are prime candidates for yeast infections.

- Men who like sweet snacks or foods – like candies, chocolates, licorice, etc. This may also be cookies, cakes or any sweet foods or drinks like soda drinks.

- Men whose wives suffer from vaginal thrush or yeast related problems, the problem gets passed from one to the other.

- Men who are typically troubled by recurrent digestive problems like abdominal pains, diarrhea, constipation, bloating, heartburn and flatulence (gas).

- Men who have taken recurrent courses of antibiotics for prostatitis, acne, sinusitis or for other similar circumstances.

- Psoriasis – check to see here if the man has any other typical or not so typical signs and symptoms of candida. If a man comes to my clinic with psoriasis the first thing I check for are digestive problems and treat accordingly. There is research now strongly linking psoriasis with candida. Show me a person with chronic psoriasis who hasn't got serious dysbiosis and candida, you will hard pressed in finding one, I guarantee it.

- Prostatitis – I have seen time and again that the male's prostate problems often disappear entirely once his yeast infection has been thoroughly cleared, and you will find this too especially if you treat the cause of the yeast infection. Guys with prostatitis or urinary issues respond very well to candida treatment, treat aggressively, these cases can be especially hard to solve if compliance is poor, are they beer drinkers?

- Poor motivation, depression and anxiety or any one of many different disorders may develop in men (like my father) who remain without a firm diagnosis for candida. Low moods make it harder to bust a yeast infection, because various eating problems can be found in guys with self-esteem or mood issues, especially if they have a problem with their sex life and can't perform when they would like to. Food, drink and sex are some of the biggest likes for the big boys, apart from sports, hunting, fishing and football or course.

Candida and the Immune System

Once in the bloodstream, candida acts as a typical allergen and is capable of creating typical various types of allergic reactions. There is no doubt, candida and allergies are commonly found together, and this is one of the major ways in which candida can cause many of the potential health complaints. Section 2 of chapter 7 will explain about the connection between stress and your immune system and is certainly worthy of a read. Not everybody with candida has an allergy, though most candida patients I have seen have food and environmental allergies or sensitivities to some degree. You will often see food allergy test (ELISA blood test) results in candida patients revealing an allergy to one or even several foods. Allergic sensitivities to molds and fungi often develop in those with candida overgrowth in their intestines, and for this reason, some have reactions in damp or moldy environments.

For this reason also, a reaction to alcohol can be the result of both a candida infestation and an allergy to the yeasts used to ferment the alcohol particularly if wines, beers and ciders are being consumed. Alcohol is the most important thing to eliminate first from your diet, and it proves for most yeast sufferers also to be the most difficult. I've said it before and I'll say it again a few more times before you are through reading this book. Many people with candida have a strong desire for it, but alcohol must go, yeasty foods like breads need to be stopped for a while and sweet treats like chocolate and candies need to be stopped as well. These food items encourage yeast proliferation that in turn will encourage immune dysfunction.

Do you react strongly to alcohol? Then candida alone is often the main culprit, especially if your skin or digestive system flares up within a day. This problem is often compounded by the other sugary and fermented foods you consume, such as breads, cheeses, yoghurts, commercial (cheap) vinegars and moldy foods like mushrooms, dried fruits and melons.

Most people know that drinking too much alcohol causes a hangover. But what about the many patients I have seen whom only drink small to moderate amounts and experience reactions the following day out of proportion to how much alcohol they consumed the previous day? If you are becoming increasingly reactive to alcohol, then seriously consider doing the Candida Crusher Program.

You will see with the candida diet later on that it is not a good idea to eat left-over foods from your refrigerator the next day for the same reason I mentioned above, molds and spores can proliferate on these foods overnight in your refrigerator.

In my observation, the typical candida patient has multiple allergies and they can in addition also develop multiple chemical sensitivities as well as inhalant allergies. These allergies and sensitivities improve dramatically and eventually disappear as the yeast and sugar-containing foods and drinks are withdrawn, the candida population is reduced and balance is once again restored to the digestive system in particular. When the small intestine is healed, their immune system is healed as well and a person's sensitivity to many substances drops.

Another common occurrence of elevated antibodies findings is with a stool test (CDSAx3), and I regularly find a reduction or an elevation of sIgA, (an antibody commonly found in the mucosa and digestive system) which also indicates a heightened immune response potentially revealing an underlying allergy. Many patients with chronic digestive problems who have had a stool or blood test performed will often have increased antibody markers as part of their test results, more so the blood based tests though than with the stool tests. You can read a lot more about the ELISA blood test for the IgG/IgA antibody levels and the CDSA x 3 stool test in "Laboratory Testing for Candida Yeast Infections" later in this chapter.

Case History # 9
Wendy, 48 years

Wendy was a woman in her forties who used to be our babysitter about fifteen years ago. Wendy called me up with urgency one evening to tell me that something in our lounge room was making her physically sick and that I had to come home at once, she had the windows all wide open and felt physically ill when I rushed home. When I spoke with her further about this it also became apparent that she had become super-sensitive to any household cleaners, aerosol sprays, perfumes and felt absolutely terrible anywhere near cigarette smoke. She could only drink water that was bottled in glass and her diet was limited to a handful of foods. This lady also had a bowel problem that she had been trying to control for a few years and had a long history of the oral contraceptive pill use.

About twenty years ago, Wendy returned from India with a severe case of diarrhea. Her doctor placed her on several rounds of antibiotics and she has not felt well since. After almost nine months on the Candida Crusher Program, Wendy's diet became far less restrictive and she hardly reacted to her environment like she used to. And now Wendy can even drink tap water and enjoy wine again, something which was inconceivable several years ago!

Perhaps you can relate to Wendy, is your diet very restricted, are you limited in what you can eat, do you react violently to many foods and have inhalant allergies? Maybe its time you considered treating your potential yeast infection that could be wrecking your immune system and ultimately your life.

Children and Yeast Infection Related Problems

A child with candida can be mislabeled hyperactive or learning disabled by a practitioner who does not fully understand or comprehend the true significance of the pediatric yeast syndrome. Dr. William Crook who authored The Yeast Syndrome certainly did, he was an excellent pediatrician who noticed that many of his young patients would improve significantly once their yeast overgrowth was eradicated. It is a pity that many pediatricians today do not have the same level of clinical experience with intestinal dysbiosis and children's health that Dr. Crook had.

Children who have candida may manifest multiple allergic syndromes that can affect them on many different levels. These children can even display behavioral and learning difficulties as a result of their individual reactions to foods, chemicals, and preservatives that may well be linked to a candida yeast infection. In my clinical experience, many children do not need drugs like Ritalin after all, particularly if they are first assessed and treated for allergies and carefully screened for candida yeast infections or SIBO (small intestinal bowel overgrowth).

Like Dr. William Crook, I have certainly noticed over the years that children who have both behavioral or learning disabilities as well as a yeast infection display a marked reduction of symptoms once the candida is eliminated, much to their parent's relief.

Behavior and candida

A small, but nevertheless significant percentage of todays children diagnosed as autistic may in fact be victims of a rather severe form of a candida yeast infection.

If the candida infection was successfully treated in these few cases, the symptoms of autism may well show dramatic improvement. It is not uncommon to find that a child with a behavioral problem was treated routinely with antibiotics in the past, for example an ear infection, a cough or a sore throat, and often times they will have been recurrently. Soon thereafter, changes may begin to occur. There could be developmental delays, speech development may stop, and within a few weeks or months the child may become unresponsive and lose interest in his parents and surroundings. The concerned parents then take the child to various specialists, and finally come up with a diagnosis of autistic spectrum disorder.

Worried mothers may have their children in and out of medical clinics and unfortunately there are still doctors who still routinely prescribe antibiotics, despite the fact that not only the malevolent bacteria are destroyed but also the friendly bacteria such as Lactobacillus acidophilus.

The yeast remaining behind now thrives, as they are not susceptible to the influences of antibiotics, and with recurring prescriptions the bacteria left behind become more increasingly resistant to antibiotics.

In addition, children love to eat sweets, and plenty of them including ice creams and all the sugary and yeast promoting foods and are thus a prime target for a candida overgrowth. In the 21st century, your child may be eating foods high in sugar more than at any other time in history. Is it any wonder that many of our children go on to develop all manner of immune and behavioral problems?

A very important part of candida treatment for children is getting them away from sweets as much as is possible, and a good way to start is by limiting all soda drinks, candy (sweets) and unnecessary food and drink items. This can present a challenge and you will find it an easier task with younger as opposed to older children, believe me. I have four children and know how difficult it can be, but it is achievable, especially if you can offer your child nice fruits such as oranges, bananas, stone fruit like apricots and plums, etc., to get them away from the highly processed sweets. Give them diluted juices to get them away from those sugar laden soda drinks. This is step one, and then you progress over time by giving them fruits that are not quite as sweet like apples, pears and kiwi, and dilute fruit juices down even further. Eventually you switch them to vegetables and herbal teas. It IS possible but takes time, patience and commitment on your behalf as the parent or caregiver. My kids just drank water, flavored with a splash of fruit juice.

How To Recognize The Child Candida Patient:

- The case history will often tell you if you are dealing with a child who has candida or not. I regularly have naturopathic students who sit in for observations in my clinic, and I like them to be aware of the importance of case taking when it comes to children in the clinic. A case well taken is a case half solved. "What happened in the past" is probably one of the most important questions you can ask the child's mother.

- It is surprising when you ask the mother when her child was prescribed antibiotics in relation to her child's health problem, time and again you will see the relationship between the cause (the antibiotic) and the effect, the bowel, skin, immune, behavioral or other health problem.

- Look for the child who has a strong sweet or sugar craving, careful questioning during the case taking will elicit this crucial information. Whilst it is not true that all children who crave sugar will have candida, it is true that most all children with candida will strongly crave sugary foods.

- Don't just look for a craving or strong desire for candy or sweets, look for the desire to consume plenty of oranges and orange juice, soda drinks, dried fruits like dates, figs, sultanas or chewing gum, biscuits and a host of other foods high in sugars.

- Look for the child who eats many pieces of fruit each day, especially fruits high in sugar. Fruit has plenty of sugar in it, some more than others.

- If there has been a history of re-current antibiotic use before the onset of the digestive health problem, you can almost guarantee that there will be candida to some degree.

- A child with recurrent worm infestations. Does the child have an itchy anus or complain about "sore tummies" routinely? There could be a sweet craving underlying here again. Suspect a yeast infection as I have often seen these problems combined in children – worms and yeast infections.

- Children who live with one parent, and then spend every second weekend with the other parent. This is often the case with separated or divorced parents, therefore always ask this question: "Does Johnny live with both parents?" It is surprising how many times I have heard: "Oh, no, in fact he lives with his father half the time". In cases such as this you may find that one or the other parent will spoil the child, and sweets, ice cream or chocolates are high on the list. Sometimes this may occur out of guilt, sometimes out of trying to buy the child's affection over the other parent, and this is more common than you may think, especially if the split wasn't amicable.

- Be aware of grandparents. They sometimes feel it is their right to be able to give the child special treats, especially sweets. I have found that when a child stays with their grandparents, or is taken out on excursions to the movies by the grandparent for example, that sweet treats or generally given, like ice creams, soda drinks, sweets, etc. Your child may be told to "not tell your mother or father", as some grandparents feel it is their right to treat their grandchild to a sweet treat. There may be a behavioral change and a worsening of symptoms when the child is returned to her parents, and in such a case you will want to carefully assess the child's diet when they have been to stay at grandma's and ask straight questions.

- Abdominal pain which is "undiagnosable" by the bowel specialist. Think about dysbiosis including parasites and/or yeast infections, once you have concluded there is no fecal (stool) loading or a case of bad constipation, treat for a yeast infection. An abdominal x-ray or ultrasound may be necessary to determine any serious obstruction. Take your child to a certified colon therapist as well, and listen for the feedback. I have more faith in the feedback from a highly experienced colon therapist than a GI medical specialist when it comes to many issues affecting the large bowel, just my experience.

- A child living in a cold, damp or moldy environment who is always sick. He will need to be moved to a better environment before you begin work on the candida eradication. In New Zealand, we have all too many children who live in such homes with drafts, a leaky roof and damp bedrooms with condensation on the windows and a tin layer of almost invisible mold on the ceiling, especially near the window. This is a recipe for a candida yeast infection, and you may find various strains of yeasts, molds and bacteria in such cases in the room, as well as in the child's body.

- Any child on drugs long-term. Does the child take any asthma drugs like salbutamol (Ventolin) and/or a steroid preventative? Perhaps a recurrent prescription of an analgesic, antidepressant or other medication? I routinely have seen such children with drug-induced illness and suspect that yeast infections are much more common here as well.

- A child with a recurrent bladder or urinary tract infection. Obviously you will want to rule out diabetes of other blood sugar issues, any underlying urinary issues that can be ruled out by an urologist, etc. But, if there are recurrent urinary tract infections or bladder issues then you may want to treat for a yeast infection. You can bet that antibiotics will have been used here routinely, and whenever they are used, a yeast infection is sure to follow.

- A child in a wheelchair or using a catheter regularly. A very much overlooked area with yeast infections is the use of an indwelling urinary catheter, and I've seen many children as well as adults with recurring bacterial and fungal issues who have to rely on these to urinate.

- A child with a recurrent ear, nose or throat, respiratory or sinus infection. Once again, suspect antibiotic use and in some cases you will be quite surprised to learn that the child has "never been well" since these antibiotics.

- A child you suspect of being celiac. Always check for a bacterial, yeast or parasitic infection long before you consider a gluten allergy or intolerance, because it is more likely that the child will have an issue with yeast rather than gluten. Does this child crave sweet foods or drinks, is there any history of antibiotic use, has this child travelled or been on holidays before the diagnosis of celiac? Was the celiac diagnosis made based on a small bowel biopsy?

- **A child who was breast fed for a several weeks only and then placed on a powdered cow's milk formula.** I've seen far too many cases of young children who didn't get the right amount of immune-boosting breast milk they may well have benefitted from early on in their life, and then went on to develop a respiratory or bowel infection as a result of an allergy. The child was then placed on an antibiotic and consequently developed dysbiosis leading into a yeast infection. Naturopaths see these children daily in their practice.

- **The child with the terrible attitude.** I have often seen children in my clinic presenting with behavioral problems, no doubt like many naturopaths have, and I am certainly not suggesting that all children with behavioral issues have a candida yeast infection, but a surprising number certainly do! So how do you distinguish between a child with a yeast infection who does not appear to fit in with the family dynamics and a child who for example has autism?

What I do is look at the child's diet and how strongly that child craves certain food items as a starting point. Many yeast-affected children will have a craving for certain foods as strong as their attitude, they may even "rule the household" and simply demand certain foods. These are the children with food allergies as well, and an allergy towards sugar. As I mentioned previously, Dr. William Crook (The Yeast Connection) wrote extensively about children, behavioral problems and yeast infections back in the 1980's, and today this connection is as strong as ever, if not even more so. Today we have high fructose corn syrup that Dr. Crook never heard of, and this stuff has permeated into too many foods, and kids love it. It feeds candida like you wouldn't believe like fuel feeds a fire.

Children today drink more soda drinks than at any other time in history, their diets are often high in processed and sugar containing foods and it is therefore important that you consider this if your child is simply "impossible" at home. Is your child controlling you? Try withdrawing all sugar from their diet and see what happens, you will notice over time a definite change in their attitude as well as an improvement in their ability to think more clearly, remember that brain fog we spoke about previously?

Case History # **10**
John, 6 years

John is a pleasant young boy with a friendly smile. His mother brought him to my clinic after spending over a year trying to ascertain what was wrong with him. He was having recurrent digestive pains and constipation as well as asthma. As a baby, John was breastfed for only six weeks before being placed on an infant formula containing cow's milk powder. John could not tolerate this formula too well and was then placed on an infant soy formula that was less problematic. He developed colic at around 6 months of age and received his first round of antibiotics a few months later for ear infections. By the time John was three years old, he had received over a dozen rounds of antibiotics for recurring ear, nose and throat infections and now needing an inhaler (Salbutamol, aka Ventolin) and steroid inhaler as a "preventative" because his pediatrician told his mother he now had "asthma". This drug-merry-go-round is unfortunately all too common with children; I have seen it one thousand times at least.

I first set about getting John's diet right, and placed him on my low-allergy diet that you will find in the book. What typically occurs is that sweet cravings occur after antibiotics, as many beneficial bacteria have been destroyed and yeasts start to multiply rapidly. The yeast wants feeding and their host has no option but to give in to their demands. And so the sugar-laden diet begins, whether it is soda drinks, fruit juice, candy or sweets, biscuits, snack bars, or any one of many sweet foods children like. It makes no difference; as long as it contains sugar it will be food for the yeast. Then they thrive and multiply and get to be an increasingly bigger problem over time.

Parents often give in just buy these foods for the child who demands the most. The "squeaky hinge gets the oil" really is true, and being a parent myself with three boys I can tell you, kids can really wear you down until you just give in. It will usually be the one child who does it, and as you become increasingly tired you just say "OK".

Then we started to use various products and probiotics to get John's immune and digestive system right. The asthma drugs were the first to go, and I asked John's mother to avoid ALL antibiotics in the future, unless John suffered from a major bacterial infection such as pneumonia or septicemia. After four months of treatment, all of John's digestive symptoms were gone entirely, his bowel is back to normal and all the pains are gone. John's mother is very grateful, but her doctor is not impressed at all with my recommendations of no asthma drugs or antibiotics, it was seen as "irresponsible". Is it ego with these guys or just plain ignorance, I'll never hnow I guess, because they never call me, even when a patient under their care for years becomes well again under my care after a few months.

And Johnny? He is drug-free at last and in fine health today and I'm happy for him.

Candida Is Often Seen As Irritable Bowel Syndrome By Conventional Medicine

I have worked in conjunction with medical practitioners on and off for many years, and when required referred patients with chronic gastrointestinal distress to gastroenterologists for an initial bowel screen to rule out anything obvious, such as a polyp, stricture, prolapse, diverticulitis, haemorrhoid or possibly even bowel cancer.

All too often though the person would come back with the diagnosis of NAD (no abnormal diagnosis) - nothing abnormal, no diseases, just "irritable bowel syndrome" (IBS), and the recommendation that they should make dietary changes, increase fiber in their diet and use psyllium hulls. In most such instances, these changes brought the patient very little relief.

One of my favourite writers is Dr. Liz Lipsky Ph.D, author of "Digestive Wellness", Liz states that in irritable bowel syndrome, there are four main causes:

1   Infection (yeasts, bacteria, parasites)

2   Lactose

3   Food allergies and food intolerances

4   Stress

I once heard Dr. Alan Gaby say (past-president of the American Holistic Medical Association) that he calls irritable bowel syndrome a "garbage can diagnosis"; and that most medical doctors just go and dump people in there when they can't figure their health problems out, and hope that somebody else will collect them and take them and their health problems away with them. It doesn't sound very nice, and I can assure you that not all doctors would do this, but the reality for many practitioners when faced with a patient who has IBS is to simply refer them on or to prescribe them a drug after a ten minute consultation.

This is very much like a patient who presents to a doctor with a pain in her behind which eventually turns out to be a thumbtack, and the doctor calls it "thumb tack disease" and promptly prescribes paracetamol for this painful disease with no known cause. Why don't we get the patient to pull that thumb tack out of her behind, and find out where she sat down at the time of the thumb tack problem?

My concerns are that some practitioners who are consulted by patients with digestive disorders have little or no understanding nor training in functional digestive complaints such as candida albicans, food allergies, leaky gut syndrome and irritable bowel syndrome. "You have nothing wrong with your digestive system that we can find" is what is typically said to the patient. Candida is a condition often caused by antibiotics, some of the most common drugs prescribed by medical practitioners.

I have several medical colleagues in both Australia and New Zealand who now can recognize and treat candida effectively, but unfortunately this number is only a fraction in comparison to the many orthodox medical doctors who believe that anything but orthodox Western medicine is absolute quackery.

You have to be the judge of this yourself, but it has always been my belief as a naturopath that it makes good sense to make the correct lifestyle and diet changes first which assist in the healing of your digestive system well before opting for any drugs or surgery. In other words, the cause needs to be addressed.

Having worked in different medical and natural medicine clinics over the years, I have had the opportunity first hand to observe many chronically sick patients, and most have had some degree of dysbiosis and/or candida yeast infections.

The candida yeast infection was not always the primary cause of their chronic ill health; rather it came along and developed in a stressed digestive system, as part of their lowered resistance, and had likely contributed in some way to the very illness itself. I have found that by working with the chronically sick patient and helping them improve their gut function, it is possible to turn the case around, but it can become difficult when there is a diagnosable disease, especially advanced pathology.

If the irritable bowel disease has not been treated satisfactorily in the first place, then it may actually be of an advantage to me, because the patient and doctor have no clear path to follow to cure the patient's health problems, and if a patient has not responded well to any previous therapy, they may well be considerably more open to making changes to their diet and lifestyle, to see if their health can change for the better. The more compromised their digestive health and affected their lifestyle has become, the higher the degree of motivation they will have to want to make the right changes and the better the compliance will be. If the diagnosis is clear-cut however, then in some instances the patient may be interested in only treating the symptoms of the condition itself, rather than working on any underlying causes.

The drawback unfortunately is that the longer a person has been unwell with IBS for, the greater the chance that some pathology (disease) will develop, and often silently in the background. It may take therefore much longer to achieve that turn-around to great health the person is looking for, and when this is the case, compliance will not be that great and drugs and surgery may be a better option, especially if a great deal of pain or pathology is present. Not what you expected me to say, but patients want to have a full range of options open to them if they are really sick, and they should too. That's what integrative medicine should be all about, the best of both worlds.

Conventional Laboratory Testing For Candida

I have not found the standard medical pathology laboratory testing to be of much use in determining a patient's level and severity of yeast infections. What you will find is that most lab tests are designed to discover "diseased" states of the body, and a yeast infection is not a disease necessarily. In addition to this, there has not been a reliable test designed to discover or very accurately diagnose the very mild or onset forms of candida yeast infections or dysbiosis (bad bacteria) in the human body.

Lab tests are based on a population of so-called healthy people. The fundamental flaw is that these healthy people were themselves never screened for mild yeast infections. They were only screened for the severe forms, or full blown or what is known as a systemic yeast infection.

The second problem with standardised lab tests for yeast infections, bacteria and parasites is that the lab tests are defined and standardised according to statistical norms instead of physiological norms. That is to say, the test scores are based on math rather than typical signs and symptoms of yeast infections experienced by a wide range of people. For example, when the yeast infection of a population is tested, all the individual scores are taken and averaged out together. The resulting group is called the "mean" and is used to calculate what is called a "probability distribution". And, in this case, the probability distribution is a statistical prediction of how often each score will occur when stool samples of a group of people with a yeast infection are evaluated.

Home Testing is Low Cost Or Even Free

> " *The only source of true knowledge is experience* "
> *Albert Einstein*

That is not to say that standard current laboratory tests for candida albicans are not useful for determining and diagnosing candida yeast infections, but is important for you and your physician interpreting to understand their limitations and appropriate uses. Listed below are several tests I use to determine yeast infections in the patients who come to our clinic. Some of these tests may be familiar to you, others you will have probably have never heard of. It is the accumulation of how many of these tests you can relate and give you the information you are looking for that can make the difference as far as the diagnosis of your yeast infection is concerned, and a good starting point for you are the eight home tests you will read about a little later.

Can't afford expensive functional diagnostic tests or they are not covered by your insurance company? Don't panic, the various home tests I just mentioned are either free or low-cost, and by doing all of these you will have a good understanding of whether you have a yeast infection or not.

The Candida Crusher covers many different home based tests which I have found most useful, and this book even includes The Candida Symptom Tracker, a chart which was designed so that you can accurately assess your level of improvement of your yeast infection over a period of several weeks. By tracking your symptoms over a period of time, you will be able to determine what results you are getting, if the treatment plan is effective and if you are staying on track or not.

Diagnosing Candida Albicans Over-Proliferation

Until only quite recently, there was a lack of reliable laboratory investigation techniques to assist health-care professionals in diagnosing candida albicans overgrowth. This lack of credible and scientifically validated candida testing has now changed and physicians no longer need to rely only on detailed symptoms questionnaires which can be somewhat unreliable to use as a sole diagnostic aid.

As my level of experience grew as a clinician, I found it less important to test each and every suspect yeast infection case. But I have completed well over a thousand stool tests over the years performed by many different companies and this information has served me well, you can certainy learn by your experiences, especially clinical experiences. Once you have seen many yeast infected patients, you will have seen candida in its many manifestations and understand that there are many faces of this condition.

You get to understand that candida isn't purely a digestive or vaginal disorder, like some physicians believe. Many practitioners still haven't figured out that a yeast infection, particularly when chronic, can affect many areas of the body, including a person's mood, behavioural patterns as well as their cognition and ability to even think straight. If you are a person who really wants to know if he or she has an underlying yeast infection, then understanding about the different tests available to detect any underlying yeast infections or to diagnose a candida yeast infection is certainly a good thing. I encourage you to carefully read this chapter a few times and learn about all the different types of tests available at your disposal. And promise me not to laugh! You may find my home tests a bit strange at first, but they are based on patient observations of many years and over time you will see that they can make a big difference if you put them to good use in your own situation. And best of all, they are mostly all free.

Won't A Vaginal Swab Be Sufficient To Detect My Yeast Infection?

Women are often used to their doctor taking a vaginal swab to determine the presence of a yeast infection. It is important to remember though that a swab does not differentiate between a candida infection and a vaginal colony of normally occurring vaginal candida, because the cotton swab is sampling the surface of the vaginal wall, it will not tell you if the immune system actually is or has been producing antibodies against candida itself. This test will only indicate what is going on locally, and certainly not systemically. The other problem with vaginal sampling is that if the patient has used a vaginal pessary or a douche then the area will have been sanitized to a degree and a swab will return a false negative reading, as the numbers may prove too low for detection. You didn't think about those points, did you? Most people and many practitioners don't, and this is why you need to be particularly careful when interpreting candida tests or any tests for that matter, you can easily get false results resulting in poor or wrong treatment. Can you see the problems and false assumptions that can arise from taking a vaginal swab to determine whether you have a yeast infection?

I'd like you to be aware of the totality of symptoms before you assume you have a major vaginal yeast infection based purely on the results of a swab. You may have a digestive yeast infection as well which may be re-infecting your vaginal area, and this could be a reason for recurrence of symptoms.

The Three Main Conventional Ways To Test For Candida

There are many ways you can detect a candida yeast infection in somebody, and there is certainly not one sure fire way which will guarantee 100% for certain that you have a candida yeast infection or not. Here are the three common ways and main ways which yeast infections can be detected, by way of the blood (A), the stool test (B), and the urine test (C). Now, let's look a little more in depth into these three main methods by which candida is detected and I'll give you my opinion, as I have used them all.

Blood Testing For Candida

1   Candida Antibody Blood Test. The standard candida test is a blood test to determine the level of candida specific antibody production in the body, the IgG test or the combined IgG/IgA and IgM test. During a candida yeast infection, the body produces specific antibodies as part of its defense mechanism and these antibodies are different from those produced initially when a host is first exposed to candida usually at birth. Therefore we can pick up these specific antibodies as they circulate freely in blood and as you will see in a moment, different types of antibodies can give us a clue as to when the infection most likely took place.

Some say this test is no good, because an early exposure can give you a positive reading even many years down the track when you don't necessarily have a rampant, but a very mild yeast infection yet have a higher than average antibody count. Others say that this test accurately reflects the degree of sensitivity your immune system has towards a yeast infection right at the time of testing. I think it is valid, but should be used in conjunction with other tests I'll outline shortly.

2   Gut Fermentation Blood Test. This is a bit like a drink-driving test, a person's BAC (blood alcohol concentration) is assessed, it sounds crazy but a similar blood test can be performed to see if you have a chronic case of candida. You may recall from reading chapter 2 that acetaldehyde plays a role in yeast infections and that a person who suffers from a yeast infection, particularly a chronic case, in some cases may appear intoxicated.
Alcohol and toxins are released into the bloodstream which can produce all manner of symptoms, and these chemicals may lead to the characteristic "brain fog" and in extreme cases may even cause a person to become a "drinkless drunk" (a person who is showing signs and symptoms of having a high blood alcohol content and appears to be drunk yet who has not consumed any alcohol). This is how I felt when I was in my twenties and suffered with a bad yeast infection, but the worst thing was that nobody believed me! I even asked a police officer to do a breath test once on me and he said "you are free to go", but I felt I couldn't be in charge of my motor vehicle at the time.

This is how the gut fermentation test is performed, first a resting blood alcohol level is measured, and then a second sample is analysed after the person consumes some sugar. If any alcohol appears in the blood, and the person has not been drinking any alcohol previously naturally, then this suggests fermentation is taking place, which is an indication of candida albicans over-proliferation.

The test has been further refined to look for a number of different fermentation by-products in the blood or urine. However, this test does not give any information regarding what is actually doing the fermenting itself, as there is increasing evidence that many bacteria can provide such a fermentation reaction in addition to candida. And as I have mentioned previously, yeasts are often found inconjunction with elevated levels of bad bacteria and various parasites.

This type of test however is not always positive for individuals with a confirmed candida infection, and I find it therefore an unreliable test to perform on the average candida patient. It is a good test to perform form however on those people who literally feel drunk or spaced out and who do not drink alcohol, as it may help point out which foods or beverages are contributing towards fermentation. I wish I would have known about this test in the mid 1980's when I felt spaced out for no reason, I can understand why some people with a chronic yeast infection literally think they are going crazy. You have to see it to believe it with your own eyes, I have seen patients who were so spaced out they could hardly walk, and have not witnessed this with any other condition to this degree. It is rare, but if you have treated yeast patients for as long as I have you will occasionally come across a person who appears at first to be in a state of acute intoxification, and you will swear at first glance that they have been drinking.

Conventional Stool Testing For Candida

I have not found it common for a medical doctor to authorize a stool test for a patient to determine whether they have a yeast infection of not, and if they did authorize it, it would only to "prove" to their patient that the very existence of candida in the stool is baloney. If the doctor has become enlightened however, and has had training in functional medicine, then he or she will probably run a stool test including not only an analysis for candida, but for levels of various bacteria, beneficial micro-flora, and pathogens such as parasites as well. That is not to say that conventional stool testing for candida is not available, it is, but is not something commonly performed and I very much doubt if their methodology would be the same that the very best functional labs run.

Conventional pathology labs will most probably not culture yeast to grow candida from a stool sample, and especially not with three separate stool samples the way the Doctor's Data from Chicago would do. Conventional testing has no interest in detecting for candida infections in a person's stool, because the medical model does "not believe" in the existence of this condition in the first place. If you are interested in this area, you will need to go the functional testing route.

Urine Testing

Like the vaginal swab, this test is only really valid to detect a local presence of candida in the body where candida has caused a UTI (urinary tract infection) or the urine sample has picked up candida due to a case of vaginal thrush. With this test, the laboratory technician looks microscopically for the actual presence of a candida yeast infection and may also attempt to culture candida in a small dish.

This test again is pretty much a waste of time to detect a more widespread and chronic case of candida albicans in the body. It is a good test however to diagnose and treat the urinary tract locally if the patient suffers from the typical pains of a UTI, as it will soon detect if and what bacteria and yeasts are present. This may be a good test however to perform on a guy with chronic prostatitis, as he may well have a hidden and undetected yeast infection, something I have commonly seen and confirmed as well after talking with Dr. Dr. Geo Espinosa, Director of the Integrative Urological Center at New York University Langone Medical Center. Dr. Espinosa is one of the rare few naturopathic doctors specializing in urology.

Functional Laboratory Testing For Candida Yeast Infections

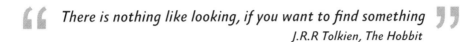

There is nothing like looking, if you want to find something
J.R.R Tolkien, The Hobbit

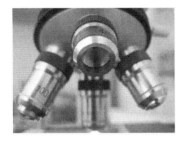

Functional laboratory testing is different from conventional pathology based testing in that it can discover any changes in the body's function which are a deviation from the norm. Conventional medical testing on the other hand concerns itself primarily with assessing if there is any pathology (disease). Functional testing concerns itself with assessing any deviations from the normal healthy body which can then be rectified before pathology begins. Doesn't this make sense? It sure does to me, yet most all medical practitioners concern themselves with disease and not wellness anyway, so testing for the function of the body becomes irrelevant because the person is not yet sick to actually require treatment.

Depending on the particular functional test and their respective results, the main points which become relevant and which I raise with a patient after a careful consideration of their case-history along with their results are the following:

- Diet modification

- Lifestyle modification

- Specific probiotic and nutritional supplementation recommendation.

- Oral (or local) anti-fungal or anti-bacterial medications.

- General supplements such as omega 3 fish oils and antioxidants.

- Initiate detoxification protocols – when it is necessary and how.

- Follow-up testing – when and which test.

TEST RESULTS ARE IMPORTANT TO CONSIDER, BUT NEVER RELY ON THEM EXCLUSIVELY Remember, it is more important in the end to consider the patient rather than purely the test results, and this is where some practitioners potentially get confused in my opinion, believing that it's all about the test results rather than the patient. But what if the results are incorrect or the integrity of the sample was compromised? I have seen this on numerous occasions when I have been asked to assist in interpreting results for a practitioner.

For example, with a Hair Analysis the patient submitted colored or dyed hair. With a Food Allergy Test (blood), the patient was taking an antibiotic right up until the blood was drawn or omitted every single food they believed they had an allergy , with a Stool Test the patient was taking probiotics during the test, etc.

I worked alongside a British medical doctor in Australia some years ago who taught me a valuable lesson. This doctor had some of the best clinical skills of any doctor I have ever worked with, his bedside manner was impeccable and so was his ability to diagnose a patient. He always used to say that one should never get "paralysis from analysis" and not to rely a great deal on any test results in order to treat a patient.

To demonstrate this point, Neil would regularly have his practice nurse draw blood from a patient and then send the blood samples from exactly the same person to two separate laboratories, and much to my surprise the results that came back were different, and this occurred on more than one occasion. The blood was the same, from the same patient, yet the results were different! I asked the doctor how this could be, and he said that there are many potential weak links in the testing chain, but the most common are:

- If urine or stool was collected by the patient, how it was collected and handled.

- How the sample was drawn and handled by the nurse at the doctor's end.

- The time and distance the sample travelled to the lab from the medical centre, and under what conditions the sample travelled in.

- The handling of the sample by the nurse and in the laboratory.

- The actual laboratory assay of the sample, i.e.; how they got the results.

- The actual experience the lab technician (or perhaps the lack of).

- The fact that some results belong to an incorrect patient, sad, but it happens.

The bottom line is not to rely exclusively on any test result, there are just too many variables why the test results may not be quite perfect but rather form a reasonably good guideline as to where to go as far as treatment is concerned. The other point I'd like to make is that the first test results obtained form a yardstick or baseline to compare subsequent results to.

I have found in some cases that a patient will come back in several years showing a similar result that she originally presented with, a confirmation perhaps that the treatment was not vigorous enough initially or that she didn't commit to the changes recommended to her diet and lifestyle.

Now I'd like to tell you of the different functional tests that are available to you to assess your yeast infection as well as the advantages and disadvantages of these tests. I have used them all in my clinic for many years, and you may be familiar with some of these tests and not so familiar with others.

Functional Test # 1
The Candida ELISA Test (Blood Or Saliva)

According to some experts, the ELISA candida test represents the most reliable means of detecting candida albicans over-proliferation at this point in time.

Once the candida yeast infection starts to cause disease in your body, it will begin to provoke an immune response, and one of the main effects of such a response will be the production of elevated levels of specific antibodies to candida.

Your white blood cells begin to make antibodies specific against the candida infection, and these antibody levels are measured by way of this test. Some say that it is not a good way to determine if you have an active and/or current candida infection, as the antibody levels can remain elevated for some time (in some cases, months or even years) after a bout of candida, and in some people, evan the slightest exposure can increase the antibody levels. Others say this does not really matter, because if your levels are high right now, it means that you still have an immune system which is very much being affected by candida. As the activity drops off, so should the level of antibody activity, but for some people they can remain high for several years.

The technique used to determine these antibody levels in the blood is called ELISA (enzyme-linked immuno sorbent assay), which is a very powerful and sensitive tool for the measurement of antibody levels in a person's blood or saliva. The way this test is performed is that a small sample of the patient's serum or saliva is coated onto a special plastic plate. The patient sample is diluted and anything in that blood or saliva sample is then grown on this plate.

If any antibodies that recognise the candida are present in the sample they will strongly bind to the candida; all remaining sample that is not bound can then be washed away and a special substrate is added. This is a colourless solution that will cause to produce a coloured sample. This colour can then be very accurately measured by something called a "spectro-photometer". If an exact known level of candida antibodies is accurately determined, then the colour that this produces can be used to produce a standard curve. A computer can then analyse the test sample's colour to give an exact value of how many candida-specific antibodies were in the original sample, now how clever is that!

The Three Main Antigens -
Delayed And Immediate Immune Markers

It is worth pointing out that there are three antigens which can potentially tag the candida specific antibodies in your blood; they are immunoglobulin G (IgG), immunoglobulin A (IgA) as well immunoglobulin E (IgE). Your body produces these three antibodies in order to fight the different strains of candida. Don't confuse this Candida Antibody Test with the IgE/IgG ELISA Food Allergy Test, I'll talk a lot more about food allergy testing in chapter 7, section 1, Understanding Diet And Nutrition.

The importance of this is that the IgG-type antibodies tend to reflect a long-term or an older, more established candida yeast infection. IgG can also reveal that your candida infection may be a lot more severe if this marker is elevated at the same time as the other two.

The IgE antibody represents a present or a more recent candida yeast infection. And an elevated serum (blood) IgA level indicates a more superficial infection, especially if the IgG and IgE levels are low to normal. An elevated IgA on its own will also tell you if the exposure is mainly limited to the mucus membranes (digestive tract, vagina and/or skin) and if you do a stool test (in the case of a CDSA as you will see in a minute) it will reveal a heightened immune response inside your digestive system, generally a food allergy, inflammation or even point potentially towards inflammatory bowel disease if the inflammatory markers are elevated in this stool sample as well.

So, if you can do an IgG/IgA/IgE candida antibody test than please do it. You will then know a lot about not only the direction the yeast infection is going in your body, but will also be able to gauge the severity of the response.

For example, was it bad a while ago (IgG) and now more recently your candida symptoms are not as bad? (IgE). The good thing about doing this test up front is that you will have established a baseline as well, meaning, a starting point for treatment.

Be Careful When Interpreting Allergy Test Results

I have read in the scientific literature that there have been occasions where IgA class antibody levels have been found in excess of one hundred times that seen in a normal population, particularly in those with a history of long-term antibiotic use and in those with recurrent and chronic bacterial or fungal infections. Having a strong family history of allergies can also make a person more likely to have a heightened level of the IgA class of antibodies in particular, so careful case-taking is necessary when performing this test to uncover such a history.

One of the major drawbacks of relying solely on a blood test to diagnose candida is that in a small percentage of candida cases there may actually be evidence of an IgA deficiency in a patient, which could lead to a falsely lowered reading or a negative result. This problem may be compounded by the fact that such patients are more likely to suffer from recurrent bacterial or fungal infections of the very nature that are being tested. You should not rely solely on the outcome of any one single test, and it is best you verify a candida yeast infection by looking at several ways to assess your condition.

The same goes for many different complaints you may suffer from, regardless of any form of testing, as you may now understand that are many unknown variables which can account for a false positive or a false negative test result.

Mucosal Antigen Levels Versus Serum Antigen Levels

You can determine candida antibodies by either the blood, the stool or by the person's saliva. Always remember that candida is in essence an infection of the mucosal surfaces of the body (mouth, digestive system, vagina, etc) and that saliva in this regard therefore represents a more suitable medium for the detection of these types of infections than blood samples.

Blood-based antigen levels will tell us that the infection is more systemic, meaning more widespread throughout the body, and can literally travel anywhere the blood can go, and high serum antibody levels are therefore much more indicative of major systemic infections. Now you can see why I recommend the serum antibody levels over the saliva levels for the reasons mentioned above.

ELISA (Blood) Test Or Saliva Test Collection Requirements

Be sure to avoid all non-essential medications and ALL dietary nutritional supplements for at least a week before the blood is drawn (or saliva produced) before you complete this test. I am surprised how many patients I have seen over the years who take supplements and drugs and even antibiotics right up until they complete the food allergy (or any) test, what a waste of money. In addition, I would prefer that you eat and drink all the foods and beverages you desire. Yes, that's right; eat what you feel like eating for a seven day period before this test, and the reason for this is to establish the true level of antigens in your body based on your cravings and desires. This instinctive diet will reveal what is really going on inside your body and will accurately reveal the antibody level based on the diet which your body is screaming out for. Your candida antibody levels will be a reflection of what "taste's good" to you, and those with candida generally like or crave the sweeter foods. Every person's treats are a little different, so eat what you really want to eat for seven days and then complete the test.

Unless you feel absolutely terrible for eating the foods you desire, just eat what you want to eat for about a week and then perform the test. As soon as you have completed the test then go back to the anti candida diet you were before.

Functional Test # 2
CDSA Test x 3 (Comprehensive Digestive Stool Analysis)

The identification of abnormal levels of yeast species, bacteria and parasites in the stool is an important diagnostic step in therapeutic planning for patients in our clinic with chronic gastrointestinal and other symptoms that may be linked with a candida yeast infection. The CDSA test provides me the clinician with a wide array of the most useful clinical information to help me plan my most appropriate treatment protocol that is quite specific to the individual patient.

While this test is not for everybody (it is expensive around several hundred dollars) it can help to solve the most difficult cases by providing me with all the answers I am looking for. The CDSA x 3 with parasitology is the most comprehensive and commonly ordered functional stool test, assessing the widest range of intestinal conditions. This test will provide information on your ability to digest, metabolise, and absorb nutrients, as well as report all bacterial flora (beneficial, imbalanced and disease causing, all yeasts, and all intestinal parasites (worms, eggs, larva, and protozoa).

It is important to analyse both the intestinal digestion/absorption functions as well as the levels of yeast, bacteria, and parasites because symptoms of mal-digestion or mal-absorption often mimic those of chronic bacterial, yeast, or parasitic infections. Additionally, chronic bacterial, yeast, or parasitic infections may have adverse effects on the body's metabolic and absorptive processes, which can all be assessed using this most comprehensive test.

As you probably aware by now, an overgrowth of yeast can infect virtually every organ system, leading to an extensive array of clinical manifestations. Most patients I have seen over the years that have had a candida yeast infection present with some kind of digestive symptom which often includes varying degrees or different kinds of abdominal pain, cramping, bloating, gas, diarrhea or constipation and/or various forms of digestive irritations. When investigating the presence of yeast in a stool sample, disparity may exist between the culturing of yeast and any actual microscopic examination.

Yeasts are not uniformly dispersed throughout the stool, which is a good reason why you should insist on three stool samples, and by only having one sample performed it may lead to undetectable or low levels of yeast identified by microscopy, despite a cultured amount of yeast. Conversely, microscopic examination may reveal a significant amount of yeast present, but no yeast cultured. Having three stool samples assayed, and NOT all mixed together and assayed as one sample, something many labs do, you are increasing your chances of yeast detection.

While candida does not always survive transit through the digestive tract rendering it unviable, the microscopic finding of yeast in the stool is helpful in identifying whether there is proliferation of yeast or not. Although some yeast may be normal; yeast observed in higher amounts is considered abnormal.

My Personal Choice Of Testing For Candida Is Functional Stool Testing

Personally I like the CDSA test the best out of all the functional tests because it goes right to the heart of the problem, the digestive system. The CDSA give me the most useful information of all the tests, and here are the main points this test reveals:

- Bacteriology culture

- Yeast culture

- Parasitology microscopy

- Giardia and cryptosporidium assay

- Digestion & absorption markers (elastase, fat stain, muscle & veg. fibres, carbs)

- Inflammatory markers (lysozyme, lactoferrin, white blood cells, mucus)

- Immunology (secretory IgA – sIgA)

- Short chain fatty acids (the end product of bacterial fermentation of beneficial bacteria in the bowel)

- Intestinal health markers (red blood cells, pH, occult blood)

- Macroscopic (visual) appearance

The CDSA test in my opinion is the Rolls Royce of candida tests, and if you can afford the rather hefty price tag then you should definitely do this test, no question about it. I have solved an amazing amount of difficult right through to "impossible" cases with this test, when all else failed the patient.

Here is a real case study to illustrate the relevance of a CDSA x3 with parasitology:

Case History # 11
Jean, 63 years

Jean saw me several years ago and came from England to settle down in New Zealand. When this patient first came in, what struck me was how thick her file of hospital notes was from London, it was over three inches thick. This patient had been suffering with multiple digestive complains for over forty years, including cramping pains, bloating, nausea and continual diarrhoea (up to ten motions a day). Her main problem was her increasing intolerance to food, and Jean's diet had become so restrictive that she could only eat a handful of foods including chicken, fish, spinach and beans. Most foods would set off the terrible stomach pains she was experiencing, and this caused the patient to eat less and less.

Jean was one of those patients who ticked every condition box on my case-taking form as positive, she had headaches, insomnia, migraines, arthritis, anxiety, depression, urinary tract infections, in fact Jean had the lot. This patient had been to over two dozen doctors and several specialists, not including herbalists, naturopaths and physiotherapists, osteopaths and more.

The main concern was Jean's weight, it has dropped to 39 kilograms (less than 80 pounds) and at five foot six in height this concerned her bowel specialist greatly so he recommended that she eat more "potato chips (called crisps in England) and chocolate" to gain more weight. What tests were performed on Jean? Apart from the usual blood tests, this poor woman had over one dozen colonoscopies performed and each time "all was normal". The last visit this patient had to her gastroenterologist stated: "Our findings indicate that Mrs. X has no significant disease". No other tests were ever performed, no stool culture tests, no food allergy tests, just the bowel examinations and the odd endoscopy (the camera down the throat test).

Whenever I see a case such as this, the very first thing I recommend is the CDSA x 3 test with parasitology. And guess what we found? We found multiple issues as can be expected, but in particular we found a 3+ level for candida in all three stool samples. This was a significant finding for this patient, for the first time we had answers and the patient and her husband were absolutely delighted, but they were also both equally annoyed at the fact that it took so long to find an answer.

How did Jean end up like this you may ask? Well, that is quite simple to answer – through the medical system. When Jean was 18 she suffered from a terrible sore throat, so her doctor prescribed penicillin. After three weeks, the throat was still painful so more antibiotics were prescribed, and then more and then more. Jean developed a bowel problem and back then in the late 1950's nobody really understood the significance of re-populating the bowel with friendly bacteria. And so the patient suffered. Jean's recovery too approxximately nine months which is a lot quicker than I thought it would take, and this was mainly due to her following all the suggestions, including the necessary lifestyle changes like relaxation, deep breathing, Tai Chi, daily supplementation and adhering strictly to the Candida Crusher Diet principles in general. Jean now weighs a healthy 61 kilograms and has one normal bowel motion a day.

We used a particular probiotic product, a candida eradication formula, a special multivitamin, digestive enzyme and omega 3 supplement. Some months we made significant progress, other months it was more difficult, but we got there in the end. The best thing about our business is seeing patients turn the corner, and Jean certainly did. Perhaps you can relate to Jean's case? If you can, then ask your health-care provider for a CDSA x 3 with parasitology, and if you have no satisfaction, then please contact me. There is no need to suffer for forty years before you can expect optimal health, you just need the right information, and about 500 or 600 dollars for this test. Is your optimal health worth this kind of money?

With The CDSA - Should I Do 1, 2 Or 3 Stool Samples?

I recommend that you always consider the x 3, especially if you are chronically unwell. The 3 day collection period is considered the gold standard by most gastroenterologists, and the scientific literature suggests that three-day collections give maximum sensitivity and specificity for parasite and candida yeast detection because many parasites do not shed from the host at even intervals, and yeasts have varying growth cycles as well. One day's sample may produce negative results, while the following day's sample may be positive, and the day after that the stool may be absolutely loaded with bugs. As I've mentioned previously, the effects of this optimal collection are diminished by the unscrupulous practice of some laboratories which unfortunately blend the three samples into one and perform only one analysis.

There are only a handful of labs that do not pool samples and perform separate analyses on each sample submitted for testing, and I reveal the lab I work with in chapter 8, FAQs and Appendixes, it is Doctor's Data in Chicago. You can also just do a parasitology test and even a stand-alone candida test through the same company, and if your results have come back positive with the CDSA x 3, you may just want to repeat the candida test as a follow- up to save on costs.

Because candida albicans is present in the gastrointestinal tract, it is possible to culture (grow it) from a stool sample. Using a special culture medium and the right anaerobic conditions (reduced oxygen), candida albicans can be grown and identified this way. David Quig Ph.D, technical manager from Doctors Data Labs (Chicago, USA) said to me that if you can culture candida albicans from a stool sample, then you have a pretty bad case of a yeast infection. Other say that this is fine, just look at the numbers, and if all three samples come back as positive (especially 3+ count like Jean, the case study I just outlined to you) then you have a real problem on your hands. You should not be able to culture a significant viable yeast population from a motion you have passed, if you can, it means you have a significant candida overgrowth in your large bowel.

Some specialist laboratories are even able to identify the different species of candida present, and such a result could be quite significant, as some strains have a tendency to be harder to eradicate (such as candida tropicalis) than candida albicans.

It's Not Just About A Positive Candida Result, What Is Your Level Of Beneficial Bacteria?

The other thing I look for in a CDSA test is the actual level of other bad bacteria in the sample and in particular the level of beneficial bacteria. Is there a 1, 2 or a 3+ of good and/or bad? You may be concerned for example if you have a positive result with candida after a stool analysis, but have failed to look at the amount of beneficial bacteria, only to discover that you have a 3+ Lactobacillus acidophilus level. You should be concerned if there is NG (nil growth) in terms of Lactobacillus acidophilus, and some of the chronic cases this is exactly what I have found, yeast in all three stool samples and NG in terms of the lactobacillus species.

I want you to remember that it is not always about killing candida; it is about restoring digestive harmony, and by assessing your level of the good and bad bacteria as well as yeast you will be in a powerful position to restore this harmony. No other pathological or functional test can give you this incredible level of information, now you can see why I believe this to be the best test you can do if you are serious about getting rid of your yeast infection permanently.

Microscopic Yeast In Stool Samples

A CDSA will reveal whether yeast will be in the stool samle or not, and microscopy will be most helpful in finding if fungi like candida are present. Yeast is commonly found in very tiny amounts in a healthy intestinal tract, and while small quantities which are reported as "none or rare" may be normal, any yeast observed in higher amounts, "few, moderate, or many" is considered abnormal.

In a healthy individual, any candida overgrowth will be prohibited by beneficial flora, the intestinal immune defence (secretory IgA) as well as intestinal pH.

Acids like lactic acid are produced by lactobacillus species which lower the pH and thereby create an environment which is unsuitable for yeast to thrive in, a good reason to have a 2 or a 3+ of beneficial lactobacillus in your stool counts. It is most beneficial to have excellent numbers of lactobacillus, because they also produce natural antibiotics themselves like hydrogen peroxide, acidolin and lactobacillin.

A significant and much over looked problem with culturing yeast from a stool sample is that they are colony forming agents and are therefore not evenly dispersed throughout the stool sample, so even though yeast may well be found microscopically, it may not necessarily be cultured successfully even when collected from the patient's same bowel motion.

CDSA Inflammatory Markers

Inflammation in the digestive system can significantly increase your chances of intestinal permeability, indicating an underlying leaky gut and compromising your ability to absorb nutrients. The extent of this inflammation, whether caused by bad bacteria or candida or inflammatory bowel disease (IBD), can be assessed and monitored by examination of the levels of biomarkers such as lysozyme, lactoferrin, white blood cells and mucus.

These markers can be used to differentiate between inflammation associated with Crohn's disease or ulcerative colitis (IBD - inflammatory bowel disease), and less severe inflammation (IBS – irritable bowel syndrome) that can be associated with the presence of bacteria or yeast overgrowths.

Lactoferrin

In the CDSA stool test, you will find that a marker called lactoferrin is only markedly elevated prior to and during the active phases of IBD, but not with IBS. Therefore, monitoring stool levels of lactoferrin in patients with IBD can therefore facilitate timely treatment of IBD.

Lysozyme

Lysozyme is another stool marker some labs perform; it can be detected particularly during an acute attack of Crohn's disease. It is one of the best inflammatory markers to detect this kind of IBD.

Calprotectin

Calprotectin is a protein found in white blood cells called neutrophils that make up three-quarters of your white blood cell counts. Some stool testing labs use calprotectin as their inflammatory marker, and some experts consider calprotectin to be the gold standard measurement of intestinal inflammation. The main diseases that cause an increased excretion of fecal calprotectin are Crohn's disease, ulcerative colitis and neoplasms such as bowel cancer. Levels of fecal calprotectin and lysozyme will be found to be normal in patients with irritable bowel syndrome (IBS). Although a relatively new stool test, fecal calprotectin is regularly used as indicator for inflammatory bowel disease IBD during treatment and as diagnostic marker.

The SIgA Marker: Candida, Infection, Allergies And Leaky Gut

Since the vast majority of the antibodies called IgA (sIgA, or secretory IgA) normally resides in your digestive system where it prevents binding of bad bacteria and yeasts to the mucosal membrane, it is essential to know the status of sIgA in the digestive system. I have discovered that SIgA is quite possibly the only bona fide marker of immune status in your digestive system.

There are several different immunoglobulins in the various tissues of your body, but secretory IgA is the main one found in mucous secretions. In my practice, I have found that a person's SIgA levels is one of the first factors I look at when it comes to the stool test, it allows me to see how strong that person's gut immune health connection is, and in particular, how capable their immune system is in fighting any intestinal infection.

IgA is produced in your blood and transported across the mucosal layer in addition to your intestinal cells, which produce an incredible two to three grams of this antibody everyday. SIgA production appears to peak in childhood, declining after about sixty years of age. When it comes to mucous, people are all too aware of this about their nose or throat, but in fact the whole digestive system is coated in the stuff.

A healthy layer of mucous is the gut's first line of defense against pathogens like ingested viruses, parasites, bacteria, yeast in addition to any foreign food proteins and toxins.
It is important to know that your mucosal barrier doesn't only consist of the lining of your entire digestive system, it also makes up the lining of your mouth, eyes, nasal cavity, sinuses, upper part of your lungs, the urethra of men and women and the vagina in women. Everywhere there is a mucosal system you will find that it is covered in a fine layer of mucous, and in this mucous you will find secretory IgA.

You may have you noticed, these are also key areas where you will find a yeast infection and therefore it is important for your body to maximize this antibody's production and heighten its activity if you are you are to win the fight and crush your yeast infection, or any infection for that matter.

The main role of SIgA is to defend the surfaces of the digestive system and other systems coated in mucous and to prevent these potential toxic substances from biding to cell surfaces, becoming absorbed by cells lining the mouth, throat, lungs, urethra, vagina and intestines, and ultimately invading the body. SIgA has the ability to cling or adhere to these foreign substances and neutralize them along with their toxins which may be released, and help to remove these foreigners by ensuring they get excreted out of the body in the feces.

Low SigA Levels

Low SIgA levels can signify that there is a progressive or underlying developing food allergy occurring, and if levels remain too low or are borderline, you will find that it can take considerably longer for the body to heal and repair any leaky gut.

When a patient has a consistently low SigA level in her stool or saliva, it tells me why she can't seem to get on top of her chronic yeast infection or food allergy. But it also reveals that her immune system generally is having a hard time coping, and can reflect in a poor recovery from psoriasis, rheumatoid artthritis or any other auto-immune condition.

It's more important and intelligent to fix the gut when it comes to the immune system than to worry about rubbing coal tar on a person with psoriasis or treating a patient with rheumatoid arthritis with steroids to reduce their inflammation.

SIgA levels which persistently remain low for years can eventually result in some of the most severe cases of systemic candidiasis I have ever seen, because the mucosal barriers are no longer effective in protecting the body against yeast and its metabolites. If you take the IgA soldiers away from their mucosal borders, what is ultimately protecting your body from being over run by free loading bacteria and yeasts?

A person with chronic candidasis will need to get their SigA levels UP, and this is often the key when it comes to healing that leaky gut quickly and permanently. A sustained higher SIgA level will mean more immune fighting power internally.

Research has revealed that children with autistic tendencies and celiacs have low SigA levels and SIBO (small intestine bacterial overgrowth), and so do people with irritable bowel syndrome and inflammatory bowel syndrome (ulcerative colitis and Crohn's disease).

I always try to establish why a person's SIgA levels are low and remain low, and it could be as simple as one food the person is routinely eating which is challenging the body (see the Low-Allergy Diet sheet in section 1 of chapter 5). What are their levels of beneficial bacteria? It is surprising how many stool tests I have seem that "NG" (no growth) when it comes to lactobacillus acidophilus, and sometimes a probiotic can make all the difference for this reason. Do they have a significant parasite or bacterial overgrowth that could be reduced through diet and supplementation?

If your SigA levels don't seem to come up to speed inspite of your very best and sustained efforts, consider looking at the "Obstacles To Cure" in section 5 of chapter 7. You may have a diseased tooth or a low-grade inflammation elsewhere in the body, and there is a specific panel of blood tests that can be done to establish this inflammatory response. A bit of investigation can go a very long way towards resolving the low SIgA, and ultimately your yeast infection once and for all.

Perhaps you may have an established yet undiagnosed auto-immune disease? I've seen this occur on numerous occasions. Any chronic low-grade inflammation will be an immune-drain and will need to be addressed before you can expect a healthy rise in SigA levels, and then watch what happens to the unresolved yeast infection. The longer and more severe and compromised the SigA levels remain low in your digestive system, the more drain on the adrenal gland function that occurs, and you may slowly slide into adrenal fatigue. For this reason, I like a patient to complete the adrenal fatigue questionnaire if they have had their yeast infection for some time, and most will have some degree of adrenal fatigue as a consequence of an ongoing leaky gut and low SIgA levels. It is very important for you to understand the relationship between your immunity and adrenal fatigue, and for this reason I have written plenty on this topic. You will find more information on adrenal fatigue and immunity in chapter 7, section 2 - Understanding Immunity, Metabolites And Stress.

Key Causes Of Low SIgA

- **High Antigenic Load.** A high load of circulating antibodies from food allergies can significantly depress SIgA levels, even in people who don't really have many overt symptoms. Check carefully for leaky gut syndrome, and be sure to follow the Low-Allergy Diet as outlined in the Candida Crusher Diet in the first section of chapter 7.

- **Certain Pharmaceutical Drugs.** A little known fact is that certain drugs can induce a temporary IgA deficiency which will generally resolve after the drug is removed. These include anti-inflammatories both steroidal and non-steroidal, sulfasalazine, hydantoin, cyclosporine, gold, fenclofenac, sodium valproate, and captopril.

- **Certain Viral Infections.** Viral infections such as congenital rubella infection, Epstein-Barr virus (EBV) or Coxsackie virus infection, may result in persistent IgA deficiency. I am always on the lookout to see if the person had these infections in the past, as they can be a cause of continual low-grade SIgA levels for many years. Treat the adrenals and see what happens, get that cortisol UP.

- **Poor Nutrition.** A person with nutritional deficiencies may have difficulty mounting an appropriate SIgA immune response, deficiencies like zinc, vitamin C, iron, folate and various other deficiencies can hinder the production of SIgA. This is just one of the reasons to take a top quality multi like the Candida Crusher Multi.

- **Inflammatory Bowel Disease.** Lower sIgA levels are frequently found in those with ulcerative colitis or in those whose first degree relatives have the disease. A diagnosis must be made, has the person had a colonoscopy and appropriate blood testing?

- **Stress.** Lower levels of SigA are frequently found in those with excessive cortisol production, so decreasing stress may lead to higher sIgA levels. These are the people more prone to developng adrenal fatigue, and I recommend most with a yeast infection of long duration do the adrenal fatigue test and get treatment when appropriate.

- **Chronic Low-Grade Infections.** Lower SIgA levels may also be found in those with chronic infections which may last for many years and remain undetected. They may have undetected bacteria or parasites because their mucosal defence mechanism may be weak or very poor. The allergic response may be increased as well, and they may have a potential tendency towards multiple food allergies. This is why I am careful in quetioning patients about any hidden focal infections, and you can read a lot more about this in section 5 of chapter 7.

High SIgA Levels

I more often will find a lower level of SIgA when it comes to stool testing, but occasionally discover an elevated IgA in a stool test. An increase in SIgA will generally mean a heightened immune respone which usually signifies inflammation. It will generally be an acute immune response, ongoing infection or significant food allergy.

An elevated SIgA along with an elevated lysozyme, calprotectin or lactoferrin level will tell you that there is inflammatory bowel disease (Crohn's disease or ulcerative colitis), an elevated SIgA with low or normal lysozyme, calprotectin or lactoferrin levels will tell you that there is either IBS (irritable bowel syndrome) or a significant food allergy or infection.

I have noticed that patients with markedly elevated SigA levels often feel quite ill, and some can feel really sick. An upregulated immune respone can create many different clinical scenarios and can affect many different systems of the body. Microbial and mircoscopic studies of the stool are useful in identifying if bacteria, candida or parasites are present, and as you can now begin to see, this information can significantly aid in formulating a plan of succesful yeast infection treatment. It is important to remember however that elevated SigA levels have been found in the absence of bacteria, candida and parasites in people with atopic conditions like food allergies, urticaria and dermatitis. Again, testing will reveal what is really going on inside the gut, and will take all that guesswork out of the equation.

Best Nutritional Way To Increase SigA – My 4-R method

There are different things you can do to elevate SIgA, but one of the best ways is to use the Candida Crusher Diet and take the Candida Crusher dietary supplements specifically formulated to enhance the Candida Crusher Program.

Here is my 4-R method of nutritional supplementation, an excellent method to significantly enhance your SigA levels:

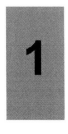

Remove offending foods, crush candida and correct nutritional deficiencies: Follow the 3-Stage Candida Crusher Diet as outlined in section 1 of chapter 7. Consider antimicrobial, antifungal, and antiparasitic treatment in the case of opportunistic/pathogenic bacterial, yeast, and/or parasite overgrowth (the Candida Crusher Formula). Take the Candida Crusher Multi to correct any underlying nutritional deficiencies.

Replace what is needed for normal digestion and absorption: Take the Candida Crusher Digestive Enzyme to significantly improve digestion and absorption.

 Reinoculate with favorable microbes: Take the Candida Crusher Probiotic to enhance the growth of the favorable bacteria, supplement with prebiotics such as the correct fibers in your diet.

 Repair digestive system cells: Repair the leaky gut and the immune system. Reduce the inflammatory response by taking the Candida Crusher Omega 3 and the Candida Crusher Probiotic.

More Ways To Increase SIgA Levels

- **Colostrum** has also been shown to increase SIgA levels. Colostrum is the first milk that contains a significant amount of immunoglobulins (antibodies) which helps confer additional immunity to an infant cow or human straight after birth. Colostrum has been shown to stimulate the production of SIgA and is certainly a good supplement to try.

- **Prebiotics.** Make sure you eat plenty of healthy dietary fiber, you can read a lot more about fiber in section 1 of chapter 7. This is an overlooked area, because most people are too busy taking probiotics to worry about eating healthy prebiotic foods which feed the probiotics in their digestive system!

- **Cayenne pepper** has the ability to stimulate B-lymphocytes into manufacturing more SIgA. By taking 2 cayenne pepper capsules a day you will be increasing your levels.

- **Saccharomyces boulardii** is a beneficial yeast and one of the few probiotics which not only helps to fight a yeast infection, it can assist in boosting SIgA levels.

- **Lowering stress levels** has been shown to increase SIgA levels by lowering the stress hormone cortisol. Elevated cortisol levels have been proven to suppress the production of SIgA. Be sure to study section 5 of chapter 7 to more fully understand why rest and relaxation is one of the best kept secrets when it comes to crushing your candida for good.

- **Following the Candida Crusher Diet principles.** By following my dietary recommendations you will be ensuring your that you are doing everthing right diet-wise to repair the leaky gut and elevate lowered levels of SIgA.

- **Take the Candida Crusher Supplements.** Be sure to follow the 4-R dietary supplement program, it will ensure that you will increase your SIgA levels in the shortest possible time. It could mean the difference between inhibiting yeast and reducing the severity of your symptoms to permanently eliminating your yeast infection in the shortest possible time.

Whenever I get test results back, I immediately wonder what the immune panel of this patient's CDSA test looks like; are there high levels of sIgA in the test results, indicative of a lot of antibody production in the digestive system? If there is a high level, then I know that I have to work quite hard on the Hypo Allergenic Diet up front with this patient, because the higher the level of sIgA, the stronger the immune response will be towards allergenic foods that person is consuming right now. The Hypoallergenic Diet by the way is the second stage of the Candida Crusher Diet, you can read about it in section 1 of chapter 7.

Positive Test Results: 38yr Old Male With Major Yeast Problem

Here you can see a colorful section of a CDSA test result, showing the yeast panel. If yeast is positive then a yeast susceptibilities panel will be shown on your CDSA test results. The following panel is the test results from a 38yr old male who had been experiencing major digestive issues for several years, including a bad case of diarrhoea. He was diagnosed as having "irritable bowel syndrome" and placed on several drugs, including a pharmaceutical drug commonly prescribed for diarrhoea, an anti-anxiety drug as well as an anti-depressant for the past few years due to his increasing despondency.

He used to work for a major telecommunications company, but had to stop work and eventually go on a sickness benefit due to his poor bowel function. The result of his CDSA was strongly positive (3+ on all 3 stool samples) for candida albicans, and here below are the results of the sensitivity panel included with this test. We treated Paul (not his real name) for over 3 months before we started to notice significant results, but it took almost 6 months before we started to see a 90%+ improvement in his condition. It has been now 2 years ago, and Paul is now back at work and most grateful for the help he has received. And his bowel function? We are pleased to say that Paul is back to one or two motions daily, instead of up to ten bowel motions daily.

CDSA Test Collection Requirements

- Eat the foods as you normally would. Just like the food allergy tests, I would prefer that you eat what you WANT to eat, follow your desires as the test results will then be a more true reflection of not only what is going on in your gut, but what digestive issues got you to this point where you now seek treatment. What is the point of testing the stool of a person who a month ago went onto a super strict healthy dietary approach for example, after they spent years drinking alcohol a few times a week, eating fries and following a processed and refined supermarket diet in general. I want the patient's stool test results based on the diet which they followed before they decided to clean up their act. This is the best way to ascertain what is really going on. You go back onto your healthy diet as soon as you have performed the stool test, but for the week leading up to the stool test you eat whet you like and want to eat.

- Avoid probiotics and preferably ALL dietary supplements for up to three days (but preferably an entire week) prior to the test. You may otherwise get a false negative result, especially with candida, bacteria and parasites.

Yeast Susceptibilities: Candida albicans

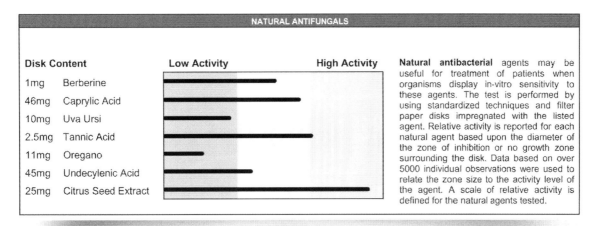

NATURAL ANTIFUNGALS

Disk Content		Low Activity — High Activity
1mg	Berberine	
46mg	Caprylic Acid	
10mg	Uva Ursi	
2.5mg	Tannic Acid	
11mg	Oregano	
45mg	Undecylenic Acid	
25mg	Citrus Seed Extract	

Natural antibacterial agents may be useful for treatment of patients when organisms display in-vitro sensitivity to these agents. The test is performed by using standardized techniques and filter paper disks impregnated with the listed agent. Relative activity is reported for each natural agent based upon the diameter of the zone of inhibition or no growth zone surrounding the disk. Data based on over 5000 individual observations were used to relate the zone size to the activity level of the agent. A scale of relative activity is defined for the natural agents tested.

NON-ABSORBED ANTIFUNGALS

Nystatin — Low Activity / High Activity

Non-absorbed antifungals may be useful for treatment of patients when organisms display in-vitro sensitivity to these agents. The test is performed using standardized commercially prepared disks impregnated with Nystatin. Relative activity is reported based upon the diameter of the zone of inhibition or no growth zone surrounding the disk.

AZOLE ANTIFUNGALS

	Resistant	S-DD	Susceptible
Fluconazole			S
Itraconazole			S
Ketoconazole			S

Susceptible results imply that an infection due to the fungus may be appropriately treated when the recommended dosage of the tested antifungal agent is used.
Susceptible - Dose Dependent (S-DD) results imply that response rates may be lower than for susceptible fungi when the tested antifungal agent is used.
Resistant results imply that the fungus will not be inhibited by normal dosage levels of the tested antifungal agent.

Standardized test interpretive categories established for Candida spp. are used for all yeast isolates.

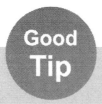

Good Tip

Stay in touch with your practitioner

Once you have started to improve or fail to improve after a few treatments, it is important to keep in touch with your doctor or naturopath. He or she will be interested in your progress and be keen to see you get well. I have noticed many times that whether a patient improves or aggravates, their visits to the clinic tend to taper off, and some people just stop coming, failing to show for their follow-up visit. Your practitioner has invested a considerable amount of time in helping you with your recovery, and by regularly keeping in touch, your practitioner will know if you still need to come in for follow-up visits, need further tests or assessments or any further treatment. Some patients just don't turn up after several visits, leaving practitioners wondering if they have improved to the point that they don't require any further treatment for the time being, or that they have aggravated and decided to take their health-care somewhere else. Let your practitioner know, because this communication will allow him or her to fine tune their future treatment protocols with you and other patients. Unmet expectations are one of the biggest reasons for "no shows" in the clinic, and are frustrating to both patient and practitioner alike.

Functional Test # 3
The Organic Acids Urine Test

I have only started to use this form of urine testing more recently, and have found it an excellent way to assess dysbiosis (bad bacteria build-up).

Urinary organic acids are assayed in a patient's urine and come from the metabolic conversion of the person's dietary protein, fats and carbohydrates intake, in addition to compounds of bacterial origin, this test can provide a unique chemical profile of a patient's cellular health. The organic acids urine test measures the actual overflow or build-up of organic acid products in a person's urine. There are various organic acid tests which can assess quite a wide range of different physiological processes including intestinal dysbiosis, energy production, nutrient cofactor requirements and even a person's neurotransmitter (brain hormone) metabolism. Like all functional tests, I have found that by carefully evaluating a patient's case history as well as their test results, in this case it is their urinary organic acid levels, I can pinpoint their particular metabolic dysfunction and then tailor-make a comprehensive, customized treatment plan for each individual patient.

The main yeast and fungal dysbiosis marker in the urine I check for elevation in particular is D-arabinitol. Here is a brief overview of this organic acid urinary marker and what it means. The treatment consideration for a urinary elevation of D-arabinitol is as outlined in chapter 7 of this book, the Candida Crusher and involves the diet, lifestyle and supplement recommendations.

D - Arabinitol – A Reliable Marker For Urinary Detection Of Invasive Candida

Evidence from multiple studies by independent investigators has led to the recommendation that high urinary levels of the sugar alcohol, D-arabinitol, be used as a reliable biomarker for the more invasive forms of a candida overgrowth.

D-Arabinitol is a metabolite (A substance necessary for or taking part in a particular metabolic process) of candida, and a high level of this marker is associated with invasive candidiasis. D-arabinitol is produced from dietary carbohydrates when yeasts are rapidly growing in the low oxygen (anaerobic) environment of the small intestine.

Because D-arabinitol is a sugar found in sweet apples, grapes, and pears, these fruits and their products are best strictly avoided 24 hours prior to urine collection to avoid any false positive test results. Can you now understand why sweet fruits are not the best of foods to consume when you commence the Candida Crusher Program, in particular those who have a severe case of a yeast infection?

Organic Acid Urine Test Collection Requirements

Collect a spot urine or a first-morning void urine specimen, or take a specimen from a 24hr urine collection container. Then transfer a 10ml sample of this specimen into clean container supplied for preservation and transportation to your functional laboratory. Avoid all dietary supplements for two days before you complete this test.

Functional Test # 4
The Urinary Indican Test

Indican is produced as a by-product by the dietary breakdown of an amino acid called tryptophan. Bacteria in the upper bowel facilitate this conversion from any unabsorbed tryptophan. Indican is normally low in healthy people and increased levels indicate small intestinal bacterial overgrowth (SIBO) or intestinal dysbiosis. Patients that may be at greater risk for indican overproduction include those with poor diets or refined diets, those who drink too much alcohol and those with hectic and stressful lives. Elevated indican levels may also commonly indicate maldigestion and hypochlorhydria. (an underactive stomach) Indican excretion is reduced when the intestines are populated with strains of beneficial bacteria, and the higher the level of beneficial bacteria the lower the level of indican is likely to be.

While the urinary indican test is not a test that is specific for a yeast infection, in my experience most patients who present to my clinic with a yeast infection are positive for urinary indican, signifying dysbiosis, high levels of bad bacteria. Those with yeast infections, especially when chronic, often have high to very high levels of dysbiotic bacteria as well.

This test is an accurate, simple and yet an inexpensive screening tool to allow the quick identification of the putrefaction of protein in the gastrointestinal tract. A positive test reflects a state of intestinal bacterial dysbiosis that almost always accompanies a yeast infection.

This test is often performed by your naturopath or functional medicine doctor, and can be performed quickly in their clinic. The urinary indican test will give you an immediate indication of how much dysbiosis you have ranging from 0 to + 4 depending on the color of the dipstick soon after it has been placed in the urine sample. Ask your health-care professional if he or she can perform this test for you, chances are that she may be able to simply get this test from his or her supplier of products or tests. Your local chemist or pharmacy may be able to tell you who does this test in your area or if they know who can supply it to you.

Some Causes Of A Positive Urinary Indican Test

- Intestinal overgrowth of anaerobic bacteria (dysbiosis)

- Intestinal mucosal permeability (leaky gut syndrome) due to damage from an infection, an anti-biotic, a toxic or reactive exposure, or nutritional deficiency.

- Protein maldigestion or too much protein.

- Alcohol consumption or a diet high in sugary and refined foods

- Constipation.

- Bile duct obstruction or gallstones.

Common Micro-Organisms Contributing To Positive Indican Tests Include:

Salmonella, Shigella, Campylobacter, Yersinia, Citrobacter species, Klebsiella pneumoniae, Pseudomonas, some strains of Escherichia coli, Staphyloccocus aureus, Bacteriodes, Clostridium, Candida albicans, and many other Candida species.

Urinary Indican Test Collection Requirements

- No alcohol the night before

- Avoid probiotics for three days prior

- Preferably a high protein meal the night before

- No iodine, bile supplements taken 3 - 4 days prior to testing (these may create a false positive test)

- Avoid all enzyme and digestive enzyme formulations 3 days prior

- Sample preferably from a second urination of the day

Frequency Of Urinary Indican Testing

This urine test is best performed every two weeks, and the mesurement recorded on your Candida Home Test Tracker which you will find near the end of this chapter.

The 8 Different Home Tests For Yeast Infections

Candida overgrowth can be difficult to diagnose in laboratory tests as it lives naturally in the intestines. The Urinary Indican Test is one lab test I do in my clinic, particularly if I suspect candida or dysbiosis in general in the patient. While you can do the Urinary Indican Test at home, you will probably have this performed by your naturopath or doctor in their clinic during a consultation.

There are other tests you can do at home to determine you status, and the more that are positive the higher the chances you have a candida overgrowth. Most of these tests can also be performed at weekly intervals to determine how successful the treatment is and if you are staying on track with your diet, lifestyle and supplementation.

Test And Measure

By using common sense with these home tests, you will be able with reasonable certainty to determine which direction you are heading with your yeast infection. First establish a baseline with your tests, i.e; before you start any treatment, complete the online Candida Questionnaire at yeastinfection.org and the 8 home tests I recommend in this chapter and write the date you test and the results all down in your Candida Symptom Tracker. Then, start the Candida Crusher Program (chapter 7) and measure your results weekly. By repeated testing over a period of several months, and with fine tuning of the Candida Crusher Program, you should be noticing that the signs and symptoms steadily decrease. This test and measure process is a very successful way to permanently eradicate your yeast infection, because you will be able to work out if your treatment is working or not and make the right adustments accordingly.

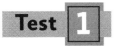

Test **1**

The Itch Test

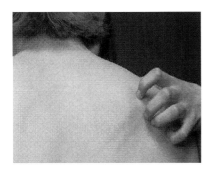

Become much more acutely aware of your body, do you have an itchy scalp, itchy groin, itchy eyes, and itchy patches anywhere in or on your body?

Do your ears need a good scratch on the inside? Do your feet or toes itch? Write down when you need to itch, you may even like to include ANY part of your body and when in your diary, or smart phone nowadays!

You will be amazed at how often you touch your body without even being aware, particularly if you have a candida problem. You become so used to itching your body that you actually become totally unaware of its presence. Does your anus itch? Do your feet or hands itch? Look for recurrent itching anywhere and record these hot spots for three days. When you are out it is interesting to observe people, and when you become aware you will be surprised to see how many people have a good scratch or itch.

If you go to a bar or out to a social gathering involving food and alcohol, you will see male beer drinkers who seem to adjust themselves or touch their private area. Many guys are so used to these adjustments that they are totally unaware, and it is surprising how many women need to itch their genital region as well, they are much more discreet however! It is any wonder, because beer and wine in particular are one of the classic candida inducers. When you go out to the shopping mall, especially where foods are served, watch those around you and see how people itch their bodies.

The lady in the corner with the cup of coffee and a sweet baked treat is scratching her head and itching her ear. The child with a pocket full of sweets complains to his mother of a sore bottom which is probably a rectal itch. You may want to observe your partner for a few days without mentioning anything, especially if he or she has flatulence (gas) or burps a lot, drinks alcohol and consumes the foods which allow candida to thrive in their bodies.

Itchy hot spots include the vaginal or scrotal region, anus or rectal area, armpits, scalp, ears, feet and toes, especially between the toes, under the breasts and folds of skin around the abdomen. In fact, anywhere where the skin is warm and covered in particular.

Frequency Of Itch Testing

The itch test is performed weekly, and the measurement recorded on your Candida Home Test Tracker which you will find near the end of this chapter.

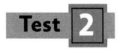

The Craving Test

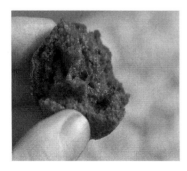

Become more aware of what you eat, but particularly what you LIKE to eat, how often and when. Those with yeast and especially a fungal overgrowth may well crave sweet foods without even knowing it. Do you want something sweet routinely after your evening meal? Do you want something sweet between meals? We could be looking at breads (especially white and refined) biscuits (any – they all contain sugar). It never ceases to amaze me how many people I speak to love sweet stuff and yet say to me "But I don't eat any sugar!" or I'll hear: "I don't have sugar in my coffee or tea" but then an hour later they have a muffin, a cookie, a muesli bar or a fruit drink which all contain sugar. When a person tells me that they "like the taste" of a food or a drink, they generally mean the sweetness.

These folk may even have a glass of wine each night yet they don't have "any added sugar" in their diet. At the turn of the last century, around 1900, the average person consumed less than one kilo of sugar in one year. And today the average person eats twice their bodyweight in sugar. Is it any wonder we have bugs in our digestive systems when we are busily feeding these bugs up several times daily?

Try this trick, eat NO sweet foods for three days and see how you feel. I am not talking about fruits and vegetables, but do avoid oranges and especially dried fruit. Just keep away from these sugars or any foods or drinks containing them for three days: all breads, pancakes, sugar and other quick-acting carbohydrates including sucrose, high-fructose corn syrup, fructose, maltose, lactose, glycogen, glucose, mannitol, sorbitol, and galactose. Also avoid honey, molasses, maple syrup, maple sugar, and date sugar. Look at labels and packaging and STOP these foods for 72 hours. Did you crash, develop a headache; feel tired or funny in any way? Then you were too dependent on sugar and may have an addiction here. A sugar fix most days to me spells a candida population that need feeding inside you.

The craving test may make a real candida sufferer feel terrible, they may literally feel like climbing the wall to get to their sugar fix on the other side, and the stronger the craving and withdrawal, the bigger the problem and the more need for self-restraint with the offending food or drink will be required.

Try it, you may be quite surprised and know exactly what I mean. Three days is all you need – but you have to be very strict and just focus on fresh vegetables, lean meats, whole grains like quinoa and brown rice, nuts and seeds and water.

In Chinese medicine they say that a person either likes sweet or likes bitter foods, if you love sweet foods you are less inclined to like bitter and the other way around. Try eating more bitter foods such as endive, chicory, silver beet, radicchio, Cos lettuce (outer leaves), mustard greens, dandelion leaf, dandelion root coffee, grapefruit and olive oil. Swedish bitters or bitter herbal medicines like gymnema, gentian or any of the liver or gall bladders herbal medicines are also good to take for a few weeks.

The more bitter foods you become to like the less sweet foods you will begin crave, that is my experience with patients in the clinic. And do you know what? Bitter foods stimulate digestion, improve bowel flora and allow your liver and gallbladder to function optimally. You will excrete more waste and toxins, burn more fat and kill more bad bugs in your digestive system as well.

Today we need to take digestive enzymes, because we prefer eating sweet foods to the bitter ones and these sweet foods stimulate the proliferation of bad bacterium and yeast. Once you get to like increasing amounts of the bitter foods in your diet, your digestion will finally turn the corner and you will be amazed at how your sweet cravings diminish, bloating and gas disappear, weight will just seem to magically drop from your butt, hips and thighs, energy will improve and your health will go to a whole new level. But why you ask? Because you took sweet foods out of your diet and started to eat bitter foods that stimulate rather than inhibit digestion. You began filling your gas tank (your stomach) with high performance bitter foods rather than kerosene, the sweet stuff. Can you now see why probiotics and enzymes are so widely prescribed and sold the past ten years in particular?

Frequency Of Craving Testing

The craving test is performed weekly, and the measurement recorded on your Candida Home Test Tracker which you will find near the end of this chapter.

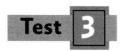

The Spit Test

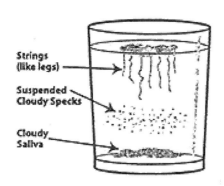

Here is a saliva test you can easily do at home, some say it is not effective but I have found it to be accurate for many patients presenting with a yeast infection. Whilst I have found a small percentage of people with candida issues who test negative with test, most with chronic infestations of yeast in their system will come up positive with this saliva test so give it a go.

First thing in the morning, before you put anything in your mouth, get a clear glass fill with water and work up a bit of saliva, then spit it into the glass of water. Check the water every 15 minutes or so for up to one hour.

If you have a problem with yeast, you will see strings (like legs) travelling down into the water from the saliva floating on the top, these look a little like the subtle strands you see hanging from the ceiling of a cave which glow worms produce. With a major candida problem you may also see suspended cloudy specks of saliva that will (eventually) sink to the bottom of the glass, becoming a small blob of cloudy saliva.

If there are no strings and the saliva is still floating after at least one hour, you may well have no yeast problem. But do make sure you eat NOTHING before you do the spit test or you will not get the results you are looking for. Repeat this test a few times and on different days in case you get a "false negative" on the test. I have also found with candida infections with many people that as soon as they eat something very sweet like a small amount of refined sugar, they rapidly will have a build-up of some saliva in the mouth, the tongue can feel also irritated by refined carbohydrates as well. An almost instant mucus production occurs in some yeast infection patients who have the slightest amount of sugar in their diet, and this will often disappear as their intestinal yeast overgrowth is halted and reversed, I have verified this with many patients over the years.

As the person's SIgA levels improve, the spit test will slowly begin to normalize, I have verified this with countless stool tests.

Forget all those folks who say this test is "fake" and worthless, when you get a positive here and are positive to the several other tests I've outlined here, your chances of having a yeast infection are a lot higher. Just watch, as the months roll on by and you notice improvements, so will your saliva and along with it your SIgA levels will come up and your food allergies will go down.

Frequency Of Spit Testing

The spit test is performed weekly, and the measurement recorded on your Candida Home Test Tracker which you will find near the end of this chapter.

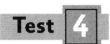

The Smell Test

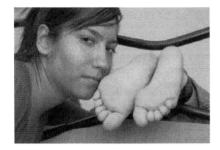

Medical research at the Imperial College in London has proved that some people with body odor have imbalances affecting the 'friendly bacteria' that live inside all of our digestive systems. Having a bad or offensive body odor can be a key to having a candida problem, and so can be overheating and easy sweating of the body. Smelly feet, smelly armpits and body odor in general is linked with candida.

There is a high degree of fermentation going on in the person's digestive system and this will produce odors and heat as a by-product. Many yeast infection sufferers I know complain of excessive perspiration and flushes of heat at night. Some women even mistake these flushes for menopausal hot flashes. I've noticed that quite a few have told me about a body odor and bad breath, sometimes even a fecal breath! The armpits can release lots of toxins through the sweat glands, and eventually the entire body. Don't worry, this will generally change for the better when you start cleaning your body and eradicating the yeast, but don't be concerned during the initial stages of cleansing because your body could initially release many toxins, which may cause more body odor and also bad breath, rest assured, this is only temporary.

Body odor is caused from the release of toxins through the pores. Have you ever noticed that if you do a lot of exercise and are not stessed, you smell less?

Have you ever opened a jar of jam or marmalade that has been fermenting in the back of your cupboard for some time, it was pretty putrid wasn't it? Have you smelled those moldy cheeses or foods that have a little mold on them? A yeast problem affecting the external body has a characteristic smell and is easy to recognize, think about athlete's foot, which is not unlike a moldy cheese. However, when a yeast infection affects the skin and is combined with a person's unique biochemistry including their residue of body oil and sweat, it can smell more like body odor, and it then may be hard to distinguish between body odor resulting from poor personal hygiene and a yeast-related problem.

What I look for are any underlying digestive problems, which will generally clinch the diagnosis, especially when combined with a stool test. If you have lots of gas, burping, bloating and digestive discomfort then you are probably fermenting bugs in your gut and producing gas as a by product, and in this case the Candida Crusher Program is well indicated. Do you smell and sweat easily? It could be a yeast infection.

Frequency Of Smell Testing

The smell test is performed weekly, and the measurement recorded on your Candida Home Test Tracker which you will find near the end of this chapter.

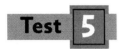

The Tongue Test

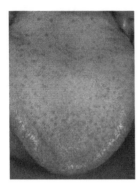

Look at this tongue; do you see the white covering across its surface? Now go and check you tongue in the mirror, is it always coated a faint white or yellowish color? Is it coated more in the middle or towards the back? Is your breath offensive? This could be a key sign of bacterial or yeast overgrowth in the digestive system. Your breath should not smell putrid in the morning let alone taste or smell like the bottom of your birdcage, yet some candida patients I've seen complain of bad breath ranging from mild right through to literally having a fecal breath.

But don't immediately jump to conclusions, you may just have gum disease or gingivitis, but if your teeth and gums are perfectly fine and don't bleed then you may well have a bacterial issue somewhere in your digestive system. Get your teeth checked out by a dental hygienist or dentist, these people are professional and can immediately tell you if you are suffering from a problem affecting the health of your teeth and gums or not.

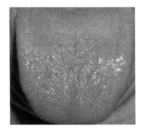

The more towards the back of your tongue the discoloration is the more likely it will be bacteria or candida in your large intestine, and if the discoloration is at the very back of the tongue, your dysbiosis is likely to be in the sigmoid colon, the part of the large intestine closest to the rectum. Healthy people with great digestive systems and proper bowel flora generally have a clean pinkish tongue, like the image of the tongue you can see to your left. Look at you dog's tongue, dogs don't often drink soda or beer or eat donuts or chocolate, their breath is sweet smelling and they have minimal bloating and if they do have gas it's because you fed them the wrong stuff!

Can you say the same about your health, and do you pay much attention to the color of your tongue and your digestive health? A tongue that is white in the middle will have dysbiosis affecting the small intestine, and the closer to the tip of the tongue the discoloration occurs, the closer to the stomach the dysbiosis is occurring.

Some people may also notice with toxins clearing from their body that they may begin to have an increasingly white-coated tongue or white spots or rashes on the skin; this is a good sign, and will soon pass.

As you go through the different stages of the Candida Crusher Program, you will notice that your tongue may at first become somewhat more discolored and furry, but over time it should clear up significantly and after you have re-populated your digestive system with lots of beneficial bacteria, you will find that your tongue will once again be a nice clean pinkish color. Your tongue can be your guide to a clean and healthy digestive system, and judging by the color of many tongues I've seen, I think that this has become somewhat of a rarity nowadays.

So don't forget, your scores of the tongue test may in fact worsen before they get better. It may happen, and with some it may not, so don't worry if it does occur because it is a good thing.

Frequency Of Tongue Testing

The tongue test is performed weekly, and the measurement recorded on your Candida Home Test Tracker which you will find near the end of this chapter.

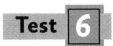

Test 6

The Sound Test

Does you digestive system make funny sounds regularly? Many candida sufferers have digestive problems to the degree that they or somebody close to them can actually hear their digestive processes, this may be particularly so at night in bed or when it is quiet.

The production of excess gas in the digestive system with bloating and a loosening of the waistband is one of the cardinal symptoms of candidiasis. Anybody who knows about brewing wine or beer will tell you that gas is a by-product of the fermentation process, much in the same way the digestive tract will also produce plenty of gas as a by-product of fermentation or dysbiosis.

A healthy digestive system is virtually silent, you feel nothing and you hear nothing. People who experience rumbling, bloating, flatus and a waistband or belt which needs loosening after a meal or the supper at night may be experiencing an underactive stomach and a poor digestive capacity, often due to low digestive enzyme production. Many people with a yeast infection will have some degree of digestive discomfort along with impaired enzyme production, and experience one or several of the symptoms I have just mentioned. While it is natural to have digestive sounds, excessive noises along with digestive bloating and gas to me spell an intestinal yeast infection, especially if this occurs after meals and in particular after sweet foods or drinks.

People who can tick positive to the sound test need to carefully assess the other tests, and it is a combination of the totality that will govern not only the presence but indeed the severity of your candida overgrowth. As your gut improves during the Candida Crusher Program, farting and excessive gas will diminish and you will hardly even notice this to be a problem as the bad bacterial and yeast levels reduce and are kept in control by the beneficial lactobacillus species. This is why you will need to take both an enzyme formula and a probiotic when you have lots of gas and bloating. The probiotic formula will increase the beneficial bacteria, and is a must.

I always recommend a top quality digestive enzyme formulation when you have a yeast infection; this supplement can help significantly with most forms of digestive discomfort as a result of a yeast infection, especially gas, bloating, and various digestive noises. Digestive enzymes are also a wise choice because they help reduce digestive discomfort caused by food allergies commonly associated with candida. I have developed my own formulation and only use the best enzymes in the business; you can read more about the Candida Crusher Digestive Enzyme formula in section 4 of chapter 7.

Frequency Of Sound Testing

The sound test is performed weekly, and the measurement recorded on your Candida Home Test Tracker which you will find near the end of this chapter.

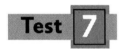

Low Carbohydrate – Biotin Test:

This test can be performed in conjunction with other tests I have recommended for achieving optimal results if you want to know if you have a yeast infection or not.

You can read all about blotin and candida in section 4 if chapter 7, later in this book.

Avoid carbohydrates and take 2.5 mg of biotin for 3 days and see if any of your yeast infection symptoms improve. If symptoms improve, especially if they improve significantly, then you are probably suffering from a candida overgrowth in your intestines. Take the biotin for this test in divided doses and with foods.

Frequency Of Biotin Testing

The low carb/biotin test is performed monthly, and the measurement recorded on your Candida Home Test Tracker which you will find near the end of this chapter.

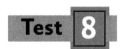

Test 8 - The CanDia-5 Home Blood Test

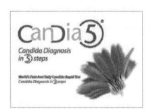

CanDia5® Is the world's first and only professional (blood-based) home test for candidiasis. This accurate test utilises just a small drop of whole blood taken from a finger stick to provide accurate diagnosis within 5 minutes. I like this test because it is accurate (90% specific for IgG), easy to do and you will have an answer within a few minutes.

This test is easy to use and will quickly yet accurately test for the detection of candidiasis. CanDia5 is the only known test which can accurately detect the presence of not only candida albicans, but for antibodies of the four common candida species C.albicans, C.glabrata, C.tropicalis and C.parapsilosis.

Why Blood Test For Candida?

With this simple test, you will be able to tell within 5 minutes if you have a candida yeast infection or not, it's that simple. You will be able to diagnose yeast infections accurately to help determine the most appropriate treatment, and after treatment you will be able to confirm effectiveness or continued need for treatment. I recommend that you re-test after 2 months. Comprehensive, easy to follow instructions are provided with this kit.

This test does not test for the yeast candida itself, but rather the antibodies created by your immune system after they have detected this little fungus and have prepared to mount a defence (antibody production) to counter it. Used by doctors, hospitals and natural health practitioners internationally, CanDia5 is the only candida diagnosis test of its kind. CanDia5 is now available to you as an affordable, non-invasive way to accurately diagnose candida infections without the need for a doctor's appointment or a full blood test. You will find a supplier online.

Frequency Of Candia 5 Testing

This finger prick blood test is performed every eight weeks (two months), and the measurement recorded on your Candida Home Test Tracker.

Candida Home Test Scoring

Here is a graph that you can use to score your weekly test results over a 12-week period. A score of Mild is 1, Moderate is 2 and Severe is rated as 3. Just write the appropriate number in the box below and follow your progress over a 12-week period. It is a good practice to assess these tests weekly and rate your progress at the end of each week over a 3-month period.

Some tests like the smell and itch test will be harder to monitor over a 3-month period, and my advice is for you to have somebody you know very well to monitor you if you can't do this yourself.

Other tests such as the spit and urinary indican test will prove a lot easier to self-monitor. In my experience, the tongue, urinary indican and sound test are all closely connected, as they are all indicative specifically of a digestive yeast overgrowth. The craving test is subtle, but with a bit of care and introspection it will not be too difficult for you to judge just how much you crave sweet foods.

Candida Test Tracker Scoring*

0 Not a problem, you don't experience any problems here.

1 Mild, something you may experience once or twice a week and is reasonably under control.

2 Moderate, it annoys you but is tolerable and you experience it several times a week or even daily.

3 Major, This is annoying you considerably and you want it gone. Chances are the reason you bought the Candida Crusher book was to learn how to get rid of these problems.

* You can also place ½ point scores for partially improved complaints, e.g. 2 ½

Candida Home Testing Frequency

Test 1 – The Itch Test	every week
Test 2 – The Spit Test	every week
Test 3 – The Craving Test	every week
Test 4 – The Smell Test	every week
Test 5 – The Tongue Test	every week
Test 6 – The Sound Test	every week
Test 7 – The Low Carb/Biotin Test	every month
Test 8 – The CanDia 5 Test	every two months

The Candida Test Tracker

TESTS	Wk 1	Wk 2	Wk 3	Wk 4	Wk 5	Wk 6	Wk 7	Wk 8	Wk 9	Wk 10	Wk 11	Wk 12
Itch Test												
Spit Test												
Craving Test												
Smell Test												
Tongue Test												
Sound Test												
Biotin Test												
CanDia-5 Test												
SCORE												

Candida Home Testing Tips

■ Avoid taking very high dosages or unnecessary nutritional supplements for 1 day before you complete the home tests, 24 hours will often be sufficient. You may otherwise get a false negative result, meaning that the results you obtain are false because they were affected by high doses of the dietary supplements. Low dosages are best the day before; you can always increase the next day.

■ The supplements most at risk of adversely affecting the results are; the probiotic (CanDia 5 test) and Candida Crusher Formula (the tongue, sound test & urinary indican), chromium or blood sugar supplements (the craving test).

■ Try to test on the same day each week, example each Sunday morning or evening.

■ Do one 12-week block then no more for testing eight weeks, then repeat another 12-week block. This will prove most beneficial in terms of tracking your progress and assist in helping you avoid any setbacks.

■ Antibiotics and the oral contraceptive pill will negate the whole testing procedure and if you have taken antibiotics or the Pill, wait for at least three weeks of probiotic treatment after you cease your round of antibiotics or Pill before you start this testing regime.

■ You don't need expensive medical laboratory stool tests, these eight tests I have used for many years and have found them all you need to determine your level of problem as well as your level of progress.

■ The CDSA x 3 is the gold standard, this is the best test but is also the most expensive, be especially sure to stop ALL supplements and drugs for up to a week before you do this test. Don't blow your money.

■ Don't forget to add the dates to the testing page!

■ You can partial score as well, for example you may have found a reduction from a grade 3 to a grade 2 score is too much, then give it a 2 ½ score.

The Candida Questionnaire and Candida Symptom Tracker ©

Besides completing the various functional medicine tests and home tests and utilizing the candida test tracker, there are other useful tools you can use to determine whether you have a yeast infection, the severity of it and track your recovery rate.

The Candida Crusher book comes complete with the candida symptom tracker, which can be of much assistance in evaluating the severity of your individual symptoms and their improvement as you work your way through the Candida Crusher Program.

The candida questionnaire, otherwise known as the candida survey, is best completed online at www.yeastinfection.org I'll now explain the relevance of both the questionnaire and tracker, and how and why you should use them.

The Candida Questionnaire

Dr. William Crook developed the original and still the best candida questionnaires in the early 1980's, and our candida questionnaires have been adapted from these. You will find an Adults Questionnaire, suitable for men and women, and there is also a Children's Questionnaire as well.

These questionnaires cover most of the signs and symptoms that are an indication of a yeast infection. Your answers to the questions will create an excellent picture of whether you have mild, moderate or a severe case of a yeast infection.

The candida questionnaire is for your benefit, the more accurate and objective you can be when you answer the questions, the more valuable will be the results. If you answer the questions honestly, the questionnaire will not only help you determine the degree of your yeast infection, but will give you most useful information and an insight into your present condition. Dr. Crook did not have the advantage in the mid 1980's of having any questionnaires online, today we do and it makes sense for you to go to www.yeastinfection.org to complete either the men's, women's or children's yeast infection questionnaire online.

The Candida Symptom Tracker

After treating many candida patients over the years, I found it pointless to ask them how they feel a week or two after treatment because I know what most are going to say. Not much better!

Chronic candida patients generally have been feeling bad for several months or even several years, and most will tell me at their initial follow-up visit "Eric, I don't feel much better, in fact I feel even worse".

People don't generally recover in a linear fashion from bad to good, there are lots of ups and downs along the way, and you will have read this before when I spoke of fantasy land (how wishful thinkers expect to recover) and of the reality check (how people actually recover in the real world). And, every candida patient I have seen has a different expectation of a recovery. You did read "How people think they get well, and how they actually get well", didn't you?

It is really handy to **always test and measure the effectiveness of your treatment**, just like it is when you plan anything in your life, whether it be an extension you are building on your house or an overseas holiday, start by writing it down and planning it, the preparation and timing are most important.

If you get things right and plan your course carefully, you will be able to track your rate of progress and make adjustments along the way to keep you right on target.
What is the point in recommending a treatment, and then having no system in place to measure the patient's response with? What are the mini and major milestones a patient is making along the path to recovery?

If you are going off track it will be more easy to get back on track if you have some method to help you guide the way. When you start to treat candida, you need to see what symptoms get better and which ones get worse. This will naturally allow you to understand which direction you are heading and will allow you to fine tune your treatment and get those positive results you are looking for faster.

I have found that some practitioners are just happy to adopt a "let's just treat the patient and see what happens" approach. This is fine, but you may or may not get the results you are looking for. But by initiating a treatment and then tracking the patient's responses over the course of several weeks, months or even years, you will really understand what is going on. And so will the patient, and their confidence will grow in their treatment program as they can actually see what is going on. This will increase compliance and keep somebody on track longer, rather than relying on a hit and miss approach. I have found the Candida Symptom Tracker to be an excellent motivational tool, and nothing is more important for patients to understand, experience and witness for themselves that their symptoms are actually improving.

If you want to measure you progress and fine-tune your prescriptions and optimize your treatment program, then you will want to adopt some sort of system whereby you can measure and track your progress, and also your lack of it. And that is where my Candida Symptom Tracker comes in handy.

List you major symptoms on the left-hand side of the sheet. Now, enter a score in column A, ranging from 0 – 3. This is how the grading works:

0   No problem, you don't experience any problems here.

1   Mild problem, something you may experience once or twice a week and is reasonably under control.

2   Moderate problem, it annoys you but is tolerable and you experience it several times a week or maybe even daily.

3   Major problem. This is really annoying you and you want it gone fast. Chances are the reason you bought the Candida Crusher book was to learn how to get rid of one or several grade 3 symptoms. This could be vaginal thrush, debilitating fatigue or it could be an itch or a terrible stomach pain and indigestion.

Just photocopy the Candida Symptom Tracker and use it accordingly, This sheet has the common symptoms down the left column, and down the bottom there is a space for your own particular symptoms. At the top of each column, you enter the date and at the bottom leave a row empty so that you can add the scores up for that particular day to see how you are going. Scores increasing mean no improvement, scores decreasing mean improvement, simple.

Some patients also like to keep a food diary and others like to correlate a particularly high (or low) score with an event like going to a wedding (where they consumed cake, alcohol, etc.) that caused an aggravation. Here you can add special short notes like "menstrual cycle started" or "started to take probiotics" or "got a cold", "my teen crashed my car", "argument with husband", etc.

These are the factors that influence the total scores and can give you a good indication of what influences the way you feel and how you have responded to treatment or lifestyle. If you find that your scores are increasing which correlate with stressful events in your life, then I'd like you to read section 5 in chapter 7 again, "Understanding the Healthy Lifestyle", in addition; you may want to address any underlying adrenal fatigue that may be relevant.

Keep the Candida Symptom Tracker on your refrigerator under a magnet so that it is always handy and learn to fill in the sheet for convenience sake at about the same time each week, fortnight or whenever you complete the test.

I cannot emphasize the importance of tracking your symptoms on the Candida Crusher Program; it is one of the most important aspects of your recovery. By tracking your treatment including any dietary and lifestyle changes you have made, you will be able to accurately judge the impact of your treatment on your individual symptoms by looking at the scoring as time goes by. If you are on track, you should notice that the grade 3 symptoms will eventually become 2, and then finally a grade 1 as the weeks roll by and turn to months.

This will tell you that as the candida yeast numbers decline, major symptoms are improving and will eventually turn to minor symptoms. Your self-confidence and compliance to the program will increase a lot which will help you improve even quicker.

On the other hand, the Candida Symptom Tracker is also a handy tool to let you know if things aren't working out the way you had hoped for. If your scores are not declining, then this could well be an alarm signal that either your health problems are not candida related, or you are not committing adequately to the program or the treatments and/or products you are using are inadequate. You have invested your time and money into wanting to conquer yeast, and this is one powerful way to track your results.

I would like to mention again, at the risk of repeating myself, that you should not be expecting a miracle cure within a few months of starting the program if your condition is quite severe or of a very long duration. Your scores may even go from 1 or 2 to a 3 with some symptoms as you could aggravate initially with treatment, especially if die-off occurs and maybe with a detoxification you undertake as well.

So remember, in an ideal world your symptoms are bad and getting better. In the real world however, your symptoms may initially go from bad to worse before they improve. I just thought I'd remind you again, there is nothing wrong with repeating myself; I just want you to understand this crucial point because at some stage you may become disappointed or disillusioned if your yeast infection is chronic.

This is one of the reasons I wrote the Candida Crusher, I wanted to be able to place this book in hands of a patient in my room, or a practitioner who specializes in treating patients with yeast infections or digestive problems, and for them to know that in many cases just as they are about to give up, if they just went that extra mile their patient could turn the corner.

I can remember on more than one occasion telling a candida patient to hang in there and that the light at the end of the tunnel does not necessarily signify the head lamp of an oncoming train, but rather a glimmer of light in the distance which signifies hope of an eventual full recovery. When you do recover, and eventually you will, you will have learned a few skills along the way, and one of them is not to give up that easily on yourself. This will hold you in good measure in the years ahead as you age and face and no doubt will then face plenty more health challenges to come.

Using The Questionnaire And Symptom Tracker Combined

Most patients who have been chronically unwell with a yeast infection are understandably impatient when it comes to the recovery process. It can appear that recovery is so slow that it is unlikely to ever happen, especially when you have been so strict with your diet, taking all the supplements and making lots of sacrifices along the way. Remember, everybody gets discouraged, and it is important to get plenty of moral support during your recovery. This is one of the reasons I developed the Candida Symptom Tracker, it was designed to measure the effectiveness of your treatment program over a sixteen week or four month period. If you follow the Candida Crusher Program carefully, you will notice that your Total Score will descrease as the weeks go by.

The candida questionnaire is different in that it does not track or measure how effective your treatment is, it was designed to determine if you have a yeast infection or not and how severe it is at the onset of treatment, remember to complete it online, it is a lot easier and within a minute you will know your score as it automatically calculates your score.

By completing the two-weekly Candida Symptom Tracker over a four month period, you have started to track your symptoms and can see what is improving and what is not, then you can adjust your treatment accordingly. Monitoring your specific symptom scores over sixteen weeks allows you to really understand what is getting better and what isn't, this will allow you for example to see if your digestive system is improving, or your skin, etc. Your commitment to the Candida Crusher Program will grow and deepen as you start to notice a reduction in scores over time. I have used this tracker with my patients and they email me their results with each monthly follow-up visit. You will find the Candida Symptom Tracker as well as the online questionnaires on www.yeastinfection.org

By utilizing the candida questionnaire and the Candida Symptom Tracker together, along with the Candida Test Tracker and perhaps the CDSA x 3 test if you have a chronic problem, you will have developed a very accurate picture of your yeast infection at the beginning of treatment by having established a very good baseline and with both my Trackers will have plenty of useful information to measure your progress by (or lack of) and make any adjustments accordingly.

The Candida Symptom Tracker ©

For each symptom, please enter the appropriate score in the point score column. *Don't forget the dates*

- **Mild** or an occasional symptom - 1 point
- **Moderate** or frequently severe - 2 points
- **Severe** or disabling symptom - 3 points

Please write the date and complete one column each fortnight. Don't forget to add the score and write the total at the bottom. This will give allow you to most effectively track your progress of the Candida Crusher Program over a 4 month period.

Candida Complaints	Date →								
Fatigue and lethargy or drowsiness	Score →								
Feeling of being drained									
Poor memory, feeling "unreal"									
Feeling of head swelling or tingling									
Poor coordination, can't concentrate									
Depression or anxiety									
Numbness burning or tingling anywhere									
Muscle weakness or paralysis									
Pain and/or swelling in joints									
Abdominal pain or indigestion									
Constipation or diarrhoea									
Coated tongue or bad breath									
Abdominal bloating and gas									
Vaginal discharge, itching or burning									
Prostatitis									
Loss of sexual drive or impotence									
Endometriosis diagnosis									
Menstrual cramps, pre-menstrual issues									
Recurring Itching anywhere									
Skin rashes									
Nasal congestion or discharge									
Postnasal drip, nasal itching									
Cough, pain or tightness in chest									
Wheezing or shortness of breath									
Urgency or urinary frequency									
Burning on urination									
Poor vision, burning or tearing eyes									
Recurrent ear infections, pain or deafness									
Toenail fungus, discoloured nails									
Other Symptoms You May Have →									
Total Symptom Score →									

The Three Groups Of Patients

> *The three great essentials to achieve anything worthwhile are, first, hard work; second, persistence; third, plain common sense.*
> *Thomas A. Edison*

I've discovered that there are three types of patients when it comes to recovering from a yeast infection.

1   Group one experience the shortest recovery time. The first group is happy to work with my recommendations and know that it is important to follow the different stages of the program; they track their scores, do the home tests and come back regularly for follow-up visits. They always take their supplements diligently, ordering more before they run out. Group one has the quickest recovery rate; they also appear to be the quickest learners, adopting their new diet and lifestyle habits and end up with a permanent resolution of their yeast infection. This group is where I get my best results and plenty of referrals from too!

2   Group two will take more of a hit and miss approach and jump ahead with the program and skip a few steps here and there. They may be enthusiastic at the start but soon stop tracking their symptoms because they either get "too busy" or are easily distracted. They break the diet due to buzziness of their life or haven't really committed. They don't do the tests nor turn up regularly for follow up visits, and may come twice or three times at the most then just appear to drop off. They take the supplements here and there when they remember and contact my office manager very infrequently, usually when they aggravate. This group has still plenty to learn about cause and effect and I find that after a prolonged period of feeling quite unwell they may re-commit and become group one, or go the medical route and become one of the "walking wounded" and drop out altogether.

3   The third category will see me once only never to return for that all-important follow-up visit. They probably only came to see me to see if I could help them get rid of a category 3 symptom, and had no desire to follow any diet or take any supplement, let alone track their symptoms of complete some tests to determine whether they have candida or not. Many of these patients unfortunately appear to be stuck in the middle of a river called the Nile, (denial) if you know what I mean. This group never really recovers, and I have seen quite a few of these patients over the years.

Are You Receiving Professional Care?

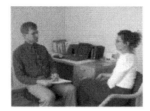

During my travels throughout Australia, New Zealand and America, I have had the pleasure of meeting with many practitioners who are true health-care professionals of many different healing modalities. They are professionally trained to very high levels, maintain professional registration, undertake regular professional continuing education and maintain excellent practices.

You may not meet or know the same people I do, so in that case here are ten simple tips to guide you in what to look for when choosing a natural medicine health-care professional. If any of these raise questions then you should discuss this openly with your natural health-care professional.

1 Spends Enough Time With You

A typical initial consultation with a natural health care practitioner is anywhere from 45 minutes up to 1 ½ hours. You should have enough time to describe all your complaints, as well as being able to ask all the questions you have. Your practitioner will be relaxed and make you feel at ease, not keeping a constant eye on the clock. Does he or she make or take personal calls, or appear to be very preoccupied with a computer screen or other business?

2 Takes A Complete Medical History

On your first visit, your practitioner should ask extensive questions on your medical history and take your case thoroughly. Your practitioner should be competent enough to at least have a greater knowledge of your disease and their treatments than you yourself, the person actually presenting with the complaints. Does she enquire into what medications you are taking; ask for blood-test results and perhaps even check out any specialist reports you may bring with you? This shows a high regard for your current medical care, and will certainly put you more at ease right from the beginning.

3 Is Professionally Qualified And Registered

Does your health care practitioner have any professional registrations? These should be displayed, along with the appropriate certificates, diplomas or degrees of qualification. Feel free to enquire where he or she qualified from, if they are professionally registered and how long they have been in practice for. You have a right, after all, you are entrusting them with your most precious asset: your health.

4 Performs A Basic Screen Each Visit

Basic health checks such as blood pressure and weight are important. It is surprising to me that some patients have never even had their blood pressure checked by their natural health practitioner. Avoid practitioners who fail to write things down or who don't take any notes each and every time they see you. They should be able to present your file in a few seconds and be familiar with what they recommended previously. Does she keep neat files; is the room neat and tidy? What is their appearance like? Your sixth sense will tell you if something doesn't quite add up here.

Help Explains What Is Wrong, Takes The Time To Answer Your Concerns.

5

Your practitioner should be willing to discuss all aspects of your illness, helping you to understand what is going on, what the diagnosis means if one has been made and help to allay any fears or anxieties you may have. Be aware of instant or snap diagnoses, claims of a cure, or practitioners who ridicule other practitioners or other treatments in the health care field.

Can See You In Emergency Situations

6

A good and caring practitioner will keep some time free for patients who need attention with urgent health problems. Can you call him or her two days later with a concern regarding the treatment, and have a quick word about a strong effect from something prescribed? Are you not even giving two minutes on the phone to allay your concerns, and told rather to make yet another appointment? Do you find that he or she won't return your call, not even after a few weeks? It may be time to look elsewhere for your healthcare.

Keep Track Of All The Medications You Take

7

Your practitioner should review all medicines you are taking, including any prescribed or over the counter drugs like acetaminophen, NSAIDS, blood pressure medications, pharmaceutical, herbal as well as nutritional medicines. Any conscientious practitioner will understand drug-nutrient or herb interactions and will always be on the lookout for potentially harmful interactions and ask you if you are experiencing any side effects. Does your practitioner do this? This is a very important aspect of any natural medicine practice. I find regularly in my practice that patients on several drugs approach me with strong symptoms, of which many are the side effects from their prescribed drugs. What a waste of time and their hard earned money when they try to counteract these drug-induced complaints with vitamins and mineral supplements.

It is prudent to remember that the fourth leading cause of death in America is from the conventional Western medical health care system and particularly from pharmaceutical drugs. (Journal of American Medical Association July 2000) Do we have any reason to believe that these statistics are any different in other developed countries?

8   Makes Fees Available, And Is Willing To Discuss All Of The Charges

You should be able to obtain a list of all the charges for various procedures, appointments and tests. If there is any reluctance or confusion when you enquire about fees, this is a warning sign that your practitioner may not be right for you.

9   Arranges Follow Up Visits Periodically

Not every health problem is solved the moment you leave your practitioner's office. A caring practitioner should like to see you periodically so that he or she can monitor your progress. Follow-up appointments are important and should be scheduled regularly until you show good improvement in your health. If you have not shown any progress in your condition after several treatments, you should be able to discuss this freely and decide with your practitioner if their treatments are really right for you. You are not obliged to book ahead for several treatments and expect to pay fees upfront for treatments you have not had.

10   Is Always Willing To Work In With Your Medical Doctor

Professional natural health therapists embrace medical science, rather than ridicule it. By willing to work in with or alongside your medical doctor, your natural medicine practitioner is showing you that he or she is a true health care professional. Many professional natural therapists today have Bachelor of Health Science degrees and even Masters degrees and higher. This is quite different from the days when diplomas were sufficient. However, you may find that your doctor could show reserve or perhaps even mock your treatments with your natural medicine health care practitioner, and it is important to remember that "condemnation without investigation is the highest form of arrogance". Don't let your doctor put you off; you decide what healthcare is right for you. You may need to find a doctor who is willing to accept your stand to embrace the healing powers of nature. The choice is ultimately yours.

CHAPTER 4 THE QUICK START Candida Crusher Guide

Crushing Women's Yeast Infections

Many female patients we see want to cure their yeast infection once and for all. They have most probably been to their medical doctor before seeking relief, and it is usually instant relief they are looking for. They want it fixed and they want that annoying problem fixed now.

Some have visited their doctor just once, some twice, and yet others have gone to their health care practitioner literally dozens of times repeatedly trying to find the magic cure for their yeast-related problems. I would question the motive as to why any health-care professional is happy to see a patient routinely over and again, often giving the same advice and not seeing much improvement, let alone a permanent cure. This chapter is about a QUICK improvement, but not about a permanent cure in most cases. If you are looking for a permanent answer you will need to adopt the Candida Crusher Program. By following my 3-step male or female fast relief plan outlined below, you will get quick relief and sometimes within a few hours. You can do this mini program over and again and each time you will most probably find even more relief.

The best and permanent results will come to those who adopt the lifestyle and diet procedures outlined in my book The Candida Crusher - The Permanent Yeast Solution.

Quickly Crush - Female Yeast Infections

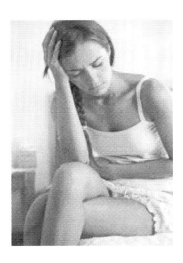

I have always found that the women most often wanting a quick solution for yeast related problem would be generally referring to a vaginal yeast infection.

If it is a *permanent* cure of your yeast infection you are after, then it is important to follow the Candida Crusher program outlined in my book in addition to following the plan I have outlined below. The female fast relief plan is a part of my Candida Crusher protocol, the same protocol I have recommended and fine tuned over the past twenty years in my clinic. I know it works particularly well for most all women who follow it, because that is the feedback I nearly always get.

Important Note: Women who are experiencing a mild case of vaginal thrush will find this chapter most useful. If you condition is severe, then it is important to get the right diagnosis rather than to keep on treating a condition that may later turn out to be bacterial vaginosis or even an STD. For these reasons, be sure to visit your doctor to get the right diagnosis.

If you have been diagnosed and are sure you have chronic vaginal thrush then you will get relief by reading chapter 5 of the Candida Crusher and adopt the measures I have outlined there, because this chapter was written just for you. It contains all the information you need and explains in detail all the different natural vaginal treatments for chronic thrush I have found to be effective over the years.

Women's yeast infections are easy to treat at home and you won't need to take any drugs or creams from the doctor either. I will outline the quick program below and give you all the instructions you need; this is one problem you can easily fix yourself.

Here are a few hints and tips:

- Expect great relief (*but not a cure!*) within 12 hours.

- Follow the 3-step permanent vaginal yeast solution as often as you like.

- Commit yourself to following the protocol regularly and as required for ninety days (3 months).

- Have everything in house to start the protocol.

- Avoid prescription suppositories, antibiotics, drugs, sprays, etc.

- Follow the protocol carefully; don't deviate from the outline too much.

- Follow my Candida Crusher Program simultaneously.

- Be careful with sexual relations, ensuring excellent hygiene at all times.

- For chronic ongoing vaginal yeast infection of long standing I recommend you do the two vaginal implant protocols in the Candida Crusher book, you will find them in chapter 5.

- Tell yourself that you you will come right, it is just a matter of time.

- Positive self-talk will get you through when you feel down and out.

If you have a menstrual cycle, it is important to commit to the program even *during your menstrual period*. Candida yeast infections can multiply rapidly during your flow days and particularly just coming into the cycle and just when it finishes. Many books I have read say to stop any treatments during your period, and that you may "cause harm" if you treat during your period. This is simply not true, and some women will wish to continually treat, even during their flow days, whereas others will wait until their period is finished, ultimately it is up to you but there is no reason why you can't continue treatment.

3-Stage FAST Relief Plan for Vaginal Yeast Infections

Here is a quick solution that will give you almost instant relief from your vaginal yeast infection, sometimes in a matter of hours. Follow each of the three steps in succession for the best results. You can repeat this series of treatments as often as you like. The quick vaginal solution is in three parts. There is a reason why there are three stages that I will explain. Sure you can just do a douche like many books recommend, but from experience in treating many women with this annoying problem; I have found my 3-step protocol to work the best. Skip stage 1 if you feel uncomfortable about it or just can't access the Manuka honey, but I do urge you to try it at least once. You will be pleasantly surprised at just how amazingly effective this 3-stage protocol is.

Why a 3-Stage Approach?

Because it works very well and gives immediate relief. The three stages are best used in succession, try not to skip a stage and you can increase or decrease the duration of each stage depending on how much time you have, the severity of the condition and your experience level of using this effective protocol.

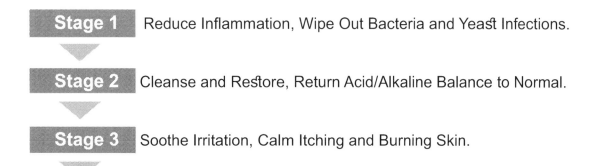

Stage 1   Reduce Inflammation, Wipe Out Bacteria and Yeast Infections.

Stage 2   Cleanse and Restore, Return Acid/Alkaline Balance to Normal.

Stage 3   Soothe Irritation, Calm Itching and Burning Skin.

STAGE 1

Anti-Fungal & Anti-Bacterial Douche
Reduce Inflammation, Wipe Out Bacteria and Yeast Infections.
(Time - leave for 30 minutes)

Main Benefit: The Manuka honey and fresh garlic treatment can give significant relief from the itching and burning of vaginal yeast infections. Manuka honey is native only to New Zealand, but is available in America and Canada, as well as many other countries and is the *only* true medicinal honey. This amazing honey reduces inflammation, wipes out bacteria and with the addition of garlic even yeast infections. Manuka honey heals cuts, burns and is now even being used in hospitals in various parts of the world.

What You Need: One to two tablespoons of New Zealand manuka honey, preferably with a high UMF rating. (Read below about UMF). For best results, add one or two finely chopped cloves of fresh garlic to the honey.

The Method: Warm the honey gently in a cup, jar or bowl suspended in hot water; this takes only a few minutes. For quick relief, I recommend that you try manuka honey and insert it vaginally, after warming it a little. After gently warming it, insert the manuka honey and garlic and let it sit on the skin in and around the vagina and pubic area for as long as possible. Lie down and relax for 20 minutes or if this is not possible, wear a sanitary napkin. After 30 minutes or longer (longer is better) have a warm douche with apple cider vinegar – (*see Stage 2*)

Why **Manuka Honey?**

Manuka honey comes from the white flower of the New Zealand tea tree oil tree named Manuka (*Leptospermum scoparlum.* Manuka honey has been shown clinically to be strongly anti-inflammatory in addition to being anti-bacterial and anti-fungal by nature.

Some scientists and leading medical experts have rated manuka honey as one of the best skin healers because it heals without harming even the most delicate skin of your body, including your vagina. Many studies have shown that manuka honey not only kills bacteria but that it is great for yeast infections and any inflamed skin in general. What about the sugar, won't it feed the candida yeast infection? No, it won't, it will only do this if you eat the honey and let it pass through the digestive tract.

Where do you get Manuka honey from? You can buy it readily online at Amazon or in the whole foods section of your health food store.

What type of manuka honey should you get? You should get the one with the highest UMF® rating (Unique Manuka Factor) you can afford, which is essentially this unique honey's non-peroxide antibacterial/anti-fungal activity level, the higher the UMF level, the more antibacterial and anti-inflammatory the honey is. A manuka honey with a 15 – 16 UMF rating is very good, but one with a 30+ rating is superb. The higher the UMF number the better and the higher grades are priced accordingly and may be harder to get.

STAGE 2

The Cleansing Douche

Cleanse and Restore, Return Acid/Alkaline Balance to Normal.
(Time –10 minutes)

Main Benefit: The cleansing douche has a pH balancing, cleansing and tonifying action on the vagina. Use a vaginal applicator or a baster and carefully irrigate most areas, without adding too much pressure as you squeeze the contents of the applicator or baster. This douche that finishes off the treatment cleanses and restores, it returns the acid/alkaline balance back to normal.

What You Need: A vaginal applicator or baster, 2 to 3 tablespoons of a quality apple cider vinegar, one teaspoon of colloidal silver and a small bowl.

The Method: In a small bowl of water, mix in 2 to 3 tablespoons of ACV and one teaspoon of colloidal silver. Either insert this mixture into the vagina with an applicator, baster, or by way of a douche, and/or splash/thoroughly rinse the region of the vulva liberally with this wash. Gently dry the area with a soft cotton hand towel then use a hairdryer to ensure a more complete dryness afterwards. Use fresh cotton underwear changed regularly throughout the day; and sleep preferably with no undergarments. When you are finished, place the cloth in a bucket or container with water containing a bleach and water solution to sterilize.

STAGE 3

The Soothing Yogurt Douche

Soothe Irritation, Calm Itching and Burning Skin.
(Time -leave 2 to 3 hours)

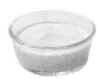

Main Benefit: The soothing yogurt douche can offer significant relief from any heat or burning sensations of vaginal yeast infections. Yogurt soothes irritation and calms any itching and burning skin in and around the vagina. This great treatment will round off the different stages as it calms and settles any irritated skin.

What You Need: A small carton of plain, unheated low-fat yogurt free of additives, colors, fruits or sugars. A syringe, spatula and small bowl.

The Method: use either a spatula to spread a layer of soothing cool yogurt over affected areas of skin, or use a syringe to inject the vagina with yogurt. Another common method is to roll a tampon in yogurt and insert. Have a good rinse and wash after you have left the yogurt in place after a few hours.

The Soothing Yogurt Douche

Many women will have heard about a yogurt douche, and quite a few will have tried this method. There are several different ways you can do this and I will explain the different methods and techniques. Women have used yogurt in Third World countries for many years and for many this is the only way they can get relief from their vaginal yeast infection.

Yoghurt is rich in lactic acid, because the process of growth from milk into yoghurt involves the conversion of lactose into lactic acid. The lactic acid helps digest lactose. In other words, yoghurt provides the enzyme required to digest milk and various dairy products high in lactose. Candida yeast infections cannot thrive in a lactic acid rich environment, and because yogurt is so rich in lactic acid, it makes sense to eat yogurt and use it regularly as a douche. You may want to use this method when on holidays or if you travel, because you need minimal equipment and it is very simple to do.

Make sure you buy top quality organic natural yoghurt, and leave some out until it gets to room temperature, because you will not want to place refrigerated temperature yogurt inside your vagina.

Making Your Own Yogurt

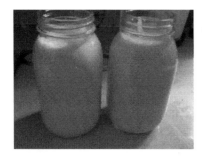 I have included my yogurt recipe in this book just in case you want to make a regular supply for yourself, this is the recipe I have recommended for many years and if followed carefully you can create a very high quality naturally soured yogurt at home, teeming with billions of beneficial lactobacillus acidophilus bacteria. There is no need to spend lots of money at the health food shop or supermarket on those expensive containers of yogurt – make your own yogurt right at home.

Don't let anyone tell you that "brand X" is the best brand and has more beneficial bacteria than "brand Y". The best yogurt is the one you make at home because it is fresh, and if you follow my recipe you will have the best yogurt that tastes better than any yogurt you can buy. For douching, you may want to omit the whole milk powder from my recipe, that way the yogurt will be less thick and creamy and easier to insert and rinse after treatment.

Douching

The first thing you will want to get is an irrigating syringe or vaginal applicator. Your local pharmacy or chemist should be able to supply you.

Vaginal Applicator

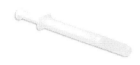

You may find the applicator from the chemist more user friendly, as they tend to have a rounded smooth end, but I have seen some kitchen-type basters which are perfectly acceptable, so find a gadget for this job that suits your own needs.

Turkey Baster

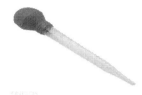

I know several women who have successfully used a turkey baster, one those plastic syringes some people use to baste poultry with gravy at Christmas. You can buy one at a good kitchen shop, and there are many different types available.

Using a Vaginal Applicator

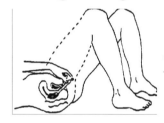

Using an applicator is not that difficult, do observe hygiene and ensure the applicator is inserted as far as possible without applying too much force.

1. Wash your hands.

2. Draw sufficient yogurt (or douche mixture) into the applicator.

3. Lie on your back, draw your knees up a little and spread them apart.

4. Gently insert the applicator with the tablet in front into the vagina as far as possible, do NOT use force.

5. Depress the plunger so that the yogurt (or douche mixture) is released.

6. Withdraw the applicator.

7. Clean both parts of the applicator thoroughly with soap and boiled, lukewarm water (if not disposable).

8. Wash your hands.

Yogurt Douche Method

You will require up to two tablespoons of room temperature yogurt and an applicator. The technique is very simple; you just pull out the plunger (or squeeze the bulb if you use a baster) and fill with sufficient yoghurt, then gently insert the tip into the vagina and squeeze the contents gently inside. Get yourself in a comfortable position you normally would if you were going to do a douche.

Do not rinse the vagina afterwards, just rinse the outside gently and pat dry. You will want to wear a maxi pad generally to minimize any possible leakage, and most women will do this before bed and leave in overnight.

In the morning you will want to have a good wash in the shower or bath naturally and preferably wear a mini pad that day to prevent any residual leakage.

The three basic treatment options for the yogurt douche are:

- Use pure natural organic low fat plain yoghurt.
- Use a mixture of purified water and yogurt to thin the mix.
- Use the whey liquid – most powerful way
  (the liquid on top of the yogurt)

Tampon Treatments

Some women will use a tampon they have rolled in yogurt, but after recommending this form of treatment for some time, I don't find the yogurt tampon as effective as the tea tree oil tampon, which is what I now recommend. To make a tea tree oil tampon work the most effectively, use the pure oil or use the water-soluble form of tea tree and make a strong solution of five parts of water and one part of water-soluble tea tree oil, soak the tampon and leave overnight.

The strongest tampon treatment is when you use grapefruit seed extract (GSE). Try this for very stubborn vaginal thrush: Soak a tampon in 1 tablespoon vegetable oil like organic sunflower oil and add from 5 – 10 drops of GSE, make sure you mix the vegetable oil and GSE very well. Insert the tampon and leave overnight. Repeat for 3-4 nights. This is one of the most effective local vaginal thrush treatments you can do, try it, you will be surprised. I've seen it shift even impossible cases. Start with the water-soluble tea tree oil tampon treatment first for 3-4 days; if it fails then try the GSE or alternate treatments.

Vaginal Pessary Recipe:

A tea tree oil tampon will clear up many vaginal fungal problems, sometimes even within a day or two.

To make a vaginal pessary you will need:

- 1 tampon
- Several drops of tea tree oil.

Remove tampon from its wrapper and pour a few drops of tea tree oil across the top and sides. Insert the tampon, as you would do during your periods. As when you have your period, change the tampon after a few hours.

Some women may be sensitive to pure tea tree oil, although I have not found this to be the case in 90% of women. Try a drop on the inside of your wrist first. If you don't want to use the pure oil, soak a tampon in a tablespoon of warm water to which you have added ¼ teaspoon of the water-soluble tea tree oil, and you can use a one part water-soluble tea tree oil to five parts of water if you wish.

Various Vaginal Douche Protocols
Apple Cider Vinegar (ACV)

Use an apple cider vinegar (ACV), which is unfiltered and not pasteurized and made from whole organically grown apples, is the best type to use for vaginal douching and will give you superior results. Apple cider vinegar can be found in most local health food stores and you will even find a good apple cider vinegar in some general grocery stores.

Avoid white vinegar from the supermarket, and avoid commercial apple cider vinegars that have been pasteurized, filtered, refined, sterilized or distilled in order to make the product look good and more appealing to the general public. Unfortunately this extra processing destroys much of the lactic acid content, most of the benefits that were in the product in the first place. A quality ACV will look cloudy. In the USA and Canada I recommend that you purchase a certified organic apple cider vinegar made by Bragg, I can highly recommend this brand. We have an ACV in New Zealand called Coral Tree, the product is certified biodynamic and like Bragg's, one of the best to use. Please avoid the white vinegar; this simply won't give you the same results that a naturally fermented ACV will.

Once opened, a good quality apple cider vinegar does not need to be refrigerated and has a minimum shelf life of 5 years. It is best to store it with the cap tightly closed and not in direct sunlight. Would you believe it, I have some Coral Tree vinegar which is more than twelve years old, and it is still highly useable ACV!

The Colloidal Silver Douche

Colloidal silver is a mixture of microscopically small pure silver particles suspended in water. When applied topically to the vaginal area, colloidal silver when diluted in water can provide immediate relief as it has a marked anti-fungal action. The usual dosage is to mix ½ - 1 teaspoon of colloidal silver with a glass of tepid pure water (250ml) and use the mixture to douche the vaginal area. Colloidal silver works well when used in this way, or when added to apple cider vinegar as a wash.

A stronger concentration can be used after several hours if you feel no change or improvement. Silver is a powerfully effective anti-microbial that is able to destroy bacterium and various fungi, and I have seen this treatment work when others failed, especially when the colloidal treatment was rotated with the water-soluble tea tree oil douche.

Calendula Douche Or Cream

Here is a great douche, which is particularly effective around childbirth, or any time the vagina has been affected by any kind of trauma. This douche is very effective for any ongoing issues after an episiotomy or any vaginal tears. Calendula herbal tincture, and be sure to get the low-alcohol extract version, is one of the most anti-fungal of liquid medicinal herbs and is well known for its ability to heal skin rapidly. Use one dessertspoon of calendula tincture per 250ml tepid water and use this mixture to douche the vaginal area. Use a suitable applicator to irrigate the vagina deeply if possible. Just speak with your naturopath or herbalist who will be able to supply you with liquid calendula of a low-alcohol content.

Don't want to use liquid herbal medicines or find it all too much? Another option is to use calendula cream or Kolorex (Horopito) cream. Kolorex cream or capsules is a New Zealand product that is available in USA. Here is yet another effective solution for you;

you may want to consider a feminine cream based on tea tree oil, Horopito or calendula.

What About Intercourse If I Have Vaginal Thrush?

It is probably best that you avoid sex for some time if you have severe vaginal thrush, or at least during the bad flare or acute stages, because you will only irritate the skin and prolong the healing.

Be most diligent about hygiene and re-infection. You may like to try coconut oil as a lubricant if you want to have sex but don't want the pain; it works well for many people. Coconut oil is an antifungal as well as a good lubricant. Even better than coconut oil is jojoba oil, a kind of a liquid wax almost, it is probably the best sex lubricant you can get and is anti-fungal too.

If you want to have intercourse when you have vaginal thrush, then I would recommend you do a yogurt douche immediately after. In addition, if your partner is not careful, you may pass the infection to your partner and then back to yourself. Later in this book you will read a case history about a 27-year-old male who contracted a yeast infection from his girlfriend who had a severe case of vaginal yeast infection. This man developed a chronic case of prostatitis that eventually cleared up after several months of treatment.

Especially avoid sex in the week leading up to your period if you have chronic candida, this is the time when most women who have a yeast infection have discovered that their yeast infection is at its most severe. I can highly recommend you study chapter 5, a chapter devoted entirely to chronic women's yeast infections.

Tea Tree Oil Douche To Remove Any Traces Of Spermicides

Some women have found that the spermicidal covering a condom contains preservatives that may cause irritation to the vagina. You may notice that you can be especially sensitive to condoms when you have a vaginal yeast infection or thrush.

If you do suffer from any vaginal irritation after using condoms, you can either switch to using the non-spermicidal variety of condoms, or you can douche to help remove the traces of spermicidal and help your vagina return to normal. Using a tea tree oil tampon each night for about two to three nights until the vagina has healed works surprisingly well.

The Importance Of Following The Candida Crusher Program

It is very important for you to remember that not only are you trying to kill the candida in the vaginal and vulva areas, you are trying to eradicate an overgrowth of a candida yeast infection in your digestive system (mouth, stomach, small and large intestine, rectum) as well as other parts of your body where a yeast overgrowth may be lurking, whether it be your ears, groin, feet or toes and anywhere on the surface of your skin in general. Bearing this in mind, the following points will make sense to you:

- Forget thinking that a vaginal infection is purely a local problem. Wrong thinking.

- Start thinking that everything you eat and drink can and will influence the health of your female reproductive system.

- Never forget that a healthy and balanced lifestyle, reducing the stresses and following a regular program of relaxation can make all the difference.

- Use an anti-fungal soap and shampoo regularly such as a tea-tree oil containing product.

- Write down and memorize this quote: "The definition of insanity is doing the same old thing over and over and expecting a different result."

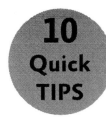

10 Quick **TIPS** for Female Yeast Infections

To reduce your chances of developing and maintaining vaginal thrush, I highly recommend that you follow these ten rules. You will notice that quite a few of the lifestyle recommendations (like avoiding tight clothing, certain sports, spa baths, etc) are based on the fact that vaginal thrush thrives in an environment which is warm, dark and moist and is fed on sugars and yeast foods in the person's diet. Knowing this, think about increasing the air flow around the vagina and perineum, wear cotton and loose fitting garments and take away the food supply that thrush likes to feed on - the sugar and yeast foods.

1 Avoid wearing tight clothing -
like jeans, nylon panties or nylon underclothing.

2 Avoid hot baths and jacuzzis -
(whirlpool baths and spas), especially if you have existing vaginal thrush.

3 After swimming, shower and then change into a cotton underclothing
and wear a cool dress or skirt (avoid nylon underclothing, always wear cotton).

4 Avoid alcohol -
especially if you are prone to thrush, even more if you have it. Other good advice is to be aware of the treats you like the most, is it alcohol, bread, or confectionery like chocolate or candy? Many women with recurring vaginal thrush enjoy a sweet treat that will have to go if the yeast infection has to go.

5 Follow the Candida Crusher Program -
adopt the correct diet and especially avoid sugars and yeasty foods in your diet (like chocolate, cookies, breads, candy, etc)

6 Have you been on an antibiotic, even a long time ago? –
If you absolutely must take an antibiotic then do follow-up with a probiotics for a long time. The rule in my clinic is that for each week you take an antibiotic, you take a probiotics for a minimum of six to eight weeks. Why this long? If you spray a weed killer (antibiotic) on your lawn (digestive system) how long does it take for the grass (the friendly bacteria) to grow back? It can take 3 months, 6 months or even longer. You may need that probiotics for several months, especially if you have a history of taking antibiotics. Some of my patients take them for a year or two during and after treatment. One day, probiotics may become even more important than multivitamins.

7 Avoid the oral contraceptive pill - or any other prescribed drug that caused thrush or even coincided with an episode of your vaginal thrush. No point trying to cure your thrush if you don't remove the cause and that oral contraceptive pill may well be underpinning your thrush.

7 Avoid becoming overheated through sports - such as squash, tennis or even by way of having a sauna or sunbathing.

8 Be aware of your posture when you sit - sitting with your legs crossed or continually on the edge of a chair does not allow adequate ventilation. Sit back and allow your vagina to breathe.

9 Do the vaginal douche protocols - in particular the anti-microbial and probiotic protocols regularly. These work very well, especially if you follow the other rules.

10 Forget the quick-fix approach - you will risk having recurrent thrush like so many women do that I've seen in my clinic over the years. Do the diet AND lifestyle AND local treatment and keep on doing it until you get well and stay well for at least six months.

Case History # 12
Sharon, 43 years

Sharon contacted me almost two years ago seeking help with vaginal thrush which had been bothering her for over fifteen years. She had consulted several practitioners over the many years and received all types of advice. She had read one of my online articles and was desperate for a solution. One of the first things I ask patients like Sharon is this: "Are you willing to do whatever it takes to get well, or are you going to leave my room with the idea that you will just "give it a go". I knew that Sharon had what it takes to get the permanent solution she was seeking, you can see it in somebody's eyes that they have been through enough suffering. They know that there IS a solution, and by the time they visit me they are well and truly committed and are focused enough to stay on track. Sharon's vaginal thrush was chronic and unremitting, she had a terrible itch that was embarrassing and just wouldn't go away. Although the drug she was taking controlled the symptoms, it was just holding and she was at the stage of wanting to go onto something stronger or finally committing to getting rid of this thing – once and for all.

The problem was, the recommendations given to her by other health-care professionals would only work for a few weeks at most and then the yeast infection would come back with a vengeance. Sharon is a coronary care nurse who works at a large hospital; her husband is an experienced pilot who is frequently away overseas, flying big jets long haul between Asia and New Zealand. Sharon works several different shifts and frequently works long hours and at unusual times, leading to sleep and energy issues. This in turn has resulted in her often skipping at least one meal per day and relying instead on foods from vending machines at the hospital. My concern here was the amount of processed food, including sugar that Sharon was consuming.

By the time she came to my room looking for a permanent yeast solution, she had been taking Fluconazole (Diflucan) an unbelievable once per week for the past five years, which apparently was keeping the condition under control. My second concern was that when her husband was home, they would engage in intimate relations quite frequently in the short time he was home which was a major cause of discomfort and aggravation for her. My third concern was that her diet and lifestyle were at fault and were in dire need of an overhaul if a permanent change in her yeast infection was to be affected.

What Sharon and her doctor were blissfully unaware of was that she still had the primary complaint of vaginal thrush, but had in addition developed side effects from taking Diflucan for over a five year period each week. And these side effects included low-grade nausea; pale colored stools and an annoying red skin rash around the tops of her thighs and upper back. She was prescribed a hydrocortisone cream for the skin rash and took an occasional laxative for the bouts of constipation she was getting regularly. Incredibly, she had learned to live with the nausea, just accepting it as a part of her life and was entirely unaware that it was a Fluconazole side effect. What a miserable life this lady had been living for the past few years, and her case is not that unusual. The primary complaint present but suppressed with a drug or cream applied regularly, inducing several side effects.

So how did Sharon fare, what recommendations did I recommend? Our first consultation was for almost one and a half hours and we got a few things straight, particularly the point that something had to change if she wanted her vaginal yeast infection to eventually disappear forever. Remember that "definition of insanity" quote? Doing something over and over and expecting a different result, have you memorized it yet? Sharon was ready to commit to change; and we agreed that she would only take day shifts for the next six to nine months while she worked on her recovery. She also promised herself that alcohol and regular snacking of chocolate, potato chips and junk would stop entirely until her discharge and itch were gone completely, we agreed on that too. Sharon started to use the Vaginal Implant Protocol and stayed with the Candida Crusher program recommendations for over six months. (The comprehensive Vaginal Implant Protocol is in chapter 5 of this book)

Tough going at first

It was tough going the first month because I wanted her to go cold turkey on the Diflucan (Fluconazole), but the nausea soon stopped to her amazement and she became more committed than ever, especially once her skin and bowel cleared up after about six weeks into the treatment. I had monthly phone-call consultations with Sharon and noticed with many patients who are serious about getting well, is that their emotional health will get as strong as their physical health. Sharon was a delight to work with because she was ready to fully commit to change, and not only has she no more vaginal yeast infection, she has lost over forty pounds in weight and looks fantastic today!

I wouldn't trade my occupation for anything else, even after tens of thousands of patients and almost twenty-five years in the clinic, it is the enjoyment you get from helping somebody go literally from a physical wreck on the scrapheap to somebody who is happy, healthy and ready to begin a new life. Are you ready to commit to permanently curing your infection? When you are ready, it will be worth it because like Sharon, your results can be as good as what she has experienced. Getting rid of a chronic health problem will give you a whole new lease of life.

Quickly Crush - Male Yeast Infections

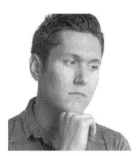

When men want rapid treatment for a yeast infection, they are generally referring to a yeast infection involving the penis, prostate or the skin around the inner thigh or scrotum. But it may also include a yeast infection of the toenail, digestive system or occasionally the mouth or throat, and these are covered later in this chapter.

Men and boys who experience a chronic yeast infection of the genital region most often experience digestive problems, toenail yeast infection or athlete's foot as other related symptoms.

Some practitioners may see yeast infections in both men and women primarily as sexually transmitted diseases, when in fact a yeast infection will have the tendency to much more commonly occupy the digestive tract and cause major issues there. Nevertheless, yeast infections do commonly affect males and females in their genital region and are amongst the most common reasons both why sexes seek help for their yeast infection.

It is unfortunate that yeast infections commonly seems to be thought of as primarily as a "women's" complaint. A male patient who came to our clinic for treatment some time ago for yeast infection treatment of the penis had consulted a medical doctor only to be told that "only women get yeast infections because they have a vagina".

Male yeast infections are in fact quite widespread and commonly misunderstood. There is an effective and rapid natural treatment option available for men who experience yeast infections, and this solution exists without having to resort to pharmaceutical drugs such as antibiotics that only produce unwanted side effects.

Causes Of Men's Yeast Infection

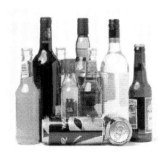

From personal experience in dealing with many men who have a yeast infection, the causes can range from alcohol, chronic ongoing stress, antibiotics or a diet high in the foods that yeasts thrive on like sweet foods.

Most guys with yeast infections tend to snack more indiscriminately and have diets high in refined carbohydrates (sugars, alcohols, breads); they may have larger portion sizes and are less fussy about the quality and quantity of what they eat. These factors can easily account for an overgrowth of candida in the digestive tract.

A male's yeast problem may have started because a partner who had an existing candida problem infected him. A lesser-known cause of penile skin yeast infections, especially in uncircumcised males, is poor hygiene after sex.

Medical Treatment Of Male Yeast Infections

Like women, men who go to their doctor with a yeast infection will often be prescribed Diflucan (Fluconazole) in either a tablet, capsule or in a cream form to apply to the affected areas. I've yet to meet a guy who was told by their doctor to stop alcohol or any sweet foods if he wants to recover fully from his yeast infection, with a drug being prescribed instead. Some men may even treat themselves with an over the counter preparation like Monistat which women commonly purchase from their drug store to treat their vaginal yeast infection. The problem with self-prescribing is that the results are usually only temporary, because in most instances the yeast infection comes back as the cause is not addressed.

Preventing Recurrences And Permanently Curing Your Male Yeast Infection

Always treat a yeast infection promptly and never let it get to a point that it becomes chronic recurring problem requiring continuous treatment. If you begin to rely on the Azole type of prescribed drugs or creams you may develop resistance to these drugs and you will then find it considerably more difficult to get rid of your yeast infection. The smartest thing you can do in preventing a yeast infection in the first place is by observing proper hygiene, diet and lifestyle practices.

Some believe that using a topical fungal preparation (treating the skin locally) is sufficient while others insist that for a faster and more complete treatment, a more systemic approach may be necessary for complete eradication of a yeast infection. I tend to agree with the latter, local treatment gives temporary result whilst local and systemic treatment gives a permanent result.

Yeast Infection Hygiene

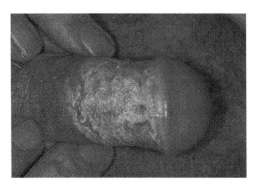

Are you an uncircumcised male? If you have a penis yeast infection you will generally find that if you roll back your foreskin that the infection is most likely to be present here, because this is the most common place for the yeast infection of the penis to be. Circumcised males do not usually get an infection here, because the glans penis in these men is exposed to the air and represents a considerably less favorable environment for the yeast infection to thrive. It is important to remember that a yeast infection requires a warm, moist and dark environment to thrive, and now you can understand why a woman's vagina is the perfect place for yeast to thrive. Hygiene is very important because a man can get a penis yeast infection from having sex with a partner that has a yeast infection; or from having oral sex from a person with genital thrush, and even from anal sex with an infected partner. It is very important to use a condom if you are unsure and to observe a high level of personal hygiene at all times to prevent the spread of a personal yeast infection.

Prostate Involvement

More rarely, a male may experience a yeast infection internally. This is much less likely to occur in a male due to the length of his urethra, in comparison to a female's urethra. Men who have an internal genital-urinary tract yeast infection may experience symptoms similar to that of a female who has a vaginal yeast infection which may include a burning or stinging pain on urination or a feeling of an intense itch inside the penis which can be most uncomfortable, irritating and persistent. On a rare occasion the prostate gland can even be affected by a yeast infection and there may even be a discharge from the penis.

Case History # 13
Paul, 27 years

Paul is a drummer in a leading New Zealand rock band. He came to see me a few years ago complaining about his nighttime urination issues. He was getting up at least three to four times most nights to urinate. His other complaints included night sweats and stabbing pains in the groin, down the inner thigh, insomnia, gas and bloating as well as depression.

With no previous history of bladder or urinary symptoms, I was rather intrigued and referred him to a urologist friend who found no abnormalities. I suspected prostatitis, an inflammation of his prostate. I also requested a complete blood count that was normal, in fact, all of Paul's results and tests were normal, yet he continued to complain of stabbing pains and night sweats. I started to question him about his relationships and discovered that the problems only started after he began a new relationship with a girlfriend about six months prior.

I suspected that Paul had an STD (sexually transmitted disease) but this was ruled out after extensive testing of urine, blood and a thorough physical examination by the urologist. This led me to conclude that he had an undetected a yeast infection, which was affecting his prostate gland, and this is where the stabbing pains down the inner thighs and groin were coming from. After a return visit, I convinced Paul to have his girlfriend visit a female doctor friend of mine, and it was discovered that she had a severe case of vaginal thrush. My suspicions were correct, Paul had contracted a yeast infection from his girlfriend and it had travelled up his urethra and infected his prostate gland. These infections are more common than you think, and if you are a male with unexplained pains in the groin and running down the inner thighs, along with bloating, gas or any other digestive complaints, then you may well have a yeast infection of the prostate as well. Does you girlfriend or wife have vaginal thrush? You may want to encourage her to get it sorted or it may affect your prostate gland.

Paul was placed on a strong candida killing formula in high doses for nearly six months, along with consuming three cloves of raw garlic each day. I had him take a powerful probiotic every three hours (up to eight to ten capsules daily) and we also used the Candida Crusher Diet principles. I was very tough on him in terms of his alcohol consumption, as he was a big beer drinker, but he really wanted to beat this thing and complied one hundred percent with my tough recommendations. It took over six months, but Paul did overcome his problems and now enjoys normal health once more.

Jock Itch

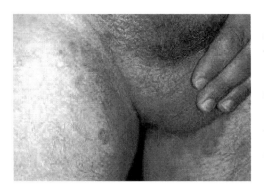

I have seen this on many occasions, and it can be a particularly persistent and embarrassing problem for many men. Yeast infections affecting the skin need to be treated internally as well as externally in order to eradicate them permanently and jock itch is no exception. Follow the 3-stage FAST relief plan for male yeast infections program outlined below simultaneously along with the Candida Crusher Program for more permanent results. The Candida Crusher Program is outlined in chapter 7.

Once the yeast has chronically infected the skin in and around the scrotum, upper inner thighs and around the perineum the skin may harden and crack at times causing extreme discomfort and pain. These chronic types of groin skin yeast infections can be notoriously difficult to completely eradicate. I have always found that it is much easier to get rid of a male's yeast infection in the early stages rather than in the later stages, after he has used many lotions and potions from the doctor for many years with only a temporary result. A chronic male yeast infection will require a significant level of dedication and commitment on the guy's part. I have seen some seemingly impossible cases fully resolve within six to nine months, and some of these patients had been plagued for twenty years or more.

Case Study # 14
Kevin, 47 years

Kevin is a laid-back guy who likes a bourbon and coke with his friends, enjoys football and going out hunting for pigs and deer whenever he can. He drives a big logging truck and is involved in felling huge trees as well. This guy is big; he weighs over 300 pounds and stands over six feet six inches tall. I really enjoyed our consultations, because Kevin had such a great sense of humor and was keen to get rid of the jock itch that he had for "as long as he could remember".

The itch was affecting his sex life because his wife was not very happy in getting close to him in case she got infected as well. His primary motivating factor was that he wanted his sex life back and was very keen to do whatever it takes. I always find that the best results come to those who have a strong PMF, or primary motivating factor behind wanting to clear up their health complaints.

Kevin was not changing his underclothing daily, and he was perspiring a lot in the cab of his truck. I discovered that a lot of his sweating was coming from a bad case of fermentation dysbiosis, and his take-out diet and the copious amounts of Coca Cola he was consuming daily weren't helping either. My instructions were for him to stop drinking all soda drinks and to just drink water in which he had dropped 5 drops of grapefruit seed extract per liter of water. We changed his diet and he was to eat a kebab or a salad and chicken for lunch instead of a McDonald's drive-through meal each day.

Kevin was also to take a candida killing formula (nine to twelve a day because he was a big boy) and a significant amount of probiotic capsules, a multivitamin and a digestive enzyme tablet with each meal. He was to buy two to three dozen pair of new cotton briefs and to change twice daily – after each shower. He also started to take a shower twice daily (instead of once every two days) and applied a tea tree oil cream to the affected areas twice daily, after his shower routine.

The hardest thing for Kevin was to give up his bourbon and coke drinks with his friends several times a week, but he was more interested in getting his relationship with his wife back on track and fully complied. Kevin's jock itch only took five months to clear, and the difference it has made has been truly amazing, he is a transformed man who has lost over fifty founds and has vowed to never go back to the lifestyle he once led. And his sex life is fantastic, because not only is his yeast infection cleared up, his body odor has vanished and his wife is more than happy to get close to him once more.

Herpes

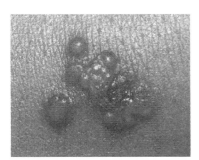

Some men and women have a genital skin rash that is in fact a Type 2 genital herpes infection (HSV-2) that may be confused with a yeast infection. Results of different studies show that genital herpes infections are relatively common.

For example, in the United States it has been estimated that about one out of every six people have genital HSV-2 infection. Genital herpes infection is more common in women (approximately one out of five women 14 to 49 years of age) than in men (about one out of nine men 14 to 49 years of age).

Herpes is a viral condition that you will not be able to eradicate but you will be able to reduce the likelihood of an outbreak significantly by following my advice on herpes in chapter 8. I have heard some very good reports from a practitioner who has recommended that patients use jojoba oil as soon as any lesions appear and to thoroughly rub jojoba oil into the lesions twice daily. He claims that the oil not only eradicates the acute manifestation of herpes infection, but that the oil it travels to the source of the infection and eradicates it permanently. You may like to try it and give me some feedback.

3-Stage FAST Relief Plan For Male Yeast Infections

Here is a quick solution that will give you almost instant relief from your male yeast infection in a matter of hours. Follow each of the three steps in succession for the best results. You will be pleasantly surprised at just how amazingly effective this 3-stage protocol is. Please read the 3-stage FAST relief plan for female yeast infections to get additional information.

Men's yeast infections are easy to treat at home and you won't need to take any drugs or creams from the doctor either. I will outline the quick program below and give you all the instructions; this is one problem you can fix yourself. Here are a few hints and tips:

- Expect great relief (*but not a cure*) within 12 hours.

- Follow 3-stage FAST relief plan for male yeast infections as often as you like.

- Commit yourself to following the protocol for ninety days (3 months).

- Have everything in house to start the protocol.

- Avoid prescription creams, antibiotics, and any drugs where possible.

- Follow my protocol carefully; don't deviate from the outline too much.

- Follow the Candida Crusher Program simultaneously.

- Be careful with sexual relations, ensuring excellent hygiene at all times.

- Tell yourself that you will come right; it is only a matter of time.

- Positive self-talk will get you through at times when you feel down.

Why a 3-Stage Approach?

Because it works very well and gives immediate relief. The three stages are best followed in succession, try not to skip any stage, and you can increase or decrease the duration of each stage depending on how much time you have, the severity of the condition and your experience level of using this effective protocol.

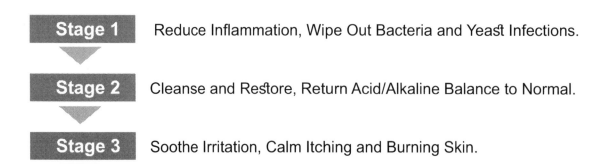

Stage 1	Reduce Inflammation, Wipe Out Bacteria and Yeast Infections.
Stage 2	Cleanse and Restore, Return Acid/Alkaline Balance to Normal.
Stage 3	Soothe Irritation, Calm Itching and Burning Skin.

STAGE 1

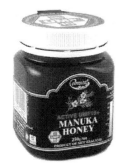

Anti-Bacterial & Anti-Fungal Treatment

Reduce Inflammation, Wipe Out Bacteria and Yeast Infections.

Manuka Honey is best

(Time - leave for 30 minutes)

Where do you get Manuka honey? You can buy it online at Amazon or in the whole foods section of your (good) health food store.

What type of manuka honey should you get? You should get the one with the highest UMF® rating (Unique Manuka Factor) you can afford, which is essentially this unique honey's non-peroxide antibacterial activity level, the higher the UMF level, the more antibacterial, antifungal and anti-inflammatory the honey is. A manuka honey with a 15 – 16 UMF rating is very good, but one with a 30+ rating is superb. The higher the UMF number the better and the higher grades are priced accordingly. It is not always possible to get a manuka honey with a rating higher than 18 – 20, and this level of UMF is generally plenty.

(Please be aware that about twice as much manuka honey is sold worldwide than is produced in New Zealand, and that a lot of manuka honey sold in the U.S. is likely to be counterfeit, either because the activity is lower than stated on the label or because it is not pure manuka honey. Therefore, it is important to purchase honeys produced by apiaries listed on the Unique Manuka Factor Association website and that carry the UMF certification).

Main Benefit: Manuka honey treatment can give significant relief from the itching and burning of male yeast infections involving the penis, scrotum, the perineum and the inner thigh.

What You Need: One to two tablespoons of New Zealand manuka honey, preferably with a high UMF rating, add one finely chopped clove of fresh garlic. Warm the honey gently in a cup, jar or bowl suspended in hot water, which takes about ten minutes. Mix in the honey and leave it for five minutes.

The Method: For quick relief, apply the manuka honey and garlic mix and apply it to the affected areas of skin. Apply it liberally to the affected skin and let it sit under the foreskin (if you are uncircumcised), in and around the scrotum and/or the upper inner thigh region.

Manuka honey has been shown clinically to be strongly anti-inflammatory in addition to being anti-bacterial and anti-fungal by nature. Some experts have rated manuka honey as one of the best skin healers as it heals without harming even the most delicate skin of your body, including your penis and scrotum. Many studies have shown that manuka honey not only kills bacteria but that it is great for yeast infections and any inflamed skin in general. You will find it most pleasant on the delicate areas of skin affected by yeast.

After 30 minutes or longer, wash the affected skin areas with an apple cider vinegar and water solution. *(See stage 2)*

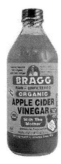

The Cleansing Wash Treatment

Cleanse and Restore, Return Acid/Alkaline Balance to Normal.
(Time –it takes 10 minutes)

Main Benefit: The cleansing wash has a pH balancing, cleansing and tonifying action on the penis, scrotum, perineum and upper inner thigh region. This wash finishes off the treatment and cleanses & restores, returning the acid/alkaline balance of the skin back to normal.

What You Need: A small clean cotton face cloth, 2 tablespoons of a quality apple cider vinegar. A small bowl of tepid to warm water (about 250ml or 1 cup), and one half teaspoon of water-soluble tea tree oil. The addition of the water-soluble tea tree oil is clever as it ensures an anti-fungal action to finish off the treatment.

The Method: Mix the ACV and water-soluble tea tree oil in the bowl of water. Soak the small face cloth or hand towel in the mixture and rinse the affected skin well. Be sure to rinse and wash the area under the foreskin and under the scrotum and upper inner thighs. Gently dry the area with a soft cotton hand towel then use a hairdryer to ensure a more complete dryness afterwards and sleep preferably without undergarments. Use fresh cotton underwear changed every day; avoid nylon underwear or nylon/cotton blends. When you are finished, place the cloth in a bucket or container with water containing a bleach and water solution to sterilize it.

STAGE 3

The Soothing Treatment

Soothes Irritation, Calms Itching and Burning Skin.

(Time -leave for 30 minutes)

Main Benefit: Yogurt can give significant relief to an inflamed penis, scrotum or inner thigh region, especially from any heat or burning sensations of men's yeast infections. Yogurt is cooling and helps soothe any irritation and calms itching and burning skin in and around the penis and scrotum.

What You Need: A small carton of plain, unheated low-fat yogurt free from additives, colors, fruits or sugars. A small bowl to place the yogurt in.

The Method: Spread a thin layer of soothing cool yogurt over affected areas of skin around the penis, scrotum and thighs. Men only need to leave the yogurt on the affected areas for 30 minutes, whereas women who apply yogurt internally are best to leave it there for a few hours.

Probiotics for men's yeast infections – If you have a burning or stinging pain you will find the cool yogurt treatment to be perfect because it calms and soothes inflamed skin rapidly. Some men may find yogurt too messy, you can introduce lactobacillus acidophilus powder directly to the skin under the foreskin and dust the skin-affected areas down with a good pro biotic powder. Leave the powder on the affected areas for a few hours and then try stage 3 – the cleansing wash. For optimal results, take a problotics capsule or powder twice daily before meals and use a little of the powder on the affected skin areas regularly.

Anti-Fungal Products For Men's Yeast Infections:

Gentian Violet - (Crystal Violet Solution 1% solution) is an old fashioned type of anti-fungal treatment yet most effective. This form of treatment was around before the discovery of the Azole class of drugs used by the medical profession. I have had very favorable reports that this treatment works very well indeed. Ask your pharmacist or chemist for Gentian Violet. Take care, this treatment can stain clothes a purple color.

Coconut Oil - Organic Coconut Oil is a medically proven anti-fungal agent that can also be used as an excellent and pleasurable personal lubricant for sex. By using coconut oil this way you will help prevent recurrences and yeast infections in yourself as well as your partner. Include coconut oil in your diet as well, and try to have one to two tablespoons per day which will enable you to gain coconut's anti-fungal benefit internally as well as externally.

Colloidal Silver – Colloidal silver has been found to kill male yeast infections quickly and efficiently and is completely safe. Buy a quality product and be aware of inferior brands made by amateurs at home and passed of as a quality product. Follow the manufacturer's instructions; your health food shop should be able to guide you when it comes to colloidal silver. You only need a small amount, about a half a teaspoon per 250ml of water.

Pure Tea Tree Oil or Water-Soluble Tea Tree Oil – Get the Australian Tea Tree Oil (Melaleuca alternifolia) if you can. You will find Tea Tree Oil so effective that it can sometimes clear up the entire yeast infection. Read a lot more about Tea Tree Oil in chapter 7, section 4.

Oregano Oil – This can be quite a powerful approach if used topically, and I only recommend that you use two to three drops (pierce a capsule) in a dessertspoon of flaxseed, coconut or olive oil. Rub on affected areas of the penis, scrotum and upper inner thighs. You will find in most all cases that tea tree oil will work wonders, but in really stubborn cases of a male's yeast infection you may want to try oregano oil. Never use oregano oil straight on sensitive skin, it may burn or sting the affected areas considerably. Read a lot more about Oregano Oil in chapter 7, section.

Apple Cider Vinegar (ACV) (Read more ACV in the Female section)

Never apply ACV neat to the skin of the penis or surrounding skin, you will find that it can sting or burn and may cause a strong burning sensation. Avoid the use of white vinegar, especially the commercial supermarket variety. Dilute AVC one part to ten parts of water and bathe the affected area twice daily.

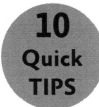

10 Quick TIPS For Male Yeast Infections

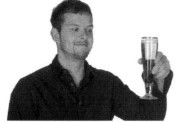

Prevention of a man's yeast infection is not unlike preventing a woman's yeast infection. To reduce your chances of developing and maintaining a yeast infection around the penis and scrotum, I highly recommend that you follow the following ten rules. You will notice that quite a few of the lifestyle recommendations (like avoiding tight clothing, certain sports, spa baths, etc) are based on the fact that a men's genital yeast infection can thrive in an environment which is warm, dark and moist and is fed on sugars and yeast foods in the diet. Knowing this, think about increasing the air flow around the penis and scrotum, wear cotton and loose fitting garments and remove the food supply that yeast likes to feed on: sugar and yeast laden foods.

Avoid wearing tight clothing - if you have a penis or scrotum yeast infection. Wear loose fitting clothing made from natural fibers like cotton.

Temporarily avoid hot baths and jacuzzis (whirlpool baths and spas), especially if you have existing yeast infection.

2 After swimming, shower and change **into cotton underclothing** and wear cool, loose fitting clothing. Always wear cotton.

3 Avoid alcohol - especially if you are prone to a men's yeast infection, you will need to keep right away from alcohol if you have it. This may well be your single and biggest obstacle, and a maintaining cause I have verified with countless men.

Follow the Candida Crusher Program adopt the correct diet and especially avoid sugars and yeasty foods like chocolate, cookies, breads, candy, etc. My book Candida Crusher contains a large amount of lifestyle and diet information.

4 Avoid antibiotics for any type of illness – Antibiotics are one of the biggest causes of yeast infections; avoid them as much as possible. And if you absolutely must take them, be sure you take a course of a probiotics to follow-up with.

5 Trim pubic hair - Keep the pubic hair very short and trimmed around the genital region because if your hair is too long it may increase body heat in that area and ensure that the moisture is kept close to the skin. Long and bushy pubic hair may ensure that you maintain an ideal breeding ground for a yeast infection.

5 Avoid becoming overheated through sports – this may occur if you play active sports such as squash, tennis, or football. Having a sauna or even sunbathing can aggravate your skin condition if you have an active infection. If you get warm after playing sport, then have a cool shower afterwards and ensure complete dryness and clean cotton undergarments.

6 Treat for 3 months continuously – if you have a penis or groin rash make sure you treat it for at least 3 months (ninety days) continuously. It is common for a man to treat a yeast infection, eliminate the symptoms temporarily, and then have the condition come back with a vengeance several weeks later.

7 Swim in salt water – In summer, try to swim in the ocean regularly and if possible, allow sunlight on the affected areas. Your skin will respond very well because you are exposing the yeast infection to salt water and sunlight, two things that candida cannot tolerate.

8 Treat you partner too - It is highly recommended that you treat your significant other so they do not give it to you again; it is best to avoid "passing the parcel".

9 Forget the quick-fix approach - you may end up having recurrent penis, groin, toenail fungus and digestive candida yeast infections like so many I've seen over the years. Do the diet AND lifestyle AND local treatment for ninety days without fail, and then keep on doing it until you get well and stay well for at least six months. Your reward will be well worth the effort, I guarantee it.

10 Coconut oil is a great lubricant – Use pure organic coconut oil as a personal lubricant. It is not only fragrant and most effective as a lubricant; it is also a very effective antibacterial and anti-fungal agent. This will ensure that you don't easily pass a yeast infection from one partner to another.

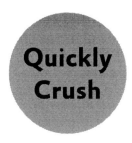

Quickly Crush

Nail Yeast Infections
Introduction

Candida yeast infections can also commonly affect the nail, nail bed and the surrounding soft skin tissue of the finger or toe nail. I have seen this condition in cooks, laundry workers, dairy farmers, market gardeners, meat workers, hotel cleaners and people who frequently immerse their hands in water or cleaning agents, or who work in damp environments. One of the worst cases of a fungal nail infection I have ever seen were the toe nails of a middle-aged man who cleaned windows full time in Wellington, NZ. He wore sneakers and his socks were always damp or wet, look at picture of his toenails of his right foot and imagine how embarrassing it must be for him to wear sandals with feet like that!

This section will deal with QUICK solutions for nail infections caused by yeast. These infections can be both most annoying and unsightly, and those who have infections here want them gone particularly fast.

Paronychia and Onychia

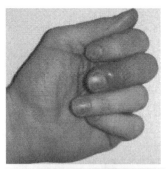

Paronychia - otherwise known as whitlow, is basically an inflammation around the *margin* of a toenail or fingernail that may also include the formation of pus. This is commonly due to the introduction of a bacteria or yeast into the skin.

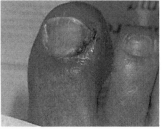

Onychia - on the other hand is an inflammation of the *nail folds* (surrounding tissue of the nail plate) of the nail with formation of pus and shedding of the nail. Onychia results from the introduction of a microscopic pathogen such as yeast or a bacterial infection through a small wound.

Causes Of Yeast Infections Affecting The Nails

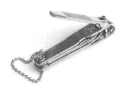

Like any other candida yeast infection, a fungal nail condition rarely affects a very healthy person, and there generally has to be an increased level of susceptibility and decreased resistance for a fungal nail condition to become established and thrive in a person. There are several potential causes for a yeast infection to affect a nail,

and one which may be less commonly thought of is the low production or output of hydrochloric acid in a person's stomach or small intestine.

A common cause I have seen is the cutting of finger or toenails. Do take care when you cut your nails, especially toenails. If you cut a nail or too much of an angle it may grow into the skin surrounding the tissue of the nail, puncturing the skin and leaving a small wound behind which may readily become infected. If you already have athlete's foot, the fungus can easily enter a small wound such as this and cause an infection.

Biting fingernails can also make you prone in particular to onychia. Another condition that may predispose one to a fungal or bacterial nail infection is thumb sucking.

Other conditions associated with fungal nail problems are diabetes, liver disease, respiratory illness and nutritional deficiencies (often due to decreased levels of hydrochloric acid produced).

Fungal Nail Disease Treatment

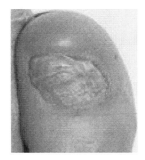

It is not hard to cure a fungal nail disease; the nails are easily accessible, small and easily treated and respond very well to treatment. Toenail fungus can be considerably more difficult to permanently eradicate than fingernail fungus. This is primarily due to the fact that many of us wear shoes continually.

Here are some of the best recommendations for yeast infections of the nails:

Tea Tree Oil – In the case of a nail infection, use one drop (more is not required) of 100% pure Tea Tree Oil straight on the nail bed. Repeat this twice daily – once upon rising and once upon retiring. You will be amazed and delighted at the results, especially if you persist. Don't give up in a hurry; it takes time to kill the infection.

Oregano Oil – Oil of oregano is considerably stronger than tea tree oil, but in my experience it is not always necessary to use stronger products necessarily. Oregano oil is stronger, much stronger and if you use it be sure to get wild crafted oregano oil. I've seen the most difficult of all toenail fungal conditions clear up entirely with oregano oil, even when nothing else worked. Go easy though, it is a strong treatment.

Strong natural medicines like drugs may potentially give strong and unwanted reactions that can be quite annoying and off-putting for some. I do like oregano oil with yeast infections, and often recommend taking one or two capsules of this oil internally. If a person can handle a drop or two on their nails, then this is THE way to go. Oregano oil is a bit like clove oil, it can be very powerful and extremely irritating, but when used very carefully it can be an absolute godsend. For a toothache for example I use clove oil, one drop and the pain is gone. If you do want to use oregano oil topically then I suggest you keep it well away from the eyes. Keep all essential oils well out of reach of children.

Grapefruit Seed Extract

Rub a drop of pure grapefruit seed extract (GSE) onto the affected nail after you take a shower or bath each day. Make sure that when you apply it that a little actually goes under the nail as well. Now leave it on. Every 3-4 days use a paper nail file and gently file away a little of the nail surface gently and rub in another drop of GSE. Continue like this until the nail starts to look normal again. If the nail yeast infection is quite severe and deep seated it can take many weeks or even several months, but it will be worth it when your nails are beautiful again, won't it? If you have tried the rest, try the best, GSE. I'd like you to try tea tree oil first because it clears up many cases of toe and fingernail fungus usually within 8-12 weeks with daily application.
Another trick is to alternate the tea tree oil or oregano oil and GSE on the nails, that way you are using the combined power of two strong natural products and choosing a more broad-spectrum approach. This will increase your chances of a quicker and more effective solution.

Fungal conditions affecting the nails are a problem that affects countless people all over the world. Every month, many people go to Google in an attempt to discover how to

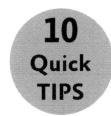

10 Quick TIPS   For Nail Yeast Infections

eradicate athlete's foot and nail yeast infections.

To reduce your chances of developing and maintaining fungal nail infections, I highly recommend that you follow these ten rules. You will notice that quite a few of the lifestyle recommendations are based on the fact that nail yeast infections thrive in an environment which is warm, dark and moist and is fed on sugars and yeast foods in the person's diet – not unlike a woman's or man's yeast infection. Knowing this, think about keeping the hands and feet clean and dry where possible, and take away the food supply that a nail yeast infection likes to feed on - the sugar and yeast foods.

Here are some of the best hints and tips I have learned which will help you crush fungal nail problems permanently. It goes without saying that optimal results come to those who follow the Candida Crusher Program outlined in chapter 7 in addition to the following ten hints and tips, especially if their condition is severe or chronic.

1   Keep your hands and feet clean and dry.

One of the best ways to avoid yeast infections of the nails is to make certain that your hands and feet are dry and dirt-free most of the time, because fungus loves to exist and grow in dark, moist and warm areas such as sweaty hands (gloves) or sweaty sports shoes.

Fingernail yeast infections often begin from hands and fingers in particular being hot and sweaty, cleaned several times daily or submerged for prolonged times in water. A fungal nail problem is more common in those who wear rubber gloves for several hours a day for example.

Toenail fungal problems often begin from too much sock and sweaty shoe use, the most common cause. Those who are more prone are office workers and especially those who play sports and end up with hot and sweaty feet. Now you can understand why locker rooms, swimming pool areas and shower rooms are notorious for spreading athlete's foot and toenail fungus.

It is very important that you keep your feet clean and dry, especially between your toes. Some people use a hair-dryer to get their feet completely dry, not a silly idea.

2   Go barefoot.

Whenever you can, kick-off your shoes and go barefoot. It is a fact that those who wear shoes and socks continuously will have a much greater chance of nail fungal problems. Going barefoot on the beach is particularly good, and you will get rid of athlete's foot and nail fungus that much quicker if you visit the beach more often.

3 Sunlight.

Place you feet in the sun, because yeast hates bright light. That's right, kick off those shoes and place your feet in the sun when you can for 15 minutes a day. This is why the beach is such a great environment and incorporates all the elements that yeast hates such as the sun, clean salty water and fresh air. I have yet to meet a person with fungal toenails or athlete's feet who loves spending time at the beach. It always seems to be the person who likes to play squash, basketball or football.

4 Replacing your socks is important.

Always use cotton socks, especially if you have an existing fungal nail problem or athlete's foot. Change your socks every day, and after you wash or bathe be sure to dry your feet carefully before you put a fresh new pair of cotton socks on. Add a little tea tree oil powder to your socks and feet.

5 Rotate your footwear and wear sandals in summer.

Avoid wearing the same closed footwear each day, rotate your footwear. Leave the pair you wore yesterday in a place where they can air or dry out. Go and buy another two or three pairs of shoes, especially sports shoes like sneakers. Do you play a sport professionally? Then you will most certainly want to have at least three if not four pairs of shoes and many dozens of pairs of socks that you can change frequently.

Drop one single drop of tea tree oil into the shoe, where the toes are, at least twice or three times each week. Wear sandals or open footwear, particularly in warmer weather, that way the air and light can more easily come into contact with your toes and feet.

6 Use natural remedies, stop using drugs.

You don't need to use pharmaceutical preparations like creams, ointments of pills to eradicate a fungal nail or foot condition. Why use something that may potentially give you a serious side effect? Natural antifungal medicines like tea tree or oregano oil will naturally prohibit the development of nail fungus and athlete's foot without the risk of incurring any side effects.

7 Foot spa or footbath.

A footbath or a foot spa to which you have added a generous amount of ACV is one of the most effective home treatments for nail or athlete's feet fungal problems.

Soak your feet in a bowl or foot spa with tepid water to which you have added a half a cup of ACV. Add one teaspoon of colloidal silver in addition and let the feet soak for at least 30 minutes, after which you should dry your feet thoroughly. Remember the hair dryer?

8 Use tea tree or oregano oil.

Tea tree oil or oregano oil are my opinion the best products to cure any nail yeast infection or athlete's foot. I have seen them cure countless nail and foot problems for many, many years. Drop the pure oil onto your nail or feet twice daily. You must be persistent and keep applying the oil each morning and each night for best results.

8 Be cautious of artificial nails and nail salons.

Artificial nails and heavily painted nails are potential breeding grounds for fingernail fungal infections. Be careful if you visit a nail salon, if they are not practicing correct sanitizing measures they can spread the fungal infection to other clients. A nail yeast infection may imbed more deeply if an artificial nail is layered onto an infected nail, and this may even be done to cover an unsightly fingernail.

9 Crushed garlic.

Peel a clove of garlic and then crush it until it is a fine pulp. Apply the garlic pulp to the toe or rub it very well into the affected area if a large area is affected. Place a large sticking plaster over the affected toe if you can, with the pulp underneath which is in contact with the fungal toe. Leave it overnight and in the morning wash the area and drop one drop of tea tree oil on the area. Repeat several times a week.

10 NEVER give up.

I always recommend persistence, because a fungal toenail will require persistence on your part if you want to eradicate it. It will not go away after just a few treatments, but will require daily treatment at times for weeks. You will eradicate this problem completely if you follow the 10 points outlined above consistently.

Quickly Crush

Mouth & Throat Yeast Infections

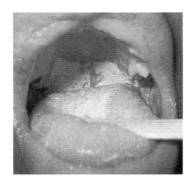

Did you know that two of the dirtiest places in your body where bacteria and fungi tend to live, are in the mouth and the anus? These areas form the entry and exit of your digestive tract. Candida yeast infections can breed readily in the mouth, throat and nasopharyngeal region (the ear, nose and throat) as well as in the large intestine and rectal area. It comes as no surprise that candida becomes a common infection of the digestive tract since the prevalence of candida yeasts in the mouth (oral cavity) can exceed 50% of the oral flora.

Oral Candidiasis – Mouth Yeast Infection

Oral candidiasis infections, yeast infections of the mouth, are most often recognized from symptoms such as burning and pain in the mouth or throat, fever and oral lesions. You may find a heavily coated tongue, whitish generally, and cracking around the corners of the mouth, a condition called angular stomatitis. I look for the tell tale signs of a yeast infection in patients with oral or throat candidiasis, which often include cravings for sugar, alcohol, bread or other forms of carbohydrates, and I generally also expect to find some degree of fatigue, depression, muscle aches and joint pain.

Common Causes Of Mouth And Throat Yeast Infections

There are many causes of yeast infections of the mouth, but here are the most common causes I have discovered:

- Poor dental hygiene
- People who wear dentures and especially poor fitting dentures
- People with diabetes
- People who take steroidal medications
- People with compromised immune systems (hepatitis, cancer, HIV, etc.)
- People under recurring stress (a lowered immune response)
- People who take antibiotics, or have a history of taking antibiotics
- People who smoke tobacco and drink alcohol

Candida Esophagitis – Throat Yeast Infection

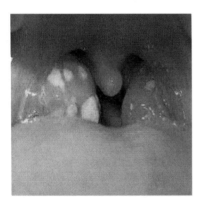

A throat yeast infection will generally result from an oral yeast infection or fungal infection that starts in the mouth and then spreads down the esophagus (throat). Yeast infections, including candida in the throat, can affect all ages and sexes. However, those with weak immune systems seem to be at a much greater risk of developing candida esophagitis.

One of the most common symptoms of a throat yeast infection is a feeling of discomfort or burning pain experienced behind the breastbone or sternum. This can be felt either behind the upper part of the sternum where the collar bone joins or it can be felt about two or three inches lower down. The symptoms of burning or discomfort can be particularly felt when alcohol is consumed, a hot drink or sometimes even after chocolate or bread. Your doctor may just prescribe an "acid blocker" medication and tell you that it is heartburn or esophagitis.

I can highly recommend that you visit a practitioner who specializes in yeast infections; you may well have a candida yeast infection that needs treatment. This is a very common complaint and I see many middle aged patients with reflux or heartburn who have in fact a yeast infection.

Angular Stomatitis – Cracks At The Corners Of The Mouth

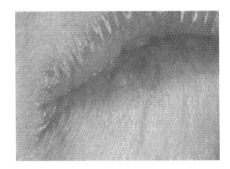

Do you notice from time to time that small and painful cracks appear at the corners of your mouth? Cracking of the corners of the mouth is a common skin complaint that is frequently seen in both the offices of dermatologists and dentists. This annoying condition is characterized by redness and cracking of the skin at the corners of the mouth and lips. There are many different reasons why this condition may occur; here are the most common causes of angular stomatitis:

Causes of cracks at the corners of the mouth

- Children and adults who drool during sleep and/or have orthodontic braces.

- In older adults, angular stomatitis can be a part of the normal aging process that causes skin wrinkling with superficial or deep lines. Skin wrinkling is the result of skin thinning from constant exposure to the environment including sun damage over many years. Ageing may cause fat and connective tissue loss, and the lips may thin as well.

- Smokers and those who drink alcohol very regularly are more prone to this condition, this will occur primarily to nutritional deficiencies.

- Denture stomatitis is a painful inflammation of the skin under a denture. Careful hygiene needs to be observed with denture wearers, and if dentures are not removed and cleaned regularly, mouth dryness and subsequent chronic yeast infections may occur. I have seen this on several occasions with elderly patients

- With the elderly, this condition can occur due to a lack of teeth; particularly the back teeth which tend to support the facial structures including the lips and cheeks. This will often lead to a bite problem and can develop into a cracking or fissuring at the corners of the mouth.

- Nutritional deficiencies are common in many patients, and deficiencies to look out for with cracking of the mouth corners in particular are iron deficiency, and especially B vitamin deficiencies. Take the Candida Crusher Multi; it contains B vitamins that will ensure you have no deficiencies leading to the problem.

- Colder weather and a drier air with a subsequent licking to keep the lips moist can increase your chances of an inflammation and infection around the mouth.

- Diabetics, cancer patients and those on long term medications may be prone to conditions which lead to changes in the health and integrity of their oral mucosa, the lining of the mouth.

Fixing Those Annoying Cracks At The Corners Of Your Mouth

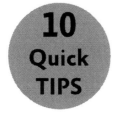

The best way to prevent crack at the corners of the mouth is to make sure you keep this part of your mouth clean and dry. Once cracks or fissures appear then saliva and food particles can predispose you towards a yeast infection. Make sure you are not deficient in the important minerals zinc, iron and the B vitamins.

Many patients will quickly overcome this condition just by taking a good multivitamin daily. You can also try sucking on a zinc and vitamin C lozenge three times daily for three to four days.

Antifungal ointments such as tea tree can also be applied liberally to the corners of the mouth several times a day to clear infection, as well as zinc oxide paste that has antifungal properties which acts like a skin barrier.

Sometimes you may find that an infection arises from inside your mouth, and it is likely to recur if you only treat the corners of your mouth. Water-soluble tea tree oil rinses or tea tree oil lozenges can be effectively used to treat minor oral yeast infections. If you have dentures, you will need to be vigilant and make sure you clean and scrub your dentures well in addition to leaving them out over night.

Brushing and flossing your teeth twice daily will help to provide optimal oral health; and proper lip support can be obtained by using an effective lip balm, especially in cold and dry weather conditions. Your dentist will be able to verify that your oral hygiene is good, and that your gum tissues are healthy and your teeth are decay free.

These methods can all help to lessen or remove the cracking and wrinkles at the lip corners. Make sure that any systemic candida yeast infections are treated on the inside as well, especially if you can relate to several of the signs and symptoms of a yeast infection you discover in chapter 3. Be sure to follow the Candida Crusher program for optimal and lasting results.

10
Quick
TIPS

For Mouth And Throat Yeast Infections

To reduce your chances of developing and maintaining a mouth or throat yeast infection, I highly recommend that you follow these ten rules. You will notice that quite a few dietary and lifestyle recommendations are based on the fact that oral and throat yeast infections thrive in an environment that is warm, dark and moist and is fed on sugars and yeast foods. Knowing this, think about excellent oral hygiene and take away the food supply that a yeast infection likes to feed on - the sugar and yeast foods.

1

Observe excellent oral hygiene.

It makes good sense to observe excellent oral hygiene, since this is the entry to the digestive tract. I recommend that you rinse your mouth first, floss and then brush your teeth. Using tea tree oil toothpaste will ensure that you eradicate an oral yeast infection. The best time to brush your tongue is when you brush your teeth in the morning, bacteria and yeasts tend to multiply more on the tongue overnight than during the day. You may be able to find a good herbal mouthwash at your local health food shop that should help as well.

To avoid re-infecting yourself when brushing your teeth, try disinfecting your toothbrush regularly by placing your toothbrush in hydrogen peroxide for a few minutes before and after each brushing. This will ensure a good level of potential yeast and bacterial reduction and will aid greatly in the prevention of re-infection.

2

Do you wear dentures?

Denture sores are a common occurrence and some estimates are that over 60% of our older denture wearers experience painful mouth ulcers as a result of an underlying yeast infection. You will know that you have a yeast infection by the redness and possible swelling, often involving the upper palate (roof of mouth) that comes into contact with the denture. The solution? Get your dentures checked to see they fit well, ensure excellent hygiene practices, brush with tea tree oil toothpaste and treat any underlying digestive yeast infections. Follow the Candida Crusher Program for best results.

3

Keep your immune system strong.

Keeping a good healthy immune system is the key to fighting any infection, especially a yeast infection. I often see patients with depressed immune systems who have a mouth or throat yeast infection, and there can be many causes for this.

Treating a yeast infection is quite straight forward with a good immune system, but for those with a compromised immune system the treatment is different and may take considerably longer. For example, those who can recognize a history of stress or those who suffer from AIDS, hepatitis, auto-immune disorders, cancer, diabetes, including those especially who suffer from adrenal fatigue or thyroid disorders, all will have one thing in common, a lowered immune response to infections, and these are typically the patients who really struggle with recurring mouth or throat yeast infections.

There are many products which can strengthen the immune system, but the first thing to take is Vitamin C, take it until you reach bowel tolerance and then work just under this dose for several days.

4

Treat mouth and throat yeast infections locally.

The best results will come when you treat locally and systemically by following the Candida Crusher Program. One of the best local treatments for oral and throat yeast infections is live, natural, sugar free yogurt. The lactic acid loving bacteria in live yogurt live thrive naturally in your mouth, and mouth thrush will often imply that your friendly bacterial levels are low. Just hold the yogurt in your mouth for about 5 minutes, and you can do this 2 or 3 times a day.

5

In addition, always treat mouth and throat yeast infections systemically. Anybody who comes to my clinic with an oral or throat yeast infection will get treated systemically. I presume they have a yeast infection in their digestive system as well. The digestive system, particularly their small and large intestine, is the major place where the yeast infection will reside. A candida yeast infection can multiply rapidly and grow out of control, leading to complications throughout the body much further afield such as the throat, the mouth and even the joints and brain.

6

Tea tree oil as a mouthwash.
Try a mouthwash made with 2 tablespoons of water to which you have added 5 to 10 drops of water soluble tea tree oil. Just wash the mouth thoroughly and spit it out. Do you have esophageal candidiasis, otherwise known as candida of the throat?

Then do the same thing, use a few tablespoons of plain water, add several drops of water-soluble tea tree oil and do a deep gargle. Rinse your mouth or gargle several times daily and please follow my Candida Crusher program, you can beat this thing. Tea tree oil is safe to use and is not as toxic as many would like to make it out. Sure, there will be some people who cannot tolerate oils such as tea tree internally, but the majority will be able to tolerate tiny amounts. It never ceases to amaze me at how the finger is pointed at natural medicines like vitamin A and tea tree oil, yet consumers are rarely if ever warned about the inherent dangers of drinking spirits like vodka or taking drugs such as Acetaminophen (paracetamol), both of which are consumed in large amounts indiscriminately, causing widespread disease and death.

I personally know a naturopath in Sydney, Australia, who took twenty drops of tea tree oil per day internally for several months with no ill effect whatsoever. Tea tree lozenges are readily available as well and I have used tea tree oil products in my clinic for nearly twenty-five years and never heard of any ill effects as a result of using this most potent antifungal medicine orally. Common sense prevails; if you are going to take tablespoons of any pure essential oil daily you will naturally end up in trouble.

7

Avoid hot and spicy foods and drinks.
If you have an issue with the skin lining your mouth and throat, then you are best to avoid placing anything into your mouth which is excessively hot, cold or spicy, which can be irritating to the oral mucosa. You will heal the skin faster by removing these obstacles from your diet temporarily.

8

Vitamin and mineral deficiencies.
Vitamin deficiencies are common in many countries. When you lack crucial nutrients like vitamins and minerals, your immune system is one of the first systems to be compromised. Immune suppression and immune incompetence commonly occur as a result of deficiencies, and the commonest of these deficiencies is iron and zinc, something I see particularly in up to 30% of women as well as vegetarians.

One of the best ways to ensure you do not become deficient in the vital nutrients is by eating a healthy and balanced diet and by taking in addition a comprehensive multi vitamin and mineral dietary supplement. This is one of the causes of mouth and throat yeast infections you can easily remedy, so be sure you start changing your diet to a healthier one, and by taking a daily multi-vitamin like the Candida Crusher Multi.

8

Iron Deficiency. It is surprising how many women lack sufficient iron in their diet. Some experts estimate that up to 30% of women in many developed countries have some degrees of iron deficiency that can have a significant impact on the effectiveness of the immune system. Wounds tend to heal slower when an iron deficiency is present, and a lack of sufficient iron is reason why wounds on the corner of the mouth (angular stomatitis) as well as mouth ulcers and throat lesions do not easily heal.

Get a blood test done to see what your iron levels are, and if low then probably the best thing you can do is to take iron supplement. By eating a small amount of red meat regularly you will be ensuring that your dietary sources of iron are met.

Zinc deficiency. Zinc has a profound influence on many aspects of immune function, and a lack of zinc in the diet can cause many problems, including impaired wound healing and chronic ulceration of the mucosal surfaces of the mouth and throat.

Ask for a zinc taste test when you visit your naturopath or nutritionally orientated doctor, and this way you will be able to determine your zinc status rapidly.

9

Try a zinc and vitamin C lozenge.
Zinc and vitamin C lozenges will heal many issues affecting the mouth, gums and tongue. I highly recommend these lozenges for a sore throat, mouth ulcers, poor immune function, and a herpes simplex (cold sore) outbreak or for colds and influenza in general. Try sucking on one of these lozenges every two hours and you will find speedy relief in many cases.

10

Avoidance of steroidal drugs and antibiotics.
One of the biggest causes of an oral or throat yeast infections is antibiotics or inhaled steroids, commonly prescribed in asthma. Pharmaceutical drugs are a commonly overlooked cause of mouth and throat yeast infections, and one major cause I have seen time and again in my clinic. Are you an asthmatic and regularly experience a sore throat, have cracked corners of your mouth or find that you experience recurring mouth ulcers? The talk to your doctor and find out if the drug you take is linked with a yeast infection, and if in doubt then go to Dr. Google.

Those who take an antibiotic will not only discover that they may be more prone to diarrhea and an upset digestive system; they will also be more prone to common problems of the mouth and throat.

Always be on guard if you have to take an antibiotic or inhaled steroid, be on the lookout for the telltale signs of a yeast infection, especially if you have been taking one or either of these drugs long-term. There are natural alternatives and all you have to do is to ask.

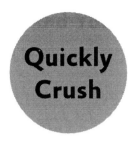

Quickly Crush

Diaper Yeast Infections

Nobody likes to see a baby suffer with a diaper rash, and if you have had children like me you will have been familiar with this condition from time to time. I have changed many hundreds of diapers when my four children were infants and can offer some sound advice.

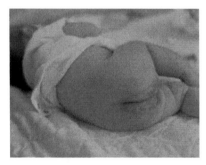

Diaper rash usually goes away on its own, and in most cases your child will cease to have episodes of diaper rash once he or she has been successfully potty trained and no longer requires the use of a diaper.

Are you determined to find a quick solution for this annoying and painful condition? Have you tried a lot of various natural cremes and ointments without success? You will find several handy hints and tips that will help you resolve your child's diaper rash quickly.

Two of the main points I like to emphasize is that it is very important to change the baby's diaper frequently and make sure that the baby's bottom is dry after you change a diaper and put a new one on. Use a hair dryer to keep the baby's bottom very dry before you place the next diaper on. Keep a hair dryer handy near the changing table for this reason, especially if your child is prone to diaper rash. Keep the dryer's temperature down and be sure to keep it well away from baby's fingers!

A Child's Yeast Infection Or A Diaper Rash?

A yeast infection tends to stay for several days and is not responsive to normal diaper rash treatments, look for a red rash involving the skin folds of the groin area and be suspicious in particular if your child has recently had antibiotic treatment or if you have if you have been breastfeeding the affected child.

It can be difficult sometimes to determine if your baby has a diaper rash, usually caused by excessive wetness, sensitivity or chafing, or a yeast infection. You can generally tell if it is a yeast infection because it will be a well-defined rash and bright red with raised borders. You may also find satellite lesions, red patches that have formed a slight distance away from the main red skin lesion. Check to see if your child has thrush or a cheesy white discharge (girl) or whitish rash around the penis (boy) that is another indication of a yeast infection.

Diaper Tips

It is best to avoid your child developing a diaper rash in the first place, and prevention is naturally the most effective way to treat diaper rash. Here are some diaper tips.

- Avoid cotton diapers and plastic diaper covers if your child has diaper rash, use disposable diapers until the rash has fully resolved. You can always go back and use pure cotton if you desire once the rash is gone.

- Today's modern diapers are very absorbent and will draw away excess moisture from the skin. Regardless, it is important to change a baby's diaper frequently, especially if baby has an existing diaper rash. This will prevent urine and feces from staying in contact with the baby's delicate skin preventing further irritation.

- Always make sure that the baby's skin is as dry as posible and clean before putting on a new diaper.

  Be careful when putting a new diaper on your child that the adhesive tape stays clear of the skin, otherwise you may irritate the skin excessively and cause a breakdown and even a skin infection.

- Avoid putting on a diaper excessively tight and allow sufficient room for a little airflow.

- Change diaper brands occasionally, some children are sensitive to certain brands and you may find that the budget brands may use inferior materials.

- Good hand washing is a must to help prevent infections of all kinds.

Avoid Chemicals On Baby's Skin – Go Natural

Be careful of what you apply to your child's skin, I have noticed various retail "natural" brands (including dusting powders) can contains methylparaben, talc and fragrance, which is a just another fancy word for chemicals called phthalates. Research has found that a baby's skin is particularly sensitive and that these chemicals are linked with bioaccumulation in humans and wildlife, cancer, endocrine disruption and hormone mimicry, allergies and skin toxicity. Some may use talc on their child's skin after a bath thinking it is a "natural" product, but did you know that talc is actually known for being contaminated with asbestos, a known carcinogen?

Avoid The Sweet And Acid Forming Foods

Of all the foods in your diet or your baby's, you will find that it will be the sweet and acidic foods that are most often to be the likely culprits when it comes to diaper rash. Should a diaper rash develop, here is a list of the most common acidic foods which you may wish to exclude from your diet if you breast feed exclusively, or from the baby's diet:

- Citrus fruits and juices. Lemon should be OK as this is alkaline.

- Tomatoes and tomato products like spaghetti and tomato sauce.

- Strawberries

- Pineapple

- Tart apples, plums and peaches

- Grapes

- Dried fruits like sultanas, raisins, dates, figs, apricots, etc.

- Do not drink alcohol if you breastfeed, especially if baby has a diaper rash!

- Eat less red meat, choosing fish and chicken temporarily instead.

Food Allergies

Diaper rash is often triggered by frequent, loose stools, so it is a good idea to avoid the foods that can potentially cause diarrhea, these may well be the foods that you (if you breastfeed) or your baby are allergic to.

Do you have a history of allergies, hay fever, asthma or eczema? Then you will want to go on an elimination diet for a few weeks to determine whether or not these particular foods are the cause of your baby's diaper rash.

If you breastfeed, you may want to adopt my Hypo-Allergenic Diet approach for a few weeks to see if the baby is sensitive to any foods you may be consuming. This is particularly important if the diaper rash is recurring and you just can't find the cause. It is important to remember that your child will become increasingly sensitive to allergens in foods from taking antibiotics, and any child who has been on an antibiotic will need extensive digestive repair to avoid becoming allergic to a food.

You can read more about food allergies and the Hypo-Allergenic Diet in section 1 of chapter 7.

The most common food allergies which may be affecting your baby include:

- Dairy products except for yogurt. (Milk is the most common allergy)
- Wheat /gluten
- Soy
- Eggs
- Chocolate
- Bananas, pineapple
- Oranges
- Fish (rare but certainly possible)
- Peanuts
- Sugar
- Legumes/beans

How do you know if the diaper rash has its origin in a food allergy? You will know by the elimination of any suspect foods for about seven to ten days. I have found that a red circle or ring around the child's anus is a good indication of a food allergy, especially if the baby draws his or her legs up to the abdomen indicating pain or cramps. Sometimes you may be dealing with food intolerance and not a true food allergy; again, this can be easily determined by a food withdrawal. See your health care professional if you are worried about any possible reactions to foods.

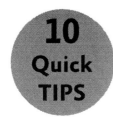

10 Quick TIPS for Diaper Yeast Infections

Prevention of a child's yeast infection is not unlike preventing a yeast infection in a woman or a man. To reduce your child's chances of developing and maintaining a diaper yeast infection, I highly recommend the following ten rules. You will notice that quite a few of the lifestyle and dietary recommendations are based on the fact that a diaper yeast infection thrives in an environment which is warm, dark and moist and is fed on sugars and yeast foods. Knowing this, think about increasing the air flow, changing diapers frequently and removing the food supply that yeast likes to feed on, the sugar and yeast-laden foods.

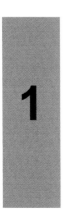

Frequent diaper changes

The first and most important step if you want a quick resolution of your child's diaper rash is to always change the baby right away if you know he or she is wet or soiled. It is important to change a newborn baby's diaper very regularly; it may be as frequent as every two to three hours. If your child is prone to diaper rash then change his or her diaper frequently regardless of their age.

Remember, urine and feces will be the greatest source of irritation if there is a diaper rash and changing and by changing frequently you will reduce this source of irritation greatly.

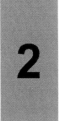

Leave the diaper off regularly.

After cleaning, the skin should be exposed to air, leaving the diaper off for several hours if possible. You will find that diaper rash will resolve more quickly by frequent airing of your baby's skin. Ensure your child is kept in a warm and dry environment and that the skin is allowed to dry sufficiently between diaper changes. Exposure to the sun in the earlier hours of the morning or late in the afternoon will also found to be beneficial.

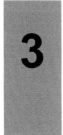

Avoid 100% cotton diapers.

If your baby has an existing diaper rash then avoid 100% cotton diapers no matter how soft, fluffy and environmentally friendly they are! Mothers who use pure cotton diapers also tend to use a plastic diaper cover that will cause even more aggravation by prohibiting adequate ventilation of the affected area. It is best to switch to the modern synthetic variety, as this type of diaper tends to draw any moisture away from the skin.

Cleanse well

Clean and carefully wipe the baby's bottom at each changing. Be gentle and take care because the irritated skin will be quite sensitive and rubbing may contribute to the rash. Use unscented wipes and preferably low allergy wipes or just use plain tepid water and a soft cotton cloth. Wash the skin with a very mild soap like a goat's milk soap, leave it air dry or lightly pat the area down.

Change Diaper and diaper wipe brands

If you use disposable diapers, try different brands. Use non-irritating or "low allergy" brands and select diapers that fit your child well with less overall friction. If you consistently find that diaper rash occurs regardless of the brand diaper you try, then consider using cloth diapers if there is consistent trouble with disposable diapers. Rinse cotton diapers with a half-cup of apple cider vinegar in the rinse cycle and add 1 teaspoon of water-soluble tea tree oil to this mixture.

Diaper rash cream

I have found in most cases of diaper rash that a quality calendula cream works best. Always use a 100% natural diaper rash cream that does not contain any chemicals or irritants. A high quality cream or ointment can stop rashes of many kinds, so be sure to use the cream with each diaper changing if your baby is prone to having rashes. Avoid petroleum based jelly (crude oil derivative) or steroid creams or ointments as a preventative daily cream. Could the rash be caused by a contact or allergic dermatitis? Stop using any new soaps or detergents that may be causing the rash. Incredible, but sometimes you will find those chemical skin concoctions your doctor recommends may even be the very cause of your child's skin rash or aggravate an existing skin complaint.

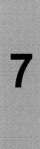

Special treatment for severe diaper rash

Start by gently cleaning baby's bottom, then soak in a large bowl of tepid water to which you have added 1 teaspoon of water soluble tea tree oil. Pat the skin gently dry rather using a soft cotton cloth than using a wiping motion. Be sure to let the area dry thoroughly, use a hair dryer turned to very low heat to ensure a complete dryness. Allow the skin to air thoroughly before applying a small amount of cream. For heavy-duty use, use a white zinc oxide cream that is thicker and may be necessary for rash-prone babies. Your chemist or pharmacy will be able to help here. Be very careful with the diet and ensure all acid forming and sugary foods and drinks are removed from the diet.

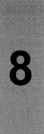

Certain foods may worsen the rash

You may have read what I wrote just previously about food allergies and food intolerances. Are you breastfeeding exclusively? Then you will want to be particularly careful with what you eat and drink, because everything you eat and drink will affect the quality of your breast milk and consequently your child. If this is the case, avoid the key allergenic foods (see above) until the rash has cleared, and in addition, take a probiotic. I'm a huge fan of recommending women to take a quality Omega 3 supplement before, during, and after pregnancy, especially when they breastfeed.

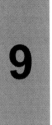

Diaper rash caused by a yeast infection

Has your child recently had a course of antibiotics or have you if you are breastfeeding? If the child has a fungal diaper rash be especially careful of sweet foods and do follow my Candida Crusher Diet. Calendula or tea tree oil cream will be found to be very effective as they are both antifungal. Be sure to give your child a probiotic capsule or a small amount of powder daily. If you breastfeed, take a probiotic twice daily yourself, and don't forget that Omega 3. You can read more about supplement recommendations in section 4 of chapter 7.

Treat systemically, not just the diaper rash

Just like any form of yeast infection, treat your child systemically as well as locally to get a quick and permanent result. If your child develops diaper rash and is breastfed by you then you are best to change your diet and follow the Candida Crusher diet and program for optimal and lasting results.

CHAPTER 5 Crushing Chronic Vaginal Yeast Infections

Introduction

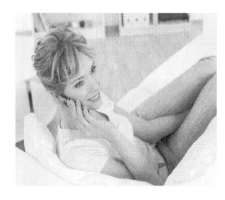

Many health problems which women face are yeast related. Most all the patients we see as naturopaths are women, in fact women they make up over 75% of our client base, and many women we see are commonly burdened with complaints of their nervous, digestive or reproductive systems in particular. Women are particularly prone to vaginal yeast infections, and this is one area I have been specializing in with regards to treating yeast infections in particular. I started to notice that many women responded positively to the yeast protocols I was beginning to formulate in my clinic in the mid nineties, but it wasn't until the late nineties that I came up with the Candida Crusher concept and started to finely tune my protocols.

Getting rid of a yeast infection can change a woman's life completely, I can still recall patient telling me this: "I was terribly difficult to live with until I completed your treatment. After I stopped taking the oral contraceptive pill, cleaned up my system and changed my diet it all changed, and who knows, it may have even saved my marriage". I have found that in most situations by following the Candida Crusher vaginal implant protocol I will outline very shortly, as well as the Candida Crusher dietary approach outlined in chapter 7; you can almost certainly cure yourself of this extremely annoying complaint. This has been achieved by many hundreds of women I have treated for candida yeast infections over the past twenty years, and it can almost certainly be possible for you as well.

This fifth chapter of the Candida Crusher will focus primarily on women's vaginal yeast infection, especially the chronic complaint of vaginal yeast infection and the related genito-urinary system afflictions as well. Naturally, women can also experience yeast infections in many other ways, and you will be able to read about these other manifestations of a yeast infections in other sections of this book.

The vagina is quite a complex ecological environment with a high concentration of many different microorganisms. Between forty to eighty percent of women are found to have at least five to ten different organisms which can be cultured from their vaginal fluid, including lactobacilli, corynebacterium, and streptococci.

A normal healthy vaginal discharge is generally whitish and milky in appearance and consists of secretions from the cervical glands and various cells that line the vaginal and cervical surfaces. The discharge can vary widely during the menstrual cycle depending on the hormonal levels. Normally the discharge will be found to be more profuse and thicker just before ovulation and will be found to be thinner and scantier in the luteal phase, after the period. In my experience, it is from one week through until just before the menstrual period that a candida vaginal yeast infection can become particularly aggravating, and is at this time when the implant protocol can put to its best use. The anti-microbial treatments utilizing either the garlic method or the tea tree oil method will be found to be most effective.

The normal healthy vaginal pH (acid/alkaline level) is around 4.5 or lower, and this is due mainly to the lactic acid level that is primarily due to the beneficial lactobacilli species. In a healthy vagina, the lactobacilli bacteria and other beneficial species will inhibit the overgrowth of potentially disease-causing organisms such as candida albicans, yeast, or gardneralla vaginalis, bacteria.

By altering this delicate and complex balance, the likelihood is increased of the development of disease causing organisms. There are many possible infections and inflammations possible, including the common vaginal yeast infection known as vaginal thrush, which is experienced by a surprising amount of women worldwide.

Vaginal thrush is one of the commonest reasons many candida patients have consulted me over the years. It has been estimated that world-wide, around seventy-five percent of women at some time in their live have vulvovaginitis, and over half of them have more them one episode. Some experts believe that 15 to 20 percent of all women in the world have chronic and recurring vaginal candidiasis.

There are a number of names given to this condition, and the most common are: vaginal yeast infection, vulvovaginal candidiasis, moniliasis, vulvovaginal thrush or thrush, a yeast infection or a monilia infection or also terms used by many women to describe this annoying complaint.

Get The Right Diagnosis

> " *If you trust Google more than your doctor then maybe it's time to switch doctors.* "
> Cristina Cordova

Before commencing this or any treatment aimed at a vaginal infection, it is important that you have a diagnosis by a qualified health-care professional in order to establish whether your symptoms are in fact being caused by a yeast infection. As you will read further ahead in this chapter, there are several reasons why you may have an infection and you need to know what you are dealing with before you can effectively treat it. If you are certain you have a vaginal yeast infection, then treat it but do seek expert help if there is no change in a short period of time.

Furthermore, there is a possibility of re-infection by transmission from one sexual partner to another, so do take precautions and get yourself checked out if in doubt.

An Annoying And Irritating Discharge

Vaginal thrush is quite annoying for most women to experience; it is a milky looking discharge that can have curd like threads. This problem can really wreck a woman's sex life and cause a tremendous amount of discomfort as well as anxiety.

Some women I have spoken to are ashamed of having vaginal thrush, believing that it is due to uncleanliness, but given the right set of circumstances, just about any woman can develop thrush. It doesn't matter what your income level is, how clean you are, what level of education you have, your social standing or whether you have an active intimate relationship or not either, thrush has no respect for any aspect of a woman's lifestyle. Some women may only have yeast vulvovaginitis once or twice in their life, yet others may experience this women's complaint over and over, with some having it monthly and others having it almost continually. An itch that drives you crazy and an annoying discharge are two of the key signs that you have joined the vaginal yeast infection ranks.

Signs and Symptoms of Vulvovaginitis

After you have treated vaginal yeast infections for a few years, you will find that there are several different presentations of vaginal yeast infections. It is easy to assume that they are all vaginal, when in fact some women do not have a vaginal problem but an infection just involving the vulva (the area surrounding the vagina) or the perineum (the area of skin between the anus and the vagina.

A woman may have a yeast infection only in the vagina (vaginitis), she may have it on the skin surrounding the vagina (vulvitis) or she may have it in and around the skin of the vulva (labia minor and major) in addition to the vagina, and in that case it is called vulvovaginitis. I have found this to be the most common (and most annoying to the female) presentation.

Vaginal yeast infections can cause symptoms that are not really specific, which means that aside from the yeast infection, other conditions can cause the identical symptoms that we will look at in a moment. The most common symptom of a vaginal yeast infection however is that uncomfortable, embarrassing and really annoying itching in the vaginal and/or the vulvar area.

Other Symptoms Of Vaginal Yeast Infection And Vulvitis Include:

- Burning or stinging

- Soreness

- Pain during intercourse

- Pain during urination

- Vaginal discharge. Vaginal discharge is not always present, but when it does occur, the discharge is generally odorless and typically has a whitish, thick appearance and texture, like cottage cheese.

Vulvitis can also cause local pain in addition to the above symptoms. Pain in the vulvar area is referred to as vulvodynia. As I mentioned earlier, for up to 15 or 20% of women, yeast vulvovaginitis may cause a recurring problem. A recurrent yeast infection occurs when a woman has four or more infections in any one year.

Your doctor may tell you that recurrent yeast infections are related to an underlying medical condition and may require more aggressive treatment. Others doctors may be quick to tell you that an antibiotic will "not be the cause" of your recurring yeast infection and the fact that you developed thrush after an antibiotic was purely "coincidental", when in fact you will find the opposite to be the case, and many instances of vaginal thrush will began soon after an antibiotic has been prescribed. Try some common sense here.

How Are Vaginal Yeast Infections Diagnosed?

In most cases, you can treat this complaint in the privacy of your own home and will soon know if you are suffering from a yeast infection or not by the improvement, or lack of, you are likely to experience. To firmly establish the diagnosis and to rule out any other underlying causes of the symptoms, your doctor will take a specimen, a smear test, scraped from the affected area for microscopic analysis or for culture in a laboratory. Identification of yeast under a microscope, when possible, is the least expensive and most rapid and accurate way to establish the diagnosis and in chronic cases I always recommend identification.

Early detection is important because you may have another condition that may present just like a yeast infection for example such as gardnerella, which is a bacterial infection and not a yeast infection.

The 10 Main Causes Of Vaginal And Vulval Yeast Infections

There are many potential causes of vaginal infections and inflammations, and here is a list of the 10 most common reasons why vaginal yeast infections strike women:

1   **A diet high in refined carbohydrates.** This is most likely to be one of the commonest causes, too much sugar, soda drinks, candy, alcohol (especially wine), white bread and cookies and other convenience foods high in sugar.

2   **Pregnancy and childbirth.** This is a time of hormonal turmoil and many women complain of vaginitis during their pregnancy.

3   **Menstrual dysfunction.** A menstrual cycle that is irregular, particularly in the week leading up to the menstrual period, may encourage the proliferation of a yeast infection.

4   **Diabetes.** Diabetics tend to pass more sugar (glucose) through their urinary tract than they should, and wherever there is an abundance of glucose in the body, a yeast infection is not far behind.

5 Stress. Stress has a way of weakening the immune system, thereby creating a higher level of vulnerability for many types of infection, including a yeast infection. You can read a lot more about the link between stress and candida in chapter 7, section 2.

6 Pharmaceutical drugs. Birth control pills and antibiotics in particular have been positively linked with candida yeast infections, but so have steroidal drugs.

7 Nutritional deficiencies. Deficiencies in trace elements and vitamins can predispose a person to an increased vulnerability of a yeast infection. This is also tied in with a diet high in refined carbohydrates. These diets have a tendency to be calorie rich but nutrient poor.

8 Chemical contamination. Vaginal tissue is very sensitive and vulnerable to the effects of certain chemicals, and the use of vaginal sprays and deodorants, colored or scented toilet paper may irritate the area decreasing the resistance of the immune system to yeasts and bacteria.

9 Sexual intercourse. Excessive intercourse in a short period of time or insufficient lubrication may cause vaginal irritation and inflammation leading to a yeast infection. I find this a particularly common cause for women in their mid forties to mid fifties.

10 Clothing. The use of certain undergarments such as nylon panties or pantyhose or tight-fitting clothing such as jeans can lead to insufficient ventilation, and may help to provide a more suitable breeding ground for a yeast infection to develop.

The 3 Main Causes Of Vaginal Inflammation

It is important for you to know whether you have a yeast infection or not, and if your symptoms are not significantly improved on my treatment recommendations then you will certainly need to go to your doctor for diagnosis. There are a number of inflammatory conditions that can affect a woman's genital area, and I will explain the most likely presentations.

There are three main types of vaginitis:

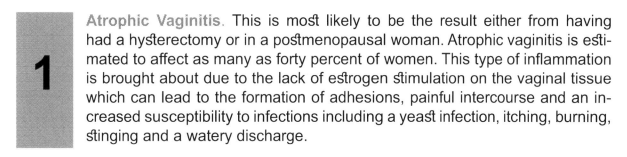

1 Atrophic Vaginitis. This is most likely to be the result either from having had a hysterectomy or in a postmenopausal woman. Atrophic vaginitis is estimated to affect as many as forty percent of women. This type of inflammation is brought about due to the lack of estrogen stimulation on the vaginal tissue which can lead to the formation of adhesions, painful intercourse and an increased susceptibility to infections including a yeast infection, itching, burning, stinging and a watery discharge.

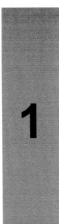

Atrophic vaginitis is a condition that you will more commonly find in older women because it refers to a thinning on the skin lining the vagina. It is caused because of a decrease presence of hormones such as estrogen that are vital to help nourish and thicken the skin lining. This condition can also affect the vulva and cause shrinkage or thinning on the skin in these areas as well. The symptoms may include an inflamed, dry, red and burning vagina and vulva. Atrophic vaginitis is responsible for causing many menopausal women to experience symptoms such as painful urination, itching and burning and painful sexual intercourse.

The problem with vaginal atrophy is that it can leave the vagina and vulva more prone to developing other conditions such as a yeast infection, making the area more susceptible to any type of skin infection.

The Solution: Conventional treatment will generally include a vaginal estrogen cream temporarily which will be prescribed and monitored by your doctor. You do not necessarily need to take synthetic hormones to get a good result with atrophic vaginitis. Go and see your naturopath or herbalist if you want a more natural and side effect free option here. You can try natural Vitamin E oil and rub it in nightly, it works wonders for many women. Herbal medicines worth mentioning are vitex agnus castus as well as motherwort, and black cohosh (cimicifuga racemosa) is one of my favorite herbs for a woman around the peri-menopause and menopause.

Black Cohosh

Women with menstrual or menopausal problems have used this herb for well over century.

Black cohosh lowers luteinizing hormone levels and appears to have a positive and balancing effect on the hypothalamus and pituitary glands and helps to regulate the body's temperature more favorably and is perfect if you have hot flashes and vaginal dryness. In Germany, up to three quarters of medical doctors have used this herbal medicine and it is even considered even a viable alternative to estrogen replacement therapy today by many enlightened doctors.

Women who are pregnant, wanting to conceive or who are nursing should not use black cohosh. You can take black cohosh as an herbal or homeopathic medicine, and I recommend that if your symptoms are primarily of a physical nature to take the herbal medicine, and if your symptoms are mainly mental or emotional use the homeopathic medicine.

While you can use both combined, and I do with excellent results, you should seek the assistance of your natural medicine healthcare professional, because there are different strengths of homeopathic medicines and a person with experience will be able to guide you best. I generally use the 6c, 30c or 200c. I have used this homeopathic medicine in the higher strengths especially well in a few cases of quite severe anxiety and depression with menopause.

Cimicifuga an excellent herbal medicine indicated for women who experience vaginal symptoms like dryness, atrophy of tissues, burning, itching and tearing. I have also found it good for women who experience tension in their neck and upper back and who may experience pain in the smaller joints of their body, like the hands, wrists, ankles and toes.

Use the homeopathic medicine in particular if you experience the mental or emotional symptoms around the peri-menopause or menopause itself. It can help you significantly if you have been suffering from headaches, depression, hot flashes and night sweats and mood swings with your peri menopause or during your menopause.

2 Irritant Vaginitis. This is most likely to be the result of an irritation or an allergy. There may be different physical agents (tampon usage for example) or chemical agents.

The Solution: Switch to pad use and be sure that if you do continue to use tampons that they are natural products and contain no chemicals or irritants. You may want to switch brands, contact your local health-food shop and enquire about a good quality natural tampon.

3 Infectious Vaginitis. You guessed, this type of vaginitis results from some type of infection, like a yeast infection, Gardnerella (bacterial infection) or an STD (sexually transmitted disease) like Chlamydia, Trichomoniasis or Gonorrhoea.

The Solution: Make sure that you get the correct diagnosis and determine what is causing your infectious vaginitis before you decide on the treatment.

The Medical Treatment Of Vaginal Yeast Infections

Your medical doctor will treat vaginal yeast infection and vulvitis almost always with an antifungal medication. These medications will be applied either topically in and around the vagina or orally with antifungal medications.

Sometimes your doctor will recommend both of these methods, but I have rarely found a doctor to recommend any dietary or lifestyle modifications that you will find in this book. I have often seen patients who drink alcohol and eat foods high in sugars even on a daily basis when taking antifungal drugs, yet have not been instructed or recommended to stop by their doctor.

It is pointless taking any treatment if the maintaining causes are not addressed, otherwise you will only experience a likely return of the symptoms not long after the treatment is stopped.

Other treatments are recommended at times, and if a swab returns several pathogens (as in mixed infections with more than one microbe) then combination of treatments will be recommended.

Topically applied antifungal creams may include:

- Butoconazole
- Clotrimazole
- Miconazole
- Terconazole

Many times a woman will try to gain relief by using OTC (over-the-counter) topical treatments. However, it should always be borne in mind that an infection other than a candida yeast infection may cause similar symptoms, and I have described some of the most common presentations above. If over-the-counter products do not eliminate symptoms, I always recommend that you see your doctor for a thorough evaluation.

Oral antifungal medications may include:

- Clotrimazole
- Miconazole
- Terconazole
- Fluconazole
- Nystatin

Diflucan (Fluconazole)

Another popular oral medication for candida yeast infections includes Fluconazole (Diflucan). I am amazed how many women I have seen who have been prescribed Fluconazole weekly on an ongoing basis to counter vaginal yeast infections, sometimes for years, yet with no further recommendations in terms of dietary or lifestyle modifications. Incredibly, some of these women have taken Diflucan for five years or more, one tablet per week. I have helped many women who have taken this drug, and have found that most all can discontinue its use after a period of eight to twelve weeks, even those who have been taking Diflucan for several years.

Side Effects

Get emergency medical help if you have signs of an allergic reaction to Diflucan such as hives; difficult breathing; swelling of your face, lips, tongue, or throat.

These are the more serious side effects of Diflucan, see medical aid if you get any:

- Nausea, upper stomach pain, itching, loss of appetite, dark urine, clay-colored stools, jaundice (yellowing of the skin or eyes);
- Fever, chills, body aches, flu symptoms;
- Severe blistering, peeling, and red skin rash;

- Easy bruising or bleeding, unusual weakness; or

- Seizure (convulsions).

More common Diflucan side effects include:

- Mild stomach pain, diarrhea, upset stomach.

- Headache.

- Dizziness.

- Unusual or unpleasant taste in your mouth.

In my experience, most doctors would prefer to treat vaginal yeast infections with vaginal tablets or suppositories rather than oral medications. But, saying that, they are quick to prescribe an oral antifungal medication or anti-biotic if they notice little result with the topical treatment. Remember, while vaginal treatment is unlikely to cause these side effects, the same cannot be said of any oral antifungal or antibiotic medications. Be sure never to take Fluconazole if there is any likelihood of becoming pregnant.

This drug is not recommended for use during pregnancy. If you have been using this drug and have experienced any untoward side-effects, or if you have been on it for some time, then I would highly recommend an herbal treatment to clean up your liver for at least three to four weeks, because the liver can be affected significantly whilst taking this drug.

Good Tip

Avoid The Repeated Usage of Drugs

Unfortunately, the use of prescribed pharmaceutical antifungal drugs and creams, especially if repeated or chronically used, can only lead to the development of stronger strains of yeast that eventually become drug resistant. Higher dosages or stronger drugs are then required which only escalate the problem even further. Many doctors now no longer use Nystatin or even antibiotics because they only weaken a person's immune system and can damage certain organs like the liver and kidneys. If you ever treat yourself with any over-the-counter preparations and symptoms continue or recur within two months, it is wise to seek the advice from your health-care professional.

Endometriosis And Candida

A female medical doctor I know well went to a health conference in Canada several years ago and the topic was endometriosis. She said that both two days was spent discussing candida albicans infections, and there were many discussions on how to identify and treat yeast overgrowth in women. It is about time that we are finally starting to see more medical doctors who are practicing natural forms of medicine, because when I started to see patients it was something of a rarity to hear of a medical doctor who had much regard for natural forms of healing, and those that did profess to use natural medicines were treated as quacks, charlatans and snake oil peddlers.

Whilst I have met women with endometriosis who do not have thrush or a candida problem, I have not often met a woman with endometriosis who does not have some type of history of candida, and then who has generally suppressed the condition with a cream or antibiotic. She may have had the thrush many years ago, and this was then supposedly "cured", which only serves to drive it further into the endometrium, thereby potentially causing eventual endometriosis. Are you a female with vaginal thrush? Then my advice is to adopt the treatment plan outlined in the Candida Crusher to successfully eradicate the condition. It may be difficult or stubborn to cure when you first start treatment, but your persistence will pay off and you can eradicate this problem in time.

Your persistence will eventually pay off, and eradicating rather than suppressing an internal yeast infection will save you plenty of discomfort and misery in the future, and for you it may even be the difference between conceiving a child and remaining infertile. Let me enlighten you with a typical example of how a young girl can eventually develop endometriosis later in life, this is a real case except for the patient's name change.

Case History # 15
Jill, 22 years

I first saw Jill when she was about three years of age; her mother brought her in with eczema, an itchy skin condition. Jill was breast fed for only about one week, her mother was simply too tired and stressed with her two other younger children to breastfeed and placed Jill on a cow's milk based formula. Jill had already been prescribed a few rounds of a broad-spectrum antibiotic by the time she was three. She presented with dark circles under her eyes, was lethargic and had multiple skin lesions up her arms and on her torso and legs were scratched raw. We successfully treated her skin complaints with a diet change and special pro-biotics.

I saw Jill back when she was 15yrs old, but this time for post-viral fatigue. Jill was very tired and complained of headaches and falling asleep at school. Her mother had taken her to the doctors, where she received more antibiotics, all to no avail. She had menstrual cramps and occasional outbreaks of vaginal yeast infections.

I then saw Jill last year when she was 21, this time she presented with endometriosis, which her doctor had diagnosed the year before. Jill came to me concerned about her fertility as she had just become engaged and was regularly getting urinary tract infections. She had undergone surgery to remove several cysts and had experienced a low-grade pain since. This time we placed Jill on the Candida Crusher program, and the results have been fantastic – no more headaches, no more bowel or urinary problems and plenty of energy.

Here is a testimonial I received in the form of an email some time ago:

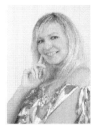 "Hi, my name is Karen Parker, I'm 39 years of age and I have been on your Candida Crusher Program for a little over three months now and the difference is amazing. Normally I have to have 2 or 3 days off work every month because of the pain with my endometriosis, but this month I was able to work through and only take pain relief medicines once over an entire day (as opposed to every 3-4 hours).

I've been trying to conceive for over 2 years now and have fallen pregnant 5 times but have suffered many miscarriages - I've also done 3 IVF cycles all to no avail. Candida Crusher makes sense; I now understand the link between endometriosis and thrush that I have suffered with for so many years.

I was a vegetarian and on a fairly strict diet, so cutting the rest out wasn't such a big change for and your diet advice made it easy to follow. Overall, I just feel so much better and have loads more energy, less pain and a renewed sense of hope. Thank you so much for your wonderful program." *Karen, London, England*

Vaginal Thrush Or Something Else?

Vaginal thrush infections are caused by yeast infections, the most common cause of vaginitis and are a cause of huge irritation and inconvenience for many women. Symptoms are itching in the groin area and in and around the vagina. Increased discharge is not necessarily present in this condition.

Remember, you are most likely at risk of developing candida fungal vaginal infections (thrush) increases if you:

- Have diabetes.

- Are pregnant.

- Habitually use an antibiotic.

- Take the oral contraceptive pill.

- Have a defective immune system.

These are some of the most likely causes, and they may lead you straight into a diagnosis of a vaginal yeast infection. A vaginal yeast infection is almost always caused by a change in the vagina's acid balance, which leads to an increase in yeast and an over growth. Yeast infections are often seen *after* a person takes antibiotics. Sometimes however, there may not be an obvious reason as to why a woman has developed a thrush infection. Diagnosis is straightforward however and can be confirmed by taking a swab from the vagina. Conventional treatment is either with pessaries (tablets in the vagina) or tablets by mouth. But is it vaginal thrush or is it something else? In just a moment we will look at a chart I put together which outlines the different kinds of vaginal problems you are most likely to experience, and their typical signs and symptoms.

Suppressive Treatments Don't Cure Vaginal Yeast Infections

Your doctor may prescribe topical therapies, and the first application may cause burning as you place a cream or vaginal suppository into your vagina. This mode of treatment is very effective and using these conventional methods cures seventy to ninety percent of thrush. But is it really cured, or has this form of treatment just suppressed the yeast because the cause was never addressed?

My belief is that this form of treatment is very suppressive indeed, i.e.; the condition is driven back into the body and because the causes remain untreated and thrush may recur at anytime. I tend to find that many women with endometriosis (and many other chronic "women's problems") can relate to having treated their vaginal yeast infection many years ago just like this, with local vaginal treatment and antibiotics, and believe they have "cured" it, only to discover in time that they are diagnosed with endometriosis or some other chronic women's problem.

The Whole Person Needs Treatment And Not Just Their Vagina

I've found from experience that an imbalance in the vaginal micro flora is most always indicative of a similar imbalance in a woman's digestive tract and further afield. Therefore, when a patient presents to my clinic with a recurrent vaginal yeast infection I always recommend that she follow the entire Candida Crusher Program. If the vaginal yeast infection is acute and not a recurrent problem however, an isolated instance can effectively be treated locally as I describe below without having to resort to systemic (diet and lifestyle) treatment. But if the problem resurfaces or is chronic, then the Candida Crusher Program is best followed for a complete resolution thrush of the thrush.

But What If It Is Not Vaginal Thrush, What Then?

Here are five other presentations besides vaginal thrush, and it is important that you know what you are dealing with before you commence treatment. As usual, it is always best to seek the help of your doctor when it comes to diagnosis, once a firm diagnosis is made and you know what you are dealing with you will be able to know how to treat it.

1

Trichomoniasis

Sometimes called "trich", trichomoniasis is different from the other complaints in that a small organism called a flagellate causes it. It is common to experience an abundant greenish-yellow discharge, an itching which can range from mild to extremely intense and even a strong burning sensation or pain in the vagina. Diagnosis is performed by analyzing a swab of the discharge. Treatment is generally a short course of (strong) antibiotics, after which I recommend to take a powerful probiotic product for four to six weeks thereafter.

2

Bacterial vaginosis (BV)

This condition is known as gardnerella vaginalis, and is caused by the growth of bacteria that causes the acidity of the vagina to become much more alkaline. Contributing factors are poor hygiene, poor health in general, birth-control IUD use, and in particular the transferring of E.coli bacteria from the rectal area to the vagina due to poor hygiene or sex.

The abundant alkalinity with this condition causes a fishy or brine-like smell and a grey foamy discharge. Diagnosis is carried out once again by analyzing a swab from the discharge, and the treatment is once again a short course of antibiotics.

Bacterial vaginosis is one of three common types of vaginitis (BV, vaginal yeast infection and trichomoniasis), and possibly the most common vaginal infection. Maybe you thought that vaginal yeast infections are the most common vaginal infection, well they are not, because BV is in fact the most common. A link between BV and low levels of vitamin D was discovered in June 2009 and reported by The Journal of Nutrition in *The New York Times.* My advice is to have a blood test for vitamin D and see what your levels are, you may be quite surprised to know that most of the population are borderline to low in the crucial immune boosting fat-soluble vitamin. Ensure good hygiene with sex, because many cases come from not enough care taken during sex.

3

Gonorrhea

Gonorrhea is an STD (sexually transmitted disease) that is caused by the gonococcus bacteria. You can have gonorrhea without experiencing any symptoms, but some people experience burning pain when urinating. However, gonorrhea is rarely seen these days. Diagnosis is confirmed by analyzing a swab from the cervix, urethra (entrance to the bladder) or back passage. Treatment is with very powerful antibiotics. Sexual partners should also be traced, tested for gonorrhea and treated accordingly.

4

Chlamydia

Chlamydia is likewise a sexually transmitted disease and is an unusual cause of vaginitis, because infection often does not produce symptoms unless pelvic inflammatory disease is present. Diagnosis is made by analyzing a sample taken from the cervix or the urethra. Treatment is with antibiotics. Sexual partners should be traced, tested and treated.

Genital Herpes

Genital herpes (Herpes type 2) is caused by the herpes simplex virus and is almost in all cases a sexually transmitted disease. It is possible to infect the genital area with the virus via contact with a cold sore (herpes type 1, part of the same family). Herpes is seen at the entrance to the vagina as small blisters. The first time a person has herpes, it is common for them to develop a fever, and night sweats may occur, swollen lymph nodes in the groin on the affected side, general discomfort is experienced, urination is painful, and the lips and entrance to the vagina may become swollen and red.

Eventually the herpes infection settles down, and the person experiences flare-ups ranging from very occasionally to very rarely. The skin in the affected area will become more sensitive and signal an imminent case of herpes.

A tingling sensation can be felt and then the blisters may appear which can itch intensely, and may even create a burning sensation if ruptured. It is in the herpes sufferer's best interests to discover how to improve their health to the point where they rarely experience these flare-ups. In conventional medicine, a diagnosis is made by a doctor based on the appearance and with special swabs sent for analysis. Antiviral treatment is often recommended, but you will find in this case that natural medicine has a lot to offer this patient. If you have herpes, especially if it is severe, I can highly recommend a course of natural medicine treatment for at least six to twelve months, because, unfortunately, doctors view herpes infections as "incurable" disease requiring a lifetime of drugs in order to suppress the symptoms.

Signs and Symptoms of Vaginal Infections & Inflammations					
Infection	Pain	Discharge	Odor	Itching	Lesions
Yeast Infections (yeast infection)	Not generally	Thick, white like cottage cheese	Yeasty or musty smell	Can be very severe	Red lesions or pimples
Herpes Type 2 (Genital) (Viral infection)	Yes. Small sores can burn or sting	No	No	Yes, can be severe after blisters form	Small blisters filled with clear fluid
Trichomoniasis (STD – Parasite)	Burning urine Painful sex	Copious grey to green, frothy	Foul or strong smell	Yes	Small red ulcers on vaginal wall or cervix.
Gardnerella (bacterial infection)	Usually without irritation	Thin, watery gray or green	Fishy smell	Not generally	No
Atrophic Vaginitis (hysterectomy or menopause)	Painful sex	Could be watery or burning discharge	No	Yes	Reduced estrogen can lead to adhesions
Chlamydia (STD – Bacteria)	Pain on urination Abdominal pain	Yellow discharge	Strong smell	May cause anus to itch & bleed	Complications include fallopian tube scarring
Gonorrhoea (STD – Bacteria)	Pain on urination Abdominal pain	Creamy or green, pus-like or bloody vaginal discharge	Odorless	Itchy or irritable vulva	Complications include pelvic inflammatory disease

Both parties need treatment

Whenever you are diagnosed with any kind of vaginal infection or inflammation, it is important to understand that your partner could (almost probably does) have the same infection too. Why play "pass the parcel;" you and your partner should be treated at the same time to keep from re-infecting each other again. Be sure to tell any recent sex partners as well, so they can get tested and treated. This is a key to prevent re-infection, and unless you pay attention to this most important point there is very much the risk of a continual infection.

The Vaginal Implant Protocol For Chronic Vaginal Thrush

Introduction

Here is a local treatment I have been recommending for many years with great results. It is in two parts, the "kill" phase and the "build" phase. I recommend that you employ this treatment for at least three months (twelve weeks) on a regular basis for best results. You will get the results you are looking for a cure by following my Candida Crusher dietary approach, taking the Candida Crusher supplements (outlined in chapter 7, section 4) and following the local vaginal implant protocol to the letter.

Yes, it is highly possible and most probably likely that your vaginal yeast infection will be completely eradicated by doing this the right way. You will get out of a program exactly what you put into it, if you are diligent and follow this protocol correctly you will be delighted with the results, I can vouch for the many women I have helped with this condition over the years, and I'm sure that most would agree with me on this with many of these cases being quite severe and of long duration.

When Should I Do The Treatments And For How Long?

The anti-microbial treatment can be used from one up to five days in a row in general, and it is up to you how long you wish to treat for. It depends on your level of comfort/discomfort and basically the effort you are willing to go to. Remember to always alternate between the antimicrobial and the beneficial implant protocol.

I have noticed that some women get more results when they do two or three anti-microbial treatments before their period, and then do several pro-biotic treatments after their menstrual cycle, whereas others just do them as a sets (the anti-microbial and pro-biotic) several times both before and after their menstrual cycle. I now prefer that women work out what is best for them, and this is because some get more relief with one part of this treatment phase, for example, anti-microbial versus the other.

You will soon work out what is best for you, the duration, what and how to use it and gauge the effectiveness of the treatment based on the results you are getting. And, always remember - treatments locally work the most effectively when they are employed along with the Candida Crusher Diet. Yes, I do repeat myself but I do it to really place emphasis on certain points.

Here is the implant treatment protocol I recommend for various conditions affecting the vagina or vulva. This is the protocol I have recommended for over fifteen years and with great success, women report that they get fantastic results – some in as little as 24 hours. There are two phases here that I recommend, and this is what makes all the difference. You will be changing the pH level of the vagina by doing so and will get results that much quicker.

Some programs I have seen just recommend the build stage (using yogurt) and others recommend the kill stage (garlic) by I recommend that you employ BOTH of these stages periodically, especially if you have chronic or recurring thrush. Do you use Fluconazole regularly (Diflucan)? Then you should most certainly do the following protocol, along with the Candida Crusher program.

STAGE 1

The Kill Stage

I have found from experience that the Kill stage works best in the week leading up to and including the menstrual period itself, and it is important to continue the implant during the menstrual stage, although you may want to omit the heaviest flow day. Continue until the flow has stopped completely.

Wait for two days before you commence with the Build stage. This will allow the vagina and its surrounding vulva skin environment to build up the beneficial flora it requires to maintain ideal health.

You may need to experiment here with the Kill Stage, some women may experience a change in their flow or even an increase in their premenstrual syndrome symptoms if they start too strong with the Kill Stage, if you have a history of premenstrual difficulties (PMT or PMS), endometriosis, polycystic ovarian syndrome (PCOS) then you may need to be cautious in your approach to any Kill treatments leading up to your menstrual period.

That is not to say that you should avoid it, just be more careful and start with a mild treatment the first month in particular.

It takes about three menstrual cycles in chronic cases to really notice the difference, so don't give up after the first month! You may well find that after completing these Kill and Build cycles for 4 – 6 months along with the Candida Crusher Diet, Lifestyle recommendations and Candida Crusher dietary supplements, that there will be a noticeable improvement in your premenstrual complaints and endometriosis. This is what I have noticed after working with many women, the feedback has been great.

This protocol can most successfully be used for:

- Chronic vaginal thrush
- Candida vaginal yeast infections
- Bacterial infections such as Gardnerella

The KILL Stage - Antimicrobial Treatment Protocol

- A - 1 crushed clove of garlic. Buy organic and use fresh. Kyolic ™ aged garlic extract can be used if you travel a lot, but I prefer to recommend fresh as it gives outstanding results most every time, I have verified this with hundreds of cases. Fresh garlic is *always* best when it comes to thrush.

- B - 1/2 teaspoon of apple cider vinegar (use a quality product like Bragg's)

- C - 1 tablespoon of yoghurt. (Buy the best natural yogurt you can find)

- Insert A, B and C at night before bed. Wear a sanitary napkin or panty pad to bed.

- Be aware that garlic is bactericidal, and may affect the beneficial bacteria that were introduced with the initial implant program.

- Some women just use the garlic and yogurt, others use the garlic, yogurt and vinegar. Do what best suits your needs.

- Always re-introduce beneficial bacteria using the Probiotic implant protocol for one week after completing the antimicrobial protocol.

- Follow the KILL & BUILD protocol several times a year to help maintain a very healthy vaginal environment.

- During the KILL phase, take the recommended probiotic by mouth: 1 capsule twice daily. You want to improve immunity and plant good bacteria in the digestive tract, reducing the chances of transferring too many bad bacteria from the perineum to the vaginal area. Always remember to wipe front to back.

- Always use this protocol in conjunction with my Candida Crusher Program recommendations. You will have a much better chance of an excellent outcome that way.

- Best Results: do the local treatment, do the diet, maintain the lifestyle, and take the Candida Crusher supplements as recommended.

- For a really good kill, alternate this Kill Stage with Boric Acid Vaginal Suppository Treatment, you can read all about this at the end of this chapter. By doing this you will get a 99.99% chance of success and will knock out even the worst of cases.

- When you have intestinal candida (like when you have bloating, gas, diarrhea, etc.) and at the same time have vaginal thrush, I want you to do the Kill stage in conjunction with Grapefruit Seed Extract Vaginal Treatment, and not the boric acid treatment. GSE is more indicated because it will greatly assist in reducing any vaginal/fecal contamination from occurring.

- Using this protocol and this alone while ignoring diet and lifestyle - while maintaining the cause - will give you temporary results at best. And that's NOT what you bought this book for– you wanted a permanent result with your vaginal thrush. Just do it!

Simple Kill And Build Phases

Garlic tampons, capsules or fresh garlic can be inserted intra-vaginally in the morning (kill treatment) and then lactobacillus capsules can be inserted in the evening (build treatment) to create a plan that both inhibits growth of the offending organism and re-populates the delicate vaginal micro-flora to its normal healthy state.

STAGE 2

The BUILD Stage

Always follow the Kill Stage with the Build Stage. Some women may complete a few Kill Stages and then do the Build Stage, as they experience more relief that way, whereas others will get a good result by just rotating these Stages. You will need to experiment to see what works best for you.

Wait at least two days after you have completed the Kill Stage before you commence this Stage, you need to get the beneficial vaginal bacteria built up a bit more.

Do not complete this stage during the period itself; the Kill Stage is OK during your period however, but do skip treatments on your heaviest flow days.
If you want to avoid any aggravations, you don't need to be as careful with the Build Stage as you do with the Kill Stage if you have a history of premenstrual difficulties (PMT or PMS), endometriosis, or polycystic ovarian syndrome (PCOS). But you will need to use common sense, and if you have experienced and serious genito-urinary complaint then you should always go very slow at the start until you gain more confidence and experience.

The BUILD Stage – The Pro-biotic Implant Protocol

Mix together:

- High potency Probiotic powder 1 teaspoon

- Low fat plain yoghurt 10 ml or the whey on top of the yogurt (straw like fluid).

- Use a 10 ml syringe or applicator to insert the mixture well into the vagina, in the evening before bed.

- Wear a sanitary napkin (maxi is best) or panty pad to bed.

- My advice is NOT to use a tampon here; the best feedback I get from women (several hundred) is when they use pads.

- In the morning, cleanse with a douche of 300-400 ml of boiled or filtered water mixed with 1 level teaspoon of powdered probiotic.

- Repeat *each evening* for 7 days.

- Is the infection not clear after 7 days of this regime, then consider other organisms such as Chlamydia or Trichomoniasis that may be present. You may want to visit your doctor and have a pelvic exam to determine what is going on.

- In some cases a stronger antimicrobial treatment is required.

- Follow the KILL & BUILD protocol several times a year to help maintain a healthy vaginal environment.

- Always use this protocol in conjunction with the Candida Crusher Program recommendations. You will have a much better chance of an excellent outcome that way. Do the diet, maintain the lifestyle and do the local treatment.

- Using this protocol and this alone (while maintaining the underlying cause) will only give you temporary results. And that's not what you bought the Candida Crusher, I expect that you want a permanent result.

The Pro-Biotic Powder And Whey Douche

There are a few options and variations to this yogurt douche protocol, and some very effective ones too. One of the best douche protocols is the pro-biotic powder and whey douche (Build). This is a variation on the plain yogurt douche, and can be used even more successfully if alternated with the Tea Tree oil douche (Kill) mentioned below. You will notice that this method like the vaginal implant protocol has a build phase (the pro-biotic powder and whey douche) as well as the Tea Tree Oil douche (the kill phase). Using this two-step kill and then build protocol is the key to success in chronic vaginal thrush, and is not emphasized enough in most all books I have read on this topic.

Instead of using yogurt, use whey liquid; try Molkosan from Bioforce, a Swiss company. It is a particularly rich source of lactic acid and a great natural product you can use to most successfully eradicate a vaginal yeast infection. Simply mix a level teaspoon of a top quality pro-biotic powder (Lactobacillus acidophilus) in about a half-tablespoon of whey solution and a little tepid water. Be sure to use tepid or room temperature water as well as whey solution, as this will be your vaginal douche solution. Insert using an applicator and use a pad as mentioned above. Leave overnight preferably like the yogurt douche.

The Best Aromatherapy Oils To Use In Vaginal Thrush

According to one Salvatore Battaglia, who wrote the textbook widely regarded as one of the world's best books on the subject of aromatherapy, (The Complete Guide to Aromatherapy, The Perfect Potion, 1995) the best essentials oils to for a yeast infection are German chamomile, geranium, lavender, lemongrass, myrrh, petit grain, tea tree and thyme.

Aromatherapy Treatment

The treatment Salvatore recommends is baths and local applications of essential oils. The oils mentioned above have been selected because of their antiseptic, antifungal and immune-stimulating properties. A sitz bath is very effective for vaginal irritation; 2-3 drops of the essential oil should be added to the bidet or large bowl of warm water and used twice daily if symptoms persist.

The Aromatherapy Douche For Itching And Soreness

Valerie Ann Worwood (The Fragrant Pharmacy. MacMillan, London, 1990) recommends a douche using whole milk yogurt containing live acidophilus cultures.

German chamomile	5 drops
Lavender oil	5 drops
Tea tree oil	5 drops

Add the above oils to a 100-gram carton of fresh yogurt. The yogurt combined with the essential oils has the dual action of antibiotic and antifungal properties. Use valerie's method if there is a considerable amount of soreness and incessant itching. Use either an applicator for inserting pessaries or a tampon applicator.

Another way of using yogurt is by diluting it with warm spring water until you have made a thin fluid. Then the essential oils are added and this mixture is used in a douche, washing the vaginal tract twice daily.

The Tea Tree Oil Douche

Tea tree oil is one of the best natural medicines you will ever use with a yeast infection, but please be sure to get the Australian Tea Tree Oil. , I have recommended Tea Tree Oil for over twenty years for yeast infections and am never disappointed with the fantastic feedback I routinely get from patients. The best maple syrup comes from Canada and the best Tea Tree Oil comes from Australia.

Vaginal Douche – Get water-soluble Tea Tree Oil (water miscible)

Remember that Tea Tree oil is an Oil, but you can also get this product in a water miscible (water soluble) form, and this is the one you want for the douche. Many books and articles regarding yeast infections will tell you to use the oil in water. While you can use the oil in douche protocols, the oil will only float on the water and you simply won't get the same amazing results than if you use a product which FULLY dissolves in water, it may work for some and some swear by it, do try both and see what suits you best.

Get the pure oil for stubborn skin areas, especially on the feet and toes as well as toe nails. It is totally safe to use on nails, and unlike thyme or oregano oil, there is little risk in this oil causing any burning sensations.

Place about 300mls tepid water into a shallow bowl, add 1 teaspoon water miscible (water-soluble) Tea Tree Oil and mix well. Fill a douche bag with the tea tree solution and apply as required to the vagina. The tea tree oil is anti-inflammatory but also an effective anti-fungal. Tea Tree Oil Vaginal Pessary And Douche Combo – Even Better

Tea Tree Oil Vaginal Pessary And Douche Combo – Even Better

Australian Tea Tree Oil is one of the best things you can use when you have a vaginal yeast infection, its just one of those medicines that works consistently time and again. A Tea Tree Oil douche has been used and recommended by alternative medicine doctors for over 50 years now for vaginal yeast infections, literally since the discovery of the remarkable natural anti fungal.

Use from eight to ten drops of the pure Australian Tea Tree Oil in 500 milliliters (or 1 pint) of tepid purified or distilled water. Douching in between pessary applications seems to be the best solution in ridding your vagina from the discomfort including the burning and incessant itching of a candida vaginal yeast infection.

Try Water- Soluble Tea Tree Oil

For women who want to use Tea Tree Oil in a douche will need to get the water-soluble Tea Tree Oil, you can use the pure oil or you can get a water-soluble Tea Tree Oil, see what works best for you. I have known several people over the years that have successfully treated their own cracked heels, tinea, athlete's feet with a warm foot spa, and including in the water plenty of water-soluble tea tree oil.

Those of us who use essential oils and know them well will tell you that apart from oregano oil, tea tree essential oil is the best anti-fungal used straight on stubborn areas of skin, jock itch, fungal nails. Use the Tea Tree Oil as spot skin, scalp or nail treatment, and use the water-soluble tea tree oil for when you want to do a douche or wash areas of skin in general.

Tea tree oil can be applied directly to candida skin problems (especially the toes or with athletes foot) or add to bath water. The water-soluble Tea Tree Oil is perfect for candida yeast infected patients; use a small amount (about 1/4 - 1/2 teaspoon to 1 cup of tepid water) as a douche or to wash the skin, feet or other areas of the body. This is the one time I do recommend that you use a tampon – make up a solution of water soluble Tea Tree Oil and water (you can try a weak solution first, like ¼ teaspoon of the water soluble oil to 1 cup of tepid water) and if all is well go stronger, such as 1 teaspoon of the water soluble oil to a quarter cup of the water. I know some women who use the Tea Tree essential oil neat on a tampon, but I do not recommend this for you until you gain sufficient experience with Tea Tree Oil and understand how it affects you in different ways. I believe that Tea Tree Oil is possibly the best product to use vaginally, besides oregano oil or fresh garlic. Try the probiotic & whey douche and alternate with the Tea Tree Oil douche. You will be quite surprised.

Two Most Powerful Treatments

Here now are two of the most powerful vaginal treatments which will be sure to work, even if ALL other treatments fail, that's why I've kept the best two treatments until last, the Grapefruit Seed Extract Vaginal Treatment and the Boric Acid Vaginal Suppository Treatment.

Grapefruit Seed Extract (GSE) Vaginal Treatment

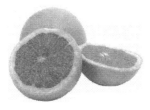

This is a good treatment to use especially if you have more than a vaginal yeast infection. If you have digestive problems AND vaginal thrush, do this one. If the boric acid treatment fails (it is successful in most cases) then try this treatment. Boric acid treatment is perfect for local thrush, whether it be acute or chronic. You can also alternate the GSE treatment with boric acid, and this I recommend for the "impossible" cases.

Treatment Method

<u>GSE Tampon</u>: Soak a tampon in 1 tablespoon of vegetable oil and 5 drops of grapefruit seed extract which have been mixed together very well. Insert the tampon and leave it overnight. Repeat for 3 – 4 nights.

<u>Vaginal GSE Rinse</u>: Add fifteen drops of Grapefruit Seed Extract to sixteen ounces of room temperature water (use only boiled, filtered, or distilled water) and shake well in a closed jar. Douche once per day for three to four days. (For greater retention of the solution, douche in a reclining position.) Repeat every seventh day thereafter.

Caution: If an uncomfortable level of vaginal irritation occurs, reduce mixture to five drops per pint (600 mls) of tepid water. Discontinue if irritation persists. Avoid douching if pregnant or menstruating unless advised by your health-care professional.

Boric Acid Vaginal Suppository Treatment

Some people get concerned when I talk about an acid when it comes to vaginal treatment, thinking that it will burn and cause a lot of pain, but this is untrue. It is important to remember that vinegar and lemon juice are kinds acid too and are equally safe to use.

Boric acid is a safe and non-toxic white crystalline powder that has anti-fungal and anti-bacterial qualities and is available without a prescription. It is has many different applications and is a very effective insecticide as well, mix it with oil and it will attract ants and roaches that will die after eating it. A good remedy for oral thrush in infants Is homeopathic remedy Borax 6 c.

Boric Acid Vaginal Suppository Treatment is particularly effective for stubborn and resistant cases of vaginal yeast infection when used in conjunction with the two phase Build and Kill stages you just read before.

How To Make Boric Acid Vaginal Suppositories

It is really easy to make your own boric acid suppositories, just get some 00 gelatin capsules and fill them with boric acid, about 500 to 600 mg. You can get boric acid and the gelatin or cellulose two-piece capsules from your chemist (drug store) or good health-food shop.

Make a lot of them up at once because they will keep for a very long time if stored dry and cool for at least a year. When you store them, place them in a container (use an old vitamin container) and drop in a sachet or two of those little packets of silicon which will help to keep your caps free of moisture and potentially harden up over time. Don't keep in the refrigerator.

Treatment Method

Insert one capsule at bedtime for a seven to ten day period. Alternate with lactobacillus acidophilus treatment in the day and boric acid at night. For recurring and stubborn cases treat for 30 days straight and after the month treat two days out of seven for even up to one year. Best results in the impossible cases are when you alternate this treatment with the GSE treatment, AND use the two-phase protocol outlined above. Treat even during your period, but stop on the few days when your flow is the heaviest.

Caution: Avoid these kinds of treatments if you are pregnant. Like GSE, keep boric acid away from children.

The Best Herbs For A Vaginal Yeast Infection

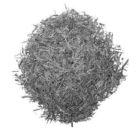 There are many ways you can use herbal medicines when it comes to vaginal thrush, but the most common ways are to make a strong decoction (simmering and using the solution) or infusions (making a tea) of these herbs to ease itching and burning; use either internally as a douche or apply externally with pads or tampons that have been soaked in the solution. It is always best to treat internally (The Candida Crusher Program) as well as externally with any yeast infection.

Andrographis, Aniseed, Chaste Tree, Echinacea Root, **Garlic** (topically), **Oregano** (topically), **Pau D'arco** (topically), **Tea Tree Oil** (use the essential oil externally), Thyme (use the essential oil externally)

Pau D'arco Vaginal Treatment

Pau D'arco is an herbal medicine that comes from the inner bark of a tall rainforest tree. It is very important that you get the real deal and not some fake product, which is often the case when it comes to the high-demand herb.

The precise dosage I recommend is based on a lapachol content of between 2 – 4 percent. Boil 15-20 grams of the inner bark in 500 milliliters (or 1 pint) of pure water, don't use tap water, for 10 to 15 minutes. Bring to the rolling boil then cover and *very gently* simmer. Do not use an aluminimium saucepan, use stainless steel.

A tampon that has been soaked in this tepid solution is perfect to most effectively treat any vaginal infection. Insert the tampon and change every 24 hours until resolution. This treatment works, especially if you get the real Pau D'arco and not a fake product. You can read more about the remarkeable herb Pau D'arco in chapter 7, section 4.

Conventional Medical Yeast Treatment

Natural Versus Conventional Medical Treatment

> *The good physician treats the disease;*
> *the great physician treats the patient who has the disease.*
> Sir William Osler

Less than one hundred years ago all health complaints were treated with natural methods, which is today seen as an alternative to science based healthcare.

What was once normal and even practiced by conventional doctors of the day is now frowned upon as fringe medicine.

Modern science and the expensive marketing of powerful and profitable pharmaceutical drugs have ensured that the modern approach is in favor of the drug-based approach. This trend has been slowly but surely reversing the past two decades, as many people are now demanding a more natural and side effect free approach towards their healthcare. While I firmly believe that the conventional science based approach to medicine has its place, conventional treatment relies on powerful chemical based medicines that only suppress symptoms. Natural treatments work more indirectly by strengthening the body's innate healing responses and in finding the actual causes rather than just relying on treating the symptoms. Many patients come to us seeking assistance with their yeast infections because they have not only become disillusioned with a lack of permanent results, they have become concerned about the risks and potentially serious side effects of the drug-based approach and want to finally get to the root cause of their health problems.

Your health can be improved profoundly with the help of an experienced practitioner of natural medicine or medical doctor who has a good working knowledge of natural medicine. If you want to stay remain under the care of a conventional medical doctor, it is preferable that your doctor has had formal training in natural medicine, and doctors who have had this kind of training have become medical practitioners initially, and then furthered their studies to include nutritional medicine and maybe even herbal medicine and homeopathy.

You should be able to find an alternative doctor online in your country through a professional association. I have worked in medical clinics for fifteen years and come to know many alternative medicine doctors during that period of time. I can highly recommend any naturopath to spend a few years working alongside doctors to understand the medical system and to learn valuable skills they would otherwise never gain. In addition, it is also preferable that your natural health-care professional has a good understanding and respect for the conventional medical system and will know when to refer you on when necessary.

Today in the 21st century, many people are interested in the best of both worlds, i.e. the benefits that medical sciences as well as natural medicine have to offer combined.

People have become a lot more informed through the Internet these days, and more gentle forms of treatment are generally preferred with the least amount of intervention before powerful drugs or invasive procedures are employed. In this sense it is good to work in conjunction with an experienced naturopath who has undertaken high-level health science based training, or a medical doctor who has undertaken post-graduate natural medicine training. The ultimate is for you to form a relationship with both of these health-care professionals so that you can get a more balanced viewpoint when it comes to the treatment of your yeast infection and associated health problems.

Which ever way your candida yeast infection is treated, it is important for your practitioner to individualize your treatment, because bio-individuality is one of the major factors in achieving a successful course of yeast infection treatment with long lasting benefits to you, the patient.

Although people may share similar signs and symptoms of a yeast infection, some practitioners may try to give all patients with a candida diagnosis virtually an identical form of treatment. I have learned that yeast infection is similar to adrenal fatigue, there is often no single way that even two persons can have exactly the same signs and symptom patterns and therefore be treated identically. Even identical twins have been found to have a different expression of the same illness. That is why they call a yeast infection a "syndrome", which is a collection of signs and symptoms that can vary from person to person. And this may create more problems for the medical practitioner than it can for the natural medicine practitioner, because the doctor will treat the disease and its symptoms as individual illnesses, whereas the naturopath will treat the person as an individual and his or her symptoms as a whole.

Seek Out An Experienced Clinician

There are many variables to consider and this is where the experienced practitioner will succeed when the inexperienced practitioner may fail to help you. If you are looking for a natural medicine health-care professional, then go to the end of chapter 3 and read the ten simple tips to guide you in what to look for when choosing a natural medicine health-care professional, and then ask your practitioner if he or she has experience in treating cases of intestinal dysbiosis and candida. If he or she does not appear to be confident, then find somebody who is. You practitioner should be able to emphatically say, "YES, I can help you, I have experience with yeast infections!"

There are many reasons why patients seek out a more natural treatment for their yeast infection problems in the end, and I have found in most cases it is because the conventional treatments have to be applied continually, and at times for many years on end, and still there are symptoms which occur as soon when the treatment is reduced or discontinued. Seeking conventional treatment can be scary for some; because drug based treatments for yeast infections can potentially have many side effects, and there is no guarantee of any cure either, just symptom control.

I never make any guarantees with patients; I only tell them that if they guarantee to do everything as right as they can and for as long as it takes, then this kind of resolve can only end in eventual success, outstanding health free from any yeast infection.

And I have proven to be correct in many instances of chronic yeast infection cases, with most patients remaining free of a candida infection many years after they first came to my clinic.

Why Do Many Medical Practitioners Miss Candida Infections?

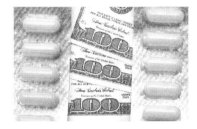 This is really quite simple to answer, since the effective treatment of candida requires a strong element of dietary intervention and immune system buildup, prestigious mainstream medical journals such as the New England Journal of Medicine and the Lancet have not much interest in this condition as a disease entity. What is happening in much of the Western developed world is that the pharmaceutical drug industry is setting the standard of medical practice.

Because pharmaceutical drug companies have dominated the academic institutions, you aren't likely to see articles published in medical journals on candida yeast infections, and the medical practitioner who relies on medical journals therefore will most likely miss the candida connection with patients. If you find this hard to believe, just read the mainstream medical journals yourself, and you will soon realize that pharmaceutical interests dominate them.

The conventional medical journals have helped to create and sustain over the years a scientific environment that is dictated by the profit-filled interests of the drug industry, busy promoting its own financial welfare. It is important to remember that the sales of pharmaceutical drugs have become more profitable than any other industrial product globally. Do you think I am cynical? I have been involved in natural medicine for over half my life and worked with countless practitioners of both natural and Western conventional medicine disciplines and know this to be a fact. You need to have your own interests at heart when it comes to your own health and have a good degree of common sense as well.

Here are the four key reasons I believe that the mainstream medical practitioner miss the boat when it comes to candida:

1

Doctors Prescribe Drugs That Can Cause Candida

One reason I feel that many medical practitioners virtually ignore yeast infections in their patients is that they prescribe antibiotics which are the very drugs that are most often implicated in the causation of candida in the first place. How can you recognize and treat a condition that you could have helped to initiate in your patient? This to me is like the person who sells alcohol and then turns a blind eye to the violence and other social problems that develop as a consequence to alcohol. The profits are certainly there but the responsibility isn't. It may seem a cynical statement at first, but antibiotics are the root cause of many health problems globally, particularly yeast infections and antibiotic resistant bacterial infections. My recommendations are for you to think carefully before you take any antibiotic, especially if you already have a candida yeast infection. The same goes with many different kinds of drugs which may be implicated, and you can read a lot more about these drugs in the chapter about causes.

2

Patients Have To Be Diagnosed Before Treatment

Another reason why candida is overlooked is that patients need to be diagnosed by the doctor before treatment can be started, and if you can't accurately diagnose the disease, then you can't treat it according to the evidence based medical practitioner.

Many candida patients I see will have already been to their doctor who will have dismissed the patient's concerns because no diagnosis of candida can be established. This is not the fault of your doctor by any means, conventional medical practitioners focus on treating the symptoms and the disease and not on health and wellness, so you may not get much joy here complaining of burping, bloating, food allergies and a whole host of other non-descript signs and symptoms associated with poor digestion, so common in candida.

You may either end up with a prescription for a pharmaceutical drug, possibly an antibiotic, further impeding digestion and adding to the maintaining cause, or be referred to a gastroenterologist who will in turn poke you and prod you with the various tests on offer and once again conclude that "all is well" and send you back to your doctor. This is my experience regarding doctors with regard to many different digestive disorders that people complain of; patients are often diagnosed as "NAD" (No Abnormal Diagnosis). This is the area where naturopaths make their bread and butter, we don't necessarily have to diagnose, and we just treat. The experienced naturopath will request an advanced stool test and/or refer to a gastroenterologist when treatment is unsuccessful or the patient is not responding to natural treatment methods. I talk about functional medicine testing (Comprehensive Digestive Stool Analysis) in chapter 3, and if you have skipped this chapter then I'd suggest that you read it now after you bookmark this page. Personally, I tend to skip and skim through medical books myself, picking out what I need and when I need it and eventually end up reading the entire book. Don't be afraid to underline something important in the Candida Crusher, because if it is important enough for you then do highlight it, it's your book!

Doctors Disallow A Patient's Subjective Feelings

I always find that the major foundation for determining the presence of candida and for monitoring the treatment of a candida yeast infection is the patient's important subjective feedback. Most busy doctors tend to have quick five to ten minute consultations that don't really allow the patient to elaborate on their problems, and in some sense the patient has almost become almost a bystander in the process of their treatment. Amazing, but the side effects derived from pharmaceutical drugs are actually seen as collateral damage when it comes to the treatment. Naturopaths take their time and spend a full hour and sometimes even an hour and a half with their new patient. This is how much time you really need to allow the patient to express how they feel.

One conventional doctor I know told me that he has become tired of practicing with one hand on the doorknob, and one eye on his computer screen watching to see who is in the waiting room, all while a patient is sitting in front of him. Dr. Wilson, the adrenal fatigue expert, mentioned to me once that he employed a new receptionist in his clinic many years ago. She said how much she enjoyed working in her new job because; unlike the medical clinics she has worked in previously, the patients in Dr. Wilson's clinic were actually "getting better".

These are but two of many examples that make me realize why I had my doubts about becoming a conventional doctor many years ago. Could I have helped patients more or achieved better clinical outcomes by having been conventionally medically trained? I doubt it, in some sense it probably would have handicapped me and made me more disease-focused rather than patient-centered, and that would have been a tragedy in terms of the patient outcomes I now achieve.

It is incredible how many times we see patients as naturopaths who tell their doctor that something is not right with their health, they communicate these subjective feelings, yet all their test results come back OK. What is the doctor to do in these instances? In most cases, the patient will be told that nothing is wrong and that it may be a case of depression and an antidepressant may be prescribed.

Doctors Work Within Normal Ranges Of Tests And Prescribe For Symptoms

I have found that a "normal" range in terms of blood and stool and other tests can vary considerably from patient to patient. Physicians practicing orthodox medicine always focus on the lab results, in the belief that by pushing the results back to normal they will resolve the signs and symptoms of the illness, all while the difficulties continue to arise from the root cause, which is rarely if ever fully addressed. It is more likely that they cover up the real problem, and often jump from one symptom to another, depending on the severity of the complaint at the time.

For example, a doctor may treat a patient's vaginal discharge with local treatment such as an applicator and a cream, ignoring the totality of the signs and symptoms the patient presents with all in the belief that these are all separate conditions and not inter-connected. While it is correct that the discharge certainly requires local treatment, it should always be treated as part of a holistic approach to get the true results the patient is longing for, a complete cure of all signs and symptoms of a candida yeast infection.

Can Conventional Medical Treatment Cause Vaginal Yeast Infections?

Absolutely, and amazingly, this is very often the case. Vaginal yeast infections occur when new yeast is introduced into the vaginal area, or when there is an increase in the quantity of yeast already present in the vagina relative to the quantity of normal vaginal flora (beneficial vaginal bacteria). For example, when the normal and protective bacteria are eradicated by antibiotics, which can be commonly prescribed to treat a urinary tract, respiratory, or other type of infection, or by immunosuppressive drugs, the yeast can multiply, invade tissues, and cause irritation of the lining of the vagina, a condition called vaginitis. Worse still, patients on massive amounts of immune-suppressive drugs, like those who are HIV positive for example, may even succumb to disseminated candidiasis, which we talk about in a minute.

Vaginal yeast infections can also occur as a result of injury to the inner vagina, such as after chemotherapy. Also, women with suppressed immune systems, for example, those taking cortisone-related medications like prednisone, can develop vaginal yeast infections more frequently than women with normal immunity.

Other conditions that may predispose women to developing vaginal yeast infections include diabetes mellitus, pregnancy, and taking oral contraceptives. The more frequent use today of douches or perfumed vaginal hygiene sprays may also increase a woman's risk of developing a vaginal yeast infection.

OTC (Over The Counter) And Prescriptive Pharmaceutical Drugs

" *To believe that sickness results solely from the visitation of some itinerant germ or virus and to accept treatment by some poisonous drug is to be found guilty of the most naive superstition.* "
Dr. D. Phillips

The tragedy I have found is that a patient can experience many of the typical signs and symptoms of candida infection, like itchy skin, bowel complaints, fatigue, dizziness and a host of other complaints, yet when all the tests are performed nothing can be found by their doctor. This often leads the patient down the road of OTC drugs; they may visit a chemist and buy a cream or a tablet on the advice of the pharmacist.

Doctors are more prone to treating women than men when it comes to candida yeast infections, I have discovered that many conventional doctors are not really convinced that males too can suffer from a yeast infection, and believe that is solely a "woman's problem".

So what then is the treatment for vaginal yeast infection and vulvovaginitis? Vaginal yeast infections may be commonly treated with antifungal medications that are applied topically in and around the vagina or with antifungal medications taken by mouth. Sometimes, mixed infections with more than one type of microbe can require combinations of treatments. And what about guys, what treatments are they offered if they see their chemist? A man will most likely be offered similar drugs a woman will.

Topically Applied Antifungal Creams

- Butoconazole, Clotrimazole, Miconazole, and Terconazole.

The over-the-counter topical treatments are an option for some women when yeast is the cause of the infection. However, it should be noted that infection other than yeast could cause similar symptoms. These include bacterial vaginosis and sexually transmitted diseases such as chlamydia and gonorrhea. Be sure to read chapter 5 as it will give you a good overview of the different problems you are likely to encounter which are very similar to a vaginal yeast infection.

If you cannot eliminate the symptoms yourself with over-the-counter products, then good advice is to see your doctor, obstetrician or gynecologist for a complete medical exam and evaluation. At least then you will have a formal diagnosis and it is then your choice to decide if you want to treat your condition by pharmaceutical or natural means. An obstetrician is a doctor who is further specialized in the area of women's health during pregnancy, whereas a woman will see a gynecologist for all her uterus/vaginal related issue if she is not pregnant.

Anti-Fungal Medications
That Are Also Available As Vaginal Tablets

- Clotrimazole (Lotrimin, Mycelex)

- Miconazole (Monistat; Micatin)

- Terconazole (Terazol)

- Nystatin (Mycostatin)

Oral medications for yeast vaginitis and vulvovaginitis include Fluconazole (Diflucan). Most doctors prefer to treat vaginal yeast infections with vaginal tablets, vaginal applicator medications or vaginal suppositories rather than oral medications. Oral antifungal medication such as Fluconazole can be hard on the digestive system including the stomach and liver and can cause many debilitating side effects such as headache, nausea, and abdominal pain, while vaginal treatment is unlikely to cause these side effects. Oral antifungal medications are also not recommended for use during pregnancy.

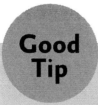

Good Tip

Liver Cleansing After Drug Treatment

Here are a few good tips for clearing any stubborn drug residues from your liver after you have received a pharmaceutical drug from your doctor. I routinely see many patients who have never felt quite well since taking a drug. How do you know if your liver is suffering?

Here are the telltale signs that your liver needs a tune-up:

- Fogginess in the head, feeling spaced out.

- Recurring headaches or a dull feeling in the head.

- Feeling sick all over, queasiness, and nausea or not right in the digestion.

- Poor or a listless appetite, could feel like being hung-over.

- Poor tolerance to alcohol, fatty foods, chips or spicy foods.

- Fatigued, tired, lack of stamina, prefer to stay in bed.

- Hard to get up in the morning, unmotivated, anxiety and easily angered.

- Drugs don't work anymore in spite of high dosages.

Try this approach: follow a liver friendly diet, eat freshly grated beetroot and carrot combined, fresh garlic, partially steamed broccoli, cauliflower, Brussels sprouts, radish, Chinese vegetables such as Bok choy, artichoke hearts, capers, olives, fresh lettuce. Drink roasted dandelion root coffee. Take a mixture like Swedish Bitters three times daily before meals and in particular take aged Kyolic Garlic as a dietary supplement at least three times daily. Be sure to drink NO alcohol for at least a month or two during liver treatment.

Still feeling unwell after a drug treatment?

Then be sure to follow the 3-stage detoxification program I have outlined in section 3 of chapter 7 Understanding Cleansing And Detox.

What is Disseminated Candidiasis?

Acute disseminated candidiasis, or invasive candidiasis, is quite a major fungal infection of candida. It usually progresses to several different organs such as the liver, kidney, spleen, eyes, brain, and heart and can certainly cause death. Candida is among the most common causes of an actual candida yeast bloodstream infection, which is typically introduced from the gastrointestinal tract or from venous catheters such as in the hospital system.

Clinical manifestations of candidiasis can be nonspecific but may include unresolved fever and may progress to sepsis, otherwise known as blood poisoning.

A definitive diagnosis requires confirmation by way of blood testing, and a presumptive diagnosis is generally used in high-risk immune-suppressed patient. Intravenous drug intervention is most always required with a confirmed positive culture, and catheter removal is recommended for suspected infections.

The most common causative yeasts found in disseminated candidiasis are

- Candida albicans (41%-65%)

- Candida parapsilosis (15%-24%)

- Candida glabrata (10%-15%)

The Four Key Antifungal Drugs Your Doctor May Use

" Doctors give drugs of which they know little, into bodies, of which they know less, for diseases of which they know nothing at all. "
Voltaire

You doctor may well prescribe an antifungal drug if he or she suspects a fungal infection, and a drug of this nature will only be prescribed if a fungal infection is diagnosed after a swab is returned positive. Here are the four common "zole" drugs your doctor may prescribe but I'd also like to mention another drug called Nystatin which doctors may recommend for yeast infections, especially natural medicine doctors. Nystatin was popularized in the 1980's by Dr. William Crook who wrote extensively on its use for candida yeast infections.

1. Intraconazole - Weakest

2. Ketaconazole - Medium

3. Fluconazole - Strong

4. Fungizone - Strongest

Itraconazole (Sporanox) appears to be at least as potent as ketoconazole and some say may be as good as fluconazole, but not in my opinion. It needs stomach acid to be absorbed, so it should be taken with food. The dose is 200 mg per day. If not enough drug is being absorbed, blood levels may need to be checked so the dose can be increased. An Itraconazole oral solution is more effective and puts higher levels of the drug in the blood than the capsule.

Ketoconazole (Nizoral) is taken at 200 or 400 mg once per day. It also needs stomach acid to be absorbed, so it should be taken with food. Antacids should be avoided. It may not be well absorbed in people with digestive problems or who cannot eat very much.

Fluconazole (Diflucan) is taken at 200 mg the first day, then 100 mg once a day thereafter. Treatment typically lasts from ten days up to two weeks for oral or skin candidiasis and three weeks for esophageal infection (or two weeks after symptoms clear up, whichever is longer). The dose may be increased to 400 mg per day if the lower dose does not work. I have found this drug to be quite hard on the digestive system, particularly the stomach and liver and can make some who take it quite nauseous indeed.

Studies suggest that fluconazole is more effective than ketoconazole, and I can vouch for the effectiveness of Diflucan in the clinic, it certainly works for many, but is not always successful because like most drugs the causes are never really addressed adequately by the doctor. Some doctors still prefer to treat aggressive fungal infections with other drugs in order to save the potent fluconazole for later use, if necessary.

You will most certainly need to take a good probiotic for several weeks, twice daily – on rising and retiring, after you take this drug. Resistance to fluconazole is well documented, and once it develops, then treatment options are very limited. In addition, I highly recommend that you naturopath prescribe you a liver supplement for three weeks to clear any Diflucan drug residues from your liver. It will make you feel much better, try it and you will see, this is my experience after having seen many hundreds of women over the years who have been treated with this strong anti-fungal drug. A good herb to take after Fluconazole is St Mary's thistle, ask your herbalist. Imagine now how ridiculous it is for a woman to take Diflucan once per week for years on end, this is exactly what one of my patients did. Yeast is clever and will develop resistance, and over time will become increasing virulent in strength and more difficult to eradicate.

Fungizone This potent drug is also known as amphotericin B, and is injected directly into a vein via injection or the patient is placed on an intravenous drip in the hospital system. It is used to treat severe disseminated candidiasis when other systemic therapies fail or when the infection is likely to be very aggressive. This drug used to be the standard treatment for systemic or serious fungal infections and the treatment phase lasted for 8-12 weeks, but often gave quite severe side effects including extensive kidney damage and anemia.

People are now usually given amphotericin B until they start to improve, usually for only two weeks, and then they are switched to fluconazole at 200-400 mg per day for about ten days. If you have had any intravenous anti-candida treatment then listen up, make sure you book in to see your Naturopath or nutritionally orientated doctor for some cleansing and rejuvenating treatments. You will pick up much faster and reduce your chances of a recurrence of any yeast related problems. Ask for a liver and bowel detoxification program as well as an extensive probiotic treatment regime. Just do it, you will be glad you did.

Nystatin

Nystatin is a prescription anti-fungal drug that kills many different kinds of yeasts and yeast-like fungi, including candida. This drug is different from the zole drugs in that it has the gentlest action of all prescriptive anti-fungal drugs, but it is nevertheless implicated in causing some major aggravations in a few patients.

Dr. Crook was a big advocate of Nystatin therapy in the 1980's, and it is still a very valid form of anti-fungal therapy today, but I am not a big fan of this kind of therapy and I will explain why shortly. Some doctors even see Nystatin as some kind of natural anti fungal treatment because of its low ability to cause toxicity. This drug was widely promoted by Dr. William Crook in the 1980's, and like most pharmaceutical drugs, the main promoters have most always been medical doctors. Dr. Crook even recommended Nizoral, a prescriptive anti-fungal that has the ability to create liver toxicity.

Nystatin is available in powder, tablet, capsule, a cream, as an injectable and even as vaginal pessaries.

Like many other antifungal and antibiotic drugs, Nystatin was originally developed from a bacterium and was isolated from Streptomyces noursei in 1950 by researchers Elizabeth Lee Hazen and Rachel Fuller Brown. They named Nystatin after the New York State Health Department Laboratory where it was discovered in 1954. Nystatin is often used today to prevent a full-blown yeast infection in patients who are at risk for fungal infections, such as AIDS patients and patients receiving chemotherapy, but it is routinely used by doctors in countries like England for oral thrush. Nystatin is generally regarded as one of the safest of all prescription anti-fungal drugs because unlike other anti-fungal drugs, it is poorly absorbed from the intestinal tract. Nystatin is therefore used for yeast infections of the mouth and throat, but also in the intestinal tract.

It is also used for yeast related problems affecting the skin and vagina. In small amounts and when used locally, Nystatin is probably a valid therapy but these treatments are then only symptomatic by nature. Many people will try and use Nystatin internally and in very high doses in some cases, and that is where you will need to be particularly careful if you want to avoid die-off reactions.

Herxheimer Reactions Are Common With Nystatin

I do have some experience with Nystatin and used to prescribe it when I was working in different medical clinics years ago, and while it is true that Nystatin is virtually non-toxic and tolerated by most people even with prolonged use, I discovered that it could easily cause Herxheimer (known as die-off) reactions in patients ranging from mild to extreme and even debilitating. Nystatin kills yeast by rupturing the cell membranes of candida, and by doing so on a large scale it allows the mass release of yeast antigens which can trigger a strong immune response. And in some people I have noticed, the response can be quite overwhelming indeed.

Dr. Crook mentions in his book The Yeast Connection that "as long as Nystatin can causes symptoms, then it is probably killing candida" and recommends to "Take Nystatin at increasingly higher dosages to kill the yeast at deeper levels". He states that while patients take Nystatin, they may experience headaches, depression, fatigue, muscle aching, vomiting, diarrhea or skin rashes and that these symptoms may occur during the first two weeks of treatment but stop on discontinuation of the drug. Each time you increase the Nystatin dose, there will often be a temporary aggravation of your symptoms.

While it is difficult for all patients to avoid die-off entirely when any candida kill product is recommended, I have found that severe reactions seem to be more common when Nystatin is prescribed than when any other herbal or herbal and nutritional anti-fungal combination is recommended, and believe that one of the main reasons for this is that Nystatin in not absorbed by the digestive tract and kills yeast on direct contact in the digestive system, starting in the throat, moving through to the small intestine and continue killing in the large intestine.

The powder seems to cause the more severe kinds of aggravations, more so than the tablets. Once you have used Nystatin in the clinic and have also used other natural products to reduce yeast infections, you soon realize the different side effects are associated with different medicines used. I don't tend to recommend Nystatin anymore because of the potential for aggravations, because I have certainly witnessed major reactions with several chronic yeast infection patients over the years and a few of the most violent of these aggravations have included shaking chills, night sweats, vomiting and diarrhea, major skin breakouts and depression and anxiety.

On the other hand, I don't want to frighten anybody from taking Nystatin, because there will be many people who take this anti-fungal drug with good results, but good advice is to go slow when it comes to dosage and not to be in a hurry to step dosages up by any means. That way you will be in a better position to slow down or stop if you experience any untoward side effects before they develop into major aggravations.

Taking a high dose of an antifungal such as Nystatin when you commence yeast infection treatment to me is like prematurely increasing the speed of a large oil tanker to its maximum velocity, once a high speed is achieved and maintained and if then a slower speed is then desired at any given time, it may take many miles for the huge ship to reduce speed due to the sheer momentum and energy it has picked up along the way. Likewise, once the strong action of a high initial dose of Nystatin begins to work on the yeast infection, it is almost impossible to halt the momentum and energy of the aggravation rapidly, and it can take many days or even a few weeks for this momentum to slowly ease up. It therefore make sense to go slow with Nystatin treatment to begin with and to slowly increase the dose, that way you will have much better control and will be more able to quickly slow down any potential reactions.

In my experience, the dosages that people have aggravated on ranged from moderate to high dosages and not low, but in saying that I have seen some quite severe aggravations with several patients even on 1 tablet twice daily.

Many who take Nystatin at a low dosage will eventually want to take higher dosages, and if you have a severe or a chronic yeast infection start on the low end of dosage at 500,000 units (1 tablet, lozenge or liquid units) per day for a at least a week before slowly and carefully increasing the dosage, that way it will be easier for you to control any aggravations before they get out of hand and get to be very uncomfortable.

Allergies To Nystatin

The secondary reason why some may react is because some people may be allergic to Nystatin. It its mildest form, this drug can produce an itchy skin rash which may occur whether the drug is used on the skin or orally. More severe forms of allergic responses may include swellings in the extremities such as the fingers, but also in the throat, face and lips. At its worst, an anaphylactic response may occur which in some people may cause chest tightness, swallowing difficulties and breathing issues.

Most people will soon know if they are allergic to Nystatin, but a small percentage may not and could pass a mild reaction off to something else, because the reactions can be very mild for some and quite hard to diagnose. If you do take Nystatin and begin to experience and changes in yourself which don't seem to go away, whether you have been taking Nystatin for one week or one month, it may well be an allergic reaction. You will soon work this out by discontinuing the drug for several days and then by resuming it. When I ask patients how long they have had certain effects on medications I have heard many say, "Now that you ask, come to think of it, since I started taking that drug".

Anti Fungal Drug Side Effects

Topical Treatments

Topical creams and ointments may cause mild burning. Some people are highly sensitive and may have a widespread skin reaction with blisters and peeling. Some creams also contain a steroid to reduce inflammation that may cause itching, irritation or dryness. Vaginal tablets do not often cause problems, but in a few women they may lead to vaginal burning or itching or skin rash. Some women experience cramps or headaches. Clotrimazole lozenges may cause minor changes in liver function, but this may not require stopping the drug.

Oral irritation and nausea are rare side effects of Nystatin lozenges. Nystatin oral rinse (Mycostatin) is almost non-toxic, but it may cause gut problems if excessive doses are taken. Stop if you notice any side effects with topical treatments and do tell your doctor.

Systemic Treatments

Side effects for the oral *azole* drugs are similar, but some studies show they're more common with Itraconazole. The most common are nausea, vomiting and belly pains. Others include dizziness, drowsiness, fever, diarrhea, headaches, rash and changes in taste. The most serious problem is liver toxicity, but this is rare and usually reverses after the drug is stopped. Nevertheless, liver function should be carefully monitored when you commence with any pharmaceutical anti fungal, particularly with ketoconazole, ask for an LFT (liver function blood test). Don't be afraid to ask your doctor for at least six monthly blood tests to assess your immune system, kidney and liver function.

Amphotericin B has many side effects, some quite strong and severe. Therefore, it is only used in cases when there's a direct threat to a person's life or all other treatments have failed. Main side effects include kidney problems and low red blood cells, known as anemia.

Others side effects include fever, chills, and changes in blood pressure, changes in appetite, nausea, vomiting and headache. These reactions occur one to three hours after an infusion, are most severe with the first few doses, and diminish with later treatments. Side effects are generally the same with all amphotericin drugs, though some forms of this drug may be slightly less toxic than others.

Anti-Fungal Drug Interactions

A lesser-known fact is that the anti-fungal drugs the doctor prescribes to you may well interact with other drugs or supplements, and here are the most common drug interactions I have discovered. There will be more clashes with azole drugs and certain drugs prescribed by your doctor, but these are probably the most common ones. Ask your pharmacist or go to Dr. Google if you are unsure. But should you use a drug or a natural medicine, what choice should you or your practitioner make?

Is your practitioner managing your drug medications appropriately? I have discovered that a considerable number of people have mild to severe adverse drug reactions. Having clarity when a patient really does need a pharmaceutical medication and when their medication is inappropriate is vital knowledge that any clinician must have, whether they are a natural medicine or conventional medicine practitioner.

Be sure to enquire if you take a drug if there is a natural alternative, and if not then enquire if there are any side effects to be expected and any interactions with the drug and any natural medicines. And thirdly as I have just mentioned, get your blood tested at least twice annually if you take a pharmaceutical drug for any length of time.

1 Antihistamines. If you take an anti-histamine, (terfenadine (Seldane) or astemizole (Hismanal) then you should avoid Fluconazole. This combination may cause serious heart problems.

2 Anti-reflux drugs. Do not combine the anti-reflux drug cisapride (Propulsid) with any of the azole drugs; again, serious side effects like heart problems can occur.

3 Sedatives. Avoid the azole type drugs with the prescribed sedatives triazolam (Halcion) or midazolam (Versed) because this combination may lead to a seriously high level of sedation leading to death.

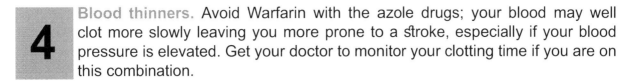

4 Blood thinners. Avoid Warfarin with the azole drugs; your blood may well clot more slowly leaving you more prone to a stroke, especially if your blood pressure is elevated. Get your doctor to monitor your clotting time if you are on this combination.

5 Oral hypoglycemic drugs. Take great care when combining an azole drug if you have diabetes and take an oral anti-hypoglycemic drug, you will need to carefully monitor and regulate your blood sugar levels otherwise severe hypoglycemia may result (low blood sugar).

6 HIV drugs. There are drug interactions that have been observed including with the azole drugs and HIV drugs, specifically efavirenz (Sustiva), nelfinavir (Viracept) and nevirapine (Viramune).

Three Points To Consider When Looking At Drugs Versus Natural Medicine

1. Firstly, in which cases are drugs inappropriate and natural medicine a superior choice in your situation.

2. Secondly, when can natural medicines be effectively and safely integrated with drugs to provide you, the patient, with the best clinical outcome.

3. And lastly, when should a drug prescription be prioritized over alternative treatments in terms of efficacy, ethical practice and the best clinical outcomes.

Most all classes of oral azole drugs share the same drug interactions. I have not found there to be any drug interactions when using localized skin creams for topical yeast infection treatment.

The Problem of Antifungal Drug Resistance

Yeast infection treatments, which fail to respond to conventional anti-fungal drug treatments, have become increasingly reported, just like antibiotic resistant bacterial infections have over the years. There are many people who just don't seem to respond to the azole class of drugs anymore, such as Fluconazole. This is partly due to the widespread, long-term use of azoles for treating and preventing yeast related health issues.

Medications do have their place at times and are sometimes useful to get rid of first-time yeast infections or major yeast infections, I have noticed that some patients over the years had a successful treatment by their doctor for their yeast infection, and never did the problem recur.

But these cases are uncommon, and in most all cases the yeast infection will recur. If you get a recurring yeast infection, then you should seriously consider not using that medication again because it could mean that you are either developing drug resistance, or that you have an underlying problem that hasn't been addressed. If you use prescription medication every time for a recurrence it means that you are covering up a problem that needs to be fixed. You need to get rid of the yeast problem at its core, the cause needs fixing and not the manifestations of the cause.

Unfortunately, the doctor's answer to fungal drug resistance may be to double or treble the dose of what he has prescribed you or alternatively to use a an even more powerful antifungal such as amphotericin B. While this drug is certainly more potent and effective, amphotericin B is considerably more toxic, especially to the kidney. If you are a person with an underlying kidney or liver disease, you will want to avoid the stronger antifungal drugs which result in changes in kidney function tests. Just like a gun with a higher caliber, the stronger the firing power the more likely you will cause more collateral damage.

Recent studies have show that exposure to azole treatment decreases the antifungal activity of amphotericin B. Two other types of antifungal drugs have also been shown to be active against azole-resistant candida yeast infections, they are Voriconazole (Vfend) which showed enhanced activity against fluconazole-resistant candidiasis and another drug called caspofungin (Cancidas) which has also shown activity against azole-resistant strains of candidiasis. No doubt there will be side effects associated with these antifungals as well.

Because of the widespread antifungal drug resistance, taking any pharmaceutical drug to prevent a candida yeast infection is ridiculous and should not be encouraged in my opinion. For example, when fluconazole is used to "prevent" a woman's yeast infections and then resistance develops, treating any potentially newer and more aggressive yeast infections becomes much more difficult and will often found to be unsuccessful until the drug is discontinued and the kidneys and liver are cleaned up. Azole drug treatments only weaken the body's immune system and toxify the kidneys and liver, creating many potential additional diseases. It is therefore best never to begin using these azole drugs in the first place, and in most all cases they will not be found to be necessary if the Candida Crusher program is adhered to.

Azole based antifungal drug treatment for chronic yeast infection treatment is certainly not encouraged in my clinic and I have unfortunately seen too many people with recurrent infections who remain on long-term azole therapy to treat and in the hope of preventing yeast infections. In these cases, side effects and drug resistance remains a concern and by the time they see me they still have the yeast infection that has become suppressed, and on top of that present with many side effects from long term drug therapy. There is a better way!

The Candida Crusher natural approach towards yeast infection eradication is the safest and most effective approach, it is drug and side effect free and will ensure a complete and permanent eradication if followed carefully.

Endoscopy

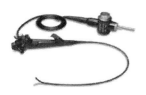

The idea behind this form of imaging is that if you see any change by way of an endoscopy, essentially a tube with a camera that goes down your throat, there is something wrong. The most commonly performed investigation on the upper digestive system is the endoscopy; a tube is placed down into the person's esophagus and continued down and into the stomach. From there it continues on into the first part of the small intestine called the duodenum, where the procedure is now called a gastroscopy.

The fine tubing includes a nifty onboard camera allowing the specialist to examine the lining of the whole upper digestive system. The specialist is on the look out for anything unusual, such as mucosal damage or a particularly red area that may reveal cancer, an ulcer or another digestive problem such as an ulcer or inflammation. The bottom end of the digestive system such as the large bowel and rectum are also viewed with an endoscope, and this area may reveal a polyp, inflammation or perhaps diverticulitis otherwise known as bowel pockets. In this case the procedure is called a colonoscppy.

Unfortunately, the small intestine is just outside of the effective range of the endoscope and colon scope, and the small bowel is the most important part of the digestive system because it is here that practically all the digestion and absorption takes place.

Yeast Infection Drug Treatment Chart

Yeast Infection	Common Symptoms	Medical Diagnosis	Medical Treatment	Medical Prevention
Oral Candida (thrush), affects mouth and throat, especially tongue.	Discomfort, burning of mouth and throat; changed sense of taste; creamy white or yellowish patches on mouth or throat.	Appearance & Symptoms. Lab tests are used if the infection does not clear after treatment.	Mouth rinses (Nystatin, Mycostatin). Lozenges (Nystatin, Mycostatin; Clotrimazole, Mycelex). Capsules (fluconazole, Diflucan 100 mg/day or Itraconazole, Sporanox 200 mg/day)	Maintain good oral/ dental hygiene. Avoid smoking and excess sugar. Weekly fluconazole.
Vaginal (vaginitis, yeast infection thrush, affects vagina and/or vulva	Odorous, white- or yellow, creamy discharge. May be burning, swelling and itching.	By appearance and symptoms. Lab tests are used if the infection does not clear after treatment.	Vaginal creams or suppositories (Clotrimazole or Miconazole). Fluconazole oral tablets.	Avoid scented soap, bleach and fabric softeners. Wear loose fitting clothing & cotton underwear. Weekly fluconazole
Throat Candida Can affect the esophagus (feeding tube)	Chest pain, nausea and painful swallowing. Usually occurs with oral candida.	Examination of oropharynx; endoscopy; culture and histology (cell).	Ketoconazole (Nizoral) 200 or 400 mg/day or Fluconazole (Diflucan) at 200 mg once a day.	If more than one case has occurred, fluconazole preventive therapy may be warranted.
Skin Yeast Infections (usually affects skin in armpits, groin and under breasts)	Bright red, uneven eruption in the folds of skin that may be coated with a white membrane; mild burning feeling.	By appearance and symptoms. Lab tests are used if the infection does not clear after treat- ment.	Creams or ointments applied 2-4 times/ day. Products include Clotrimazole Nystatin, ketoconazole, Miconazole, Econazole and Amphotericin B.	Keep skin dry.
Systemic Candida (affects organs throughout the body)		Can be difficult to diagnose. Common in AIDS patients.	Amphotericin B (Fungizone) orally or intravenously.	

The Candida Crusher Program
Permanent Yeast Solution

Introduction & Overview Of The Candida Crusher Program

Chapter seven has been divided into five sections which all build on each other, and while you can just read this book at any point, which is perfectly fine, when it comes to Chapter 7, I would prefer if you read this chapter all the way through. Please take notes or underline what is important to you and feel free to write in this book, this is your book so highlight what is important to you.

The Candida Crusher Program will help guide you through your recovery and you will find that a complete recovery program is outlined in this chapter in the five sections. By reading and implementing all of the information contained in this comprehensive chapter, you could well achieve the same great outcomes that my patients achieve when they visit me in my clinic or have consultations with me on Skype. Once you get a good understanding of the Candida Crusher concept, feel free to modify your program including the diet, lifestyle recommendations as well as the Candida Crusher supplementation dosages to suit your own individual needs.

The Candida Crusher Program has been successfully trialed and tested over many years involving several thousand patients. I know this program works because of the most positive feedback I have received not only from patients, but from naturopaths and other health care professionals I have shared several of these secrets with as well over the years. These are not "secrets" really; but like achieving most things in life that are really worthwhile, it is a matter of applying clearly defined principles and sticking with a proven plan and never giving in until you get the desired results. And what if you don't get a good outcome? Then you will need to tweak the program until you do, or discover the hidden obstacles preventing you from healing yourself and that's exactly what I have tried to do with patients over the years. I have learned from the many mistakes I made in the early years and don't think you should have to repeat these mistakes. Your success is virtually assured *as long as you stay on track*. Pay particular attention to the information contained in the boxes, many are great tips which can help you fast track your results.

As you will learn later on, if improvements don't occur long-term, or if improvements hold only temporarily and then your health quickly regresses, then you will need to look for what I call the "obstacles to cure", and you will learn all about these at the end of section 5. One or more of these obstacles may be in your way and could be preventing that breakthrough from occurring that you have been so desperately looking for, especially if you are one of those patients who has been to countless practitioners, read all the candida books, tried all the fancy diets as well as candida supplements and still doesn't get well and stay well.

My main motto has always been to *never give in in life with anything*, and this is what will make the difference, sheer persistence. Persistence eventually pays off; after all, it has taken me several years to write this very book because it was written in a time of my life with four teenagers, in the middle of adding a 120 square meter extension to my home while simultaneously operating two businesses, including my busy international naturopathic consultancy.

Almost anything is possible in your life with sheer persistence and determination, I want you to remember this down the track when the clouds roll in and cover your sun, and it looks like you will never get well in spite of your best made plans.

I have experimented with countless different candida diets over the years and found many are just too rigid for the average candida patient to follow, while others were just too plain liberal. Some books I studied did not clearly define when to re-introduce certain foods and drinks which were eliminated, and others would elaborate on a "paint by numbers" approach to the candida diet, for example – for the first two weeks you avoid this food, and then for the next two weeks you avoid another food, etc. Many candida diets were just too confusing and some were plain impossible to follow for too long. And, if a program is too rigid then the compliance will be quite poor and consequently the results will simply not be forthcoming. Is it any wonder the typical chronic candida patient is confused, bewildered and completely disappointed in the end?

In addition, some companies who strongly promote dietary supplements maintain that supplements alone will cure candida and not to worry too much about diets, because they are just too plain difficult to follow. Some supplement resellers even call the candida diet the impossible diet; yet actively promote products, paying a small amount of attention to diet while mentioning zilch about those all-too-important lifestyle changes required.

While some high quality candida dietary supplements are required, especially in chronic cases, you will get the best possible results you are looking for by a utilizing a combination of the right diet for you, lifestyle habits and high-quality dietary supplementation. All three are required if you are to beat that yeast infection, and my emphasis is on 80 percent focus on diet and lifestyle and 20 percent focus on special anti-candida foods and specialized supplements. A well-coordinated approach works beautifully, and I have proven this to be the case time and again with many candida patients. The right diet "for you" implies that no one size fits all, and that you will need to be especially tough the first few weeks but then loosen up and modify my recommendations to suit your own needs. Don't worry if this all sounds a bit confusing, I'll explain as we go along.

Each of the 5 sections chapter 7 are important, and if you want to get the best out of the Candida Crusher then I would recommend that you read chapter 7 in particular a few times over. It will be almost as good as coming to see me in private in my consultation room or having a catch-up on Skype for a yeast infection consultation.

The QUICK START Guide and FAQs

Don't forget, Chapter 4 is called the QUICK START guide that gives you many quick solutions to the most commonly found yeast infections without having to wade through hundreds of pages of information looking for your solutions. In many parts of the Candida Crusher you will find FAQs, these are the questions I most commonly get asked. In the Appendix at the end this book you will find over one hundred such FAQS and there will be many more questions answered online in my You Tube videos in time. And also, if you are now reading this book with an electronic reader, the quickest way for you to navigate and jump to exactly where you want to go in the Candida Crusher book is to go back to the Contents pages at the beginning of the book and click the link you are looking for. You will be magically transported to the information you are looking for. Hit the back button to take you back to the contents page. If we could only hit the back button in life, we would then be able to go back and address the causes of our yeast infection, and skip forward to discover that we have saved ourselves from a lot of misery!

Why A Four-Month Program?

The Candida Crusher Program, if adhered to correctly, will take about twelve to sixteen weeks (three to four months) to become really effective and this time frame is based on many cases successfully treated for this duration.

While it is possible for great results to be achieved much sooner, in some cases it can take as long as twelve months to fully clear a yeast infection. Why does it take so long for some people to recover, while others recover in a matter of mere weeks? This can easily be explained because every case of candida I see, just like every patient, is different and has developed a yeast infection under a different set of circumstances. In addition, some cases will be straightforward whereas others will be much more complex and have a hidden cause that ensures the person only ever partially recovers, because they have their own personal obstacle to cure which needs addressing. Another reason is that every patient will have his or her own reasons for wanting to recover, and this may be a partial or full recovery, as strange as it may sound.

My advice is to steer clear of any health programs that promote "instant" cures; in reality there is no such thing as instant when it comes to good health. This is a bit like getting an "instant PhD" I have seen advertised online for five hundred dollars. A friend used to tell me that it is "morally wrong to allow suckers to keep their money", and many people will unfortunately fall for such scams for the instant things in life. Whenever you act in haste in this life it often follows that you may have to repent at your leisure.

It takes time to develop outstanding health because good health is based on the foundation of learning how to lead a healthy and balanced life, and as you may be aware, learning to develop great health takes time because first there is the theory and then there is the practice of adopting and implementing these healthy lifestyle and dietary habits. The main thing is to do the best you can, and even if you can't cure your underlying health problems.

This in turn will make the Candida Crusher Program just that more effective. When I wrote this book, I wanted you to eradicate your yeast overgrowth for life, not just for a mere few months or years, but *a permanent yeast solution.*

Four Month Program – Helping Yourself Back to Health
The Candida Crusher Program – A Quick Overview

The 5 Stages To Your Permanent Yeast Solution

The following 5 points represent the five sections you will read in chapter 7. The Contents pages at the beginning of this book will give you the overview of each section in much detail, click the links in the Contents pages to navigate.

1 Candida Crusher Diet – Understanding Digestion And Nutrition. - if you want to recover quickly and completely, let's begin by recommending a good cleanse followed by the Candida Crusher Diet. Most people will benefit from a brief bowel cleanse out before we commence; I call this cleansing stage the Big Clean-Up. I'll show you what to eat and the best ways to eat as well. Eat the right foods for as long as it takes and starve out the fungus to stop it reproducing. The three-stage diet I've been using for years is proven and has been used on many thousands of patients in my clinic with great affect.

I'll explain in section 1 all about diet and nutrition in much detail and most all of your candida dietary questions will be answered. Section 1 is your top priority, it is by far the biggest section of the book and my many dietary recommendations are at the heart of this successful program.

2 Candida Crushing Immunity – Understanding Immunity, Metabolites and Stress. Many people don't know about the metabolites that candida produce, I'll explain in detail and show you what you can do about them. You will learn how to rebuild your immune system and restore the integrity of your metabolism and stress axis by understanding how stress can affect your immune system. Many candida sufferers have varying degrees of stress related health complaints that can and should be improved, and by doing so you will pave the way for a successful and permanent eradication of your yeast infection. This key information is missing in most books on this topic.

3 Candida Crushing Cleansing – Understanding Cleansing and Detox. A good detoxification program is one of the most positive health builders you can do *after* you have beaten your yeast infection. I'll show you how to successfully complete the 3-stage Candida Crusher cleansing program. This section outlines the most efficient ways to cleanse and detoxify your body, and I'll also mention heavy metal toxicity and more advanced concepts.

 4 Candida Crusher Eradication - Learn about Special Foods, Supplements and Herbs. Do you want to know the best foods to eat that aid in suppressing and eradicating a yeast overgrowth? This section shows you the most

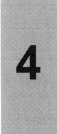

beneficial foods that help and the specific Candida Crusher nutritional supplement formulations I have researched and developed after twenty years of working with patients just like you. I'll teach you the best ones to take and explain exactly why and when you need them. Without correctly and thoroughly eradicating the yeast infection and re-populating your digestive system with beneficial bacteria, you will be only half doing the job and risk a recurrence of yeast related problems. And, you don't need to spend a fortune and take dozens of different supplements for life either.

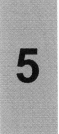

Candida Crusher Lifestyle - Understanding the Healthy Lifestyle. Some of the book's most important information is contained in this fifth and last section, as it will teach you how to remain candida-free for life. This stage explains how to reduce your current risk factors for not only candida, but for a host of other diseases as well. Section 5 explains about the importance of sleep, relaxation, exercise and meditation and shows you how to stay away from the perpetrators of candida overgrowth. This final section will outline how to put your personal candida program all together.

Individualized Treatments Work the Best

What I have found interesting is that when it comes to the treatment of candida, similar to the treatment of any other health problem a person may have, many health care professionals adopt a "one size fits all" approach. I don't mean this to be arrogant, but in most cases when a yeast infection patient comes to my clinic with candida issues who has been to somebody previously, they may well have been given a diet sheet and a bunch of supplements and that's about it.

Perhaps you are a naturopath or a health-care professional reading this right now, and if you are then I'd like to share some insights with you which I feel can help you a great deal in your quest to help others significantly with yeast related issues. Patients are all entirely unique and individual, and by understanding this unique individuality and treating people as such, you will be able to attain great and even outstanding clinical successes. If ten patients show up at a medical center with a similar illness, all ten will most likely receive the same treatment based on their diagnosis. If these ten show up on my doorstep, it would be most unusual for me to make exactly the same recommendation even twice.

How People Think They Get Well
And How They Actually Get Well

The trick with a very successful candida treatment program is that it has to be individualized to suit the individual, but what exactly do we mean by this? Simple, first it is important to look carefully at the person's presenting complaints and understand how serious the candida yeast infection has taken hold of this person.

Then we try to figure out what type of person we are dealing with to see how we can apply the treatment plan successfully to them. Are they particularly sensitive? Are they strong-willed? Are they impatient and want results today? Are they willing to apply themselves and stick with my recommendations?

It has always been my belief in clinical practice that you can offer the best lifestyle advice, the best program and the best products but if the patient is not willing to fully engage you are wasting your breath, your time as well as the patient's hard earned money. So how do you make a person engage in the Candida Crusher Program to the point where they won't just get average results, but actually get rid of their yeast infection permanently? Well, you make sure that they start to feel better sooner rather than later and that they experience only a few set-backs in their first month of treatment particularly, i.e. you need to earn their respect as a good clinician and you should be able to back up your claims you make in the clinic that they will feel better soon.

Personally, I have never offered any ironclad guarantees of a cure to any patient, but do tell them that getting better is not a smooth ride from feeling bad to feeling awesome. I will often draw a candida patient this picture:

Fantasy Land - How People Think They Get Well

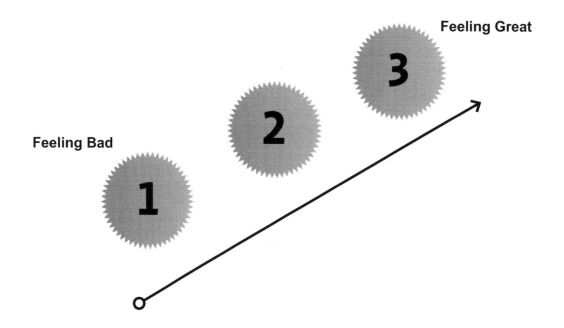

Many believe that if you have a problem wrong with your body, you take a pill or treatment and you get better, simple. Western medicine tends to make people believe that when symptoms go away, you are "cured" and are well again. I suppose if you give credit to somebody who gambles and is always poor, you take all his or her money problems away too. Note that the circles with number 1, 2 and 3 are all in a linear fashion with no ups and downs? Many people expect no or very little bumpy rides along the way to recovery. As smooth as silk. Sorry, it isn't going to happen, I have never seen a patient in all my years of practice with a candida problem who did not experience a few ups and downs along the road to recovery. This is fantasyland, we would all like to go there, but no one has come back to me and told us how fantastic this place is. It must be time for a reality check and to wake up from our dreams of an instant recovery.

Reality Check - How People Actually Get Well

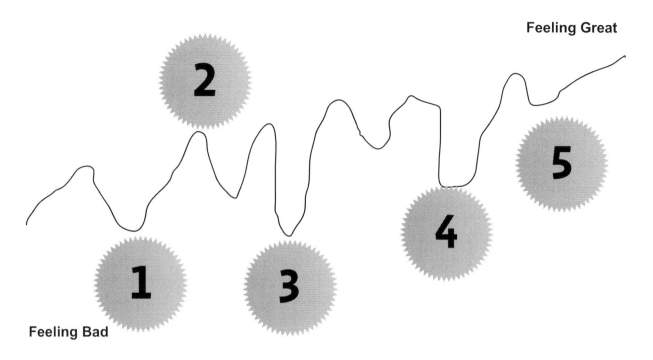

You will see from the above diagram that circle 1 is in fact almost lower than the starting point. Indeed, some patients tell me they can even feel somewhat worse in the first week of treatment. See circle 2, I call this the window of improving health.

The peak here is in fact the highest initial point on this line, and patients on the road to recovery will get a day or two within the first few weeks of treatment which almost seem like they have literally no health problems at all *just for that day*. This signifies recovery, and is a sure sign that if they keep going they will recover in time, providing they keep sticking to the treatment plan. But the window will shut, and circle 3 may prompt the patient to call or email me being disappointed because they were doing just fine, but the crashed "for no apparent reason".

It just so happens that there was a bona fide reason, but it was not apparent to the patient at the time; just don't change that treatment plan! The crash at number 3 was because the patient went to a party, a wedding, etc., and then ate or drank something that pulled them right down. They felt great until they had that food or drink, because they though they could handle it, but their digestive system was not ready yet. They may have also started to improve but then stayed up until one o'clock in the morning after coming home for a dinner and a drink or two. Either way, something made this person go downhill, and it is up to me to help them to establish what this "something" was. Can you remember that I recently spoke about education as part of improving your health and wellbeing? Well, this is part of learning to live a healthier lifestyle, learning about the cause and the effect.

Note that not long after the trough of circle 3 there is an elevation again? The window is now open for two days or more this time, more improvements and the patient may even notice that she can now all of a sudden eat a particular food which previously caused her to feel unwell. The window stays open a little longer because some lessons are now being learned now, and the patient is beginning to slowly learn about cause and effect. Some people have an "aha" moment at this stage, the light bulb goes on and they are starting to learn and apply this knowledge to their diet and lifestyle.

By this stage we are beginning to experience an improved digestive system and most probably an improved bowel flora. By the time the patient hits circle 4, she is experienced enough to understand the cycle of "feel good-feel bad" and will be less critical of her aggravation and of the actual time frame of her recovery, she knows that it will all be good in time because she is starting to feel like her old self again. There may be the odd call or email, but these tend to taper off in the first three to four months I find. After one year I don't tend to hear from patients anymore, even those who have been unwell for twenty years or more. Initially I thought it was because they went elsewhere because they weren't getting results with my recommendations, and then I started to call them up and routinely heard: "I'm OK Eric, there is no need to see you again, my health is great, in fact better than it has been for as long as I can remember". OK, thanks for letting me know…

By the time circle 5 comes around, the aggravation is very short lived and not severe and the person has accepted that there will be days when she cheats a little, she may stay up longer, get a little less sleep, drink a little too much alcohol or go back to some of her old ways of eating. The stronger the digestive and immune system has become, the smaller the aggravation that will be experienced.

This is in reality how people get well, notice that there are lots of ups and downs in the diagram above? Getting from the point of feeling bad to feeling great can take one month right up to eighteen months or more, it all depends on the following five factors. The trend is a big UP, but there are lots of ups and downs along the way. Doesn't this sound like the stock market? People panic and sell on the downturn, and then later regret they didn't hold out just that bit longer, it's human nature I suppose.

The 5 Factors Which Determine Your Recovery

1. Your willingness to stick with the program, how bad do you want to get well?

2. The severity of the candida, how bad your candida is. Mild cases will experience a much more rapid recovery; severe cases often take more time.

3. Your ability to weather the storms, the ups and downs you will face as you slowly but surely improve over time. How you handle feeling bad when it invariably happens.

4. Are you going to jump straight into pharmaceutical treatments when symptoms like headaches, skin rashes, digestive upsets and more such aggravations occur? You will take several steps back if you do and it will take a lot longer to heal. How quickly do you hit that medical panic button?

5. Your lifestyle, are you willing to do all it takes to not just beat candida, but to feel really well and avoid candida…for life? More on this will be covered in a later chapter. Many patients I see are very much "candida diet focused" and tend to completely forget about major benefits of daily relaxation, how stress affects them and adopting a regular form of exercise.

I can recall when I bought my first computer in the 1980[s], the technician who set it up for me drew me a line on a piece of paper like this:

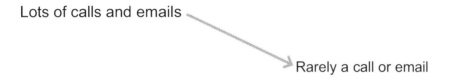

Lots of calls and emails

Rarely a call or email

What he explained was that once you buy into something new and foreign, you are in a learning mode and need to ask many questions from the person you bought that "something new" from. In the beginning you are still in the learning mode, and as time goes by and you learn more and the kind of questions you ask tend to be more difficult and complex. In the end you don't need to ask any more questions because you have learned what you need to know.

Case History # 16
Ann, 62 years

Ann is a retired accountant who had been suffering for as long as she could remember with headaches, nasal congestion, irritable bowel syndrome and several other complaints including a persistent fungal complaint involving several toenails. Six years ago Ann was diagnosed with rheumatoid arthritis. During the consultation, we uncovered two root canalled teeth that had been sensitive for several years. I referred Ann to a dentist friend who examined her mouth and mentioned that her two teeth required extraction because a low-grade infection was present. After careful extraction, the sockets were carefully cleaned and we waited until her mouth was sufficiently healed before we undertook a detoxification program that lasted about six weeks.

It took approximately four months of treatment, but her painful fingers and wrists were getting less painful by the week, and after six months the pain had gone from a scale of eight out of ten down to two out of ten. Ann had improved so much, here headaches were long gone and so was the nasal congestion. The bowel was now almost back to normal. We had Ann on the Hypo-Allergenic Diet that she had followed religiously for almost six months until one day she decided, "enough was enough". She started to drink a glass of wine with dinner each evening and then the chocolates crept back in. She was in my room two weeks later complaining that the pain had crept back up to six out of ten and was steadily getting worse by the day.

I asked Ann what had happened, and her reply: "Well, I was feeling so good I thought that a glass of wine here or there wouldn't hurt me". She said that she was "disappointed" with the treatment and felt that she was "going backwards". This is when I showed her the diagram above and said that it common for somebody who had been unwell to experience what she was going through. You improve and then think all is well, that you can go back to your "normal" lifestyle. I asked her this: "Did you improve initially?" and she said emphatically "YES, I haven't felt that well for as long as I can remember". That's when I said "Well, we must have been on the right track, the problem is that we didn't keep on the path long enough, somehow you became lost and took a side-track". Ann's husband said that his wife thought that she was "cured", and this is what I commonly find with many folk. They start out with the right intentions and want to get well bad enough to be good for several weeks to several months. But then the boredom sets in; the patient becomes frustrated and wants to resume the same diet and lifestyle they had prior to developing the complaints. What they may not be aware of is that it was probably several of these lifestyle and dietary factors that contributed to the demise of their health initially. If they only held out just that bit longer and then re-introduced the offending foods and drinks much more slowly over a prolonged period of time, starting with those items least likely to cause problems, which are most probably not their favorite foods and drinks. People often have the tendency to re-introduce their favorite treat foods and drinks – and it is these that cause spiking of their complaints, and then the disappointment sets in. That is when I get the phone call or email requesting a follow-up visit to see "what else we can do" to improve their complaints. I mentioned to Ann that I had a very quick solution that would almost guarantee to eliminate all her symptoms entirely within three months from now. She laughed when I said: "It's simple, we will just place you on a deserted island and feed you on fish, rice and coconuts"

Ann left my clinic understanding that it was all up to her. It is going to take time; there will be plenty of ups and downs. No smooth sailing. No quick fixes, no BS. Is she is going to get 100% well she has to work for it and be persistent and logical in her approach. I said that I wanted her in my room in three months with a pain level of one out of ten and showing much-improved signs of fungal toenails. I have found that as the gut improves, the fungal nails slowly disappear. You will see a clear demarcation between a healthy toenail growing out and the fungal nail above it. This is a sign to me of digestive improvement in most cases. I know Ann; she wants improvement bad enough and is that sort of person who needed to learn the relationship between cause and effect which she did. After a good talk Ann decided that this was it, she'd had enough and would return in twelve weeks with no pain.

Are you like Ann? Are you going to be patient as a patient, or do you put a time limit on your recovery? Forget it, I leave that to the medical doctor who will give drugs and expect to turn symptoms off. I want to see my patient well enough in time to never have to resort to toxic pharmaceutical drugs ever again. Taking drugs to "cure" candida is very short sighted and will never give you the result you are looking for permanently. And, you will never feel well overall in your mind, body and emotions either. The bottom line is to expect ups and downs but they will smooth out in time and you will feel better in time, better than you most probably have felt in years.

Candida Patients Often Have Addictive Behavioral Patterns

It is not that uncommon to find a patient who comes to my room with an addictive type of behavioral pattern, and this is something I have witnessed with many chronic digestive cases time and again particularly with a digestive disorder like a chronic candida overgrowth. The addiction can be to sugar, alcohol, biscuits, or a lifestyle pattern that in time may contribute to a yeast overgrowth like staying up consistently late each night, not chewing foods properly, worrying too much and not relaxing enough because of work addiction.

Stress is often a key factor; meals can be delayed or perhaps skipped in favor of high carbohydrate snacks. These patterns can continue for months depending on the person's age or even for several years. It may be a pattern a young person goes through when they are perhaps twenty years old for example. They leave home, get a job and live in an apartment and hang around their friends a lot. This may include studying, part-time jobs and all too frequent partying. It may be a male or female who works as a shift-worker at a factory, or a busy single mother with kids who works as a part-time nurse. It may be a taxi driver or an airline pilot or airline traffic controller. It may be a middle-aged woman trying to take care of her aged mother and her teenagers at the same time.

In many of these instances, their diet may leave a lot to be desired including alcohol, sweet foods, coffee with sugar, take-away meals and considerably less time or motivation to focus on nutritious well balanced home cooked meals. Whenever there is a person with a chronic case of candida, then there will often be a chronic case of a faulty diet and/ or lifestyle underpinning this.

I like to point these things out because it may be you reading this right now with a somewhat dysfunctional lifestyle or dietary habit preventing you from having a great digestive system and optimal health. Stressful patterns and hit and miss diets are a classic way to cause dysbiosis and eventual yeast overgrowth. With a stable life and a nutritious diet comes a stable digestive function. No secrets, remember, just plain common sense.

Case History # 17
Kaye, 39 years

Kaye is a single mother with three children; she came to see me a few years ago with chronic recurrent vaginal thrush. She had been having problems for several years, since her late twenties, and had been to her doctor seeking help a number of times. Her doctor had at first prescribed her a product that was applied locally with an applicator, but this gave only occasional and temporary relief. Kaye was then prescribed a powerful anti-biotic and had been taking this on/off for two years. The vaginal thrush would disappear at times, only to re-appear at other times. Her bowel had become problematic and her main presenting complaint was actually occasional "bowel leakage" which made it difficult for her to operate as a tele-sales marketing person. Kaye's problem was that she was so busy trying to earn a living and support her family that she had become totally burned out emotionally, mentally and physically. When she complained of fatigue to her doctor, the reply was naturally: "I think you have depression", and recommended a prescription for the anti-depressant Prozac that Kaye refused. At this point Kaye came to see me.

Kaye was drinking red wine most nights and having several cups of coffee throughout the day. She would often skip breakfast because she was busy getting the kids off to school. Kaye's addictions were to alcohol, caffeine and chocolate. Her sleep was erratic and she was very unhappy with her life. I found out that she was great with computers and encouraged her to start her own online business. I also treated Kaye with the Candida Crusher Program over a six-month period. The results have been fantastic, we have not only cleared up the thrush, but the brain fog is gone and Kaye now has a successful online business that is starting to earn her good money. Kaye has stopped all caffeine and alcohol and her "depression" and fatigue are all a thing of the past. This is a typical case I tend to see, a pattern of overwork, fatigue and a spiral down the slope of chronic health problems. Is this you, do you have a stressful lifestyle underpinning bad dietary habits? Maybe it is time you made some BIG changes in that case.

Many Patients End Up With Varied Outcomes

You may be a person suffering with Candida right now, and if you are then you will be able to find the answer to your problems shortly, and if you apply the principles I outline in this chapter in particular, then you are sure to get the results you are looking for, even after having suffered with yeast related issues for one, five, ten or more than twenty years.

The main reasons some don't fully recover from a yeast infection are as follows:

- The person may have been misdiagnosed and treated for another condition.

- The person may have been treated, but relapsed due to poor follow-up.

- The person aggravated after the first treatment and never came back.

- The person did not follow the plan effectively or gave up on the diet soon.

- The person thought they could beat a yeast infection with supplements alone.

- The person did not stop drinking alcohol entirely, no matter how little consumed.

- The person regularly takes prescribed drugs, maybe the Pill or antibiotics.

- The person does not adopt rest, exercise or support a healthy lifestyle.

- The person is subject continually to a low-grade stressful lifestyle.

- The person is in denial and wants to have his or her cake and eat it too.

Yes, You Can Be Cured Of A Yeast Infection

I've always said that it is the intelligent patients who are the ones who only stay sick for a short period of time; they earn from their mistakes and then move on. It is the ignorant ones or people in denial who are more likely to get sick and stay that way recurrently and sometimes even permanently, and that's just how it goes unfortunately. You may think that I'm a bit hard on people and that's OK, this is my experience based on seeing tens of thousands of patients over the years.

Those who are willing to learn why they got sick in the first place and are willing to correct their lifestyle and dietary indiscretions are the ones who come out on top a lot sooner than those who remain blissfully ignorant and are not interested in making the changes necessary. The definition of insanity is to do the same thing over and over and expect a different result. If you follow the Candida Crusher Program your outcome is certain, and if you can strongly relate to the signs and symptoms of candida yeast infection in chapter 3 and you stick to the game plan you will win, and that's all there is to it.

The Four Types Of Recovery From A Yeast Infection

Most candida patients get well in several stages; in my experience these are the four different types of recovery generally with patients who present with a yeast infection to my rooms:

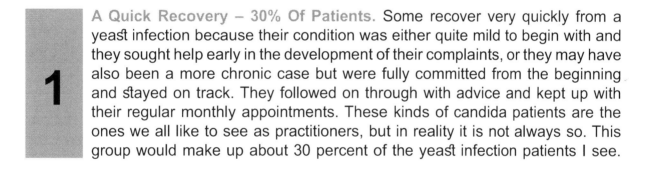

1 A Quick Recovery – 30% Of Patients. Some recover very quickly from a yeast infection because their condition was either quite mild to begin with and they sought help early in the development of their complaints, or they may have also been a more chronic case but were fully committed from the beginning and stayed on track. They followed on through with advice and kept up with their regular monthly appointments. These kinds of candida patients are the ones we all like to see as practitioners, but in reality it is not always so. This group would make up about 30 percent of the yeast infection patients I see.

2 Initial Partial Recovery – 40% Of Patients. In my experience, this is by far the biggest group. Most will partially recover and then relapse before finally re-committing and finally becoming cured of their candida and digestive issues. These are the most common group of candida patients we see, and I believe that 40 percent of people who see me are in this group.

3 Almost Recovered – 20% Of Patients. Some people almost recover, only to find they relapse several months after treatment. There are still several lifestyle and dietary lessons to learn here, or we are perhaps dealing with a hidden cause that I will cover later: "What to do if you don't seem to come right", see section 5. A surprising 20 percent fall into this group, about 1 in 5 people I see with a yeast infection have an obstacle in their way, and impediment that prevents them from becoming really well. Some stay unwell for several months, others for several years but most recover in time after their healing obstacles have been overcome.

Some Just Never Seem To Get Well – 10% Of Patients. There are two distinct groups here, on the one hand, some people are just after a pill or other quick fix, entirely ignore the causative factors or for some reason just don't want to address those obvious or hidden causes, like wanting alcohol, sodas, sweet foods like chocolate, etc. These are the people who are not willing to fully commit to the Candida Crusher Program and they will either get well partially or not at all, and I have seen many people like this over the years. But the second group belongs to the people in whom a clearly defined cause can be extremely difficult to uncover, and these are the patients that keep me on my toes. Every health-care professional can relate to this challenging group, they can be difficult but sincere people indeed, and sometimes we win and sometimes we lose.

After several years, I worked out that four months is about the right time for a candida patient to recover, but six months is more realistic for many people, and a full twelve months of healthy living will mean that not only will the candida yeast infection be completely cured, but all of your digestive and skin complaints can be entirely gone and your health should be outstanding. This is the result I would expect you to obtain if you follow the principles carefully which I have outlined. Your body's cells are continually renewing themselves, and if the conditions are just right then your body will strive towards self-heal.

I want you to be patient and understand that excellent health can't be bought, you don't "catch" good health like you "catch disease", you have to earn good health and work hard for it. The harder, but smarter is a better word, you work the easier it will become, just like success in any other endeavor in your life, if you put in the work and stick with it then it will become easier and before you know it you will have achieved great success.

Nothing good ever comes really easy, and as I mentioned before, if any book or product makes claims that sound almost too good to be true, then it usually is to good to be true. Don't fall for the hype like so many people I know have in the past. Dr. Norman Vincent Peale, a prolific author who wrote many books on positive thinking once said, "Whenever God wants to give us a big gift, he wraps it up in a big problem." The way I see it, the gift is fantastic health and the problem is your yeast infection.

You may find this strange, but a health problem like a yeast infection can be viewed more from a positive rather than a negative perspective, your yeast infection did not drop into your lap; it developed over time due to one or several causes. If you figure out these causes and recover, a huge lesson will have been learned, and your gift will be great health you long for.

Recovery - No Smooth Sailing

> *My aim in sailing is not to be brilliant or flashy,*
> *but just to be consistent over the long run.*
> Dennis Conner, America's Cup winner

There is no such thing as smooth sailing in a successful candida program anymore than there is trying to win the America's Cup. A strong gust of wind can come out of nowhere, an unpredictable storm may break your mast and your crew such as your partner, family or a friend, may even bail out on you at times finding you, the captain, just too difficult to handle. A yeast infection treatment program can cause you to become emotional and difficult to be with at times, believe me, I have verified this with so many patients so *be patient* and understand that you need to prepare yourself for some potential rough seas ahead, because you don't know what lies ahead in those murky depths.

Once you have weathered the yeast storm in all her fury you will become quite skillful to handle anything that a yeast infection can throw at you and in time will learn to develop that patience you require to hang in there and successfully complete your course of treatment. Plot your course carefully when you start your yeast treatment, the Candida Crusher Program, as outlined, make sure you are well equipped for your voyage (the right advice, the correct dietary protocol and the best dietary supplements) and most importantly, never give in, regardless of the weather ahead. You don't need to tie yourself to the mast and go down with this ship.

Just be consistent with your candida treatment over the long run, you don't need to be flashy or brilliant. Just be consistent and persistent, because your persistence will break that yeast resistance.

When you become a skilled navigator of the oceans and have finally learned to make the right diet and lifestyle choices, you will discover that you will be able to easily identify any circumvent potential upcoming bad weather patterns such as poor food choices at home or at parties, weddings, barbeques, etc., and to skillfully avoid damage to your yacht. It all comes down to the experiences you learn to build up over time, and over a prolonged period of time you will be able to cross the biggest ocean effortlessly.

The Last Resort Patient

Do you need to drink alcohol several times a week to give you an escape from reality? Maybe you need several cups of coffee a day to give you a boost, or rely on a regular chocolate bar? These are some of the addictive patterns I see which may lead you into a path of a reliance of uppers like caffeine and downers like alcohol, or even just those high carb foods in general that so many people love to eat day in and day out.

Your appetite may become disordered, your eating patterns erratic and before you know it you could easily develop a digestive problem. Some last resort patients may take 10, 20 or even 40 different dietary supplements in the belief they will conquer the bad symptoms inside, there will be a lot more on that topic in section 4 of this chapter.

And then candida comes along as an opportunistic infection and you develop a yeast infection and poor digestive health. And then you are off to visit the doctor looking for a solution that will generally come in the form of a five-minute visit and an antibiotic or an antidepressant. Problem solved you think, but wait a minute, that's when the fun begins. You keep the underlying dietary and lifestyle patterns going but now compound your addictions and compulsions with pharmaceutical drugs to conveniently switch off the problems. And you begin to feel worse, another trip to the doctor or naturopath and yet another drug or dietary supplement. And when you practitioner is finally sick and tired of you complaining about being sick and tired, you may be labeled as a difficult or non-compliant patient. I had enough of working in medical clinics after more than ten years; that's when I decided to once again set up my own clinic and work with chronically unwell patients who had enough of being bounced around, hopping from one doctor to another.

The Apple Picker

To be honest, I really don't care if I upset a few people here or there, I have lost a few patients over the years but I have had good results with many seemingly hopeless cases which were long ago discarded by practitioners who go onto easier pickings, or what one doctor friend called the "low-hanging fruit". You can't achieve quality in a brief ten-minute consultation, and the more challenging patients require much more time, valuable time a medical professional simply hasn't got.

The apples at the very top of an apple tree are the last resort patients, they are much more difficult to pick and win over than the apples at the bottom of the tree, and are probably the best apples when you finally can reach them. There is a risk of falling if you do try to reach out to them, but you get to be a skilled apple-picker after a while, and by falling I mean offending them with more direct talk, or potential strong aggravations they may receive during treatment, etc. These are often the last resort patients who end up in my clinic.

I have been known to be straight up with patients with addictive behaviors, there is no point beating around the bush. "Do you want to get well" I ask them.

"Yes I do" is the reply. "Are you willing to do what it takes to get well?" "Yes I am". "Do you enjoy feeling this terrible, having headaches, bowel problems, fatigue, etc." "No, I don't, I've had enough". "I'm willing to do whatever it takes, I've spent thousands of dollars and really have had enough, I am ready to get well". I have often thought about calling my clinic The Last Resort because that is what some patients tell us as naturopaths: "You are my last resort".

Many naturopathic doctors will have heard these very words, and the longer they practice and the more experience they gain, the more chronic and complex cases they tend to see. It is for these naturopaths that I have developed the Candida Crusher concept as well, for those who see the last resort patients.

Are you a looking at checking into the last resort hotel yourself with your chronic health problem? If you are a Baby Boomer like me, you may be familiar with a song from the American band The Eagles called "Hotel California". Remember the line from Hotel California: "You can check out anytime you like, but you can never leave"?

Some patients I have seen love being in the Last Resort Hotel, it almost suits a purpose of staying unwell, a kind of self-sabotage. Like the 27-year old patient I had who was abused as a girl and now feels comfortable at 220 pounds to avoid an intimate relationship. Like the 48-year-old work at home mother who goes to her refrigerator for ice cream a few times a day and has peanut butter sandwiches for lunch. "I can't be bothered, I've been with my man for twelve years and we have kind of drifted apart. He does his thing and I do mine". Yet another person who feels like she is permanently checked into the Last Resort Hotel.

The crazy thing is you can check out of the Last Resort Hotel any time you like, and you can always leave. It's your decision, and if you come to my clinic you will get your wake-up call, but a nice one though, unless you eat the chocolate from the mini-bar! The Candida Crusher Program contains many tricks and tips on how you can avoid becoming a last resort patient, and if you have living in this establishment, how you can check out for good.

Aggravations And How To Minimize Them

There are many different types of aggravations people experience who come to seek the help of a health care professional. Some people come in with one or several pharmaceutical drug induced side effects, such as after an antibiotic, others experience a reaction when they stop taking a drug or change brands of drugs, etc.

Many people can potentially develop an aggravation at the beginning of natural therapy treatment, and this can be quite discouraging for some. Those who are used to conventional Western medicine find the concept of "feeling worse before you feel better" a bit disturbing and some find it even downright crazy, particularly those who strongly adhere to tenets of modern medicine. Modern medicine believes that a diagnosis must first be made before treatment usually in the form of a drug that supposedly cures the complaint by way of eradicating the symptom.

Aggravations can come about for many different reasons and here are six examples of common reactions that I see occurring regularly with patients:

1. Drug side effects that we call iatrogenic disease.

2. Coming off any medications or detoxing from pharmaceutical drugs.

3. A change in diet after commencing treatment.

4. Combining several different treatments, drugs and dietary supplements, at the same time.

5. Improperly combining drugs and natural medicines at the same time.

6. Cleansing reactions of the body after commencing natural medicine treatment, often times this will be drug residues clearing from the body.

You may notice that I have not mentioned a "die-off" reaction above (Herxheimer reaction), i.e., candida yeast dying off in the body due to effective candida treatment. In my experience, many people incorrectly perceive aggravations after the commencement of yeast infection treatment as "die-off".

I have found that these aggravations are often due to a combination of several factors and cannot be blamed solely on "yeast dying-off". Many diseases often get somewhat worse with effective treatment for a multitude of different reasons.

Unfortunately, we live in an age that seems to be obsessed with speed, everything has to happen NOW, it seems as if we can't seem to wait until tomorrow for anything anymore. As technology increases and everything speeds up, so do our expectations of healing our bodies. As a result we expect a quick fix, and conventional medicine certainly comes up trumps here, it gets rid of symptoms, more likely suppresses them, so the disease goes somewhere else and gets buried deeper inside our bodies. Do you have a rash on your skin? Then take an antifungal cream, it will go deeper when you apply that cream and will not be cured by any means, but will temporarily disappear, which is a "cure" according to your skin specialist. Is it any wonder we get aggravations once we actually stop these kinds of suppressive treatments and all these hidden and buried symptoms rise to the surface of our bodies? Drugs taken even many years ago have residues which can remain deeply buried inside your body, and these toxins can and will resurface at the most inconvenient times, often when you try to improve your health by natural means. A die-off reaction is not necessarily what you are experiencing, your reaction is more likely to be a thorough house cleansing, especially if you have been on a drug cocktail in the past.

You will find this particularly so once you start the Candida Crusher Program; because it will dig deep and help the body throw off these buried poisons. Personally, I would rather not take any pharmaceutical drug that merely suppresses symptoms, upsets my stomach and puts pressure on my liver.

To examine what a disease aggravation means, let's take a look at the father of medicine, Hippocrates.

Hippocrates – The First Physician

Hippocrates was born around the year 460 BC on the Greek island of Kos (Cos), and became a famous ambassador for medicine. Essentially, he was the first Western physician and is credited with being the first person to believe that diseases were caused naturally, not due to superstitious beliefs or the gods.

Hippocrates separated the discipline of medicine from religion, believing and arguing that disease was not a punishment inflicted by the gods, but rather the product of environmental factors such as a poor or wrongful diet and of bad living habits. What you may find interesting is that an aggravation of an illness before recovery is an important concept, a concept that has been unfortunately lost in traditional Western medicine today. Likewise, the concept of looking for the cause is lost as well, because not much attention is paid today by medical practitioners when it comes to the actual cause of disease because it is all about treatment, because treatment is profitable.

In Hippocratic medicine the belief was that a *healing crisis*, was a point in the progression of the disease at which either the illness would begin to triumph and the patient would succumb to death, or that the opposite would occur and natural healing processes would make the patient recover. After a healing crisis, a relapse may follow, and then possibly another crisis. According to Hippocrates, crises tend to occur on certain days, which were supposed to be a fixed time after the contraction of a disease.

Hippocrates was a humble and passive man and based his therapeutic approach on "vis medictrix naturae", the healing power of nature. He believed that rest and immobilization were of prime importance if true healing was to take place. Hippocratic medicine was very kind to the patient, and treatment was gentle with emphasis on keeping the patient clean and his wounds as sterile as possible. For example, clean water or wine were used on wounds, though keeping wounds dry was preferable treatment. It is important to mention that the germ theory did not come about until almost two thousand years later. Hippocrates developed his theories after much observation and a lot of common sense, something sadly lacking in modern medicine today. Unlike physicians of today, Hippocrates was most reluctant to administer any strong drugs such as heavy metals and poisons which were commonly used back then, or to hastily engage in any specialized treatment that might later prove to be wrongly chosen.

If you remember what I wrote previously about "How people actually get well" you may notice that there are ups and downs, and these are the aggravations and recovery phases. The degree of aggravation depends much on your lifestyle and diet during your treatment, as well as the degree of how sensitive you are. Aggravations can be mostly avoided with careful preparation. Just like anything in this life, it's all in the planning. If you plan carefully and prepare your body when you want to change your diet and lifestyle and carefully *ease yourself* into new ways, you will find that an aggravation will either be very mild or almost non-existent. Those who seem to suffer the most with violent aggravations are those who do not ease themselves carefully into treatment.

Some patients ignore my advice and take twenty capsules a day of a supplement instead of two or three, is it any wonder they aggravate? Others make very quick and strong dietary changes, going from seven cups of coffee to zilch, or decide one day to clean up their act and made radical changes to what and how they eat. Radical people end up with monumental aggravations, mild mannered people who make subtle and slow changes end up with minimal aggravations, certainly no rocket science here.

Very shortly you will be reading the diet and nutrition section of this book, and I'd like you to read it all the way through and take your time when you implement my recommendations. Plan your strategy, and that is why I want you to do the "Big Clean Up" I've outlined in the first section on this chapter, it will get you started correctly and minimize your chances of developing aggravations.

12 Candida Crusher Perseverance Tips

Recovering from a yeast infection depends to a large degree on your ability to discipline yourself. If anything in life is worth achieving, it is worth sticking to clearly defined principles and a well-defined plan until you reach your objective.

Here are my twelve favorite perseverance tips along with some of the best quotes I know. It is good practice to read these tips several times, especially at times when you feel yourself slipping down the slope.

You will need the ability to discipline yourself.

> *If I want to be great I have to win the victory over myself - self-discipline.*
> *Harry S. Truman*

You have probably bought this e-book because you are sick and tired of your yeast related problems and want to finally get rid of them. You may have read other similar e-books or consulted one or several practitioners as well. The ability to discipline yourself in order to enjoy the greater reward of making a full recovery from your yeast infection is by far the biggest and most indispensable pre-requisite you will need to ensure your complete success. Have you had enough, are you finally wanting to really commit? Yes? Then you are already half way there in getting rid of the problem that has been plaguing you for ages, but be aware of the pitfalls and traps all along the way which may sabotage your attempts to rid yourself of candida, such as parties, BBQs, eating out, birthday parties, Christmas, weddings and similar social occasions. Plan your outings so that you don't fall into temptation. Section 5 of this chapter will outline the importance of lifestyle, and this is one key area often neglected in yeast infection recovery, making the right changes here are persevering with the changes can literally mean the difference between recovering or failing to recover.

Do Not Give up Because of Laziness!

> *Genius is one percent inspiration and ninety-nine percent perspiration.*
> *Thomas Alva Edison.*

A life without a candida yeast infection is your aim, that's why you bought Candida Crusher surely. There are no shortcuts to a perfect health. Life and optimum health is a journey and not a destination. Living a lazy easy lifestyle will never be satisfying in the long run, in fact, it usually leads to feeling of unhappiness, being overweight and out of shape, having fatigue and all this can potentially lead to anxiety and depression. Living a healthy, happy and very satisfying life is hard work initially as you learn to pick up the slack and you will come to appreciate that having a great life including outstanding health takes commitment, but eventually it will become easier and easier. Don't give up; when the going gets tough… you know the rest. Your self-esteem will soar as you begin to reach milestones and then away you go; there will be no stopping you!

Pursue Your True Desire For Optimal Health

> *Discipline is the bridge between goals and accomplishments.*
> *Jim Rohn*

Never give up on ridding yourself of a yeast infection, particularly if you have had many health challenges for years and you can't go a day without thinking about a complete recovery. A lot of the time we aren't really going after a complete resolution of all our health problems because of some underlying fear or insecurity. We end up pursuing a very average life and this way we never end up feeling fantastic and living up to our full potential. This is why you must really go after what your heart desires, an excellent state of health free from yeast infection. This can be difficult because of social conditioning, peer pressure and many of society's implied rules which you are raised with, such as drinking alcohol, taking antibiotics routinely, eating cookies, drinking soda drinks and eating ice cream. Believe me, once you are pursuing your heart's true desire of being free of the torment of a yeast infection, perseverance and stick-ability will take care of itself. You will be naturally motivated to pursue your desires, especially after any aggravations have cleared and as your health progresses.

Never Give up Due To Little Or Lack of Progress.

> *Most of the important things in this world have been accomplished by people who have kept on trying when there seemed to be no hope at all.*
> Dale Carnegie

Worried about your seemingly lack of progress? This will take care of itself if you are pursuing your true desires, because your desire will be so strong, that a seemingly slow progress will become irrelevant. However there still will be times where you might become discouraged because of the slow or lack of progress in your recovery. I'd like you to think again of fantasy land, can you remember that while in a blockbuster movie you can see a character progress or change his whole lifestyle in a mere matter of 2 hours, in real life this progress is much slower? This is why most people don't stick with their goals, because they have unrealistic expectations.

I have seen too many patients over the years who didn't feel "cured" after a month and moved on to another form of treatment. Aim for a steady slow progress, and above all, remember the ups and downs you are likely to encounter as you recover.

Success is Much Closer than You Think.

> *Many of life's failures are people who did not realize how close they were to success when they gave up.*
> Thomas Alva Edison

Your success might just be around the corner, you may be surprised how close you are to beating the beast called yeast. Even if it's not, by persevering in pursuing your goal of great health you will be building a great lifelong habit of adopting a healthy diet and lifestyle. If you give up on your goal of permanent yeast eradication, how do you know that you will not give up on your next goal or the one after that? Be careful not to make giving up a habit in life! If you hang in there and keep working at it, you are building a persistent determined character and are sure to succeed. Quitters never win, and winners will never quit.

Always be Flexible & Willing to Change.

> *How am I going to live today in order to create the tomorrow I'm committed to?*
> Anthony Robbins

If I had a dollar every time I heard a patient say: "I can't take supplements, I just forget to take them" or "I don't like to swallow any pills" or "There is no way I could eat like that", "Your diet is too difficult to follow", etc., then I'd be a rich man. Please don't let your current identity or self-image limit the pursuit of your ultimate health goals. Always be willing to make the necessary changes, to try new or different foods, and to learn new skills like relaxing, laughing, breathing deeply and more. Be willing to look like a fool every now and then! Remember that definition of insanity? You will hear this time and again in this book, in fact it has been written down more than six times – The definition of insanity is doing the same thing over and over and expecting a different result. So to achieve a new goal you must slowly make changes and try different things.

Start Visualizing the New You Today

> " *Self-discipline is an act of cultivation.*
> *It requires you to connect today's actions to tomorrow's results.*
> *There's a season for sowing a season for reaping.*
> *Self-discipline helps you know which is which.* "
> Gary Ryan Blair

Don't knock it; visualization is very powerful especially as you use it more and more. Whatever goal or endeavor you are pursuing, close your eyes and start visualizing yourself as having achieved it. Visualize how happy you feel as a result of an optimally functioning digestive system – no bloating, no constipation or diarrhea – ever. Visualize beautiful skin, a sweet breath, loads of energy, no headaches, and no vaginal thrush. Just visualize for one moment that you go from day to day enjoying your body and never have to worry about any symptoms anymore. Especially, visualize becoming a lot more successful in all other areas of your life because of the extraordinary confidence you now have obtained from achieving your goal of being completely free of a candida yeast infection. Daily review your goals, and visualize achieving them.

Add Strong Emotions to Your Goals

> " *Strong, deeply rooted desire is the starting point of all achievement.* "
> Napoleon Hill

If you set yourself a goal of "just getting better", then this is just a goal, a few words or a meaningless sentence. However, once you add a strong emotion, it starts to take on a whole new meaning and becomes a part of you. Achieving the goal of optimizing your health becomes a strong part of your character. Let's say you set the following goal "I want to cure myself of a yeast infection". This is a very plainly stated goal. What does it look like when you add emotions? "I want to get rid of my yeast infection permanently because I'm sick and tired of when I go out eating with friends that I can only eat a very limited range of foods". Or perhaps, "I want to get rid of my vaginal thrush permanently because it is causing a lot of tension between myself and my partner" Maybe this one "After ten years of digestive problems, I want to be able to be one hundred percent free of bowel problems like bloating and pain and know what it is like to have my slim waist back again" The more emotional reasons that you come up with for why you must achieve your goal of a permanent yeast eradication, the better. You should regularly review and add to your list of reasons.

Use Your Personal Network for Support

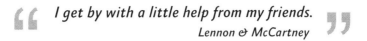

I get by with a little help from my friends.
Lennon & McCartney

The best resource is your personal network, you will have a circle of contacts and there will be friends and family only too willing to support your recovery. It's your job to communicate effectively to your network by being clear about what your intentions are and that you'd appreciate support in your quest to permanently kick your yeast infection. It helps to be specific when approaching your friends to give them information that's easy to act on, such as "I'm avoiding alcohol for the next several months, and I'd really appreciate some support guys".

Use My Multi Staged Approach

Make at least one definite move daily toward your goal.
Bruce Lee

The successful treatment of an overgrowth of Candida albicans needs a multi-stage attack, you need consistent persistence and a daily advancement towards your goal. Bruce Lee trained daily like there was no tomorrow and became a legend in martial arts. You also can become a legend in your own circles by committing daily towards your health goals. In my professional experience, all five aspects of the Candida Crusher Program I outline need to be carefully followed otherwise you will just get average results, my clinical observations have shown this repeatedly with many patients. I want you to forget that "magic pill" that will "cure" you; it is simply not going to happen. Following the Candida Crusher Program is not a walk in the park, yet it doesn't have to be a one-year hike into the wilderness either. I have found that there are some patients who have enormous difficulty sticking to the commitment they make to change their lifestyle. They are sometimes so much at the mercy of their candida-induced confusion; some have muddled thinking and a lack of clarity that at times accompanies the high levels of toxins produced by the Candida, that it can be quite difficult for them to take consistent action. I just wanted you to be aware of this important point before we launch into the Candida Crusher Program. You will get well; it is just a matter of time. Imagine a life free of digestive hassles, skin problems, it is not only a distinct possibility, it is a certainty with your perseverance.

Winners never quit and quitters never win

We must all suffer from one of two pains: the pain of discipline or the pain of regret.
The difference is discipline weighs ounces while regret weighs tons.
Jim Rohn

I want you to know that a permanent solution to your yeast infection can and will happen for you, providing you stay true to your word and follow the plan. Look for example at sports professionals, they follow the rules of the game carefully, and in your case, the rules for candida eradication as outlined in my Candida Crusher Program, they get regular and professional guidance from their coach, in your case, your health-coach, the Candida Crusher, they persist with much training and the outcome is almost always assured, success in their field. The winner takes it all, and like the Olympic athlete, you could even shoot for gold and totally surpass your own expectations by permanently shifting that chronic health problem like that weight you have been trying to permanently shift for years but gave up on. The difference between silver and gold is in going that extra mile.

There are many aspects to getting over candida and restoring your health and wellbeing, and it is absolutely possible to completely overcome candida. Please follow my five steps carefully, and most importantly, remember that there is no clearly defined time for overcoming your candida yeast infection. It is all up to you, some patients achieve amazing results in as little as three months, with others it can take considerably longer, a year or more.

Regularly Review these Words of Calvin Coolidge

> *Nothing in the world can take the place of persistence.*
> *Talent will not; nothing in the world is more common than unsuccessful men with talent.*
> *Genius will not; unrewarded genius is a proverb. Education will not;*
> *the world is full of educated derelicts.*
> *Persistence and determination alone are omnipotent.*
> *Calvin Coolidge*

The Candida Crusher Diet – Understanding Digestion and Nutrition

> *Disease can be cured through the proper use of correct foods. This statement may sound deceptively simple, but I have arrived at it only after intensive study of a highly complex subject: colloid and endocrine chemistry. My conclusions are based on experimental and observational results, gathered through many years of successfully treating patients. I have sought to prescribe for my patients' illnesses antidotes which nature has placed at their disposal.*
> Dr. Henry G. Bieler, M.D. (1965). Food Is Your Best Medicine.

Why Eating Correct Will Give You Permanent Results

Change your diet; don't feed candida on foods that yeasts love. I often tell my patients to be careful, because these foods will "call your name", they will tell you to buy them and consume them regularly and its called a craving, and in disguise many cravings are actually sugar cravings. "I like the taste of that" almost always means that the food you like contains sugar. I recently attended Expo West in Anaheim, California, in March 2013, and to my surprise, most of the fruity drinks and even vitamin C beverages contained sucrose as their main ingredient!

Avoiding these highly desired foods means avoiding as much as possible any refined carbohydrate foods like white flour, refined sugars such as corn syrup and glucose, fruit juices and honey and more, just look at the "Foods to Avoid" list in the Candida Control Diet. There are countless books and articles I have read relating to candida eradication, I have tried many diets with patients but have achieved outstanding success with the 3-stage Candida Crusher Diet which I have found actually works, and it works brilliantly. The thing is to use common sense, and not the latest diet-book fad. If you crave it, then just stop eating it. If is very sweet in your mouth and you know it is wrong, then stop eating it!

I have found that a candida patient will often desire a particular food or beverage, and this may very well be the one underpinning the condition. Think about it for just one moment; are you a person who has a strong desire or craving for a particular food or drink?

Yeast hates a healthy diet full of fresh vegetables, fruits and high quality proteins devoid of refined carbs. After many years of treating candida patients in my clinic, I have not been convinced that all patients need to strictly avoid all fruits (but NO dried fruits please!) with candida issues, but do request that those with major problems of several years duration follow my eating program as outlined below carefully. In 1986, Dr. William Crook, the author of the well-known book The Yeast Connection, did a huge amount of research into foods and candida and found out these four points after interviewing many practitioners and patients:

- Avoiding all sugar containing foods and the refined carbohydrates.

- Eating more complex carbohydrates (vegetables especially)

- Eliminating fresh fruits during the early weeks of the diet.

- Eliminating starchy vegetables during the first two weeks of the diet.

If you suspect candida, it is useful to take note of my dietary advice since it does not contradict the general guidelines for good healthy eating and has made an enormous difference in the lives of so many patients who unbeknown to them, were being made miserable by this condition. Just do the diet strictly from two to four weeks, then slowly include more fresh fruits, starchy vegetables and as you improve you will be able to eat a much wider assortment of foods, all in good time.

Many people who seek help eradicating their yeast infection routinely approach our clinic, and many of these men and women have been following some kind of dietary protocol for a long time, in some cases for many years. Unfortunately, if many of these patients fail to adhere very strictly to their diet and just for a day or two revert back to foods they could consume years ago, their symptoms return almost immediately. This does not prove that their diet doesn't work, it proves that their candida protocol isn't working for them. The diet is but a small part of eradicating candida, it is an important yet nevertheless small part, and once you have finished reading chapter 7, you will understand what I mean by this. It is more likely that the person who has had the most difficulty in recovering, will be the one most likely to be suffering from a condition such as adrenal fatigue. Other patients may have some kind of block, and eating a "perfect" diet certainly won't make the difference in such a case, I can assure you.
Just remember, you cannot eradicate your yeast infection by diet alone, you may subdue or tame it, but it will be ready to flare up and make your life miserable at the next opportune moment.

10 Golden Rules For Healthy Eating

1. Slow down when you eat. Take your time and do not rush. Your digestion and bowel function will improve.

2. Chew your foods well, Eat more slowly, chew more slowly and deliberately and be aware of what you are doing. You'd be surprised how quick you chew and swallow your foods!

3. Relax, and never eat when stressed or tired. Remember, you don't have to eat if you don't feel like it, eat when you are hungry.

4. Have at least one day per week where you eat very light, light enough to make you feel like you could have had more after your evening meal. This will keep your digestion in good shape as you age.

5. Smell and taste your foods. Savor your foods and enjoy the experience. This will ensure that sufficient saliva is produced and your digestion will be in fine form. This is a bit like priming the engine of your lawn mower, chainsaw or brush cutter before you start the engine. A stomach anticipating foods will digest more efficiently.

6. Don't watch TV, read papers, books or emails or computers while you eat. Your mind should be on the job!

7. Eat smaller portions. Buy smaller dinner plates and if you eat out don't feel that you have to eat everything on your plate. Do you really need that dessert after your meal?

8. Increase the quality and decrease the quantity (except fruit and vegetables) of the foods you consume. For example buy organic or grow your own vegetables and fruits as much as possible. Buy organic chicken at least over commercial poultry.

9. Eat a lot less red meat (beef, pork, sheep, and deer) and get more protein more from fish, legumes, nuts and seeds and fermented tofu like tempeh. Avoid all kinds of processed meats.

10. Eat breakfast like a king, lunch like a prince and dinner like a pauper. Have a good-sized breakfast, a medium sized lunch and a smaller portion with your evening meal. Your weight will become much more manageable and your energy levels will increase in the afternoon as your blood sugar levels improve. It takes time to adjust to eating like this so please be patient!

Stay on the diet especially stage 1 and stage 2 that I have recommended, for as long as it takes, which can be from 3 to 6 months or even longer. Why does it take this long you are thinking? It takes this long because you are trying to establish healthy bowel flora, and because the surface area of your digestive system is considerable and there is a large amount of bacteria present, including several hundred different species, it simply won't happen overnight. If you ever tried to start a new lawn you will understand exactly what I mean. It takes plenty of time and commitment, because you have to water the lawn, keep people off it initially, refrain from mowing it for several weeks and feed it regularly. After several months your lawn looks beautiful, because you took the time to care for it and did the right thing.

Over a period of time and commitment, your digestive system will feel great and you will have probably made some long-term changes as your health has improved in many different ways. And who wants to continue with symptoms like bloating, flatus, and itching, mental fogginess and fatigue anyway?

I have found with patients that the ones who get the best long-term results are generally the ones who are totally committed to changing the way they think about their dietary and lifestyle choices, they make the right choices long term, and more importantly, they actually stick with those new healthy choices. If you change what you eat and make healthier choices, your digestive system will improve as a result, the yeast infection will go away and your health will improve. It's as simple as that.

Caution - Confusing Candida Dietary Advice Exists

One word of caution before we go any further, you will find some confusion in the sometimes wildly and differing opinions of those who advocate various yeast control diets. Some books and websites I have studied over the years are far to "easy" on the candida diet, one well-known book even recommends that all fruit is OK, whereas others are way too strict. One well-known American website claims that nuts should never consumed by those with a yeast infection, as they are among the foods on which candida thrives. This is a myth, I can understand that peanuts are taboo as they are potentially highly allergenic and are frequently moldy, but to take almonds for example out of the diet of a person with yeast infection is plain ridiculous.

After having worked with patients with yeast infections for over two decades, I can state with absolute confidence that most all yeast infection sufferers can tolerate nuts, but common sense prevails naturally. It is not wise to allow a person to eat 200 to 300 grams of nuts every day.

You need to obviously exercise caution, and some readers of this book will be more sensitive than others to one or several of the foods I may recommend. Others with a yeast infection may even be OK with a limited range of fruits as they begin their treatment, you will find that throughout this book that I advocate trial and error. One thing is for certain, one size does not fit all and you will need to tweak this program to suit your self.

Crush This Habit – Eating The Wrong Kind Of Foods

" *If we are not willing to settle for junk living,*
we certainly shouldn't settle for junk foods. "
Sally Edwards

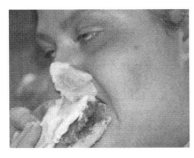

The very foods we love to eat and the ones we buy from the supermarket and the ones marketed by the fast food companies often on the television are the foods that favor the overgrowth of candida yeast colonies in our bodies. Before you are serious about starting the Candida Crusher Program, it is advisable to make the right dietary changes and to adopt the correct basic dietary habits you will soon read about. Are you guilty of eating take-out foods once, twice, or several times a week? This is the very first thing you change, stop buying those fast foods and eat more at home. Buy fresh foods from your grocery store, butcher and Farmer's Markets, you will be making healthier choices. This is the first step in the right direction as far the Candida Crusher Diet and Nutrition Program is concerned.

Junk Food Challenge, Can You Do It?

Avoid These Foods For 21 Days

- No soda drinks

- No chocolate

- No ice cream

- No sweets or candy

- No biscuits of cookies

- No donuts, muffins or cakes

- No pastries

- No white breads

- No chips

- No pizza, fried chicken or take-out foods

- No Nutella, peanut butter, jam or spreads

Crush This Habit - Eating Too Fast

> " *Some people immediately descend on the dishes*
> *the moment they have been set down. Wolves do that.* "
> Desiderius Erasmus 1536

I have spent many an hour in the clinic talking with patients not only about the foods they eat, but when and how and under what circumstances they eat them.

The people we see come from all walks of life, for example one day a patient may be a mother who is small business owner and who simply does not take the time out to eat properly and meals are often a hurried affair. She is off to work in a hurry with breakfast consisting of a coffee and a piece of toast, her child is dropped off at day care as she speeds to the office. Lunch will be quickly consumed over a keyboard, a nut-bar may be consumed in the afternoon with more coffee and on the way home from work a take-away meal is bought to be eaten in front of television along with a glass of wine or a Coke.

The hurried 21st century habits we have created and very way we eat today is probably one of the most candida predisposing factors of them all; we tend to eat on the run whilst trying to do other things. It is called "multi-tasking"; a term that never existed in the 60's when I grew up.

Today we seem to be gadget rich yet time poor and our digestive systems suffer as a consequence. The sugar and starch content of many meals today is way too high and the fiber component of our diet has become much too low, including our consumption of fresh fruits and vegetables. Convenience foods have become a quick-fix solution to our hurried and worried modern way of living.

The past five years I have focused on researching the best ways to treat stress and fatigue in my clinic and have found that this way of eating can predispose you to fermentation dysbiosis, particularly when you are stressed at the time of eating. You can read all about the effects of stress on digestion in this section 2 of this chapter.

To sum it up, many of us eat on the run, eat a highly refined diet and suffer very much from stress. Is it any wonder that yeast overgrowth and digestive problems are rampant?

Crush This Habit – Just Eating Too Much

> " *One-quarter of what you eat keeps you alive.*
> *The other three-quarters keeps your doctor alive.* "
> (Hieroglyph found in an ancient Egyptian tomb.)

The sheer quantity of foods consumed today can also dispose a person towards a yeast infection. Many of us are still conditioned to eating all the foods on our plates, we eat far too much and too often, considering the fact that many of us live sedentary lives and exercise infrequently (if at all) and increasing technology has meant that many do very little compared to as little twenty years ago before this mobile phone, tablet and computer age. There is little doubt that the best exercise you can perform is simply to push that dinner plate away from your body when it is half empty.

When I was a student of naturopathy I can remember reading an excellent book written by the Swiss naturopath Dr. Alfred Vogel, called "The Nature Doctor". Dr. Vogel outlined the importance of eating much more slowly than we do today and in particular to chew each mouthful several times slowly and deliberately before swallowing and in addition, not to eat when we are stressed or tired. Do you eat your main meal later in the evening, perhaps at eight or nine after a glass of wine? Many patients I have spoken to do just this, particularly the city folk. Remember the old saying; "eat breakfast like a king, lunch like a prince and dinner like a pauper"? How often have you consumed a meal in front of the television news or whilst checking your e-mails, perhaps reading the local weekly newspapers or skimming through the junk mail?

Many people in countries like Spain and France still take their time with meals allowing their digestive systems to work more effectively, producing digestive enzymes and digesting their foods before they resume their work. Meals are consumed as an important part of their social rituals, whereas we tend to regard eating as something that needs to be completed as soon as possible because we have more important things to do, like checking our inbox or replying to that SMS on our mobile phone.

It is a known fact now that those who live the longest tend to eat fewer calories as they age, and my dietary recommendations are for as you get beyond fifty, to increase the quality of your foods and decrease the quantity of your foods. Many of us still have the "two-dollar shop" mentality when it comes to buying foods for the family, and look at saving as much as they can on the weekly grocery bill, but then go out and blow the savings on alcohol and take-away foods each week. Isn't your health worth it? Of course it is, buy the very best foods you can afford, the very quality of your life will depend on the quality and quantity of foods you consume, especially as you age over the years.

Your blood sugar levels will be naturally at a low point when you get up, that is why they call breakfast the "break-fast" meal, as your body has rested over night and fasted and is now ready for some food. If you skip breakfast like many busy women do, your blood sugar will stay at a lowered rate and you will be operating on your reserve levels until lunchtime. By eating a sugary breakfast cereal or a piece of toast with jam, or a donut and a cup of tea or coffee your blood sugar levels will quickly rise again but then drop rapidly as well making you feel tired, jaded and even a little jittery. Sudden drops in energy will have you clamoring for the refrigerator or pantry again for something quick or sweet. If however, on the other hand you have a protein meal for breakfast you will not suffer from this problem. It becomes easier for you to resist sweets or sweet foods when you get into the habit of consuming more protein in general, particularly before lunchtime. Try it yourself and see the incredible difference something simple like this can do to your health.

Crush This Habit – Technology And Eating

Were you aware that one in five people in America have at least one meal of the day while checking their Facebook status? A question I ask my patients is if they watch TV, check their mobile phone, IPad or computer while they eat their breakfast, lunch or dinner, and around forty percent say "Yes, I do". A 2010 Nokia study found that the average person stares at his of her phone over 100 times in a day, which works out to be about 6 minutes out of every hour a person is awake. According to Nokia's 3G consultant Tomi Ahonen, a mobile phone is a faster way to reach consumers than any other digital form of communication. A study done in New Zealand found that the average email is opened 48 hours after it is sent while the average text message is opened 4 minutes after being sent. Ahonen said, "SMS is literally 720 times faster than e-mail in message-opening throughput." My concern with all this increasing technology is that this incessant need for speed is making mobile phone users way too reliant on increasingly accelerated forms of communication, which serves to accelerate stress responses in their body as well. Later on you will read about the SNS, the sympathetic nervous system, stress and digestion. How about putting those mobile phones away and only them at certain times of the day? Do you really need to check those emails every hour?

Your Stomach Is Like A Cement Mixer

I find it helpful to explain digestion in simplistic ways; people tend to remember it a lot better that way and can picture these explanations in their minds better than showing complex charts with digestive organs and using a bunch of fancy Latin names. A cement mixer to me is a lot like the stomach, you place gravel, sand and cement powder in it (carbs, proteins and fats), and you then add water and mix it. Chewing food is like running the cement mixer, it needs to be done thoroughly and properly or the mix won't be any good.

Many folks eat too quickly, chew foods once or twice and then swallow. Imagine what kind of concrete this produces! A concrete truck in fact constantly agitates the mix, a bit like a camel is constantly seen chewing food. Did you know that some people in the Middle East can chew one fresh date for more than six hours?

Your stomach produces a fluid called chyme, a liquid substance found in the stomach before passing through a small valve and into the small intestine. It results from the mechanical and chemical breakdown and consists of partially digested food, water, hydrochloric acid, and various digestive enzymes.

I was helping a friend last year to build a raised garden for his vegetables. We had to mix concrete as part of the job, and he said to only ever fill a cement mixer about three quarters full of gravel and cement powder, because by the time you add water it is still achievable to turn it and make cement. When I once tried to put more in, it didn't work and I started to realize how the stomach is the same. In fact, if you eat smaller meals and take your time eating, your digestion will be much more efficient because you break the food particles down to a much smaller size and mix the food more efficiently with saliva and digestive enzymes.

I worked out that by filling the cement mixer by fifty percent, we could mix it much more thoroughly, empty the bowl much more easily, and work more efficiently with smaller batches too. It was also easier to clean the equipment and we didn't make half the mess.

I also worked out that too much water in the mix made it sloppy and ruined the concrete, and not enough made it too dry and unusable. I feel the same about drinking with meals; you will need to work out the right amount to drink with meals. You don't add coffee, tea or beer to cement, and it really should the same when you eat; just add a bit of water. Watch the difference what comes out the next day, your motions will be better formed. With a bit of trial and error, you can get your "mix" just right.

Crush This Habit - Eating The Wrong Way Around

One of the most important measures we can take to significantly improve our internal environment is meal reversal, meaning larger meal for breakfast (king) medium sized meal for lunch (prince) and a smaller meal for dinner (like a pauper).

I have seen many patients improve on this regime where many other suggestions or treatments to improve their overall health failed. Your body, like everything else in nature, is designed to work in a time-pattern, and the Chinese gained this knowledge several thousand of years ago. Professor Kurt Richter first discovered this pattern, a well-known American bio-psychologist who died in 1989 aged ninety-four. Dr. Richter discovered in 1927 the biorhythm principle that governs body function.

A whole new science has grown from his early work now known as bio-chronology. By understanding bio-chronology, we learn that our body runs on a body clock and that by understanding the gastrointestinal peak times and troughs we can significantly improve our digestion and health in general.

Stomach – The peak performance of your stomach is between 7.00 – 9.00am, so by including plenty of proteins in your breakfast at this time you will ensure a more complete breakdown of foods rather than eating loads of heavy proteins at your evening meal. Your stomach's activity peaks early in the day and slowly tapers off until mid afternoon. This includes the digestive tract and most organs in general. Most people have a bowel motion on rising (the large intestine is most active from 5.00 – 7.00am) and the excretion of motions is further enhanced by the stomach's activity a few hours later, if you eat breakfast, that is, increasing peristalsis which is a fancy word used in medicine to describe the wave like contractions of your intestines which help propel motions through it.

Small intestine – The peak performance time of the small bowel is between 1.00 – 3.00pm, so as you can see it pays to eat your protein load like a king in the morning, like a prince at lunch and considerably less with your evening meal. Most of your protein digestion and absorption occurs from about 7.00 am until 3.00pm. That is not to suggest that no protein digestion occurs at other times, it is just more concentrated between these hours. I suggest some protein with lunch, but not as much and a lighter grade than with breakfast. I personally prefer eggs with breakfast and fish or a small amount of chicken or fish with lunch. For dinner I suggest that you eat a lighter protein meal like fresh fish or free range chicken, tempeh (fermented tofu), lentils, and beans or perhaps quinoa.

Large intestine – Your colon is most active very early in the morning between the hours of 5.00 – 7.00am. This is the time you want to head to the bathroom, have you noticed? This is a good time to drink plenty of water as well, and be sure to drink plenty of clean, fresh water between rising up until the early afternoon in particular.

21 Best Guidelines For Following The Candida Crusher Diet

Here are twenty of the best dietary guidelines for counteracting the candida yeast syndrome. Food lists are given later in this chapter as well, to assist you in your efforts to stay with these guidelines and achieve the best effect with your diet.

1 Eat real food, fresh foods with every meal. Never skip meals, and it will really pay to snack on fresh foods like vegetables, between meals. Avoid snacking on fresh fruit, too much sugar. Keep away from bread as a snack for a long time if you have a yeast infection.

2 Be sure to eat each day at least one, but preferably two of the following groups: the green leafy group: (spinach, broccoli, salad greens, asparagus, celery, etc.), the colored group (red, yellow, purple, orange like peppers, tomatoes, eggplant, zucchini, etc.) and the candida specifics (coconut, garlic, oregano, fresh yoghurt, etc.). A portion would be from one to several tablespoons.

3 You can eat vegetables in six different ways – raw, steamed, stir fried, grilled, baked or boiled. Raw is best and boiled is the worst. Start with eating small amounts of raw vegetables and plenty of steamed vegetables and start eating less baked and boiled. In time, forget boiling and eat only raw, steamed (lightly) and stir-fried. This way you will destroy considerably less enzymes contained in these foods, and eat foods higher in phyto-nutrients with less chance of depletion.

4 If you want to consume vegetable juices then I would recommend that you don't juice your vegetables with a conventional juicer. They extract the juice only, and you end up throwing away the bulk, or the fiber. The fiber content is important for several reasons, particularly for reducing the chances of constipation and giving the bowel food to grow ample beneficial and friendly bacteria. Both of these reasons are important for those with candida because candida yeast sufferers often get constipated and lack sufficient beneficial bacteria in their bowel. Get a vegetable juicer that pulverizes the whole vegetable, that way you get sufficient fiber. You will be reading a lot more about juicing and the best juicer to buy in this section soon.

5 Your bowel motions will give you a good indication if you consume adequate fiber in your diet. If you consume sufficient vegetable fiber, you bowel motions will improve and be easier to pass. They will be of good size and float more than they would sink. I learned this saying from Dr. Alan Gaby: "small stools = big hospitals, big stools = small hospitals".

6 Eat ten to fifteen serves a week of first class protein, which includes poultry and eggs, seafood including fish and shellfish, and the pink & red meats including beef, venison, pork and lamb. Choose fish, eggs and chicken instead of the pink and red meats. Eat no more than 500 grams (1 pound) of read meat a week, you will read a lot about why you will want to reduce red meats soon in this section of the book.

7 If you crave sweet foods then you are best to eat small amounts of protein foods several times a day. Your blood sugar will be better balanced and you will crave less sweet foods as a consequence.

8 Be mindful that too much protein can constipate, therefore eat plenty of (especially green or highly colored) vegetable fiber in addition. Remember, you bowel motions will be your guide to a large extent. Do the "eyeball test", i.e.; look at your motions daily to see how your digestion is. If you start seeing food particles then you will need to chew your food more thoroughly, and consider staying with the digestive enzyme supplement for some time as well.

9 Eat meats stir-fried, steamed or baked – not microwaved, grilled, deep-fried and preferably not fried. Meats cooked medium rare or medium will be better digested than meat cooked well done. Trim off the fat (but not all, you need saturated fat in your diet) but do avoid meat that is marbled with far too much fat.

10 Drink a glass of water on rising, and another before breakfast and before each meal. It is also best to have a glass of water before bedtime, unless you have to get up out of bed early in the morning. Try to drink six to eight glasses of water daily. Your digestive system will improve tremendously, and this is the most important system to improve when you have a candida yeast infection. So, drink up!

11 A very clever idea is to add one to two drops of liquid grapefruit seed extract to each liter of water you consume throughout the day. I got this tip several years ago from a doctor in America who specializes in candida infections. It works very well and is most efficient if done for 3 months; if two drops is too much, just add one. This may well be the turning point for you if you have a chronic yeast infection, just this one tip daily (when continued for 3 – 6 months) could mean you are well on the way to a full recovery, especially if you keep your diet clean and healthy. While you are at it, add a drop or two of pure oregano oil to salad dressings.

12 Add lime or lemon juice to your water, it will aid digestion and has an antifungal action. Herbal tea is acceptable, but try to reduce or eliminate coffee and tea. Use a water purifier to filter tap water, preferably a reverse osmosis purifier.

13 Use a good quality sea salt and avoid the supermarket white salt. Useful seasonings to add flavor to your meals are black pepper, caraway, chives, cloves, curry, paprika, sage, and parsley. Particularly good choices are oregano, thyme, rosemary and marjoram because they are antimicrobial by nature. It is a good idea to grow these herbs and add them to your dishes all spring and summer long. Garlic and ginger should be used daily in your cooking, fresh is best.

14 The best oils to use are extra virgin olive oil, peanut oil, sesame oil, and organic sunflower oil. Avoid canola and "mixed" vegetable oils. Keep your oils (except olive oil) in the refrigerator and preferably in dark glass bottles. Nice oils to use on your salad as a dressing include avocado, or nut oils such as macadamia or walnut oil. These are more expensive, but you only need to use them sparingly. Coconut oil and coconut milk are particularly good choices as they are anti-fungal by nature.

15 Remember to eat natural foods, and to completely avoid soda drinks, as well as snacks and sweets like candy, biscuits, cookies, donuts, muesli bars (sugars) and other hidden sources of sugars. After you have avoided sweet foods for two to three weeks your cravings will diminish remarkably, take 500mg chromium picolinate with meals if you still crave sugars, you soon will not. Avoiding sugars and hidden forms of sugar is very important in successfully overcoming your candida yeast infection. It is critical that you identify early on the key sweet foods and/or drinks you regularly enjoy.

16 When you go to the supermarket, shop around the outside perimeter, there you will find the fresh produce such as meat, fish, vegetables, and other real foods. The foods in the aisles with be processed and packaged and is best avoided by you, especially in the first month or so. The reason why the perishable foods are situated on the perimeter is to give the shop assistants better access to foods that have a much shorter shelf life; the stuff in the center aisles can last for years due to the inclusion of preservatives, colors, additives and various other chemicals.

17 Eat less with your main meals; it is a good idea to leave the last spoonful or two of food on your plate. A good tip is to buy smaller dinner plates, you can pile a small plate up and think you have a lot of food on your plate, if you pile up food on a large plate – you are eating too much. I've said it before; one of the best forms of exercise is to push your plate away from your stomach, to the middle of the table before you have eaten all the food on your plate. You will be surprised how much better you feel and how easier it will be to maintain your weight. Avoid deserts, and if you get hungry later on, you can always have a little healthy snack.

18 Eat only those foods that you know are healthy for you. We are all human and like to indulge in the not so healthy at times. It is all about balance, but why eat foods repetitively with which you have a bad relationship? If you know what food is bad for you or brings you down in some way, then simply avoid it.

19 You dietary requirements depend on several different factors such as your age, occupation, your health habits (such as smoking) or taking pharmaceutical drugs for a health condition. It is best that you work with a naturopath or a nutritionally orientated doctor to establish your needs, and it is likewise important that you regularly visit him or her for your follow-up visits.

20 Be sure to take the correct dietary supplements with meals or away from meals that you require to help eradicate candida, restore balance and suit your individual needs. You can read all about the unique Candida Crusher dietary supplements in section 4 of this chapter. Again, it is best to work in conjunction with your practitioner in this regard. This book will give you good guidelines, but for any fine-tuning, be sure to ask your physician, and be sure that your physician gets a copy of my book. I can be contacted too for Skype or telephone consultations for distance patients.

21 Last but not least, please don't get discouraged with the Candida Crusher Diet; it is only temporary and a means to an end. Tell yourself that a strict adherence is best, particularly in the beginning phases. That way you will overcome your yeast infection along with any accompanying symptoms quicker, and you will soon be on the road to full recovery. I have helped many patients recover from candida infections and have noticed that one of the most important prerequisites is persistence, the person who sticks with the recommendations and stays on track.

20 Commonly Held Myths In Nutrition

Here are a few of the commonly held beliefs in nutrition in general. Some you may well be aware of while others may be new to you. Many of these myths have been promoted by mainstream health and medical authorities and are viewed as factually correct by many members of the public.

1. A well-balanced diet supplies all of the nutrients in sufficient quantities we need for optimal health and vitality. Fact: this is not true, it is now well established that most people do NOT consume sufficient nutrients through their diet.

2. Processed foods such as bottled, packaged or canned foods contain nutrients sufficient for optimal health and disease prevention.

3. Our foods contain "safe levels" of agricultural chemicals such as herbicides and pesticide residues. The chemical companies would like us to really believe that the human body has evolved sophisticated mechanisms that will allow it to detoxify over 60,000 chemicals it is exposed to in our environment.

4. Chlorine, fluoride and many other chemical residues found in tap water are harmless in the doses found. Unfortunately, they block iodine from working.

5. Vegetarian based diets are best for everyone, and eating a predominantly vegetarian diet will prolong your life.

6. Sugar is a natural part of life, according to the sugar manufacturing companies.

7. The processing of food does very little harm, e.g.; storing, packaging, freezing, coloring, processing, flavoring, gassing and irradiating it.

8. The selection of foods from the five major food groups is good nutrition for everyone; you need no more than this to sustain good health.

9. Food allergies and food sensitivities are rare and affect less than 5% of the population, according to mainstream medicine.

10. Nutritional deficiencies are rare in modern western society; we get all we need from our supermarket-based diet.

11. Fast take-away foods are an acceptable part of a "balanced nutritional program".

12. Alcohol is safe and harmless when consumed in small quantities.

13. Milk is an essential food for the growing child, lack of it will cause bones to crumble and the person will develop osteoporosis. It is interesting to note that countries with the highest intakes of dairy products have the highest levels of osteoporosis, while countries with the lowest levels of dairy intake have in fact the lowest levels of osteoporosis.

14. Foods have little influence on behavior, learning, emotions and long-term health and wellbeing of the individual.

15. If we suspect a nutritional deficiency, all we have to do is to increase the quantity of foods we eat to correct it, or take a pill containing those missing nutrients.

16. Organically grown fruits and vegetables are totally safe to eat and contain more nutrients than supermarket purchased fruits and vegetables. What about spray drift when organic orchards are planted next to conventional orchards?

17. Taking dietary supplements is useless, a waste of money and even fraudulent according to some mainstream medical websites.

18. Real butter and eggs are bad for your heart and cause an "elevation in cholesterol", we are told to eat margarine and eat little in the way of eggs.

19. Nutritional supplementation produces expensive urine. See Dr. Linus Pauling speaking on "expensive urine" on YouTube.

20. Dietary manipulation and nutritional supplementation have absolutely no influence on diseases that have a genetic component, e.g. cancer, diabetes, arthritis, cardiovascular disease, according to one leading American medical website.

Are You Eating For Emotional Comfort?

" *Do not bite at the bait of pleasure till you know there is no hook beneath it.* *"*
Thomas Jefferson

How do you deal with feelings of anger, anxiety, frustration, fear, stress, loneliness, conflict, depression or disappointment? Do you find comfort in food? Are you a patient I've see in the clinic who is trying one weight loss plan after another, or are just constantly on a diet, but in spite of a "perfect diet and exercise program" never seem to be losing weight? When you feel frustrated or disappointed with events or people, is the answer to eat something sweet? If you answered several of these questions with a 'yes', then I may call you an emotional comfort eater. Sure there are many reasons why you are not losing weight, it may well be your thyroid gland. But in many cases, it will be how you eat, what you eat and more importantly, why you eat, and under what circumstances.

Emotional eating is the practice of consuming large quantities of food in response to how you are feeling at the time, instead of when you actually feel hungry – usually involving the comfort of junk foods. I have spoken with many nutritional and dietary experts over the years, and some estimate that many cases of overeating are caused by feelings, which means that many of us at times are guilty of using food as a prop to cope with how we feel emotionally at the time. Am I saying that most cases of obesity are caused by emotional reasons underpinning the eating problems? No, I am not, it is generally a combination of faulty lifestyle and dietary habits as well as emotional issues that cause weight issues with people. Many people today eat too late at night, don't chew their foods sufficiently, eat in a hurry, skip meals, over-eat or have too large a portion size. And others simply don't prioritize eating anymore or cook good wholesome meals like their grandparents used to. So you can see, there are many issues here that can account for a person being overweight. Take a look at your favorite treat or snack food right now. Is it chocolate or ice cream? Is it home baking? Is it licorice candy or perhaps biscuits (cookies) like my dad used to eat in large quantities? I think you may be starting to get the picture by now.

Some patients I see were overweight as kids. As an overweight child, they may regularly turn to junk food to relieve feelings he or she couldn't deal with. And we know from ample research that big kids have a much higher risk of developing obesity as adults. And as these big kids grow into big teens, overeating causes them more feelings of guilt, disgust and failure. Then there is the ridicule, the shame, the bullying and the comfort in computer games, the couch and remote control and the fridge or pantry.

Maybe you can identify with the emotional overeater, and even though you're eating and emotional thought patterns may not be as extreme – you might still be labeled as someone who eats for comfort.

What are the consequences of emotional eating? Basically, the comfort one finds from eating is only very temporary. Comfort eating does not resolve life's issues or feelings anymore than a credit card solves your financial woes. This type of eating leads to long-term consequences such as emotional instability, the guilt and shame and poor self-esteem as well as the physical problems that eating too much brings like obesity, digestive disorders like candida, blood sugar problems like diabetes and heart and circulatory problems that the increased body weight causes.

Keeping A Food Diary

So what are some practical steps you can change eating for comfort patterns? You can start for example by logging when you eat and are not actually hungry. Do this for one week, and ask yourself – what triggered my need to eat? Were there any thoughts, such as stress, conflict, disappointment, fear, or anger driving me to food?

Think about the events that took place the day before eating and write out in detail what occurred prior to eating for comfort versus eating for hunger. It may have been a while since you actually ate because you felt hungry. Eating, though an enjoyable activity should be based on being hungry, and not pleasure. When was the last time you got hungry and then ate? I prefer overweight people to go on detox programs and juice fasts; it lets them experience what it is like to feel the need to want to eat which is not based on emotions, but rather on being hungry.

Maybe you don't use food for comfort all the time. How could you begin to use the healthy coping skills you practice more often? Identify any healthy coping skills you use in response to the emotional triggers you have discovered.

Let's Explore And Deal With Feelings

> *Better to eat a dry crust of bread with peace of mind than*
> *have a banquet in a house full of trouble.*
> *Proverbs*

The next step is to implement interventions and a strategy for dealing with the anger, resentment, depression, low self-esteem, fear and stress underlying the eating for comfort syndrome. Your emotional feelings underpinning you wanting to grab something sweet are indicators that something is not quite right in your life right now. Deal with your feelings directly by asking yourself "what is the issue I am facing and is it valid?" Once you identify these core issues in your life underlying the eating for comfort, you can then begin to work on healthy coping skills. Are you ready to face the core issues? Do you really once and for all want to get a handle on those love handles? Patients with major weight issues most always have major digestive issues that go along with it, and candida is not far away when you explore the "comfort foods".

Case History #18
My Father

My dad bought several candida books in the 1980's after suffering from digestive problems for so many years; he had so many different examinations by bowel specialists (gastroenterologists) that I lost count. A family friend suggested he might have a bowel problem after watching him eat a whole packet of sweet biscuits one afternoon. But then again, dad did like his biscuits, ice cream and many cups of coffee with several sugars. And he continued to like sweet foods right up until he died in 2004, his freezer was full of ice cream and I found a several dozens cans of sweetened condensed milk in his pantry and many dozens of packets of cookies there as well. His weight had ballooned up to over 250 pounds (about 125 kilograms) yet his height was about five feet eleven inches. His blood pressure was sky high at 190/110 and he would on the odd occasion take his blood pressure medications. Dad died of a stroke at the age of 72. Like any son, I loved my dad, but I found that he had a total lack of regard to his diet; he simply ate whatever "tastes good" as he used to put it. When a person tells me that they like food that "tastes good", I have found from experience that this generally means it is something sweet and you can count on it that it will be loaded with refined sugar.

Dad continually had flatulence, bloating and complained of all manner of bowel problems like constipation and diarrhea. The foods he craved were always calling his name. And he responded by consuming them, in vast quantities. Dad was an emotional person who solved many problems by eating, and generally the foods he would consume were sweet by nature. I couldn't help my own dad, after all, he was my dad and I learned over the years not to give health advice to friends or relations that was unsolicited. It most always falls on deaf ears. I only help those who come to me and ask for advice and actually pay me for it, there will usually be a commitment then. Do you have unresolved emotional issues? Are you eating for comfort? Think about it, is there a particular food or drink right now that is calling *your name*?

The Candida Crusher Diet May Cause You To Lose Weight

After treating many patients with yeast infections over the years, I have discovered that when many adopt a strict anti-candida diet, they invariably loose weight. I often get emails from patients about their weight-loss concerns on the anti-candida diet, and I reassure them that it is nothing to worry about because their weight will stabilise over time. Most of us are too heavy and eat too much food anyway, and that's a fact. The ideal percentage of bodyfat is about 12 to 15 percent for men and roughly 18 – 20 percent for females. Remember, if you do not stay active or exercise as you age you will loose muscle size and this is often replaced by fat.

Losing weight is a struggle for most of us, but NOT for those on the anti-candida diet. Why? – simple, the key foods that the yeast thrives on are the key foods that allow you to gain weight in the first place – the carbs and sweet foods. And these are often the foods and drinks that many of us are addicted to and find it hard to reduce or eliminate from our diets – bread, alcoholic drinks, candies, cakes, biscuits, soda drinks, take-away foods, etc. I'll bet that when you look at the anti-candida diet you will be thinking: "But those are some of my favourite foods, how am I ever going to avoid them in my diet". This is a key reason why you have not eliminated candida from your digestive system until now, you probably never tried hard enough or long enough to eliminate them.

I'm not at all suggesting that all overweight persons have candida, but I am suggesting that many people who are overweight would benefit from my candida diet approach considerably. The diet is very healthy and you will lose weight if you are overweight, there is no doubt about it. The bonus is that as your weight drops off, your metabolism will begin to normalise and so will your appetite.

Health Tip:

Eat small amounts of whole grains daily to avoid weight-loss

Some people who are losing weight too rapidly on the anti-candida diet will benefit in eating small amounts of safe grains like quinoa, brown rice, millet or buckwheat to curb their weight loss. They should aim for ¼ to ½ cup per day initially, and then increase to suit if they don't aggravate. This will also make their diet more interesting and help to avoid boredom. Many people will want to lose some weight anyway, and for those that weight gain is not necessary (and especially where weight loss is desired) then I'd recommend you follow my dietary recommendations carefully, and these include taking all grains out initially and slowly adding them back into your diet.

Why No Carbohydrates, Yeasts and Sugar Containing Foods

It is a known fact that excessive carbohydrates in the diet (especially sugars and grains) in some people encourage candida infection for several reasons:

1. Eating refined sugars, in particular, depletes B-complex vitamins, as well as zinc, manganese, selenium and many other vital nutrients. This can worsen the body's immune response and other defenses against yeasts and other parasitic organisms.

2. Sugar is also the food that nourishes yeast organisms. The more of it one eats, the more fuel that is available for the growth of yeast organisms in the intestines. Some of the sugars one eats may even nourish yeasts that live in the vagina, on the skin or elsewhere.

Eliminate Sugars Of All Kinds, Including Fruits And Most Dairy Products

Candida's main food supply is a steady supply of sugar and carbohydrate-rich foods and all forms of it such as lactose contained in dairy products (except butter), honey, maple syrup, molasses, glucose, fructose, lactose, and sugar substitutes, i.e. NutraSweet, aspartame, saccharin, etc. – see list below. Eliminating sugar is the most important part of the Candida Crusher Program.

My candida dietary approach is similar to Dr. Galland's approach. Dr. Leo Galland is one of America's most experienced doctors specializing in digestive disorders, recommends the following dietary approach for candida patients:

- Low-sugar and low-yeast and a predominantly dairy free diet *to begin* with. Lactose-free milk may be OK if you are not dairy food intolerant or have a dairy allergy.

- Complex carbohydrates are allowed, but caution with the high starch vegetables initially.

- If patients don't improve, they go on a *very low-carb diet* for 2 or 3 weeks.

- Then, most people can increase their complex carbohydrates without problems.

-

How To Break The Sugar Addiction

> " *If Obama wanted to make radical changes to America's health long-term, all he has to do was treble the price of sugar.* "
>
> Jamie Oliver

If you want to break the sugar addiction, give yourself at least 3 months, because that is how long it can take for you to break away from this extremely addictive substance. Because sugars and refined carbohydrates are so addictive, the first few days of being off them can be quite difficult. There is no doubt; you will experience cravings and withdrawal symptoms. And after about 4 days the cycle will be broken, and you could try some sugar to get an idea of what it has been doing to your body. I can assure you, it isn't pleasant experience.

To repair your body's digestion to the point where it can tolerate small amounts of unprocessed sugars, it can take from 3 to 6 months. This allows you not only to wean off that sugar addiction, but it also gives your digestive system the time it needs to heal and to develop the health bacterial flora so important in keeping that overgrowth of candida yeast at bay.

One of the best ways to wean off sugar is by following a whole food plan just like I have outlined in the Candida Crusher Program. After your health starts to improve significantly, you can start testing small amounts of whole sugar foods like pure maple syrup, malt

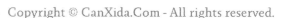

extract, and honey. If you notice the burping, bloating and gas production again, then reduce and stop these sugary foods and focus on the whole foods again. Once you begin to re-introduce these sweet foods into your diet, do it slowly and carefully. It is a good idea to remain on the probiotic during this stage as well, and this is one of the main reasons why the probiotic is the last dietary supplement for you to stop taking during the Candida Crusher Program.

Candida loves sweets, and if the yeast does not get fed on the most refined of carbohydrates (the simple sugars), honey or molasses will do. Yeast is not fussy, it will feed on the sugar you supply it in your diet, whether it be a refined sugar or a less refined sugar like the fructose in fruit which will be perfectly acceptable. The more severe your yeast infection, the higher the demand for these sugars will be, and the more pronounced the symptoms of bloating and gas will be as a consequence for most people. Sugar is also contained is most processed foods such as smoked luncheon meats, tomato sauce (ketchup), soup, etc. so reading labels carefully is very important. Reading labels can be tricky if you don't know the many names of sugar and sweeteners. Here's a partial list to help you.

Names For Sugar, The Natural And Artificial Sweeteners (Partial List)

Aspartame, carob powder, corn starch crystalline carbohydrate dextrin dextrose, disaccharides, fructose, galactose, glucose, high fructose corn syrup, levulose, malts of any kind, maltitol, maltodextrin, maltose (malt sugar), mannitol, mannitol, mono-saccharides, sucrose NutraSweet, polydextrose, polysaccharides, ribose, saccharin, sorghum, suamiel, succanat. Please note, not all sugar substitutes directly feeds candida, but all of them damage the immune system, and most are neuro-toxic (causing damage and disturbances to the brain and nervous system).

Sugar Depresses The Immune System

The fact that sugar greatly depresses the immune system has been known for many years, mainly because of the work of Linus Pauling. Pauling is the only person ever to have received two unshared Nobel Prizes, one for Chemistry (1954) and for Peace (1962). He concluded that white blood cells need a high dose of vitamin C, and so he developed his theory that high doses of vitamin C were needed to combat the common cold, the flu and even cancer.

Did you know that vitamin C and sugar have similar chemical structures so that means they compete with one another for entry into the cells? If there is more sugar around, less vitamin C is allowed into the cell, and vice versa. It is interesting that taking vitamin C also helps curb sugar, alcohol and high carbohydrate cravings.

Since our bodies cannot make vitamin C on it's own it must be obtained from foods or supplements on a daily basis. Try taking 1,000 to 2,000 milligrams of vitamin C daily if you have strong sugar cravings. You might be quite surprised to find that you no longer want that ice cream or cookie after your main meal.

A Few Of The Hundreds Of Bad Effects Sugar Has On Health

- Sugar is an addictive substance and can be intoxicating, similar to alcohol

- Sugar contributes to the reduction in defense against bacterial infection

- Sugar interferes with absorption of calcium and magnesium

- Sugar feeds yeast, and is candida's favorite food

- Sugar can interfere with the absorption of protein

- Sugar upsets mineral relationships in the body

- Sugar can increase the body's fluid retention

- Sugar can change the structure of protein

- Sugar can cause hormonal imbalances

- Sugar reduces oxygen to your cells

- Sugar makes you sick and fat

Sugar Causes Insulin Resistance

Insulin is a hormone secreted by the pancreas. It helps the body utilize blood glucose (blood sugar) by binding with receptors on cells like a key would fit into a lock. Once the key insulin has unlocked the door, the glucose can pass from the blood into the cell. Inside the cell, glucose is either used for energy or stored for future use in the form of glycogen in the liver or muscle cells.

The body's cells become insulin resistant because they are trying to protect themselves from the toxic effects of high insulin that is required to regulate blood sugar levels when the diet is high in sugar and/or carbohydrates. This causes the cells to down-regulate their receptor activity and the numbers of their receptors so they don't have to receive the noxious sweet stimuli all the time. It is like having constant loud disgusting music being played and you just have to turn down the volume or you will go insane! Insulin resistance leads to blood sugar problems like hypoglycemia and diabetes, and to high blood pressure.

Sugar Makes You Sick And Fat And Here's How

A less known fact is that insulin also stores magnesium. But if your cells become resistant to insulin you can't store magnesium, so it is lost through urination.

Intracellular magnesium relaxes muscles. What happens when you can't store magnesium because the cell is resistant? You lose magnesium and your blood vessels and muscles constrict. This causes blood pressure to increase and reduces energy since intracellular magnesium is required for all energy producing reactions that take place in the cell. But most importantly, magnesium is also necessary for the action of insulin and the manufacture of insulin. When your insulin is raised, you lose magnesium, and the cells become even more insulin resistant. It becomes a vicious cycle that begins even before you were born. This is another very good reason not to eat sugar and high carbohydrate foods.

If I Can't Have Sugar, What Sweetener Can I Have?

Stevia and Xylitol are the only sweeteners allowed for candida patients, but they should then only be consumed in *very* small amounts and not during the first three to four weeks, because like all sugar (and artificial sweeteners) it will increase cravings for sugar and high carbohydrate foods.

I have found that Xylitol is the better option; it has the ability to inhibit streptococcus bacteria and has even been endorsed by the US Dental Association as being safe for children in terms of dental caries. Xylitol has proven anti-bacterial and anti-fungal properties and is very heat stable. I use it in cooking and baking and it tastes great. It is important to remember – only small amounts of Xylitol, but do avoid Xylitol in the first three to four weeks. As you progress through the various stages and improve, you can have small amounts of Xylitol and Stevia. Whenever I see a patient with severe candida issues, I prefer they abstain from ALL sweeteners for as long as it takes for them to:

A) Break the sugar or sweet addiction cycle

B) Learn to be able to go shopping without the need to buy a sweet treat

C) Have balanced their digestive flora (no bloating, gas, etc.)

D) No longer need sugar between meals (tea of coffee) or after meals (dessert)

Sweet Tip:

Gymnema And Vitamin C For Sugar Cravings

Have you heard about an herb called gymnema sylvestre? This herb reduces the taste of sugar when it is placed in the mouth. From an extract of the leaves were isolated glycosides (an herbal chemical compound) known as gymnemic acids that exhibit quite a profound anti-sweet activity. This effect lasts up to about 2 hours after you place some of the liquid herb in your mouth, and you only need a tiny amount on your tongue. It is believed that gymnema may block sugar receptors on the tongue, so it perfect to carry a small bottle around with you if you have "killer" sweet attacks in the first month when following the Candida Crusher Program. Gymnema has no side effects, but it does taste somewhat bitter, but you soon get used to it. It does it kill any good bacteria or cause die-off; it just suppresses the sugar cravings.

Vitamin C is another good option if you have sweet cravings, and I recommend you take 1,000 milligrams in the morning and another 1,000 milligrams in the afternoon. Take before meals, and if you find that it only helps a little then increase your dosage to 1,000 milligrams three times daily. Vitamin C can be used in conjunction with gymnema. Just make sure your vitamin C powder does NOT contain any sucrose (sugar), because many do!

Grains To Eat And Grains To Avoid

After two weeks you can eat quinoa, amaranth, millet buckwheat again. I prefer it if patients stay off all wheat, oats, barley and rye products as well, not only for the first two weeks, but for a full month at the very least. This is where the real weight loss may certainly occur. You should be able to have wheat again in a month or so after you start the anti-candida diet, and if you do then only eat flat breads that have been made with only with whole meal flour, salt and water. Make sure there are no yeasts or sugars in this bread, and preferably buy high quality organic stone-ground flour and make your own flat bread.

The main grains and flours to avoid are commercial wheat, white flour, white rice and any refined, puffed or extruded cereals you get in those boxes from the supermarket shelves. They are highly refined and stripped of their goodness during the processing. They just clog up your digestive system because these "foods" become a gluey, sticky mess in your bowel. This results in a potential toxic build-up, reduces your immune function and just contributes to the candida growth.

I recommend that you eat brown or wild rice, quinoa, millet and buckwheat. I have started to really enjoy quinoa and have incorporated it into my diet considerably. You will find that quinoa can be cooked in small amounts for breakfast, lunch or dinner. It can be added to most salads, as a side dish or be included on your plate with your evening meal. It is high in very protein and gluten free and perfect for those who have a yeast infection. You read about quinoa earlier a little further ahead.

Eliminate Any Foods High In Carbohydrates

This is a difficult area, some say to eliminate ALL carbs from the diet initially, others say that carbs are ok. My experience has taught me with patients that complex carbs are *probably* fine, but the refined ones are definitely not fine.

Although some people can react very strongly to complex carbohydrates, it is a matter of trial and error really. If you find that you react to a complex carbohydrate food strongly – like potato, pumpkin or corn, then avoid most all complex carbohydrates for up to three weeks before you re-introduce.

Candida can also feed on high carbohydrate foods such as starches and grains, including breads, pasta, pizza, cereals, baked goods, beans, potatoes, peas, lima beans, etc. Some high starch vegetables must also be avoided strictly by some because they are also high in sugars and/or carbohydrates, i.e. beets, squash, corn, maize, parsnips, sweet potatoes, yams, carrots, etc. Once again, you will need to see what suits you and what doesn't. Take your time and work out the key foods which aggravate your condition, you will be able to tell pretty quickly with these potentially aggravating carbohydrates in your diet. You will either feel OK when you have them or you don't.

These high carb, or starchy, foods store their energy as complex strands of sugar molecules (starch), which acts just like sugar in the body. That is why grains are just as addictive as sugar. After taking all sugar and grains out of your diet for a few weeks you will find your craving for both of them will decrease.

A high-complex-carbohydrate diet is nothing more than a high-glucose diet or a high-sugar diet, albeit harder to digest. All carbohydrates turn into glucose (blood sugar) in the body, and 58% of protein and 10% of fat are also converted by the body into glucose. Our body can fulfill all of its blood sugar requirements by a diet of proteins and good nature-made fats alone. That is why Eskimos are very healthy on their natural diet of only meats and fats.

Why You Should Avoid Starches And Grains Initially

Eliminate all grains, seeds, nuts and legumes. Please note that legumes are plants containing seedpods, i.e. beans and peas, and by legumes I don't mean fresh or frozen green, yellow or string beans. Peanuts are legumes, and soy is too, they are highly allergenic to some people and are best avoided by those with a yeast infection as well for some time, and this includes peanut butter as well. It you like peanut butter then try tahini, it is a paste made from sesame seeds and is delicious.

Candida Patients Are More Prone To Low Blood Sugar

These are several good reasons why candida sufferers would do well to eliminate starches and grains, and in some instances the high carbohydrate vegetables. Most all grains can potentially feed candida because they have a high glycemic (GI) index just like sugar, and like sugar they feed candida and create insulin resistance within the cells. I have seen plenty of candida patients over the years with blood sugar problems, especially hypoglycemia (low blood sugar), and there are a couple of reasons why they have developed these issues, here are some of the main reasons:

- Some candida sufferers eat fruit, and plenty of it, because they have started to react to many different sweet foods which they crave but haven't figured out that many fruits are equally as bad when it comes to food reactions.

- Some candida sufferers have very restricted diets but continue to snack on dried fruits with the fallacious belief they are eating a "healthy" snack.

- Some candida sufferers skip meals or haven't quite figured out yet that small meals or snacks has a more stabilizing effect on their blood sugar levels, as well as mood and energy control.

- Other candida patients I have seen who used to eat plenty of take-out, drink alcohol or Coke every day, love chocolate bars, etc., have made an abrupt and sudden change in their diet and decided to "go healthy" very suddenly. Some of these patients have ended up in trouble with weakness, fatigue, dizziness, nausea, headaches, and the many other abnormal signs and symptoms associated with abnormal blood sugar control. For these patients I recommend a good dietary supplement (containing chromium, B vitamins, zinc and magnesium) to help them overcome these issues. Their body will adapt to the new diet in about a two to three weeks period.

Gluten May Cause Problems In Those With Candida

Certain grains contain gluten, which is an elastic gluey protein found in wheat, rye, barley, oats, spelt, kamut, and triticale, and it is hidden as well in an endless variety of processed foods. Triticale is a new hybrid grain with the properties of wheat and rye, while spelt and kamut are gluten-containing wheat variants despite claims to the contrary, and are likely to cause problems in the gluten department similar to other wheat varieties.

Gluten is a protein that is difficult to digest, and can potentially cause a great deal of intestinal damage. This damage, combined with the effects of yeast overgrowth, can make the intestines incapable of absorbing nutrients such as proteins, carbohydrates, fats, vitamins, minerals, and even water, in some cases. In my experience, many candida sufferers have become gluten intolerant, and I have seen some even being diagnosed with celiac disease prior to finding out about candida. What I have found in many cases is that these patients can go back and enjoy their daily bread once their yeast issues became resolved. In my opinion, all too many people use the "I'm gluten intolerant" line without a thorough investigation as to the main causes of their digestive issues.

It is easy to point the finger and blame one protein found in food, but there are so many causes as to why they have developed a digestive problem that it can become very difficult to work out what went wrong in the first place.

Many practitioners find it easier to make the recommendation to "avoid all gluten" for the rest of the patient's life, rather than to spend an hour or two in the clinic trying to establish the real underlying factors of their patient's digestive problems (or other health complaints) and place the blame on gluten instead.

"But hang on a minute Eric, I took my patient off all gluten products and she is feeling so much better" you may say if you are a doctor. Yes, I believe it, but remember also that this patient has become a lot more wellness focused instead of disease centered and made several other changes to her life such as drinking more water and less wine, making better dietary and lifestyle choices in general and then she tells you that gluten was the main culprit. Was it the peanut butter or sweet spread she had on her bread, did she take a probiotic around the same time she stopped gluten, thereby correcting a poor bacterial digestive issue

Many changes occur to a patient's diet and lifestyle simultaneously, and it is almost impossible to implicate gluten as being the number one cause for all her health problems. After saying all this, I do believe that in many chronic cases of yeast infection it makes a lot of sense to remove all wheat products temporarily just like any other potentially allergenic food, at least until good improvements occur at which stage they can be re-introduced later. People love wheat, and to deny them from eating bread lifelong is not right in my opinion; besides, most all people will gravitate back to the foods they love to eat regardless of who they see for their health problems. Gluten is innocent until proven guilty in my opinion.

The Gluten Allergies And Candida Connection

Some experts believe that there is a direct link between a yeast infection and a gluten allergy, and I believe there is after having noticed how many patients I've seen who were diagnosed as being gluten sensitive or celiac, who could once again eat wheat and gluten products without any aggravations after having followed the Candida Crusher Program.

There is a protein within the cell wall of candida albicans (Hwp-1, also known as Hyphal Wall Protein-1) that allows candida to attach itself to the cells of the intestine. The body's immune system does not recognize Hwp-1 as being that much different from the intestinal cells, allowing candida to remain in our digestive system. The configurations of the amino acids that make up Hwp-1 protein are very similar to the proteins α-gliadin and γ-gliadin found in gluten (wheat, barley, rye) products. Over time, the yeast cells begin to change and are not as fixed as the gliadin proteins, they die, their colonies expand and they hyphenate, sending out spores.

The immune system becomes challenged and mounts a response that not only includes an attack on the Hwp-1 protein, but also on the similar gliadin protein as well. Crossover allergic reactions begin to occur as the immune system becomes confused, and as the immune system becomes increasingly sensitized to the effects of gluten, leading to celiac disease being triggered in susceptible people.

Because the immune system is confused and cannot readily distinguish between the Hwp-1 proteins and specific gluten proteins, it can lead to a condition known as auto-immunity. And this is how celiac disease may even be caused for all we know. Have you never wondered why perfectly healthy people all of a sudden become "gluten intolerant"? There is always a cause, but it is generally never sought for, and this has lead to a whole new industry and mindset, the gluten free movement.

I have discovered in the past several years that when many people who have been diagnosed with gluten intolerance finally beat their yeast infection, they can go back to enjoying their daily bread again.

In view of the Hwp-1 protein and candida connection and the development of gluten sensitivities, does this not make sense to you? Many people with gluten sensitivities have had a digestive problem that has not been thoroughly investigated, and the person certainly did not suspect a yeast infection. Did they ever have a comprehensive stool test performed to determine what bacteria; parasites or yeasts were involved before they decided to go gluten free? Did they ever try a strict no-sugar diet while treating their digestion for bugs? Probably not, they just took gluten out of their diet, end of story. But if they had tried to commit to a yeast eradication program they would probably find that they actually could go back to eating wheat products again without any aggravation.

Over the past several decades, there has been a sharp increase in people diagnosed with gluten sensitivities and celiac disease. Ulcerative colitis cases have sky rocketed, and Crohn's disease is seven times more likely in those who are sensitive to gluten. It has been estimated that an incredible 1% of the population is celiac, with the majority not even knowing they have a problem with gluten. Some health experts believe that gluten sensitivities and celiac disease is totally understated, and in their efforts to understand why there could be such a rapid increase they have been looking for clues as to why there could be such a rapid increase. My guess is antibiotics, alcohol, pharmaceutical drugs, sugars and processed foods and the increasingly stressful lifestyles we all tend to lead. Those with gluten issues in my opinion should really try and stick with a yeast eradication program for 6 months before they give themselves a life sentence of gluten avoidance.

Best Grains Are Buckwheat, Quinoa, Amaranth And Millet

Grains that are safer to consume are more seed-like than grain-like, and they do not contain gluten. These grains include amaranth, buckwheat, millet and quinoa. Brown rice is also a safe grain for those with candida.

Some people say to avoid all grains, including buckwheat, quinoa, amaranth and millet until you have progressed far enough on a candida program so your body can handle them. This is simply not true; it may be for some of the most extreme cases (like 2%) but is certainly not a major factor for the other 98 percent in my experience.

Some candida patients I have seen have a tendency to lose too much weight rather quickly, and they will need to eat small amounts of safe grains to stop their weight loss. It is really all about trial and error here, there are no rules when it comes to buckwheat, quinoa, amaranth and millet, and I recommend that you experiment to see what is right for you. It is a great idea to avoid gluten containing foods for a period of several months if you have had severe and recurrent candida, which includes lots of digestive problems for a long time, especially if you have been attentive to eliminating any other potentially allergic foods from your diet (like milk, oranges, peanuts, fish/shellfish, etc.) but have never tried in earnest to remove all wheat and gluten products.

The stage 2 component of the Candida Crusher Diet involves removing any potentially allergenic foods from your diet, and will cover this aspect more in depth.

Quinoa

Have you ever tried quinoa? I first tried quinoa several years ago but have started to eat it more over the past two years. I love this tiny white colored seed called quinoa, and have become used to cooking and eating it, this grain satisfies my taste buds as it has its own subtle yet distinct taste which tells me that quinoa will end up becoming one of my favorite foods, just like avocado, after I began to appreciate the subtle flavors of the avocado flesh many years ago.

The Great Gluten Free Crop Of Andean Civilization

Quinoa originated in the Andean region of South America, where it has been an important food for more than 6,000 years. In contemporary times this crop has come to be highly appreciated for its nutritional value, and the United Nations has classified it as a super crop for its very high protein content (12%–18%). Unlike wheat or rice, which are low in lysine, quinoa contains a balanced set of essential amino acids for humans, making it an unusually high protein complete food. This means it takes less quinoa protein to meet one's needs than wheat protein. It is a good source of dietary fiber, is 100% gluten free and considered very easy to digest.

Quinoa is a very easy food to prepare as well, it has a pleasantly light, fluffy texture when cooked, and its mild, slightly nutty flavor makes it an excellent alternative to white rice or couscous. Once you get into the habit of eating and snacking on fresh and wholesome foods like quinoa and avocado, your taste buds and sense of smell will develop significantly. You will find that confectionary like chewing gum and even chocolate in time will lose its sparkle. Who knows, you may even end up disgustingly healthy one day.

Quinoa is pronounced "keen-wa" and is a complete protein grain, meaning it contains all the essential amino acids required each day. Did you know that quinoa contains 50% more protein that wheat? When cooked, quinoa expands to four times its volume. This amazing grain contains plenty of nutrition including lysine, iron, phosphorus, magnesium, vitamins A, E and B as well as double the calcium of most other grains.

Tips For Preparing Quinoa

Like any grain from a third-world country, always wash carefully. It is not unheard of for quinoa to contain tiny pebbles or grains of sand. While the processing methods used in the commercial cultivation of quinoa remove much of the soapy saponins that coats quinoa seeds, some people believe that it is a good idea to thoroughly wash the seeds to remove any remaining saponin residue.

An effective method is to run cold water over quinoa that has been placed in a fine-meshed strainer, gently rubbing the seeds together with your hands, or rinsing it in ample running water either in a fine strainer or in cheesecloth. To ensure that the saponins have been completely removed, taste a few seeds. If they still have a bitter taste, continue the rinsing process.

Cooking Quinoa

A common cooking method is to treat quinoa much like rice, add one part of the grain to two parts liquid in a saucepan. After the mixture is brought to a boil, reduce the heat to simmer and cover. One cup of quinoa cooked in this method usually takes 15 minutes to prepare. When cooking is complete, you will notice that the grains have become translucent, and the white germ has partially detached itself, appearing like a white-spiraled tail. If you desire the quinoa to have a nuttier flavor, you can dry roast it before cooking; to dry roast, place it in a skillet over medium-low heat and stir constantly for five minutes.

Since quinoa has a no gluten content, it is one of the least allergenic grains, but its flour needs to be combined with wheat to make leavened baked goods. Quinoa flour can be used to make pasta, and quinoa pastas are available in many natural foods stores

Quinoa Flour

Quinoa flour can be used in wheat-based as well as gluten-free baking. For the latter, it can be combined with sorghum flour, tapioca, and potato starch to create a really nutritious gluten-free baking mix. A suggested mix is three parts quinoa flour, three parts sorghum flour, two parts potato starch, and one part tapioca starch.

Lastly, quinoa may be germinated in its raw form to boost its nutritional value. Germination activates its natural enzymes and multiplies its vitamin and mineral content. In fact, quinoa has a notably short germination period: only 2-4 hours resting in a glass of clean water is enough to make it sprout and release gases, as opposed to 12 hours overnight with wheat. This process, besides its nutritional enhancements, softens the grains, making them very suitable to be added to salads and other cold foods.

Quinoa Serving Suggestions

- There are many ways you can serve up this tasty grain, I like to just simmer it in a little beef of chicken stock and have it as a side serve instead of rice occasionally.

- Vegetables and seasonings can also be added to make a wide range of dishes. It is also well suited to vegetable pilafs.

- Quinoa can serve as a high-protein breakfast food mixed with almonds, or berries; it is also sold as a dry product, much like corn flakes.

- As a snack food, quinoa can be toasted in a dry pan over medium heat until it is browned and mixed with a muesli, fruit (fresh or dried), coconut strands, or just eaten by itself.

- Combine cooked chilled quinoa with pinto beans, pumpkin seeds, spring onions & coriander. Season to taste & enjoy.

- Add nuts to cooked quinoa and serve as breakfast porridge.

- For a twist on your favorite pasta recipe, use noodles made from quinoa.

- You can even sprout the seeds in just a few hours. Sprouted quinoa can be used in salads and sandwiches just like alfalfa sprouts.

- Add quinoa to your favorite vegetable soups.

- Ground quinoa flour can be added to cookie or muffin recipes.

- Quinoa is great to use in tabouli, serving as a delicious and wheat-free substitute for the bulgur wheat with which this Middle Eastern dish is usually made.

- Quinoa Sushi - does this sound a little crazy? Try this dish, you will love it, it is not crazy at all, you will find recipes online.

Grains Are Best Soaked, Sprouted Or Leavened With Sour Dough

Grains, nuts, seeds, and legumes are best properly prepared in order to make them much more nutritious to eat. There is some talk about the benefits of preparing these foods before consumption. This is because they contain phytic acid which combines with calcium, magnesium, copper, iron and especially zinc in the intestinal tract and potentially blocks their absorption.

This is why a diet high in such foods may eventually lead to mineral deficiencies, bone loss and symptoms including dizziness, and even erratic unstable heartbeats in some.

Improperly processed grains, seeds, nuts, legumes, bran, etc. may cause irritable bowel syndrome, and various other adverse affects. I have witnessed this with several patients who have gone all out in their quest for optimal health and who moved away from the conventional grains such as white rice and wheat and introduced a diet rich in amaranth, beans and peas, buckwheat, quinoa and more. In some instances their health deteriorated and I feel it was because they did not prepare these foods properly and introduced them too quickly.

Soaking seeds and grains also removes the enzyme inhibitors that impair digestion and cause gas. It is especially important to soak grains if you have poor or weak digestion, have food allergies or leaky gut syndrome.

Sally Fallon – Nourishing Traditions

If you want to get optimum nutrition from these wonderful foods, proper preparing involves soaking that allows the natural enzymes, lactobacilli and other helpful organisms to break down and neutralize the phytic acid and their protein blocking enzymes. Therefore all of these "new" grains are best when properly soaked, spouted or better still, leavened with sour dough. This will dramatically improve their ability to be digested, and it is best that most nuts, seeds, and legumes are soaked in a slightly acidic medium like liquid whey (Molkosan), lemon juice or a good organic apple cider vinegar. I can highly recommend that you buy a copy of Nourishing Traditions by Sally Fallon; this book is simply one of the best and will teach you the best ways to select, prepare and cook healthy natural foods.

I have not seen a better book in terms of healthy cooking, you will soon find that your copy will be well used, be sure to cover it with plastic to avoid it becoming soiled like my copy has become. If you ever get a chance to hear Sally speak, do go to one of her most enlightening seminars on healthy eating.

Eliminate Dried Fruits

A common misconception is that dried fruits are a healthy addition to your diet. Dried fruits like raisins, apricots, pears, dates and figs are not only concentrated forms of sugar, they are frequently moldy as well. Avoid them strictly if you have yeast related infections. I have found that many patients who have seen me over the years love to snack on dried apricots, sultanas, figs and dates, etc. They will either eat these alone or in combination with various nuts and seeds. Dried fruits can be re-introduced in stage 3 of the diet, and should be one of the last snack foods you re-introduce because they are such concentrated forms of sugars. Be especially careful with prepackaged breakfast cereals and muesli, as they often contain many small pieces of dried fruits.

Health Tip:

Avoid fresh and dried fruits if you have candida and a sluggish bowel
The irony with some patients I have found is that a candida yeast infection in many patients can cause a sluggish bowel. Some candida patients then think they are doing the right thing by consuming lots of dates, figs, dried apricots and prunes to relieve their constipation, when in fact they inadvertently just keep the vicious circle going. And in addition, I have also seen many vegetarians and vegans develop chronic yeast infections because they ate no animal proteins and tried to obtain much of their energy from grains (breads) and other carbohydrate foods including dried fruit for snacks.

Why Raw Foods

" *To eat is human, to digest divine.* "
Mark Twain

Many people talk about eating a pH balanced diet and how it is so important to consume an alkaline and predominantly raw food diet. Raw foods, particularly raw fruits (the non sweet varieties) and vegetables are quite alkaline, whereas cooked foods, especially proteins and sugars, are acid forming. It is important to follow a predominantly alkaline diet if you have a yeast infection, this is not because an acid rich diet will favor the growth and proliferation of a yeast infection in your body, which is a myth, but because diets that are more acid forming than alkaline make it easier for candida to move from your digestive system into your bloodstream (translocation). Once this occurs, candida can proliferate in this more alkaline environment and cause serious problems.

Acidic diets have been linked to many chronic diseases such as diabetes, heart disease and various cancers. For example, red meat is one of the most acidic foods, and the consumption of more than 500 grams of red meat per week is now linked to a 30% increased risk of cancer. First let's take a look at the benefits of eating raw foods in your diet, and then explore the pH issue.

Raw Foods

I have always found it strange how many foods are promoted as healthy, organic and natural – and then they are cooked, baked or even deep fried before they are consumed. Every time you cook food you will invariably destroy some of its nutritional value. Some people even see fries (deep fried potatoes) as "healthy" because they are potatoes! Remember, it's not only about what you eat; it's about how it is prepared, and how you eat food as well.

You may well be aware of foods which are rich in antioxidants or contain other nutritional factors which confer many health benefits, but only when they are eaten in a semi-raw or raw and natural state. Take for example spinach, blue berries, avocado, bell peppers and strawberries, an example of foods packed with many kinds of antioxidants, vitamins and minerals.

Researchers have found that the brighter the color the fruit or vegetable has, the more it is likely to be packed with nutrients which help to combat degenerative diseases. But what happens to their beautiful colors after cooking? They fade away like the colors of a rainbow after the rain has stopped; so by heating up and cooking these special foods we are tampering with their special protective factors.

It is hard to believe how much food is consumed in the Western world, and many people eat like there is no tomorrow, but the strange thing is that we have an unprecedented situation in which many are actually suffering from malnutrition in this virtual ocean of food. That's right, many people have become so deficient that their cells are starved and the incredible variety and affordability of foods is contributing to their chronic degenerative disease conditions by the time they reach 50 or 60 years of age.

One of the best ways to resist the temptation of living the refined and junk food lifestyle is to develop a different attitude towards cooked food in general and adopt a more partially cooked or raw food lifestyle. Have you noticed how the trend in the past five to ten years has been towards the low GI diet, i.e.; eat a diet low in carbohydrates and more in vegetable and meat proteins? Many nutritional experts are now also advocating the paleo or cave man diet, to eat vegetables and meats foods more in their natural state. Both of these dietary trends have tendency to be more on the alkaline than acid side as well, particularly if you avoid the carbohydrate and processed foods.

I am personally not a big fan of an all-raw food diet and would find it boring and unappealing to eat most everything raw, but prefer instead to maintain a balance between raw, partially raw and cooked foods. Some foods are best consumed always raw, and no doubt you would be aware of this with for berries, most fruits and salad vegetables, but what about bell peppers, red onions, garlic, spinach, and a whole host of other foods you may have never tried to eat raw?

> *Don't eat anything your great-great grandmother wouldn't recognize as food. There are a great many food-like items in the supermarket your ancestors wouldn't even recognize as food, stay away from these.*
>
> *Michael Pollan*

Raw Dairy Products

It is true that dairy products should be initially avoided, especially in the first month; I have most certainly found that the addition of raw (straight from the cow, un-homogenized and unpasteurized) dairy products such as milk, kefir, yogurt, buttermilk, cream and various cheeses can be quite beneficial. Personally, I would be more inclined to trust the opinion of a healthy cow over a scientist in a white coat and have never believed that foods like margarine or tampered with dairy products are conducive to good health.

An important point to remember is that raw dairy products straight from the cow, or minimally processed dairy products which have been made into various products, contain enzymes, beneficial fats, probiotics, and prebiotics not found in pasteurized dairy products.

Some patients with candida can actually tolerate these organic raw dairy products all the way through their treatment, so you may want to experiment and if in doubt ask your health-care professional about an ELISA food allergy test to determine your immune's antibody status when it comes to dairy products.

Incidentally, if your blood-based IgE-IgG food allergy test results reveal very high antibody levels towards dairy products, then you should avoid these dairy products regardless of whether they are pasteurized, homogenized, 100% certified organic or even biodynamic dairy products. The proteins will be the same, so just avoid them until your digestive and immune health improves.

The Paleo Low-GI Ecology Diet

How about a new diet that incorporates high protein (paleo diet), low carb, low GI diet, and yet looks at implementing a diet rich in cultured and fermented foods (the body ecology diet)? Well, this is how my grandparents ate in the 1950's. So what's new? My grandmother kept bees, made her own sauerkraut and yogurt and my grandfather maintained a large vegetable garden and orchard, as well as kept pigs and chickens. Their diet was rich in high quality proteins such as pork, chicken and eggs, plenty of fresh fruit and vegetables, fermented and cultured foods, honey and fresh fruits from the orchard. This is certainly a far cry from how people eat and live today. My father died when he was 72 but loved to eat take-out foods, white bread, ice cream and cookies. He did eat vegetables, but these were frozen TV dinners and heated in the microwave. Both my father and grandfather smoked but granddad lived until he was 93. My grandparents never did eat take out foods or ever heard of a microwave oven, and I certainly don't advocate the use of them.

It is important to try to maintain a fresh and healthy diet rich in meats, vegetables and especially cultured and fermented foods of which I will speak about later on, these foods could well hold the key to your complete and permanent recovery.

Raw Foods Contain Enzymes – Fries Don't

One of the most important reasons why you will want to consider eating a certain amount of raw foods in your diet every day is because raw foods contain enzymes, and these enzymes are destroyed when you cook food. Without enzymes, your body has a hard time digesting foods, and it is only the living things you consume that can make enzymes. Have you noticed how a fresh food can rot rather quickly, and that a processed food can stay looking good for months, even years, without deterioration? It's all in the enzymes. Your body has two main types of enzymes: those that run your body, called metabolic enzymes, and other enzymes required for digestion, called digestive enzymes, which aid in the digestion of foods including proteins, carbohydrates and fats you consume.

Foods that are raw and which come straight from nature contain enzymes, and it is these enzymes that are responsible for the release of the nutrients from the foods we eat.

Super Size Me

 When you see the Golden Arches you are probably on your way to the Pearly Gates.
William Castelli, MD - Director, Framingham Heart Study

Super Size Me was a 2004 American documentary film directed by and starring Morgan Spurlock, an American independent filmmaker. Spurlock's film follows a 30-day period from February 1 to March 2, 2003 during which he ate only McDonald's food. The film documents this lifestyle's drastic effect on Spurlock's physical and psychological wellbeing, and explores the fast food industry's corporate influence, including how it encourages poor nutrition for its own profit. Are you a fast food junkie? This movie may change all that, my 14-year-old son was disgusted and has refused to eat take out food ever since watching this documentary.

Spurlock started to develop a rather sick liver and was advised by his doctor to resume a normal healthy diet. There are no enzymes in take-out food and his body had a hard time digesting the food he was eating, is it any wonder his digestive system started to become unwell? Only raw foods that come straight from nature come complete with their own enzymes, so be sure to consume some every single day.

The Happy Meal Project

Looking almost as fresh as the day it was bought, this McDonald's Happy Meal is in fact an incredible six months old. This plastic food was bought by New York artist Sally Davies in April 2010, and photographed at the end of September 2010. You will find photo of Sally's Happy Meal Project on www.flicer.com Note the complete absence of mold or decay even after six months, how this "happy food" can contain the slightest shred of nutritional value at all is anybody's guess. Imagine what this fake food does to your digestive system and to your health, especially if you eat it several times a week. It would have made Mr. Spurlock seriously ill had he kept on eating it beyond a month according to his medical doctor. Is it any wonder we have so many fat, sick people and half-dead people in our world today?

Heat Destroys Enzymes – The Less Heat The Better

 If you are surprised that diseases are innumerable, count the cooks.
Seneca (4 BC-AD 65)

I read a book a few years ago called Enzyme Nutrition written by Dr. Edward Howell, and was surprised to discover that heating foods about 48 Centigrade (118 Fahrenheit) kills any enzymes in the food. Without enzymes in the foods you consume, your body has to start relying on producing an increasing amount of its own digestive enzymes to satisfy the demand. Those who eat refined or processed foods regularly will find that their digestion will begin to suffer, along with their energy and overall wellbeing. Those with a yeast infection will find that it is most important to maintain an excellent level of enzymes in their digestive system because candida does not like a gut that has a high level of enzymatic activity. High enzymatic activity maintains a low pH (acid) environment in your stomach in particular, which discourages bad bacteria and yeasts from proliferating. Enzymes can also assist in busting open the cell walls of bacteria and yeasts, rendering them incapable of functioning.

Anybody with a yeast infection who is serious about recovery should remain on a enzyme formula until they have fully recovered; the difference they make is astonishing. Some of the best candida supplements contain enzymes for this very reason, and this is why I developed a product containing several different key enzymes along with probiotics to assist in not only in improving your digestion, but is destroying an intestinal yeast overgrowth directly while reducing inflammation, all at the same time. You can read all about the Candida Crusher Digestive Enzyme later in this chapter, in section 4.

Microwave Cooking Destroys Enzymes

Enzymes are not only intolerant to heat, but also to irradiation from microwaves, and this is a very good reason to avoid cooking any foods in a microwave oven. Pasteurization also kills off any enzymes, and the milk you buy from the supermarket is "dead" for this reason.

There is a big movement the past several years not only in in New Zealand, but in America and many other countries amongst the many of enlightened people who appreciate natural health, to start using real milk from the cow again just as nature had intended. I made an interesting discovery some years ago that many people who cannot tolerate milk due to food allergies or intolerances can often tolerate unpasteurized and unhomogenized fresh milk. It is because there are plenty of natural enzymes in real milk, enzymes that have become de-activated and destroyed by the heating and sterilizing process. Many raw and fresh foods such as milk contain their own highly specialized enzymes, and if these are supplied it will be that much easier for the body to process it. Another interesting observation is that human beings the only creatures that cook their foods, and over the past few hundred years we have developed the tendency to cook or heat everything we put in our mouths. Health experts now believe that many humans die below half their potential lifespan, and that much of the development of our chronic and degenerative illness and most of the premature deaths we face can be put down to faulty dietary and lifestyle measures.

When you think about it for one moment, cooking is the most profound abuse of food. But don't get me wrong, as I mentioned earlier, I'm certainly not a fan of eating everything raw. But to me, there is nothing more satisfying than biting into a fresh apple or a juicy tomato, or enjoying the smooth and creamy taste of a fresh avocado. Once we start to cook and bake foods we tend to load them up after either sugar, salt or a host of spices to bring out the flavors destroyed by cooking and make no mistake, the nutritional value will have vanished along with the color.

Isn't it interesting that many health-conscious people of today steer clear of processed and refined foods, but will not think twice about placing foods in boiling water, wrapping it in aluminum foil, place it in a styrene container, or cook their foods in a microwave or in a conventional oven? These same health-conscious people tend to forget that heating foods to very high temperatures is actually processing foods. We have been told that the less food is processed, the better. Then why process nearly everything we eat, but then tell ourselves that supermarket foods are not OK because they are processed?

Just be aware of the fact that processed foods are not just foods you buy from supermarkets in packets, boxes and cans, they are also the healthy foods you cook to very high temperatures are home when you place them in the oven or microwave. Try to eat some fresh and raw foods each and every day, your digestion will improve and you will be amazed and delighted at the difference that eating "living" foods can make. I love cats, and the healthiest cat I ever had was fed on one large, fresh sardine each day. I drove a garbage truck for several years when I was a naturopathy student and found a tiny little kitten in a garbage can on one of my rounds. I named it Wally, and fed my cat only on fresh and raw fish which I received regularly from a shop on my rounds. Everybody commented how amazingly beautiful Wally looked, his eyes and coat were the healthiest and shiniest of any cat I've ever owned, and I have no doubt it was his diet because he consumed every part of the sardine including the head, gut and even the scales. This is in stark contrast to how most people feed their cats, on highly processed biscuits or cooked canned foods. If you have the opportunity to feed your pet on fresh, raw and unprocessed foods, you will be absolutely amazed at the difference it can make. Imagine if you ate only fresh, raw and unprocessed foods, your digestive problems would be solved literally in weeks or a couple of months, and your yeast infection would soon follow.

Eating Six Or Seven Serves Of Vegetables A Day – But How?

It is a fact that most people I see in my clinic don't eat the recommended daily amount of vegetable and fruit servings. If you really eat 6 or 7 servings a day along with some animal, vegetable, and grain, nut or seed proteins you will desire little else and your digestion will function very well. You will feel full and satisfied most of the time, your appetite and weight will be controlled as well.

But how do you achieve eating so much fruit and vegetable matter? It's not as difficult as it seems, all you need to do is increase your portion size of vegetables on your plate (eat less meat and more vegetables), snack on carrots, cucumber, bell peppers, apples, kiwi fruit, celery, etc. Let's take a look at a few different ways you can incorporate more vegetables and fruits into your diet.

Eating More Vegetables And Fruits In 4 Simple Steps

I have helped many patients over the years overcome their issues of eating more vegetables and fruits and have some tips that I think might help you. Try and get away from the idea of just eating meat and three vegetables on your plate and do experiment with your vegetable intake. You may like to begin by eating a combination of cooked and semi-cooked or raw vegetables. This is why I like Asian ways of eating, especially wok cooking. This way of cooking involves high temperatures for only a very short period of time, and the vegetables are eaten partially in their raw state.

> " *Life expectancy would grow by leaps and bounds if green vegetables smelled as good as bacon.* "
>
> Doug Larson

Wash your Vegetables and Fruits Well

Besides pesticides, fungicides, and other chemicals, mold spores maybe present on the outside of fruits and vegetables, it's important to wash them well before you consume them, especially if you are very unwell with a yeast infection. The more chronic your yeast infection or digestive problem, the more important it will become for you to eat predominantly organic and spray-free produce. You can help to clean your vegetables more effectively by adding a little Bragg's organic apple cider vinegar to the water.

4 Steps To A Diet Richer In Fresh Fruits & Vegetables

First Step - First it is a good idea to tell yourself all the reasons why you should eat fruit and vegetables in increasing amounts in your diet, there are too many reasons why you should eat more of these health foods and less of the processed and refined foods, this will help you stay motivated and make you think twice about buying that bar of chocolate or packet of your favorite snack food like chips, whatever this treat may be. Watch how your digestion and bowel health improves, you will certainly notice this. Tell yourself you will be halving your risk of cancer, diabetes and heart disease. Visualize how great you will look and feel, as you get older.

Second Step - Write a list of all the fruits and vegetables that you enjoy eating and actually like the taste of and wouldn't mind eating on a regular basis. If you put a bit of thought into this, you will be surprised to find that your list will be a lot longer than you originally thought! This will help you to realize that you have many options indeed to pick and choose from, and not just the boring green stuff like lettuce, cucumber and tomatoes.

Third Step- Go to your fresh produce store or Farmer's Market and buy several of your favorite vegetables and fruits. Start by adding one new vegetable each week, which means that after a month you will have added four vegetables you wouldn't normally have eaten. Try and aim for seven to nine different vegetables that you will eat on a regular daily basis. Include two or three leafy green vegetables (broccoli, spinach, bok choy, lettuce, etc.) Two or three colorful vegetables (bell pepper, egg plant, zucchini, asparagus, corn, etc.) and two or three starchy or root vegetables (sweet potato, pumpkin, potato, parsnip, onions, squash, etc.).

You will soon notice however that we limit these starchy vegetables initially for the first few weeks as you commence the Candida Crusher Diet, but then add them back as your digestion improves. Now depending on how you like to eat these vegetables, there are seven different ways as you will see in a moment, I'd recommend stir-fry or semi raw like saute'.

Fourth Step – Understand that what you do for a twenty-one day period of time can become a habit. If you begin to incorporate more vegetables into your diet on a daily basis for twenty-one days then you may very well find that it becomes part of what you normally do with your mealtimes. When you eat out be sure to order a meal rich in vegetables, like a Thai dish or a Japanese meal. It's not hard to do and once a habit is formed it will become part of our normal routine.

Health Tip:

Avoid trying to convert other people's diets!

A good tip is to try and not enforce your dietary changes onto those you love and care about, whether they are family or friends. You don't want to become the food police after you have discovered just how good it feels to eat a healthy diet and rejuvenate your health and wellbeing. I have always personally found that the best way to get somebody to change is to change your own ways - first. Your loved ones or best friends may well change their "bad" ways over time as they see you looking and feeling fantastic. You will avoid a lot of potential antagonism and stress by looking after your own needs first. This of course does not count for young children but it does for teenagers. Trying to increase the average teenager's vegetable intake is like trying to nail Jell-O to a tree. Lead by example, it always seems to work the best.

There are many ways that you can increase your intake of fresh vegetables and fruits, depending on how you like to prepare your foods. You can eat vegetables and fruits raw, steamed, boiled, stewed, baked, or stir-fried or deep-fried ☹. When you eat vegetables and fruits in their raw state, you are ensuring that your digestive system has access to the valuable nutrients contained within. Eating vegetables and fruits in a semi-raw state is good too, and in many cases it will be a more pleasant experience. Stir-frying is personally my favorite method of cooking vegetables, but so is a partial steaming of vegetables. Remember, the more and prolonged heat you apply, the more chance you will be destroying those all-important enzymes. Casseroles, soups and stews are a favorite method for many people, particularly in the colder months. These methods are good, and even though you reduce the enzyme content, you lock in many minerals that would be otherwise discarded by cooking methods such as boiling or steaming.

Nutrient Loss When Cooking Foods

Many patients have told me over the years that they only like to eat raw foods, because any form of cooked food is inferior over a raw or fresh food when it comes to minerals and vitamins. This is simply not true. Take for example raw dried beans and most legumes; these high protein foods contain enzyme inhibitors that make it really hard for your body to digest any proteins they contain.

When you heat legumes, you disarm these inhibitors and allow the body to have access to the proteins contained inside them. Other foods are unhealthy to eat raw or uncooked, and can potentially cause much harm like eggs, chicken and meat.
It is the vitamins more so than the minerals that are affected by cooking, especially heating, and these are the nutrients most likely to be lost when you cook foods. Simple strategies like steaming foods rather than boiling, or broiling rather than frying can help to significantly reduce the loss of many vitamin and other nutrients when you are cooking foods.

If you want to preserve the nutrients in your foods, the best cooking methods are when you use the least amount of water and heat. And remember, if you cook vegetables in water, don't throw the water out because it will be rich in nutrients, use it for gravy, a casserole or a soup base. Fortunately, when we cook foods at home we have complete control, but when we eat foods out we have no control and you can bet that the vitamin and mineral content may be severely compromised. Just another reason for you to eat at home.

Minerals are virtually unaffected by most cooking methods, as they tend to be much more heat stable than vitamins. The minerals in particular which have a tendency to remain in foods whether they are cooked or eaten raw are calcium, magnesium, phosphorus, iron, zinc, iodine, selenium, copper, manganese, sodium and chromium. Potassium is the mineral that most easily escapes from foods into the liquids, but it is not affected by heat or air. Potassium broth is an excellent alkalizing and cleansing broth that I will be outlining soon.

The two most stable vitamins when it comes to cooking are vitamin K and vitamin B3, niacin. Many vitamins are easily destroyed when they become exposed to water, heat, air or even fat (cooking oil) exposure. Here is a table that highlights the vitamins and their sensitivities.

Vitamins and Minerals Affected By Cooking Methods				
Nutrients	Air	Fat	Heat	Water
Vitamin A		✔	✔	
Vitamin C	✔		✔	✔
Vitamin D		✔		
Vitamin E	✔		✔	
Vitamin B1 (thiamin)			✔	✔
Vitamin B2 (riboflavin)				✔
Vitamin B5 (pantothenic acid)			✔	
Vitamin B6 (pyridoxine)	✔		✔	✔
Vitamin B12			✔	✔
Folate	✔		✔	
Biotin				✔
Potassium				✔

How To Avoid Vitamin Loss When Cooking

Vitamin C – The best way to ensure you don't lose too much vitamin C is to use as little water and as little heat as possible. Light steaming or stir-frying is best, but most fruits and vegetables with a high vitamin C content are best eaten raw or partially raw. By not peeling vegetables, especially root vegetables when you cook them, you retain over half the vitamin C content in comparison to vegetables that have been peeled and then cooked. Serve promptly, and don't reheat after keeping in the refrigerator, most of the vitamin C content will be lost from foods which are high in vitamin C and then re-heated.

B vitamins – It is the heat and water that affect B vitamins, and I find that slow cookers are best here, just keep the heat right down and cook for prolonged periods of time. You consume the liquid that way, which is richer in minerals and vitamins. Bone broths are an exceptionally good way to get an incredible amount of vitamins and especially minerals into your diet. Don't rinse rice before you cook it, especially brown rice, because you may wash a lot of the thiamin (vitamin B1) away.

Fat-soluble vitamins A, E and D – Try not to cook these foods in too much butter, fat or oil, because you will end up loosing much of the valuable fat-soluble vitamins into the cooking medium. Baking, steaming or broiling are better options when it comes to foods high in the fat soluble vitamins.

- Never overcook fresh foods; excess nutrient loss is in direct proportion to how much heat was applied during the cooking stage.

- Eat red meat medium rare and not fully cooked, studies conducted by The National Cancer Institute have revealed a 30 percent less cancer risk in those who ate medium rare beef over those who consumed well-done beef.

- Cooking time and applied heat account for the two biggest factors when it comes to nutrient loss.

- Use very little water when cooking, steaming and stir-frying foods. It is the water that leaches the valuable vitamins and minerals from your foods.

- Avoid deep-frying and frying if at all possible.

- Cook vegetables as soon as you can after cutting them to prevent oxidation and nutrient loss.

- Remember that the four biggest factors accounting for nutrient loss in your foods are air, fats used in cooking, water used in cooking and applied heat. The less you use of these four elements the better.

Soups, Casseroles And Stews

One of the best ways to cook vegetables is by way of a crock-pot or slow cooker, and this is one of the easiest and laziest ways to prepare soups, stews and casseroles. You can make a delicious soup with just about any vegetables and legumes and some of the best things to throw into the soup or stew pot are carrots, onions, be sure to use red or purple ones.

You will find that the more colored the fruits and veggies are the more likely they are to contain higher levels of anti-oxidants. Other good choices are celery, yams or sweet potatoes, chopped spinach or other greens like broccoli, chopped cabbage, and whatever else you like.

This gives you the opportunity to throw into the pot any foods you would not necessarily cook by using other methods such as steaming or stir frying because the produce is a little older or sad looking. OK, so it might be down on nutritional value a little like this, but why waste money and toss out all that good food?

The minerals are most always maintained as your produce ages, but the vitamin content goes down rather quickly so it is always best whenever possible to consume your fruits and vegetables as soon as you buy them. Better still, you could have a vegetable garden like I have and grow your own!

Add Beans To Your Vegetable Meals

Did you know that beans are packed full of protein, are full of healthy dietary fiber, low in fat, and are a very healthy way to add protein and fiber to your daily meals? I have long been a fan of beans cooked in Mexican dishes and lentils cooked in Indian dishes. Have you ever tried cooking beans or lentils in a slow cooker with onions and tomatoes, adding some spices and garlic? Have you ever tried to make your own baked bean dishes? They taste so much better than the canned variety and you save plenty of money too. Some practitioners who treat patients like I do with yeast infections have told me that it is best to recommend the avoidance of beans like starchy carbohydrate vegetables for the first few weeks from the diet. I find that if they are introduced too rapidly into the diet that they can be the cause of a tremendous amount of gas and bloating, so go slow at first. In my experience, hold off with beans and lentils for a few weeks, or just go *really easy*. Here are some good tips on beans in your diet:

- Avoid beans and lentils for the 2 – 3 weeks, especially if you have bloating.
- Introduce as soon as your digestion begins to improve.
- Go real easy to begin with, start with ¼ cup a day and work up slowly.
- If you do develop gas and bloating, reduce the amount & take a probiotic.
- Soak beans and slow cook seems to reduce the amount of aggravation.
- Chew your foods very well, this will greatly aid in digestion, slow down!
- At first, try to avoid mixing your bean or lentil dishes with too many starchy vegetables, especially if your digestive system is sensitive.

Hummus, Guacamole And Salsa With Vegetables

Have you made hummus yet? This is a simple bean dip made from garbanzo beans (chickpeas) and is delicious when served with strips of carrot and celery, broccoli and cauliflower. Guacamole and salsa are also easy to make and taste delicious as well. These dishes are minimally processed and are eaten in conjunction with fresh vegetables. Guacamole is made with avocado, but you can also make it with a base of red onions, coriander (cilantro), lime and tomatoes.

Adding vegetables to meat fajitas is so easy and tasty, and for the vegetarians you can make vegetarian bean fajitas. Vegetables are also great in quesadillas, especially spinach and burritos. Have you tried Mexican foods? Burritos are great; you simply roll up flat corn bread which contains either a meat or bean filling which is topped with freshly cut tomato, lettuce, onion, grated carrot, zucchini, red bell peppers, mushrooms or even lightly steamed sweet potatoes.

It is easy to make a Mexican salad that is topped with guacamole and some salsa. Add a few sliced olives, sun dried tomatoes and sliced avocado and what a feast.

Pita Bread With Vegetables

Pita breads are fantastic, and it is so easy to create an excellent snack or meal with these breads. Be sure to lightly toast or grill your pita bread just before you use it, this is the trick. You can stuff a pita bread with anyone of a hundred different fillings such as shredded lettuce, tomato and carrot or what about lightly sautéing some vegetables, sweet potato and beans. Add a splash of Italian dressing (do read labels, watch the sugar content) and top with a tiny bit of grated Parmesan cheese and you have a winner.

Grilled Vegetables

The trick to tasty and tender vegetables that have been grilled is a good marinade. Just like meat, if you marinate vegetables beforehand they will be more tender and tasty. I just use olive oil, finely cut fresh garlic, a little lemon (or lime) juice and salt & pepper. You can also add teriyaki, Worcestershire or a few drops of Tabasco sauce. My personal favorite is lightly grilled Portobello mushrooms, and these taste just like meat! Be sure to marinate overnight in the olive oil/garlic and lemon juice mix. Have you ever tried grilled avocado or grilled fresh asparagus? You will love it. I know that mushrooms are taboo with candida, but try marinating them overnight with olive oil and freshly chopped garlic and presto, your mushrooms have been soaking in one of the most powerful antifungals, so relax.

Steamed Vegetables

Vegetables are delicious when steamed, but the trick is not to overcook, but rather undercook. Always turn the heat off before they are steamed, take off the heat and by the time you serve up they will have sat an extra minute or two which is enough to have them still crunchy. If your fork passes very easily through steamed vegetables then they are overcooked, simple as that. Partially steam leeks and red onions before adding them to some fresh fish fillets which you grill, and you have a very tasty dish.

My favorite vegetables steamed when picked straight from my vegetable garden would have to be broccoli or fresh string beans but any vegetable lightly steamed with some butter added is simply delicious. A meal for me would be one steamed head of freshly picked broccoli, and a portion of fresh white fish fillet grilled or steamed.

Great Health Tip:

Marinating vegetables and meats

Try marinating vegetables and meats with some olive oil, garlic, sea salt and a generous amount of fresh oregano, thyme or rosemary. These herbs in particular are anti-bacterial and anti-fungal and can help considerably in reducing the yeast population in your digestive tract. The best herb is oregano in my opinion, just grab a handful of fresh oregano, be sure to harvest the fresh herb in the middle of the day, preferably when the sun is at it's meridian at noon as this will ensure a good level of the essential oils are present. Place the oregano in a mortal and pestle and crush well, failing this you can tear the herb with your fingers until it is well bruised and you can really smell those oils. Now, place the crushed oregano in a jar and add enough extra virgin olive oil to cover. Add several fresh cloves of freshly minced garlic to the jar, place the lid on and shake well. Leave this mixture in a dark cupboard for a few days until you can taste the oregano oil in the olive oil, only then is it ready to use. Now you can marinate your chicken pieces, pork or beef overnight in this oregano and garlic infused oil. Both delicious and anti-fungal, the best of both worlds.

Vegetable Curries

Have you ever tried a vegetable korma? It is a vegetable curry, just buy some korma sauce, make sure there is no sugar in this product, or make your own and add a few cups of diced vegetables, leave to cook with the lid on until the vegetables are just tender and serve with some steamed brown rice or cooked quinoa. You can make up a vegetable fried rice or a vegetable chow mein as well.

Potatoes, Yams And Sweet Potatoes

The humble potato is such a versatile vegetable, but one starchy vegetable I keep candida yeast patients away from during the first few weeks of the candida diet. Potatoes contain lots of fiber and vitamin C, they are healthy and there is so much you can do with them. They taste great when mashed, baked, roasted and are great when served cold in potato salads. They also taste good when boiled and served with a leafy green vegetable, or served with herbs, butter and olive oil.

Sweet potatoes and yams contain large amounts of potassium and are a good alkalizing vegetable. They are a better choice for those with yeast infections over other starchy vegetables. These root vegetables are delicious when roasted with other vegetables and are great in soups, stir fry dishes, curries and casseroles.

Asian Stir-Fry Dishes

Have you ever tried to make Thai, Chinese, Vietnamese or other Asian style dishes at home? These are my personal favorites because Asian style cooking incorporates some of the best techniques that ensure you eat your vegetables in the freshest yet tastiest of ways. I highly recommend that you take a good look online and view some recipe websites to get good ideas Be sure to visit either your local library or bookstore and get a good cookbook on Thai and Chinese style cooking.

There are countless Thai, Chinese, and Vietnamese dishes that include so many partially cooked all vegetables in combination with different meats that are often marinated. Trust me, the real key to succulent, juicy and tender meat is to marinate!

Stir-frying considered one of the healthiest of cooking methods because vegetables are cooked literally without water, I add a few teaspoons to help steam the vegetables a little and use a small amount of oil and only a few minutes on high heat. Vegetables and meats should be sliced thin in order to heat and cook them fast. Because it's fast, stir-frying sears the outside of what's being cooked, locking nutrients inside.

Stir-fry dishes are just so easy to make, and the steel wok is cleaned in less than a minute. Just start with a little olive oil, some garlic, onion and fresh ginger and then add some meat of choice. Good stir-fry vegetables include broccoli, carrots, bok choy, onions, red bell peppers, baby corn, asparagus, green beans, onions, and snow pea pods. Serve with steamed jasmine rice or brown rice. Please use fresh vegetables, and avoid the temptation of using frozen stuff, it only takes a few minutes to cut up and prepare fresh vegetables.

Pizza Dishes

I'm personally not a big fan of pizza dishes, as I find that you will be consuming too much bread, fat and cheese along with vegetables that have been literally grilled to death. Even though pizza is a tasty dish, my preference is more for a kebab or pita styled bread that incorporates fresh salad vegetables to which no heat is applied.

More Tips On How To Add Vegetables To Your Meals

Why not make up your own kebabs or hamburgers at home? Choose a thin piece of flat bread and add a substantial topping of your choice, begin with a meat, bean, tempeh (fermented tofu) or whatever high protein choice you like.

Then, simply add shredded lettuce, tomato, red onion, cucumber, grated carrot, finely sliced olive, etc. The choice is yours and if you use the freshest of ingredients it will taste just great. Try substituting meat for beans when you make a burger, you will be eating more fiber and the taste is great.

- Why not make your own vegetable sauces? Just cut up bell peppers, mushrooms, tomatoes and zucchini, sauté' in olive oil, add plenty of freshly chopped garlic.

- Add vegetables to meat dishes to add plenty of texture, fiber and flavors. Shredded vegetables like carrot and zucchini, a simple process when you use a large hand grater or food processor. Shredded vegetables are so easy to hide in many different meat dishes such as lasagna, spaghetti and meatballs.

- Have you tried to marinate squash or eggplant in olive oil, salt and garlic and then bake or grill these delicious vegetables?

- Vegetables are easy to add to many different kinds of dips as well, and you can do this simply and cheaply with a good food processor. Try blending up beans, onions and garlic with a little sour cream and add some fresh herbs like basil and serve with veggie chips, pita bread or just dip raw veggies in the dip and enjoy.

- Vegetables make great side dishes; try blanched fresh green beans or asparagus for example. One of my favorites is a combination of red, green, yellow and orange bell peppers along with Portobello mushrooms, zucchini and red onions sautéed in olive oil, soy sauce (or chili sauce), and plenty of fresh garlic. Add some freshly ground salt and pepper and enjoy this side with any number of dishes you prepare.

- Roasted bell peppers taste fantastic! Just split a bell pepper into four, clean out the seeds and brush liberally or spray with olive oil and then grill until the skins just start to blister. You can also roast zucchini this way, but remember – don't roast for too long or you will kill off a lot of the goodness these vegetables have to offer.

> *It's bizarre that the produce manager is more*
> *important to my children's health than the pediatrician.*
> Meryl Streep

Fresh Fruit Ideas

Fresh fruits are discouraged for the first two weeks once you start the Candida Crusher Diet, but there is nothing wrong with eating fresh fruits as your digestive system begins to recover in stage 3 of the C.C. Program. It is important to point out that some fruits are better than others when it comes to having a yeast infection, and I have found with yeast patients that fresh fruits tend to be considerably less of a problem than dried fruits, even in the tiniest amounts. Citrus fruits and fruit juices, except for lemons and limes are best avoided until you have improved to a very high degree because they contain too much sugar. Grapefruit and grapefruit juice is probably one of your best initial citrus options, particularly if you add a few drops of GSE (grapefruit seed extract) which is extremely antifungal. You can read a lot more about GSE in section 4, later in this chapter. Remember, if it tastes really sweet and especially if you crave a particular fruit then leave it well alone until well down the track.

Fruits initially safe with candida	Fruits not initially safe with candida
Paw paw, kiwi fruit, blueberries, avocado and green apple (Granny Smith), lemons and limes.	Pineapple, stone fruits - plums, peaches, nectarines, apricots, citrus fruits - oranges, mandarins, bananas, grapes, dates, dried fruits such as figs, dates and raisins, are particularly high in sugar as well.

Whilst fruit is OK to consume during the Big Clean-Up cleanse I'll talk about shortly, do avoid the fruits I mentioned above in the right column initially which tend to aggravate those with a yeast infection during the initial phases of the Candida Crusher Diet. I'm mentioning this about fruit up now, because everybody wants to know what fruits they can and can't have and when to re-introduce them!

Apples And Candida

> *Even if I knew that tomorrow the world would go to pieces,*
> *I would still plant my apple tree.*
> Martin Luther

But isn't an apple a "forbidden" fruit if you have a yeast infection? I don't find that all varieties are, and I've yet to find a person who eats several tart or sour apples like the varieties such as Granny Smith green apples, these are more sour or tart apples. Perhaps some readers may, but generally speaking they would be much more inclined to eat several of the sweeter and newer varieties daily, bred especially for their high sugar content. People don't normally aggravate on sour or tart apples with yeast infections, and I've not seen many aggravations come about with the consumption of one green apple per day.

If your apple tastes very sweet, and in New Zealand we have very sweet varieties bred especially for the Asian market, such as Pacific Rose, then you are best advised to leave them well alone, because you may find that you end up substituting your sugar intake for this sweet treat instead.

When I wrote this section of Candida Crusher, I did some research and found that people rarely publish the sugar content of apple varieties. It looks like most commercially available varieties seem to have similar sugar content but this will be hard to judge by taste as sour or tart flavors can mask sweetness. It is difficult to standardize sugar content of fruit because there can be an enormous variation due to the climate the fruit was grown in, the rainfall, the time of harvest and how ripe the fruit is when eaten.

My guess is that the more sour or tart varieties contain less sugar than their sweeter counterparts and are a safer option. I've also noticed that those who eat one tart or sour apple a day tend to have better bowel motions and are increasing the beneficial fiber content of their diet. What many are not aware of is that one apple a day, besides keeping the doctor away, will be giving their digestive system a food containing beneficial pre-biotic fibers to build health levels of beneficial bacteria. And that's not a bad thing if you have a yeast infection.

Avoid Fruits with Stems

Be careful of fruits that contain stems such as apples, cherries, berries, grapes and certain kinds of stone fruit. These kinds of soft fruits may be more prone to harboring different kinds of molds that are very difficult to see with the naked eye. You are best to leave the softer and sweeter stemmed fruits well alone until you feel much better, particularly grapes.

It is a easier to eat a lot of sweet fruit with stems, like grapes, and that means you will be eating lots of sugar too. And do remember, at the sake of repeating myself, wash any fruits and vegetables especially well because of the possibility of them being covered in molds or spores, especially if you have kept them in your vegetable crisper in the fridge for several days. It is these kinds of small but significant things you do in the kitchen that can make all the difference.

Avoid High Fructose Fruits, Foods And Drinks Initially

Don't be fooled by fruit, some books on yeast infection I have read state that "fruit is safe to eat by those with a yeast infection". This is simply untrue, candida proliferates by consuming and fermenting sugars like sucrose, fructose and other simple sugars, that's how it lives and thrives. The less sugar you eat, the less chance candida can thrive and the sooner you will beat that yeast infection. What you will most probably know is that most fruits contain sugars, especially a sugar named fructose, a sugar which is twice as sweet as sucrose.

Caution With HFCS - High Fructose Corn Syrup

Today, most human fructose intake comes from high-fructose corn syrup (HFCS), a man-made sugar composed of 65% sucrose and 35% glucose. This abundant sugar is used to sweeten just about every processed food because it is cheap and mixes well with many different kinds of foods, many health experts are now viewing HCFS as being a toxic addition to our diets, it just increases our sugar intake needlessly, and along with it the risk of a candida yeast overgrowth. Did you know that soda drinks account for 33% intake of a person's fructose intake these days? An average 600ml can of soda drink contains nearly 36 grams of HFCS fructose, and experts tell us to limit our total fructose intake to no more than 25 grams per day.

So what fruits and sweeteners contain the highest amount of fructose? Well I'm glad you asked, because I took the time to compile a list for your benefit. Try to avoid those fruits and sweet additions to your diet with the highest fructose intake at least until you feel a lot better in your digestive tract, experience a lot less bloating, gas and irregular bowel motions. Is it any surprise that dried fruits contain the highest amount of fructose? So please do avoid all dried fruits until you feel *much better*.

As you improve, slowly increase your intake of fresh fruits first, the ones with the lowest fructose intake, and remember not to include dried fruits until much later. Be prepared to remove any high fructose fruits until you improve and drop back to the lower fructose containing frits like berries, especially if you aggravate when you re-introduce the higher fructose containing fruits during the reintroduction stage of the Candida Crusher Diet.

Higher in Fructose (mg of fructose per 100 gr)	Lower in Fructose (mg of fructose per 100 gr)
Honey – 40,900 (not a fruit, but look at the fructose!)	Apples (sour or tart) – 5,700
Dates – 32,000	Persimmon – 5,560
Raisins – 29,700	Blueberry – 4,970
Figs – 22,900	Kiwi fruit – 4,350
Molasses – 12,800	Plums – 3,070
Prunes – 12,500	Strawberry – 2,500
Grapes – 8,130	Blackberry – 2,400
Apples – 6,250	Raspberry – 2,350
Pears – 6, 230	Pineapple – 2,050
Cherries – 6,000	

Why a pH Balanced Diet?

It is important for you to understand what pH means and how when carefully balanced it can make all the difference when it comes to crushing your yeast infection permanently. What does pH mean, and how does it relate to your health when it comes to a yeast infection?

The letters pH is an acronym for the words **P**otential **H**ydrogen, and come from the chemistry formula for calculating the concentration of hydrogen ions present in a substance. The pH scale measures acidity and alkalinity and the scale ranges from 1 (most acid) right up to 14 (most alkaline) with a pH value of 7 being regarded as neutral, pure water thus has a value of 7. Foods that are predominantly alkaline by nature have a pH value above 7, whereas foods that are predominantly acid by nature have a pH value below 7. Your blood has a pH finely balanced at 7.365.

Your body not only tries very hard to maintain a constant temperature of close to 98.5 Fahrenheit (37 Degrees Celsius), it tries even harder to maintain a pH balance of almost exactly 7.365, and it achieves this by way of maintaining your oxygen levels within a fine range.

Scientists have worked out that in order for your blood cells to remain the healthiest, they require a blood-based pH level of 7.365, which is slightly alkaline. Meanwhile, your digestive system, in particular your stomach, requires a pH level of around 2, which is very acid to break down foods, especially any protein foods.

We have also discovered that if the body's capacity to absorb and retain oxygen becomes compromised in any way and the pH becomes imbalanced, that we can get sick much more easily and become more prone to diseases like infections, inflammation, heart disease, cancers and even a candida yeast overgrowth. So, when your body's pH levels fluctuate widely, and especially if they remain too low (acidic), you may gravitate from one infection to another and may be considerably more prone to all kinds of acute or chronic illness.

Many who live in the Western world tend to adopt diets that are too refined, they eat too many prepackaged foods that tend to be processed and full of sugar, salt and fat, and the bottom line is that they may develop a real problem absorbing and maintaining adequate oxygen levels.

Myth: Candida Needs And Acidic Environment To Thrive In

Your pH balance is an important factor for you to seriously consider if you want to beat that yeast infection once and for all, because pH affects the delicate balance of your biochemical health profoundly.

While it is a myth that a predominantly alkaline diet discourages yeast and a predominantly acid diet favors yeast, understanding the pH balance is important when it comes to maximizing your digestive health, and by optimizing your digestive health you will be discouraging a yeast infection. More importantly, by maximizing your digestive potential, it will be harder for candida to translocate from your digestive system into the bloodstream, where it can cause major problems.

Let me explain first about acidity, alkalinity and your body. For example, the vaginal environment is acidic. Your digestive system is a predominantly acidic environment likewise, especially your stomach and small intestine, where most of the protein digestion occurs. Lactic acid favours the production of lactobacillus species in the digestive system, and without an acidic environment created higher up in the digestive tract, the pancreas lower down will not be sufficiently stimulated to create the alkaline pancreatic enzymes and juices.

Real problems arise once candida translocates from the digestive system, a predominantly acidic environment, into to the blood stream, a slightly more alkaline environment. Yeast begins to thrive in this slightly alkaline environment because the hostile environment of the digestive system does not challenge it. The pH change that occurs with this translocation allows candida to change into its more pathogenic fungal mycelial form. Besides, your immune system will have become weakened over time and find it harder to counter the yeast infection once it has moved from the gut to the bloodstream. The more balanced your body's pH levels, the healthier you will be and the easier it will be for your system to fight off a yeast infection.

Foods and pH

Foods are categorized as being either acid or alkaline based on the residue they leave behind in your body after they have been metabolized.

Your body's pH balance is determined to a major degree by the foods you eat and the beverages you drink. If you eat too many acidic foods, you can experience acidosis. Alternatively, if you are not eating enough acidic foods, your body could have too high of a pH, and this is known as alkalosis. Raw foods are generally more alkaline than cooked foods, although there are some exceptions to this rule. Although you can find charts on the Internet describing which foods are more acidic and which more alkaline, I have supplied one here for you right here in the Candida Crusher. It is important to remember that this chart is an acid/alkaline chart and not a candida diet recommendation sheet. For example, note the dried fruits listed in the alkaline section, this does not mean that dried fruits are OK to consume if you are trying to get rid of your yeast infection! You should only consider eating dried fruits well down the track, once you have just about recovered. Fresh fruits should be re-introduced well before dried fruits are.

The foods and drinks listed in the left column represent foods and drinks that have a tendency to be more acid by nature, and those listed in the right column have more of a tendency to be alkaline by nature, it's as simple as that. The foods and drinks that have an asterisk in the left column are the ones that are inclined to be more acid forming by nature. The best balance appears to be an 80% alkaline and a 20% acid forming diet.

As a general rule, most grains, dairy products, meats, seeds, legumes and nuts tend to be acid forming, whereas most fruits and vegetables tend to be alkaline forming. Cooked foods tend to be more acid forming than raw foods. Most natural medicine health care professionals spend time educating their clients that modern Western diets generally are too acidic for good health due to a lack of fruits and vegetables, and we often stress the importance of modifying one's diet to achieve a better acid-base ratio. I want you to understand that it is not purely the foods you eat and the beverages you drink that account for a body which is more acid or alkaline, it is not that simple. There are many different factors that may account for pH fluctuations, and one simple example here is hydration, are you drinking enough water? I have found that most patients I see are dehydrated, that's right, they don't drink enough water but instead rely on coffee and tea which are acid forming drinks. A lesser-known fact of becoming too alkaline is by consuming lots of mineral water, or by taking too many mineral supplements which can also tip the balance towards alkalinity.

Lemon Is Alkaline

Did you know that lemon and lime juice are considered alkalizing by nature? These juices are acid outside the body, but once consumed the body renders them alkaline and as such are considered alkaline fruits. Most all fruits are alkaline by nature but many contain sugars and are best left well alone until your yeast infection improves considerably. Lemon juice however, discourages candida.

Symptoms Of an Altered pH

So how do you really know if you are developing signs and symptoms of an underlying pH imbalance? There are many potential illnesses that can develop as a result of an altered pH. Whether you are a woman who regularly experiences a vaginal yeast infection, a man who experiences jock itch, or if you are a person who experiences a fungal nail infection or you have a child with diaper rash, you will most always find that by addressing the pH imbalance, your diet and consumed beverages in particular, that there will be a noticeable reduction in the frequency, duration as well as the severity of your yeast infection. Get your body's biochemistry right and it will be that much easier to maintain your pH balance. Your body will be less prone to infection and inflammation, less chance of a UTI (urinary tract infection), prostatitis, acne, arthritis, candida yeast infections and even cancer.

Determining Your pH

I often get asked: "OK, I know about pH, but how can I find out what my pH is?" Simple, just go to your local chemist and ask for urinary pH test strips. These are also called litmus paper, and all you need to do is to take a midstream morning urinary sample and note the color of the test paper compared to the color on the container. You may want to test after meals and between meals. Try several times a day and write the findings down, you soon will be able to discover the relationship between what you eat and drink and the pH your body produces as a consequence. The litmus paper will tell you instantly what your pH is and thus, how alkaline or acid you are. Test strips are also available online, and with regular testing you will be able to fine-tune your diet and stay more on the alkaline rather than acid side.

Health Tip – Urinary pH

Lower urinary pH in the morning just after waking is normal, your urine will tend to be darker in color and more concentrated and the same may occur after a large protein meal, a coffee or a tea. You need to take your urinary pH at different times of the day, after different meals and different levels of hydration. This will teach you the important relationship between what you eat and drink and your body's delicate biochemistry, and ultimately your health.

Acid Forming 20% of Diet	Alkaline Forming 80% of Diet
Alcohol *	All fresh fruits (except most citrus) Lemons are alkaline
All processed foods with wheat or white flour	All raw or steamed vegetables
Black pepper	All salad greens
Bottled salad dressings	All sprouts - grains, beans, seeds, nuts
Any breads, all wheat * products generally	Apple cider vinegar
Cake *	Dates
Canned and most frozen convenience foods	Dried apricots (sun-dried)
Chocolate *	Dried figs
Cigarettes, tobacco	Vegetable juices (especially wheatgrass juice)
Coffee *	Seaweed
Complaining, anger, hatred and jealousy & envy	Fresh or dried seasoning herbs
All cooked grains, (except millet and quinoa)	Fresh raw vegetable juice. Have 1 glass/day
All dairy (butter, cheese, ice-cream, milk, etc.)	Most vegetables in general – can't go wrong here
Distilled vinegar	Herbal teas – (no caffeine)
Eggs, all junk & take-our foods	Honey – *in moderation please!*
Foods cooked with oils, deep-fried foods	Love and kindness, compassion and forgiveness
Glazed or sulfur preserved dried fruits (e.g; apricots)	Maple syrup (it has to be 100% pure – read the label!)
Red meat *, fish, poultry, shellfish (all animal meats)	Nuts and seeds
Pasta	Legumes – chickpeas, split peas, lentils
Popcorn	Lima beans
Processed cereals	Melons, millet
Processed milks (soy, rice, almond, oatmeal)	Molasses
Salt	Potatoes
Water crackers	Quinoa, raisins
Soda drinks ** and cordials **	Cold-pressed olive oil
Sugar **	Cold pressed flax seed oil
Tofu and soy products, white vinegar Foods marked with an asterisk * are the most acid forming ones	© Compiled by Eric Bakker ND.

Acid Forming 20% of Diet	Alkaline Forming 80% of Diet

Why Fermented And Cultured Foods?

Those with candida yeast infections can safely eat fermented and cultured foods without fear of eating any of the bad yeasts commonly associated with commercial bread and alcoholic beverages. This is very important point I discovered several years ago, and if you do this you are assured of a speedy and long-term recovery from your yeast infection. Foods that contain probiotics (pro-life) bacteria or are rich in lactic acid can and should be added to your Candida Crusher diet to bring back balance to the gut flora.

The Body Ecology Diet

The Body Ecology Diet is an excellent book written by Donna Gates, this book is all about foods that help to support the growth and reproduction of healthy bacteria in your digestive tract. Donna had a yeast infection herself and overcame her health problems many years ago by understanding the principles of inner health and fermented and cultured foods. She has a good grasp on this topic in her book, especially on coconut kefir.

Foods that have been cultured naturally or lacto-fermented are important additions to the diet of those with a yeast infection, because they contain enzymes and bacteria that help digest food and help the body to eliminate wastes. These foods help to cultivate friendly bacteria in the intestinal tract that in turn aids in digestion, helps to boost immunity and increases the uptake of Vitamin B12. Naturally cultured or lacto-fermented foods are particularly important to eat during pregnancy when a woman's digestive system may have slowed down considerably, and it is also during pregnancy that many women are prone to vaginal thrush.

Many women know that yogurt is good to use as a douche, but not many women are encouraged to eat kefir, yogurt, kim-chi or sauerkraut during pregnancy. Cultured foods will not only help to prevent constipation and other digestive problems, I have found them to be and most useful in preventing and treating many different kinds of yeast infections. Have you taken an antibiotic recently? Then why not consume lacto-fermented foods that will help to replace the beneficial bacteria that were destroyed by these kinds of medications.

Probiotics are also known as friendly bacteria, they are the microorganisms that normally suppress the growth of candida in the gastrointestinal tract. If they are depleted, generally through prolonged usage of certain medications like antibiotics, the Pill, antacids, etc., then the risk of a candida infection increases in proportion. Bad bacteria can also squeeze the good bacteria out, and when this occurs then an overgrowth of candida is almost assured. And how do you squeeze the good ones out? By drinking lots of alcohol and eating a sugar laden and junk diet in general.

Be sure to understand the concept of fermented and cultured foods in this chapter, and please do try to incorporate them daily into your diet, it is a very important concept of the Candida Crusher Diet and can be the difference between winning the yeast battle of just holding your symptoms at bay. This food group is generally fine in all the stages of the diet, although you may find that initially you may find it difficult to have too large a portion size of say for example yogurt or sauerkraut if there are lots of bad bacteria and yeasts in your digestive tract initially, so go slow to start and as you improve you should be able to eat more and varied amounts of cultured and fermented foods.

Have you tried to regularly eat foods that have been cultured, other than yogurt? There are many different types of foods from many different cultures that are preserved in these methods such as sauerkraut, Kim chi, sourdough bread, miso and many more. Keep an open mind and experiment, I love sauerkraut but my wife adores Kim chi, originally from Korea. But then again she likes laid back eighties music and I prefer classical. We all have our own individual tastes and it is important to bear this in mind.

Fermented foods are foods produced or preserved by the action of microorganisms. They can come about either by fermenting sugar with yeast and produce alcohol, or by way of another fermentation process involving the use of bacteria such as lactobacillus, which includes the making of foods such as yogurt and sauerkraut.

Since the by-products of digesting meat and dairy products actively inhibit the growth of beneficial lactobacillus bacteria in your digestive system, and since these congestive foods are responsible to a degree for the accumulated, impacted debris in the lower intestine and colon, fermented foods such as sauerkraut and kim chi should especially be eaten with meat and often are.

Try consuming these fermented and cultured foods regularly, and be amazed at the difference they make to your level of digestive comfort, including the reduction and banishing of candida symptoms like bloating, gas, constipation and diarrhea. If you get to include them from now on, and keep on consuming them, you are well on your way to a permanent yeast solution.

Fermented And Cultured Foods Are OK But Introduce Them Slowly

Do not make the mistake for one moment thinking that fermented and cultured foods actually cause a yeast infection; they are perfectly fine foods to include into the diet for those with a yeast infection and one of the best kept secrets. I've heard various natural medicine practitioners over the years telling people to avoid all such foods because they can actually "cause a yeast infection", but this is simply not the case.

Apart from The Body Ecology Diet, I have rarely found this information in any candida yeast infection books and it really does surprise me why not, I guess it is because most of these books were written by those who never actually see patients with yeast infections, and therefore have little experience in seeing the results of their dietary recommendations first hand like I have over the years. Donna Gates experienced first hand what these foods did to her digestive tract, and how they cured her yeast infection, and so did I, I've eating sauerkraut for many years and have recommended these kinds of foods to my patients for over two decades.

I can see why fermented and cultured foods have received a bad rap, because what you will find is that if a person has a bad yeast infection and they try to stop consuming all the offending foods at once (like alcohol, sweets, soda drinks, ice cream, cookies, bread, etc.) and then start taking probiotics, candida kill supplements and begin eating lots of fermented and cultured foods then they may be in for a rude awakening. Their digestive system simply wouldn't be able to cope, nor will their liver and they may feel pretty bad.

But to blame this kind of aggravation on the cultured and fermented foods is plain wrong. They would have experienced a lot less trouble if they had introduced these beneficial foods more slowly and gradually into their diet.

Be Aware Of Budget Fermented Products

Many pickled or soured foods are fermented as part of the pickling or souring process, but be aware that many are simply processed very quickly and cheaply with brine, white sugar, white vinegar, or another cheap acid such as citric acid. When you buy vinegar, for example, my advice is to spend a bit more and buy a glass bottle of vinegar which you may find on the bottom shelf, if you buy in the supermarket with a good selection, or ask the person at the counter of the health shop for a good organic fermented vinegar.
It pays to be choosy where you buy and what you buy, and you always seem to get what you pay for, have you noticed? It is great to see many supermarkets now offering larger ranges of soured and fermented foods such as pickled olives, Kim chi, tempeh, natto, goats cheeses, miso, and many gourmet pickled and soured vegetables in the delicatessen section. This is good news for health-conscious consumers looking to increase their digestive, cardiovascular and immune health, since these traditionally lacto-fermented foods belong to some of the best foods you can eat to build good health.

Healthy Fermented Foods Versus Commercially Processed

Fermentation is an inconsistent process, and more of an art than a science; so commercial food processors have developed various techniques to help standardize more consistent yields. Many cultured foods today are produced on a large commercial scale like cheese. If you get the chance, try a boutique homemade cheese and you will be very surprised at the incredible flavor. Commercially prepared cheeses just don't come anywhere near the flavor.

Refrigeration, high-heat pasteurization and vinegar's acidic pH all slow or halt the fermentation and enzymatic processes. If you leave a jar of pickles that is still fermenting at room temperature on the kitchen counter, they will continue to ferment and produce carbon dioxide, possibly blowing off the lid or exploding the jar, which is why, of course, all shelf-stable pickles are pasteurized.

It's probably not surprising that our culture has traded many of the benefits of these healthy foods for the convenience of mass-produced pickles and other cultured foods. Some olives, such as most canned black olives, for instance, are not generally fermented, but are simply treated with lye to remove the bitterness, packed in salt and canned. Olive producers can now hold olives in salt-free brine by using an acidic solution of lactic acid, acetic acid, sodium benzoate and potassium, pasteurized entirely differently from the old time natural lactic-acid fermenting method of salt alone. The emphasis is on quick today.

Some pickles are simply packed in salt, vinegar and are pasteurized. Many yogurts are so laden with artificial sugars and processed fruits that they are little more than sweet puddings, have you noticed? Unfortunately, these modern techniques effectively kill off all the lactic acid producing bacteria and short-circuit their important and traditional contribution to intestinal and overall health.

Get The Incredible Health Benefits
Of Lacto-Fermented Foods

As fermented foods expert Sally Fallon asks in Nourishing Traditions, with the proliferation of all these new mysterious viruses, intestinal parasites and chronic health problems, despite ubiquitous sanitation, that it may well be that by abandoning our ancient practices of fermenting and culturing foods, and insisting on a diet in which everything has been pasteurized, homogenized and sterilized from any micro-organisms, we have compromised the health of our intestinal flora and made ourselves vulnerable to legions of pathogenic microorganisms. Like those cheap two-dollar jars of dill and gherkin pickles from your supermarket, are we undermining our health by insisting on fast and cheap foods?

If you look, you can still find some healthy traditional varieties of these fermented and cultured foods. The stronger-flavored, traditional olives you are most likely to find in the Greek, Italian or Spanish shops are most likely not lye-treated, and will still be found to be alive with active cultures. So are the locally-crocked fresh pickled olives made in your local Mediterranean deli, as well as the pickles, sauerkraut and other fermented foods you will be able to buy from many of these shops or can easily make yourself at home. Generally, the stronger and more complex the flavor, not counting any added flavorings or other hot pepper flavorings, the more likely that the food will still have active and beneficial lacto-bacteria.

So how can you be sure if you are getting the benefits of these active, fermentation cultures? For one thing, you can make your own or buy from a reputable seller like a good health-food shop, for example olives, sauerkraut, miso, tempeh, or Kim chi. There are plenty of great recipes I discovered online when I did a Google search the other evening, I found hundreds of excellent websites, and so can you.

In addition to being good for our overall health, reducing carbohydrates and cholesterol, strengthening the digestion and immune systems, eradicating yeast infections and even proactively helping us fight off and prevent diseases like cancer, these fermented and cultured foods are a lot simpler, easier to prepare and enjoy than you might think. Some people seem to think that the term fermented sounds vaguely distasteful, but many others however enjoy these foods every day that are results of ancient preparation and preservation techniques, produced through the breakdown of carbohydrates and proteins by micro-organisms such as bacteria, yeasts and molds.

Recent research has found fermented foods to be extremely beneficial to your overall health, so much so that some of these functional foods are now even considered to be probiotics, which can help your health in the following ways.

Some Of The Health Benefits Of Fermented And Cultured Foods

- Increasing your overall health by optimizing your nutritional status

- Promoting the growth of friendly intestinal bacteria

- Aiding digestion and supporting immune function

- Increase in B vitamins (even Vitamin B12), and uptake of omega-3 fatty acids

- Increase in digestive enzymes, lactase and lactic acid

- Increase in other immune chemicals that fight off harmful bacteria and even cancer cells.

Have You Tried Sourdough Bread, Kim Chi, Kefir, Or Cultured Vegetables?

Probiotics are popular these days, in fact so popular that you may think that fermented foods containing beneficial bacteria will be just another one of those quick health fads like so many other diets. The fact is that cultured foods have been consumed for many hundreds and even thousands of years around the world, and those who have consumed these foods were most probably oblivious to the fact that these foods contained simply loads of pre and probiotics. These beneficial live bacteria are found in abundance naturally in fermented foods, and through observation it has been found that those who regularly consume these foods are less likely to suffer from colds or other immune problems, amongst other numerous health benefits

Homegrown probiotics

In addition to buying the many quality probiotic products today, you can make your own tasty and nutritious probiotic foods with surprisingly little effort or expense. It is well worth the effort you put in to create these wonderfully nourishing foods. Your family's health will improve and you may well have some fun in making these preparations. I have made yogurt as well as sour dough bread for many years and also enjoy making Kim chi, one of my wife's favorite condiments for many years now.

Whey

Rarely has natural product been praised so often, and for such a long time, as whey. In about the year 400BC, a Greek physician named Hippocrates recommended the "milk serum" of goats, sheep and cows to his patients. He left boiling milk to curdle with fig juice and vinegar and thereby created a refreshing and tangy drink.

Hippocrates observed that those who drank his concoction suffered a great deal less from digestive discomfort, although he had no idea of the microbial benefits of a lactic acid rich fermented food.

An outstanding commercial Swiss whey supplement you can buy is Molkosan, a supplement I often recommend for those who have a yeast infection. Molkosan is a fermented whey concentrate that was developed by Dr. Alfred Vogel in 1952. Dr. Vogel was a true herbal medicine pioneer in natural health and was the first person to bring the popular herbal medicine Echinacea from Nebraska, USA, to Switzerland in the early 1950's.

He started a company over fifty years ago called Bio force, which still produces today some of the finest natural medicines available today, including Molkosan. Alfred Vogel devoted a great deal of his time to whey and from 1947 he repeatedly reported its positive effects in his magazine, Gesundheits-Nachrichten (Health News). In his classic work, "The Nature Doctor", which appeared in 1952, he wrote at length about the health building properties of "cheese water". Indeed, had it not been for Dr. Vogel, few of us would know exactly what whey is in the 21st century.

The Valuable Ingredients Of Whey

When you make sugar from sugar cane, you are left with molasses, an incredible healthy food which is packed full of iron and minerals. Refined white sugar is useless from a nutritional perspective; it is an empty and refined carbohydrate. Molasses is very under rated nutritionally, a bit like whey.

When you make cheese you are left with liquid whey, likewise, an incredibly healthy liquid that has many major health benefits. It's not that milk is empty by any means, but milk is best consumed in its raw state from the cow, just like sugar cane juice is best consumed raw. That way you are getting from nature exactly what it intended, a food packed full of nutrition and enzymes. The whey is such an important health food that I am amazed at how few people actually really understand the true value, particularly those with yeast related health problems.

In order to obtain cheese from milk, the cheese maker must ensure that the solid and the liquid components of milk separate. For this to happen, the milk needs to be curdled by means of rennin and lactic acid bacteria making it thick. This solid component consists mainly of milk protein and milk fat is then made into cheese.

The left over liquid is whey, a fluid which still contains some of milk's very valuable ingredients and has very few of the calories. The whey products like Molkosan are then fermented with lactic acid with selected bacteria cultures and, in addition, is enriched with additional lactic acids, a physiologically valuable substance which contributes considerably to Molkosan's beneficial effect because the body can take it up directly.

The anti-fungal activity of whey is due to its acidity and buffering and alkalizing capability. It is able to re-establish the normal balance of beneficial bacteria in the digestive tract. This powerful antifungal activity can be used most successfully when applied topically against vaginal thrush, athlete's foot and ringworm. You will find that fat free and protein free whey has an abundance of excellent effects on your health and that regular consumption will influence your digestive tract and the immune system in a very positive way.

A healthy intestinal flora is not just a prerequisite for the healthy functioning of the body's naturally occurring defenses, but is also fundamental to your overall health and wellbeing. I'll talk more about how to take whey and use it externally when you have a yeast infection in subsequent chapters.

Raw, Organic Unpasteurized Apple Cider Vinegar

Before you declare that all vinegar is out of the question if you have a yeast infection, I want to make an important distinction right here and now, if you can manage to get hold of a bottle of unfiltered, raw, organic apple cider vinegar you will find it of significant help in your quest to eradicate a yeast infection from your body. As I have mentioned earlier, most supermarket bought vinegar products have been distilled, filtered and pasteurized, in other words they are "dead" and contain no natural enzymes because all that processing kills off any goodness. You simply cannot compare a dead and devitalized grocery bought item to a natural product!

I have been recommending raw and natural apple cider vinegar for over 25 years for yeast infections after reading Paul Bragg's book on the topic over thirty years ago. Paul Bragg was one of America's leading health gurus who in fact opened up America's first health-food store. Apple cider vinegar is one of those products that you can use both externally and internally with confidence, but do discontinue if it causes you any discomfort or burning. Before you stop using it however, try to dilute it because you may have taken it in too strong a dose to begin with, like many healthy foods, you may need to go low and go slow before you increase the dose.

Here are four uses for using raw, unfiltered and organic apple cider vinegar when it comes to a yeast infection:

Apple Cider Vinegar As A Wash For Athlete's Foot
Add 3 to 4 tablespoons of organic, raw and unfiltered apple cider vinegar in a bucket containing about 2 liters (2 quarts) of tepid to warm water. Soak the affected foot for at least twenty minutes, allow to air dry and use clean cotton socks. I'd recommend that you do this each evening for about two weeks.

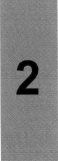

Apple Cider Vinegar As A Drink
Add anywhere from 1 to 3 teaspoons of apple cider vinegar to a glass of tepid water. Good to sip during or between meals. Apple cider vinegar is a good alkalizer of the digestive tract and is a perfect daily drink throughout the Candida Crusher Program. Some folk claim that apple cider vinegar kills a yeast infection, but this is not my experience. It helps to restore digestive harmony by alkalizing the system and it also helps to stimulate the production of digestive enzymes in the stomach, pancreas and small intestine. This is perfect for those undergoing a diet change that needs more digestive power.

Apple Cider Vinegar As A Douche

Add anywhere from 1 to 3 tablespoons of apple cider vinegar to 1 to 2 litres of tepid water. For an even better effect add ½ teaspoon of water-soluble tea tree oil. Use this cleansing recipe whenever you have a vaginal yeast infection as it will soothe any itches and reduce any irritating discharge. Use as required, more on some days and less on others. See chapter 5 for more complete information

Apple Cider Vinegar In The Bath

Draw enough water to have a bath and ensure the water is the right temperature; you don't want it too hot. Add 1 to 2 cups of apple cider vinegar and again, if you have a stubborn yeast infection or a particularly irritating one (whether it is jock itch or a vaginal yeast infection) you may want to add at least 1 -2 teaspoons of water soluble tea tree oil to a bath. Do experiment with dosages when it comes to the apple cider vinegar and tea tree oil, the dosages I recommend are suggested dosages only. I tend to recommend higher dosages generally, because I believe that by doing so you will get superior results. Ensure that you dry yourself very well after a bath and be sure to always use 100% cotton under garments.

Fermented Soy Products

Before I get started explaining more about this group, there is one myth I'd like to discuss. Is soy good or bad, should I avoid soy entirely because many websites tell me so? NO, you don't have to avoid soy. Before you decide that soy is a poison like many today claim it to be, I'd like you to do your own research and read the "for and against" arguments. I've never been a fan of soya milk; I just don't like the taste, but do enjoy organic tofu and the fermented soy products, namely tempeh and miso.

I find it most interesting that just about everybody who attacks soy does not seem to have a problem with the fermented soy products, even though they contain significant amount of soy isoflavones just like soy milk and tofu. Think about it logically for one moment, how can soy ferments be 100 percent devoid of isoflavones, genestein or in fact any other component that is present in soya milk or tofu?

Parrot Talk

I just love African Grey parrots, they are highly intelligent birds and many are good talkers. These clever birds listen with great care and then copy you word for word, verbatim, without even thinking about what you have just said. The next time they see somebody, they will repeat what they heard you say, and after awhile, even the person who hears the parrot speak will repeat what the parrot said to somebody else.

Many people I know are just are like parrots, they just keep on repeating what they have heard from others, word for word, without even thinking or researching for themselves if what they have been told makes any real sense. Some health-care professionals are guilty of this, and many tell their patients to avoid soy because of these kinds of reasons they have been told:

- Soy weakens your immune system

- Tofu wrecks your brain

- Soy turns boys into homosexuals

- Soy may cause cancer and brain damage

- High soy diet during pregnancy and nursing may cause developmental changes in children

- Soy can cause severe allergic reactions

- Soy supplements fail to help menopause symptoms

- Pregnant women should not eat soy products

- Soy can lead to kidney stones

- Soy baby formula linked to behavioural problems

- Soy formula exposes infants to high hormone levels

Anti-Soy Campaigns And Rodent Research

Soy has been trashed in the media for some time now, and I believe one of the prime reasons why this talk originally started is because soya milk sales compete head on with cow's milk sales. There was a huge interest in commercial soya milk in the eighties and especially the nineties, just about the time when all the evidence came out about how soy could poison you, cause various cancers, shrink your brain and even turn your son into a homosexual by shrinking his gonads. But, notice how there was never any mention of the bad effects of any of the fermented products, just soya milk? That's because the fermented soy products don't compete in the market place with any other foods. Soy sales in the 1980's in USA were 300 million dollars annually, and in 2008 they were 4.2 billion, money that is not being spent buying dairy or other competitive foods. Smear campaigns and dirty marketing work well, they helped margarine sales kill butter sales in the 50's and 60's, and many have woken up to this myth only recently.

I wonder whether the biased soy studies have been funded by the National Meat Institute or the National Dairy Board, the soy research I have seen appears to be a bit like university research being funded by pharmaceutical interests. Most soy studies look at rat or mice studies for a few weeks or a month or two duration, and not actual human research of populations who have been consuming soy for over two thousand years.

The people with the longest lifespan on earth currently happen to live in Okinawa, Japan, and they consume an average of 60 to 120 grams of soy protein daily. Okinawans have up to 80 percent less cancer and heart disease than Westerners. Chinese people eat on average 30 – 50 grams of soy protein daily, and both in Japan and China, where the highest soy consumption appears to be have no fertility issues. (Wilcox et al, 2004) I think I'd rather believe a living and breathing human model when it comes to studies, and not some biased rat or mouse study, these are flawed studies based on an entirely different species with a vested interest.

Soy is bad for my thyroid you will have been told. In Asian countries where soy consumption is between 50 to 100 times higher than in the Western world, there is certainly no high occurrence of hypothyroidism, and a big reason why is because these enlightened people eat seaweed, naturally high in iodine. Women living in the Western world eat no sea vegetables and have a forty percent chance of hypothyroidism. They eat foods depleted in essential minerals and a high-stress lifestyle, they are often lacking in the thyroid essential minerals such as zinc, iodine, selenium, manganese and more. The bottom line is, if you eat soy products then be sure to also include some sea vegetables in your diet, because research has uncovered that those who do eat soy regularly eat sea vegetables as well, interesting stuff but common sense, and it just goes to show that you need to take things in context.

Based on looking at both sides of the argument for several years, I do believe that the majority of adults can enjoy the taste and nutritional benefits of a wide variety of soy based foods, including tofu, tempeh, soy sauce and natto without placing their health at risk. I'm not talking about foods containing concentrated soy isolates or GM soy products, but whole organic and natural soy foods; the way nature intended them to be and the way they have been consumed traditionally for thousands of years. There certainly is sufficient evidence when it comes to infants and soy-isolate concentrated foods, but the same applies to giving infants whey-concentrated foods when they are only a few months of age as well.

Breast-feed is always the best-feed and anything else is second best, regardless whether it is soy, cow or goat's milk, and goat's milk being probably the best out of the three in my experience.

There is also sufficient evidence to suggest that soy may be a major issue for those with liver disease, major autoimmune dysfunction and intestinal inflammatory conditions such as Crohn's disease or colitis. But there is also ample evidence to suggest that cow's milk and many other such contentious foods are equally suspect in these individuals. I recommend that you consult with your health-care professional if you can relate to one of these conditions and want to make dietary changes.

Soy Is A Personal Choice – Take The Middle Path

Personally, I have been eating soy products for over 30 years, have four children and can assure you, my testicles have not shrunk, I have not developed breasts, nor am I homosexual and my brain has certainly not been wrecked. Eating soy is a personal choice, and it is up to you to decide if soy products are right for you. Before you condemn soy, I'd like you to become a lot more informed and to read for and against arguments.

Don't just automatically assume that eating soy will make you sick or increase your risk of cancer. You were probably using a mobile phone yesterday, and that is going to be potentially more of a health risk than many foods you will ever eat, and no doubt as phone charges drop over time you will be using it more prolonged, increasing your risk even further. Everything in life carries a risk, but believe me on this one - the fear of living and of eating specific foods because of what the may potentially do to your health will be found to be considerably more damaging to your health than the very food itself.

Every time you drive your car the risk of serious injury and death is always a possibility. And then you say: "No soy for me, it may harm my health". I've long worked out that there are as many nutritional fanatics as there are religious and medical ones, and some will defend their view almost to the point of death it seems. Maybe you would consider my own personal balanced approach, take the middle path and include in your diet a wide variety of foods I have outlined in this chapter, including vegetables, meats, eggs, chicken, fish, alkaline grains, nuts and seeds, soy products, sea vegetables as well as the fermented and cultured foods. How can you go wrong with this approach?

Tempeh

I can still remember when I first experienced tempeh, I was in my twenties and tried a tempeh burger at a vegetarian restaurant and was blown away by the unique flavour. Have you ever tried tempeh? It is made from soaked and then partially cooked soy beans to which a fermentation starter containing spores of the fungus Rhizopus oligosporus have been added.

This mixture is then spread out in a thin layer and allowed to ferment for a day or so and temperatures of around 30°C (86°F). In the best tempeh of the highest quality, you will find that the beans are knitted together by a fine white mat of the fungus.

Lower temperatures may result in a darker tempeh that does not affect the quality or the taste. Tempeh originated in Indonesia, and they consider it a good food once it has fermented for several days. The best ways to describe the taste of tempeh is meaty, nutty and complex. I eat tempeh regularly and sometimes find that it tastes just like hamburger meat. This is the closest thing to meat you can get in a vegetarian sense, and if you are a devout meat eater and want to move away from animal proteins than tempeh is for you. Over the years I have seen several vegetarians who gave up eating meat entirely only after discovering tempeh.

Tempeh is an unusual food that is non-meat yet high in protein and beneficial bacteria that can even produce vitamin B12. During the fermentation process, the phytic acid content of soy is reduced which allows your body to readily absorb more minerals. The rhizopus fungal culture helps to break the carbohydrate content down, especially the oligosaccharides that are associated with the production of bloating and gas and can even produce indigestion. I've noticed that those who eat tempeh once or twice a week appear to have a better digestive and bowel function than those who don't. Can you imagine for one minute if you ate tempeh regularly, as well as kefir, sauerkraut and yogurt? Your yeast infection would find it very hard to exist indeed in such a healthy digestive environment.

Tempeh In The Kitchen

What do you do with tempeh, how do you cook with it? Treat tempeh like you would a piece of chicken or beef steak, you can fry it, roast it, cut it into pieces and stir-fry it, tenderize it a little, cook it and then make a burger with it along with all your regular favorite toppings of lettuce, grated beetroot and carrot, tomato, etc. You can use tempeh in soups, stews, casseroles, salads, and sandwiches or just cook it and eat it alone. You can use it in tacos and burritos, in chili, or any one of a thousand other ways. It freezes well and you can buy it from your local health-food store either fresh or frozen. The uses of tempeh are only limited by your imagination, but just think of it as a kind of meat and then you will probably have several idea of what to do with tempeh until you get used to this most versatile, delicious and nutritious food.

Natto

Natto is not unlike tempeh, but it originated in japan and not Indonesia. In Japan, natto is popular as a breakfast food and is made from soybeans which have been fermented with bacillus subtilis.

It is usually eaten with rice and has a quite strong and characteristic flavour, and to be honest it is not for me, but you may find it OK and perfectly acceptable.

Natto has a sticky and stringy texture that some find unappealing, but you should try it at least once or twice before you make up your own mind though. Natto has many potential health benefits indeed backed by plenty of medical research. It contains an enzyme known as nattokinase that helps to prevent blood clots which may assist in the reduction of strokes, heart attacks and pulmonary embolism. Natto also contains large amounts of vitamin K_2, which assists in bone formation and the prevention of osteoporosis. Natto is the perfect food for those who have a history of blood clots or who have had a stroke in the past. Nattokinase is superior to warfarin, yet without the side effects.

Natto In The Kitchen

Natto is generally available in packs of 50 to 100 grams. The most popular way to eat natto is to place the natto in a small bowl and to stir it well, do not mash it. Stirring for a minute with chopsticks is sufficient, then add some soy sauce and Japanese mustard. Natto tastes better with the addition of finely chopped spring onions placed onto a small amount of steamed rice. Natto can also be served with miso soup or as a side dish along with some cooked wakame and steamed rice. I found many different recipes online and so can you.

Miso

Miso is another form of fermented soybean, it is a thick paste-like substance that is brownish in color and tastes very salty and tangy. Miso is one of my favorites and I enjoy miso soup quite regularly. Miso is high in protein and very rich in minerals and vitamins and the darker the paste is in color the stronger the taste will be. Miso is made by the fermentation of soybeans and aspergillus oryzae and the most common varieties are made with soy, although miso can also be made also with rice or barley.

Miso is readily available from many health-food shops and will keep for months in your refrigerator if stored well. Miso is very different from tempeh or natto in that there are literally countless varieties available. The colors range from almost white to black, and the flavors have been described as sweet, salty, fruity, earthy and savory.

Miso contains many different flavonoids and isoflavones, including daidzein, genistein, malonylgenistin and malonyldaidzin which are seen as bad for our health, yet many who condemn soy actually promote miso, a little strange?

In my opinion, miso is one of the best of the fermented foods for the candida patient. Microorganisms such as aspergillus that are used in the fermentation process help to pre-digest miso, which in turn allows your digestive system to easily digest and absorb the nutrition from this super nutritious food. Many forms of miso actually contain copious quantities of beneficial bacteria themselves, including various species of lactobacillus. Miso is one of the best of the fermented foods to consume daily because it powerfully supports digestive health, tastes great and is easy to obtain. Miso has many other health benefits, too numerous to mention, including cardiovascular and immune boosting properties.

Miso In The Kitchen

Just like tempeh, there are many ways you can enjoy miso. Here are a few quick suggestions on ways how you can incorporate this delicious fermented soybean paste into your diet.

- Miso soup is very quick and easy to prepare, just warm some water to which you have added miso paste and add a few shiitake mushrooms, some organic tofu, carrots, and a little daikon radish.

- Make a salad dressing by mixing a little miso paste with fresh garlic, sesame or olive oil, fresh ginger and a few drops of lime juice.

- Enjoy a hot miso soup drink instead of a coffee or cup of tea.

- Try a miso sandwich, just spread a little miso paste onto a piece of sourdough bread and add avocado or tahini.

- Use miso as a marinade along with an oil of choice and some fresh garlic, you can use this marinade with chicken, fish or meats of many different kinds.

Sourdough Baking

One of the main foods my patients always tend to complain about when they start on the anti-candida diet is that I recommend they stop all commercially baked breads.

I recommend this because this commercially made food is full of yeast and sugar, two of the main things you will want to avoid when you are serious about getting rid of a yeast infection. Some people say that you must avoid all grains entirely, including wheat, oats, barley any rye if you want to eradicate a yeast infection. I have found this to be not to be the case, and have helped many people eradicate their yeast infection by recommending that they stay on grains otherwise they will soon lose interest in the diet, and besides many experience fatigue and weight loss when they stop all grains, which can be quite dramatic and disconcerting for some.

There is no need to avoid wheat and other grains, unless you are a celiac, and have been positively diagnosed by way of a biopsy (not self diagnosed please), or allergic to gluten, which has found to be strongly positive with a IgG/IgE food allergy blood test.

Have you ever considered sugar and yeast free sour dough bread? Try it; it is very nice and rich in lactic acid that favors the development of lactobacillus acidophilus in your digestive system. Sourdough baking with lactic acid fermentation is much healthier than yeast baking, and is the best way to consume bread if you have a yeast infection by far. This form of healthy baking makes many minerals and inositol much more readily available than will be found in various commercially prepared breads. You can use the unheated sourdough ferment as a source of live food that is very rich in probiotics.

Many people are concerned that bread like sourdough which does contain natural and wild yeasts, will encourage their yeast infection. I have not found this to be the case with patients in my clinic, and providing a person does not have an issue with wheat or gluten, they are OK to eat sourdough bread. By being able to consume healthy and tasty sourdough bread you have made yourself, you will not be depriving yourself of that nice piece of bread for breakfast or lunch, just be sure not to put jam or honey on it, avocado or hard cheese are better options.

The Starter

The secret to making a good loaf of sourdough lies in a concoction known as the starter. Starter begins as a mixture of water and flour and is typically kept in a loosely covered container at room temperature. After several days of feedings with additional flour and water, the mixture becomes home to thriving populations of lactic acid bacteria and wild yeast, don't worry, we are not talking about candida albicans yeast here.

The process of making the starter by relying on wild yeasts and bacteria is like stepping back in time; this is how all bread once used to be made. Encouraging a mixture of flour and water turn into a living ecosystem at room temperature cultivates a greater appreciation for the microbes on which we rely so heavily for the production of fermented foods.

The type of beneficial yeasts that settles down in the starter may be *Saccharomyces diarensis and Saccharomyces exiguus,* while the bacterial organism is usually a strain of lactobacillus. Did you know that there are at least 10 different strains of lactobacillus bacteria that have been isolated from sourdough breads? Among the most commonly occurring are *Lactobacillus brevis, Lactobacillus plantarum,* and *Lactobacillus sanfranciscensis,* named for San Francisco sourdough bread, from which it was isolated in 1969.

Normally you save a cup of the sourdough starter for the next batch. When doing this for the first time then use instead half a cup of acidophilus yogurt or several acidophilus-bifido capsules or any other suitable source of acidophilus. You can also use some of the lactic acid rich water that you will find on top of natural, unsweetened yogurt. A good product to try also is Molkosan.

Honey or molasses are added as food for the bacteria to be converted to lactic acid, don't worry, the sugars will be consumed by the bacteria and won't be consumed by you and become a food source for candida.

If you are worried about gluten, try using buckwheat flour to make the bread stick together. There are many different recipes you can find online for sourdough bread, for example you may want to replace part of the rice flour with another non-gluten flour, as for instance coconut, lentil or pea flour, which you can make yourself by grinding dried coconut or seeds in a coffee grinder and putting it through a fine sieve. Just add more water as required for mixing.

Health Tip – Use A Yogurt Maker

I have experimented and found that a yoghurt maker is a brilliant way to keep the starter warm; this will accelerate the culture and is a very good method for making sourdough and keeping the starter healthy in wintertime. When the mixture becomes frothy or has doubled in volume, it is ready to use.

Remember, sourdough is a live fermented food and tastes a little sour like yogurt. You may use it with any good spreads (but no jam, marmalade, honey, etc.!!) and in addition to salads and other meals just like you would any bread. Sourdough is very nice when dipped in olive oil, try it, you may like it. Add a little garlic as well for some anti-fungal activity.

Basic White Sourdough Bread Recipe

This basic sourdough bread recipe will produce approximately 2 to 2.2 kilograms of dough which will be more than enough dough for 2 normal sized bread tins to be about half filled. What you will find is that because sourdough bread lacks brewer's yeast, it won't rise as much as commercial bread. This dough will rise very nicely nevertheless when baked and you will find that it should fill the tin.

Ingredients

- Starter - about 300 g ripe sourdough starter which is about 2 cups full, though I usually don't use this as a measurement, because starter varies a great deal in volume.

- White Organic Unbleached Flour - (or regular white flour), Use about 1.2 kg white flour. As a rule of thumb, the more wholemeal the flour, the more water it will hold, so allow for this when adding the water when using wholemeal flours.

- Water - about 600 ml of water (the temperature of the water needs to be luke warm in winter, but for the rest of the year room temperature will do).

- Salt – sea salt. Use about 25 grams.

Mixing In Flour

Use a large stainless steel or glass bowl to mix the flour and starter. Place the flour in the bowl; make a small well in the middle of the flour. Then pour in the water, starting initially with half the water and then quickly adding the rest. I always keep a little water for later, just in case the dough feels too tough. Now place all the starter in the water in the well.

Mixing The Dough And Starter

Mix the ingredients (I use one hand and keep the other clean), at this stage you do not want to knead, just mix it rather roughly together. Don't be too concerned about lumps. You will soon discover that by keeping one hand clean you can answer the phone and clean up much more easily afterwards. You will also soon learn that your kitchen will end up quite a mess if you use two hands to mix the starter! Add water as required if the dough feels too stiff or tough. Add the water with the clean hand; see how the vessel stays clean? If you mix with both hands you will soon notice just how messy the kitchen becomes.

The Delayed Method

I discovered this by reading many recipes online and trying out several, this method works really well and is the one you should try first, not after many experiments and failed attempts like me. Please ensure that you mix the flour, water and starter sufficiently so that the flour has absorbed all the water. This is very important before you place the bowl to rest the mixture after covering the bowl for an hour.

The Kneading Of The Dough

After you have let this mixture rest for an hour, sprinkle the sea salt over the mixture. Knead the dough well and in no time at all you will end up with nice smooth and soft dough. Once the dough becomes less sticky, use the other hand as well because you will find that the dough does not tend to stick to your hand.

Proofing The Dough

After this kneading, leave the ball of dough rest in the bowl for between 6 to 8 hours. It all depends on the temperature, and in winter I may place the covered bowl on the mantelpiece not too close to the fire. In summer I just leave it on the kitchen bench. You will soon get a feel for how long to leave the dough rise based on the temperatures in your house and what season it is. It can take up to twelve hours if the temperature is quite low. You want the dough to basically double in size during this first proving, but it may not be achievable due to a poor starter culture or poor temperature.

Proofing for the second time: Once the dough is ready, take it out of the bowl and cut it into two halves. Now take each piece of dough and gently make a round shape of it, placing the seam at the bottom of the loaf. Now place these unbaked loaves in a warm and cozy place so they can recover their shape once more. Again, temperature permitting, this may take only a half an hour but in winter it could be an hour.

Form The Loaves

After the second proofing, take the dough out and place it on a bench (lightly floured). Keep the seam on the bottom and gently roll the dough into a longish cylinder. Let them rest (covered) again for a few minutes to recover. Now prepare your bread baking tins.

Ready For The Bread Tins

Very gently spray or brush a little warm water onto the surfaces of the dough that you have formed into cylinders. Now lightly dust the surface (place flour in a sieve) and make a few diagonal slashes in the top of the dough, reasonably deep. Carefully pick up these dusted and slashed loaves (from underneath!) and place them into the oiled or buttered tins. It is best that the dough occupies about three quarters of the tin; this will allow them to rice nicely.

Baking Your Sourdough Bread

Finally ready to bake. Once the loaves have risen again, turn on the oven to 180 degrees Celsius. If you oven is efficiently fan-forced, you may want to reduce the temperature to 160 degrees Celsius. Your sourdough bread should bake in about an hour, maybe less, so keep a close eye on the oven. Here's a trick – the longer you bake the break, the thicker the crust will become. Don't go to far from the kitchen like I did once, or you may end up literally baking a brick like I did a few times.

Removing Bread From Tin

A hollow sound on the loaf will indicate whether it has successfully baked. When cooked, remove the bread from the tin and place it promptly in a bread rack to cool. How do you know if the bread isn't cooked properly? It will sound with a dull thud, and this is something only experience will tell you. A bit like buying a nice watermelon, a good one will sound hollow and bad one will sound hard or dull.

If the loaf sounds hard or dull, leave it in the oven which has been turned off for a further ten minutes or so.

Sourdough Recipe #2

- 2 cups of brown rice flour

- 1 cup of buckwheat flour

- 1 cup of liquid sourdough starter

- 2/3 cup of warm water

- 1 or 2 tsp.
  of honey or molasses

Cultured Vegetables

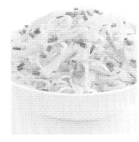 Cultured vegetables are raw vegetables that are allowed to ferment for about a week at room temperature in order for the beneficial lactobacilli bacteria to grow and are then refrigerated until eaten. Vegetables such as cabbage, carrots, beetroot and even garlic can be fermented into delicious cultured foods that maintain their lactobacillus count for as long as 6 months after preparation. Vegetables can be cultured with whey or Celtic sea salt, and taste like pickles or sauerkraut.

Some of the health benefits associated with cultured vegetables include reducing symptoms of conditions such as colic, peptic ulcers, food allergies, constipation and many other digestive tract disorders. Give your baby a bit of the juice to build up their beneficial digestive bacteria.

Sauerkraut

Ingredients

One 5 to 8 kilogram green cabbage (10 - 16 lbs.)

Salt (½ to ¾ teaspoon per 500gr of cabbage. (one pound)

1 tablespoon juniper berries, they are optional but give a great taste.

2 teaspoons cumin seeds, also optional but give a great taste.

2 bay leaves (optional)

Salt water to cover (1 tablespoon salt per quart of water)

Method

There are as many ways to make sauerkraut as there are sauerkraut recipes, but here's how I do it. Try to get a ceramic crock or you can even use a small wooden barrel. I use a round wooden lid (covered with a clean damp cloth) that sits inside the pot and rests on top of the cabbage. This lid is weighed down with a few heavy (clean) stones. I obtained a couple of clean stones from a riverbed nearby and so can you.

- Shred the cabbage finely with a serrated bread knife into a large bowl; add salt and optional spices. Gradually add mixture to a large container, crushing to release juices, I use a round untreated wooden stick about two inches wide. Place the wooden lid on top of the crushed cabbage then add the weighting stones and push down firmly.

- Top off
with salty water to cover stones by 1 inch, you will get a better result if you use chlorine and fluoride free water. Ferment 4 to 6 weeks at a reasonably warm temperature. One way to achieve the warm temperature is to place the container in your hot water cupboard.

- I check each week and clean any ferment from the wooden lid, you will soon know when it is ready and with experience will get to know the exact taste and smell which indicate it is ready to place in clean glass mason jars in your fridge. Sauerkraut tastes great cold or warm.

Kim Chi

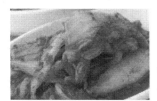

Kim chi is sometimes spelled "kim chee", but I prefer the "chi" spelling because that is the spelling of the oriental word *chi* (*gi*, *ki*) that means "natural energy" or "vital force". Of the countless varieties of kim chi that are made in Korea, by far the most common version is the one made with Chinese (wong bok) cabbage.

Just like sauerkraut, kim chi that is made with cabbage is loaded with indole-3-carbinol (I3C), a compound that is well recognized as a powerful cancer-fighting compound. Numerous studies indicate that I3C can offer protection against many different types of cancer and may even stop the growth of existing tumors.

I learned about kim chi when I was a student and completed a Cooking For Health course many years ago at naturopathic college. A great thing about this dish, like all fermented foods is that it keeps for many weeks in your refrigerator, yet still tastes fresh.
The garlic and vinegar are natural preservatives that keep the raw vegetables and fruits tasting great for a long time. If you have one of those keep warm crock or hotpots in your kitchen, then a wholesome snack or even a full meal is not far away. Kim chi is like sauerkraut, it is not only a health food, it can be regarded as a convenience food, and both of these foods can be served cold, warm or hot. An important point to bear in mind is that kim chi must be fermented properly.

Cabbage And Onions

In my opinion, two of the best ingredients to ferment for promoting beneficial bacteria in your digestive system and inhibiting the unfriendly bacteria are cabbage and onions. There is no doubt; fermented cabbage is the absolute best. Once the cabbage soaked in vinegar has had a chance to age, only a day or two in the refrigerator or a few hours at room temperature, the cabbage ferments and produces the nutrients that the beneficial lacto-bacteria thrive on.

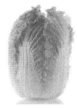 When you make **kim chi**, be sure to use Chinese cabbage, which is one of the most common Asian vegetables found in Australia, New Zealand and probably in your country, and is also known as Peking cabbage, Napa cabbage, or wong bok. It has an elongated head with tightly packed crinkly pale green leaves. Unlike the strong-flavored waxy leaves on round heads of cabbage, these are thin, crisp and delicately mild.

 When you make **sauerkraut**, be sure to use the normal round green cabbage. It has a stronger and sharper taste and suits sauerkraut better. This cabbage is a bit harder to slice because the leaves are more densely packed so be sure to use a sharp serrated knife.

Health Tip:

Raw Cabbage Cures Ulcers

I once placed a male patient with advanced digestive ulcers on a diet rich in kim chi, sauerkraut, plain steamed vegetables, fish and rice. In less than 12 weeks, the ulcers that had resisted years of medical treatment were completely healed; I know this to be true because the patient had his cure confirmed by way of endoscopy. If you eat foods like sauerkraut and kim chi, you may well heal all manner of chronic digestive complaints that have been unresponsive to conventional drug treatments. What have you got to lose except your ulcer?

Kim Chi Recipe

To make healthy kim chi that still has lots of flavor and health-promoting compounds, start with a whole head of fresh wong bok cabbage. Don't worry about the addition of the fresh fruit here (apple and pear) as the sugars will be consumed and converted into beneficial (lactobacillus) bacteria, creating a lactic acid rich environment.

Ingredients:

- One wong bok cabbage - about 500gr (one pound)
- Sea salt
- Water
- Fine red chili flakes (Asian shop)
- 1 tablespoon minced fresh garlic
- 1 tablespoon minced fresh ginger
- 3-4 spring onions (scallions), sliced
- 2 tablespoons anchovy or fish sauce (optional)
- 1/2 brown onion
- 1/2 ripe apple
- 1/2 ripe pear

Directions:

1. Separate cabbage leaves and chop into bite-size pieces.

2. Dissolve a quarter cup of sea salt in a bowl of warm water, and then pour salt water over cabbage leaves. Give cabbage a gentle toss to distribute salt water. Allow salted cabbage to sit for at least four hours.

3. Give cabbage a good rinse to remove excess salt, and then transfer cabbage to a large bowl.

4. Combine a quarter cup of fine red chili flakes with warm water, stir gently with a spoon to create a red chili paste, and then transfer chili paste to cabbage.

5. Add minced garlic, minced ginger, spring onions (scallions), and fish sauce.

6. Blend brown onion, apple, and pear with one cup of water, then add this natural sweetener to the cabbage.

7. Give everything a thorough toss and good rubdown. You want to evenly distribute all ingredients, especially the red chili paste.

8. Transfer seasoned cabbage leaves into a large glass container (which you have cleaned previously with very hot water).

9. Be sure to use firm pressure with your hands to push down on cabbage leaves as they stack up inside the bottle.

10. Transfer any liquid that accumulated during the mixing process into the bottle as well - this liquid will become the kim chi brine. Some liquid will also come out of the cabbage leaves as you press down on them, as they are stacked in the bottle.

11. Be sure to leave about 50ml (2 inches) of room at the top of the bottle before capping it tightly with a lid. Allow bottle of kim chi to sit at room temperature for 24 hours.

12. Your kim chi is now ready to eat. Refrigerate and take out portions as needed. The refrigerated kim chi will continue to ferment slowly in the refrigerator over time. So long as you use clean utensils to take out small portions, it will keep for up to a month or even longer in your refrigerator.

Cultured Dairy Products

Fermented milks had been made since early times, when warm raw milk from cows, sheep, goats, and even camels or horses was naturally preserved by using common strains of Streptococcus and Lactobacillus bacteria. With the development of microbiological and nutritional sciences in the late 19th century, came the technology necessary to produce cultured dairy products on a much larger scale, on a commercial basis. These cultures were generally obtained by including a small portion (seeding) from the previous batch. These harmless lactic acid producers were effective in suppressing spoilage and pathogenic organisms, making it possible to preserve fresh milk for several days or weeks without refrigeration. Cultured products eventually became ethnic favorites and were introduced around the world as people migrated to different countries, for example Greek immigrants started to make yoghurt on a large scale when they migrated to Australia in the 1950's, after World War 2 particularly.

Central to the production of cultured milk is the initial fermentation process, which involves the partial conversion of lactose (milk sugar) into lactic acid. Lactic-acid producing Streptococcus and Lactobacillus bacteria accomplish lactose conversion. At temperatures of approximately 32° C (90° F), these bacteria reproduce very rapidly, perhaps doubling their population every 20 minutes. Many by-products that result from their metabolic processes assist in further ripening and flavoring of the cultured product. Subsequent or secondary fermentations can result in the production of other compounds, such as diacetyl (a flavor compound found in buttermilk) and alcohol (from yeasts in kefir), as well as butyric acid (which causes bitter or rancid flavors).

Cultured buttermilk, sour cream, and yogurt are among the most common fermented dairy products in the Western world. Other, lesser-known products include kefir, koumiss, acidophilus milk, and new yogurts containing bifido-bacteria.

Cultured dairy foods provide numerous potential health benefits to the human diet. These foods are excellent sources of calcium and protein. In addition, they may help to establish and maintain beneficial intestinal bacterial flora and reduce lactose intolerance.

Be sure to make yogurt from raw milk that is available much more freely these days than it was ten years ago. There are many health-food stores than have organic milk suppliers and you should be able to obtain this valuable food. While you can use plain supermarket commercial milk to make cultured dairy products, you are not getting the benefits obtained from milk straight from the cow, like the inclusion of enzymes, prebiotics, probiotics and healthy fats. All these will have been removed or destroyed due to the process of homogenization and pasteurization.

Yogurt

Why not just buy yogurt at the store? One of the most well known and most readily available probiotic foods, many varieties of store-bought yogurt are high in sugar and not very potent in probiotic content. Homemade yogurt is likely to contain much more beneficial bacteria and less sugar, preservatives and chemicals, plus it's easy and fun to prepare. Your own homemade yogurt will be a great source of calcium, protein, magnesium and other essential vitamins as well as beneficial digestive tract bacteria without unnecessary additives.

I would like to stress once again, yogurt is OK for most people with candida, but it depends on the quality of yogurt. Don't be afraid of yogurt, butter and occasionally cream. These dairy products can be tolerated by most who have a yeast infection and should be trialed before you simply dismiss them as being to allergenic. Don't touch dairy products if you know you are very sensitive to them, otherwise you should be OK. Don't believe a lot of information you read online with regards to dairy foods and candida. The stage 2 component of the Candida Crusher Program does include excluding cow's milk from your diet for two to three weeks, and the object of this is to help heal any underlying leaky gut, because cow's milk is potentially the most allergenic of all foods, more about this later.

A True Super Food

Yogurt is a true super food indeed; it is also known as sour milk and is the result of the fermentation of milk. Yogurt is very much a pro-biotic food and that means food that contains plenty of beneficial bacteria. Based on research, yogurt has many benefits for human health. The history of yogurt as healthy drink began when Dr. Elie Metchnikoff made a hypothesis. He found that there was a strong relationship between the longevity and habit of consuming fermented milk in Bulgaria's mountain society.

An Ancient Past

While it is unclear exactly is when and where yogurt was developed, fermented dairy products were probably consumed for thousands and thousands of years, ever since the beginning of the domestication of cows. One of the first records of yogurt consumption comes from the Middle East during the times of the Genghis Khan in the 13th century, whose armies were sustained by a food similar to yogurt. Yogurt and other fermented dairy products such as kefir have long been a staple in the diets of cultures of the Middle East, Asia, Russia and Eastern European countries, such as Bulgaria. Yet, the recognition of yogurt's special health benefits did not become apparent in Western Europe and North America until the 20th century, as a result of extensive research done by Dr. Elie Metchnikoff.

Dr. Metchnikoff conducted research based on many years of work on the health benefits of lactic acid-producing bacteria and postulated that the longevity of peoples of certain cultures, such as the Bulgarians, was related to their high consumption of yogurt and fermented dairy products.

Why Is Yogurt So Good?

The nutrient rich content found in yogurt is the reason why we need to consume yogurt. Yogurt contains B complex vitamins and a higher percentage of vitamins A + D than milk. Yogurt is a natural and powerful antibiotic, helps to prevent cancer and has been found beneficial in colds and upper respiratory complaints, high cholesterol levels, constipation and diarrhea, irritable bowel syndrome, arthritis, diverticulitis, diarrhea, gallstones, osteoporosis, kidney disorders, many cancers of the digestive tract, thrush, hepatitis and various skin complaints.

Like the milk it is made from, yogurt is a very good source of calcium, phosphorus, and protein. During the fermentation, there is a synthesis process of vitamin B complex, especially thiamine (vitamin B1) and riboflavin (vitamin B2), and also amino acids. Yogurt is not only a good source of protein, it is also an excellent source of calcium, phosphorus, vitamin B2, B 5, B 12, iodine, zinc, potassium, and molybdenum. These several nutrients alone surely qualify yogurt as a super food. But probably the most important aspect of this food is the inclusion of live bacteria.

Unlike milk, real yogurt also contains pro-biotics, the good bacteria your digestive system needs to process and benefit from all the other things you eat. The most common pro-biotic in yogurt is lactic acid bacteria including Lactobacillus bulgaricus, Streptococcus themophilus, and Lactobacillus casei.

Selecting And Storing Yogurt

Here is an important point you may not of though about when buying yogurt. Did you know that some manufacturers actually pasteurize their product? Some do and some don't, and what you need to look for are products that feature "live active cultures" or "living cultures" on their labels. This is especially important if you want to not only enjoy yogurt as a tasty food, but to gain the pro-biotic benefits as well. The problem with pasteurization is that it basically kills off the beneficial lactic acid and the good bacteria, rendering yogurt useless in terms of its ability to be a true super food.

I always recommend people to avoid those small containers of yogurt that contain artificial sweeteners like aspartame, as well as colors and many additives. Avoid those fruity yogurts that taste very sweet because they often are laden with fake sugars. And of course you always check the expiry dates on the side of the yogurt container to make sure that they are still fresh, don't you?

One major American website with lots of candida information online is promoting aspartame containing dairy products as being OK to consume. When I read this kind of information, I tend to take the rest of their information with a grain of salt. Anybody who promotes aspartame as being OK is clearly ignorant, there is enough information about this toxic pseudo sugar available online, so if you must consume aspartame and truly believe that it is totally harmless, you do so at your own risk and are crazy in my opinion. A good tip is to look out for yogurt made from organic milk. Organic dairy products are becoming more widely available in an array of sizes, flavors and varieties. Make sure you store your yogurt in the refrigerator in its original container. If unopened, it will stay fresh for about one week past the expiration date.

But I Am Allergic To Milk.
Does This Mean I Am Allergic To Yogurt?

There is no doubt about it, cow's milk is probably the most allergenic all foods I have come across in my clinic. And although allergic reactions can occur to virtually any food, research studies on food allergy consistently report more problems with certain foods such as cow's milk over all other foods.

Stage 2 of the Candida Crusher Diet involves the low-allergy diet, and cow's milk is listed prominently on my Hypo-Allergenic Diet patient handout.

Note that on this diet you will see various foods in the right hand column in bold, these are the key allergy foods in my experience. And dairy products as you will note are all in bold, including yogurt. Don't worry, many with a yeast infection can tolerate yogurt as part of their diet.

It is important to realize that the frequency of food allergy problems can vary widely from country to country and can change significantly along with changes in the food supply or with other manufacturing practices. For example, in several part of the world such as North and South America you will find corn and maize allergies to be more common than other parts of the world. In Canada, Japan, and Israel, sesame seed allergy has risen to a level of major concern over the past several years, and in many Western countries countless folk now have gluten allergies.

But why would this be so? This can be easily explained due to the fact that people in these countries tend to eat more of these foods. Can you remember a statement I made earlier, that it is usually the foods you eat the most are likely to be the ones that can cause the most problems? These potentially allergenic foods do not need to be eaten in their absolute pure, isolated form in order to trigger an immune mediated reaction. For example, yogurt made from cow's milk is also a common allergenic food, even though the cow's milk has been processed and fermented in order to make the yogurt. Ice cream made from cow's milk would be an equally good example, and so is cream.

In most cases, when I recommend a temporary cessation of cow's milk I generally mean cow's yogurt as well. You can try sheep's cheese or goat's cheese like Feta, however.

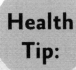

Health Tip:

Eat Butter, It Contains Butyric Acid

Butter will be found to be far less problematic than any other dairy product, as far as allergies are concerned. And because butter is high in fat and contains virtually no protein, it contains almost none of the main allergic component found in dairy product, beta casein. Butter is also rich in butyric acid, a most beneficial substance that is a food for the cells of the colon. Don't be afraid of eating a quality organic butter regularly if you have a yeast infection, it tastes great and is good for your health.

Yogurt is a rich source of not only beneficial (and yeast hating) bacteria; it is also a rich source of calcium.

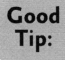

Good Tip:

Eat Yogurt

Are you worried about your calcium intake?

Many people are worried about their calcium intake and get concerned when I ask if they stop milk, a high source of calcium in the diet. Milk products encourage a yeast overgrowth due to their lactose (milk sugar) content, and this is why a natural yogurt is allowed, the beneficial bacteria feed on the lactose and create a soured product (not sweet) which has little to no lactose content.

14 Health Benefits Of Yogurt

1

Helping People With Lactose Intolerance.
Lactic acid bacteria can ferment lactose in milk into glucose and galactose, and stimulate the secretion of the enzyme lactase in the digestive tract. Those suffering from lactose intolerance can generally safely eat yogurt, even the 3-½% fat from the full-cream milk becomes defatted and soured and more easily digested. This is good information for those who are conscious of animal fat intake in the diet. However, you may suffer from casein intolerance. Be careful if you have dairy allergies, many people do, but you will soon discover this once you eat small amounts of yogurt daily. It's all about challenge and elimination.

2

Yogurt Has Anti-Diarrhea Properties And Improves Constipation.
Yogurt may prevent the activity and the growth of pathogenic bacteria that cause diarrhea. Lactobacillus bulgaricus (a bacterium that plays a role in the formation of yogurt) can produce bulgarican, a most effective antimicrobial to inhibit pathogenic organisms.

3

Yogurt Helps Inhibit The Growth Of Pathogenic (Bad) Bacteria.
Lactic acid can reduce or kill the bacterial pathogens (disease-causing bacteria) and suppress the production of potentially dangerous compounds, such as phenol, skatol, and H2S, produced by bacterial pathogens. Lactic acid-producing bacteria also produce certain kinds of natural antibiotic-like compounds that can inhibit the growth of pathogenic bacteria. Therefore, the yogurt has a value of treatment of stomach and intestinal injury.

4

Yogurt Can Confer Anti-Cancer Benefits.
Research on rats showed a doubling of cancer cells in mice that were fed with yogurt is more constrained than mice without the yogurt. The bacteria that involved in fermentation of milk may change pre-cancerous substances that are present in the digestive tract, thus the bacteria can inhibit the occurrence of cancer. Yogurt that contains live, or active cultures like L. casei may have cancer prevention benefits.

According to the National Centre for Complementary and Alternative Medicine (NCCAM), live cultures can reduce the risk of cancer recurrences. Probiotics are healthy bacteria that can significantly boost the immune system and promote digestive regularity and therefore can have a most beneficial effect in terms of helping to prevent cancer. The University of Michigan Health System's (UMHS) nutritional charts regarding calcium lists yogurt at the top of the lists, with a 1 cup serving containing 415 mg. The high calcium count of yogurt, like milk, may keep people from developing other forms of cancer as well as bladder cancer.

If you think that high-fat dairy products are not good for your health, you may want to think again. A study published in the *American Journal of Clinical Nutrition* has discovered that eating full-fat yogurt and other full-fat dairy

4

foods, such as whole milk, kefir, cheese, cream, sour cream and butter, may significantly reduce your risk for bowel cancer. Over 60,000 women aged 40-76 years were followed during an average of 14.8 years. Those who consumed at least 4 servings of high-fat dairy foods each day were found to have a 41% lower risk of bowel cancer compared to women eating less than one serving of high-fat dairy foods daily.

Although these foods are high in saturated fat, high fat dairy foods contain a number of potentially cancer-preventive factors such as conjugated linoleic acid (CLA), which has also been shown to be protective of heart and circulatory disease. We do know that research has confirmed that it is wise to limit your intake of saturated animal fat by cutting back on servings of high-fat red and processed meats in particular, but that enjoying full-fat versions of yogurt and other dairy products may actually be cancer and cardio-protective.

5

Yogurt Is Excellent For Your Digestive Tract.
Live yogurt has many beneficial effects on your digestive system. Lactic acid from the yogurt may stimulate the peristaltic movement in nearly all parts of the digestive tract. Stimulation of the peristaltic movements can maintain the body's health through improved digestion, absorption, feces disposal, and disposal of bad bacteria from the digestive tract. It is a well-known and scientifically established fact that pro-biotics in yogurt helps to restore the balance of bacteria and can eliminate the abdominal pain, gas or constipation.

6

Yogurt Is Protective Against Helicobacter Pylori
An interesting study in the *American Journal of Clinical Nutrition* found that Helicobacter pylori, the bacterium responsible for most ulcers, could be effectively inhibited by yogurt. Ingestion of yogurt containing Lactobacillus acidophilus and Bifidobacterium lactis significantly decreases activity of Helicobacter pylori after six weeks, according to the results of a placebo-controlled intervention study published in the September 2004 issue of the American Journal of Clinical Nutrition.

Consuming Yogurt Can Lower Blood Cholesterol Levels.
Do you have high cholesterol levels? Did you know that by adding a daily cup of yogurt with probiotic bacteria to your healthy way of eating is an easy way to improve your cholesterol profile? Yogurt contains factors that can inhibit the formation of LDL (bad) cholesterol so that cholesterol levels dropped and prevents clogging of atherosclerosis blood vessels that causing coronary heart disease.

7

Yogurt not only helps to lower your LDL level ("bad" cholesterol), it also assists in raising your HDL ("good" cholesterol) levels. Daily consumption of 100 g of a good pro-biotic yogurt, like my yogurt recipe teeming with health-promoting bacteria, has been shown to significantly improve the cholesterol profile in women volunteers. In this study, (Fabian E, *Annals of Nutrition & Metabolism*), one group of 17 women consumed 3 ounces (100 g) a day of pro-biotic yogurt, while a second group of 16 women were given 3 ounces of conventional yogurt (no probiotics) daily for 2 weeks. Then both groups were given 6 ounces (200 g) of the type of yogurt they had been consuming for 2 more weeks. The study ended with a final 2 weeks during which both groups of women ate no yogurt.

7

In the women consuming pro-biotic yogurt, not only did levels of LDL decrease significantly, but also their HDL substantially increased. Women consuming conventional yogurt also experienced a drop in LDL cholesterol, but not as significant as in the first group, and their HDL did not rise. This shows you that it is important to avoid those commercial yogurts and make your own yogurt or to buy a high quality organic yogurt, teeming with probiotics.

8

Yogurt Can Significantly Boost Your Immune Function.
Yogurt is an ancient wonder food, strongly antibacterial and anti-cancer. A cup or two of yogurt a day boosts immune functioning by stimulating production of gamma interferon. A study authored by Georges Halpern MD PhD, professor emeritus in the department of internal medicine at the University of California, discovered that people who 2 cups of yogurt a day for 4 months increased the level of gamma interferon, a protein that helps the white blood cells fight off disease. Gamma interferon is one of the best defenses your body has against viruses. In addition, yogurt stimulates activity of natural killer cells that attack viruses and tumors. A study published in the *Journal of Nutrition* has shown that Lactobacillus species found in cultured foods like yogurt and kefir, significantly improved the immune response including the ability to even fight off pneumonia.

9

Consuming Yogurt Can Increase Your Chances Of A Long Healthy Life
Research has consistently found that people with the highest life expectancies are often people who consume the lease amount of alcohol and highest levels of fermented and cultured foods such as yogurt and sauerkraut throughout their lives. The highest quality yogurt in your health food shop or supermarket contains a live bacterium that provides a host of health benefits, as previously mentioned. Yogurt that contains live bacterial cultures may help you to live longer, and may well fortify your immune system. Research studies have shown that increased yogurt consumption, particularly in immune-compromised people such as the elderly, may enhance the immune response, which would in turn increase resistance to immune-related diseases. Immune function declines with age, so eating a small amount of yogurt daily is a great way to ensure you keep your immune system topped up.

One study tracked a population of 162 very elderly people for a five year period, and it was discovered that the incidence of death for those subjects who ate yogurt and milk more than three times per week was 38% lower than the incidence of death those subjects who ate yogurt and other dairy foods less than once a week. You may be interested to know that those who consumed citrus, especially limes and lemons, twice a week and who had a low consumption of red meat were also associated with decreased incidence of premature death.

10

Eating Yogurt Reduces Chances Of Candida Yeast And Thrush Infections
Eating yogurt may help to prevent vaginal yeast infections. In one study, women who had frequent yeast infections ate 200 grams of yogurt daily for 6 months. Researchers reported that a 75% reduction in infections was seen in these women.

11

Yogurt Helps To Boost Bone Health Significantly

Yogurt and kefir are a lot more than just a calcium and health food rich in good bacteria, they also contain lactoferrin, an iron-binding protein that boosts the growth and activity of cells which boost bone production, the osteoblasts. Not only does lactoferrin increase osteoblast activity, it also reduces the formation of osteoclasts, and these bone cells help to increase bone turnover or bone loss. Lactoferrin has been shown to reduce osteoclast activity by an amazing 50-70%, thus helping to prevent or even reverse osteoporosis. But wait, there's more - lactoferrin also increases the proliferation of cells that build cartilage called chondrocytes.

I cannot recommend a high-quality organic yogurt high enough for your health, so it pays to enjoy yoghurt because lactoferrin's effects were found to be dose-dependent, stimulating an up to a 5-fold increase in osteoblasts at higher doses consumed

12

Yogurt Can Help Significantly With Weight Loss

You wouldn't think of yogurt as a weight-loss food, but it can help you loose weight a lot. A study published in the International Journal of Obesity revealed that in just 12 weeks, 16 obese men and women on a calorie restricted diet that included three portions of yogurt a day lost an amazing 61% more fat and 81% more abdominal fat than 18 obese subjects assigned to a diet with the same number of calories but who consumed little or no high fat and calcium dairy foods like yogurt. Not only did those in the yogurt group lose more body fat, especially around their waist, but they also retained more lean, muscle tissue than those people who were on the yogurt-free diet. The study indicated that adding one or two servings of yogurt to your daily diet could help you maximize your fat-loss and minimize loss of lean muscle.

13

Eating Calcium-Rich Foods Has Been Linked To Lower Body Fat

It is amazing at how rapidly our children are becoming obese, and this has been in part linked with low calcium diets. Australia leads the world in childhood obesity, and New Zealand is not far behind. It is good news for parents to hear about a study published in the Journal of the American Dietetic Association that revealed that calcium-rich foods were found to be negatively correlated with body fat in both children and adults. Last century, diets with calcium levels as high as 4000mg daily were not unheard of, and today an adult is lucky to get 1500mg from his or her daily diet. In America, childhood obesity has more than doubled in the past ten years according to the New England Journal of Medicine, and the International Obesity Task Force recently reported that childhood obesity in England is already three times higher in 2011 than it was in the year 2000. In late 2012, one in ten children who started preschool in England were classified as obese.

14

Yogurt consumption for fresh breath

Consuming just 90 grams of yogurt twice a day helps to eliminate those tongue-coating bacteria and helps to reduce dental plaque formation, cavities, and even the risk for gingivitis. Regular yogurt consumption also helps to lower levels of hydrogen sulfide and other volatile sulfide compounds responsible for that bad breath.

Make sure you select yoghurt's that contain those live cultures, I have found that the highest quality products will often indicate exactly how many live bacteria are contained in their product.

Different Ways To Enjoy Yogurt

Yogurt has been enjoyed in much of the world for over 4,000 years. Originating from central parts of Asia and India, and southern and central Europe, it is now eaten almost everywhere in the world. Probably no other food product apart from yogurt can claim such an amazing history while being healthy and nutritious as well as cheap to buy or so easy to make at home!

Yet there is an incredible difference between a shop bought, pasteurized, artificially sweetened and artificially colored yogurt, and a fresh, natural yogurt - preferably made at home. The taste of unsweetened yogurt can take some getting used to; I have found that many patients find it too bitter or "acidic" at first. Even natural yogurt is more commonly eaten with lots of fruit and even sugar added, or as part of a multitude of other recipes - from Indian curries to stir fry dishes and all manner of savory or sweet dips.

- Top your daily cup of yogurt with a quarter-cup of muesli, a handful of nuts, and some frozen berries for a quick, delicious and sustaining breakfast.

- Creamy yogurt, chives, and freshly ground sea salt and pepper make a great topping for cooked vegetables. Good to use instead of sour cream.

- Yogurt parfaits are a visual as well as delicious treat. In a large wine glass, alternate layers of yogurt and favorite fresh fruit.

- For a creamy salad dressing or vegetable dip, just mix a cup of yogurt with a quarter cup of extra virgin olive oil and your favorite herbs and spices. Yogurt combines with different herbs and spices quite well.

- Instead of using coconut cream in your curry, use yogurt instead.

- Yogurt has a nice cooling flavor after a hot spicy meal.

- Try yogurt on top of cooled porridge, topped with fresh green apple or kiwi.

- Make dips out of the plain yogurt and serve it with meat, chicken and rice.

- Add chopped cucumber and dill weed to plain yogurt. Eat this delicious and cooling salad as is or use as an accompaniment to grilled chicken or lamb.

- Try yogurt with a sprinkling of ground flax seeds, fresh blueberries and chopped raw walnuts.

- I like plain yogurt with cinnamon on top.

- Try and put the yogurt in the freezer for about half an hour and eat like ice cream, mix berries in first.

- Soak overnight whole rolled oats with 1/2 cup each of oats, water, and yogurt. In the morning add either fresh blueberries and ground flax seed.

- You can use yogurt in place of sour cream.

- Dip vegetables in yogurt so you don't have to add fattening sauces or butter.

- Mix yogurt with cottage cheese, fruit and slivered almonds.

- Toss cubes of cooked eggplant with plain yogurt, chopped mint leaves, garlic and cayenne.

- Yogurt is a great base for salad dressings. Simply place plain yogurt in the blender with enough water to achieve your desired consistency. Add to this your favorite herbs and spices.

Different Types of Lactobacillus Species

- Lactobacillus acidophilus - Lactobacillus Acidophilus bacterium is probably the most well known and some Lactobacillus species are used industrially for the production of cheese, sauerkraut, pickles, beer, wine, cider, kim chi and other fermented foods. It is sometimes used together with Streptococcus salivarius and Lactobacillus delbrueckii ssp. bulgaricus in the production of acidophilus-type yogurt.

- Lactobacillus bifidus - is a friendly bacteria that helps maintain healthy bacteria in the large intestine by increasing the acidity of the region it inhabits and making the area inhospitable to dangerous bacteria. This friendly bacterium is particularly important in the very young as well as the elderly.

- Lactobacillus rhamnosus - is a probiotic bacterium that was originally considered to be a subspecies of Lactobacillus casei, but later genetic research found it to be a species of its own. Lactobacillus rhamnosus inhibits the growth of most harmful bacteria in the intestine. It is used as a natural preservative in yogurt and other dairy products to extend the shelf life. It has probiotic properties. When administered orally it adheres to the mucous membrane of the intestine and may help to restore the balance of the GI micro flora, promote gut-barrier functions and diminish the production of carcinogenic compounds by other intestinal bacteria.

- Lactobacillus bulgaricus - is one of several bacteria used for the production of yogurt. It is also non-motile, and it does not form spores. It has complex nutritional requirements, including the inability to ferment any sugar except for lactose.

- Lactobacillus casei - is a transient, anaerobic microorganism of genus Lactobacillus found in the human intestine and mouth. As a lactic acid producer, it has been found to assist in the propagation of desirable bacteria. This particular species of lactobacillus is documented to complement the growth of Lactobacillus acidophilus.

The Candida Crusher Yogurt Recipe

This yogurt is made in the Greek style; it is creamy and delicious, fresh and simple to make. This recipe has been fortified by inoculating the yoghurt with additional beneficial bacteria, providing you with large amounts of beneficial bacteria unobtainable in even the very best store-bought yoghurt. If you want to make really healthy yoghurt, try using raw cow's milk, you haven't had yogurt until you have made it with organic raw milk, just try it, you will be amazed.

Those suffering from lactose intolerance can generally safely eat yoghurt, even the three and a half percent fat from the full-cream milk becomes defatted and soured and much more easily digested. This is good information for those who are conscious of animal fat intake in the diet. However, some may suffer from casein (dairy protein) intolerance, so be careful if you have dairy allergies, many people do. Just try this yogurt first before you decide that you are allergic to it, you may not be, especially if you add probiotics to it as it is setting.

Some people may tell you that adding probiotics as the yogurt is setting is silly and serves no purpose, but after having made this yogurt myself for over 15 years and noticing first hand the benefits it has made in my life and that of the many patients who now make it, I would disagree. It makes sense that there will be some benefits, lactobacillus loves an environment that contains milk sugar and is warm, it makes sense that yogurt fortified in this way will have an added punch.

Ingredients:

- Lactobacillus acidophilus capsules. (3 capsules per 4 cups of milk)

- 4 cups of full cream organic milk.

- ½ cup of full cream powdered organic milk

- 2 Tablespoons of plain acidophilus organic yoghurt

Method:

- In a large saucepan, add powdered milk to the regular milk, mix well with the wire whisk. Heat until hot, boiling is not necessary.

- Remove from heat and cool for about one quarter of an hour.
  (Until about 43 - 49 centigrade) Use a thermometer to check the temperature.

- Add the plain yoghurt to the warm milk stirring continuously. Stir well and be gentle.

- Add the three capsules of a probiotic, stir well and gently, using a wire whisk.

- Pour into plastic container and seal with a tight fitting lid. Place in a warm spot e.g. on top of a hot water cylinder. Wrap some cotton cloths around the container to insulate it and to keep its temperature constant. Leave over night & next day, creamy yogurt!

Notes:

- For your starter, use a high-quality plain and certified organic acidophilus commercial yoghurt, make sure it is free of sugar, artificial sugar or fruit. You can also use yoghurt from the last batch as a starter. Starter must be fresh, if yoghurt doesn't set, then try again with fresh starter.

- Do not disturb the yoghurt while it is setting.

- Excessive temperature (over 49 centigrade) destroys the starter. If the temperature is too cool (below 38 centigrade) ordinary sour milk bacteria will form.

- Refrigerate the set yoghurt for a few hours before you eat it.

- This yoghurt keeps for about 3 to 4 weeks in the fridge, but can still be eaten for weeks after.

- Fruit such as kiwifruit or blueberries are delicious blended with the yoghurt, but do avoid bananas with a yeast infection, best to wait until you feel much better until you add bananas to your diet, you are better off sticking with blueberries, green apple, a pear or a kiwi fruit.

Kefir

Kefir is a specially prepared, delicious fermented drink. There are 2 types of kefir- water and milk kefir; the latter can be made with sheep, goat or cow's milk. The liquid is fermented with kefir "grains"- (colonies of yeast and healthy bacteria), and the resulting drink is an excellent source of healthy intestinal micro flora, B vitamins, Vitamin E, and (for milk kefirs) complete proteins. Those who are lactose-intolerant will easily be able to digest both water and milk kefir.

Scientific research has shown promises that regular consumption of kefir leads to numerous health benefits. Some of the reported health benefits are:

- Regulating cholesterol, blood pressure, blood sugar

- Cleaning the digestive tract and regulates metabolism and digestion

- Effectively healing diarrhea, colitis, catarrh, reflux, leaky gut syndrome, irritable bowel syndrome

- Improving the body's immune system and resistance to disease

- Improving liver and gallbladder function

- Effective treating acne and various skin disorders

- Has anti-aging effect due to abundance of anti-oxidants in kefir

Making your own kefir requires nothing more than milk or water, and some basic kitchenware. Your good health food store may be able to supply you with an excellent starter recipe for kefir, and you can easily find fun, tasty variations of this recipe online. Once you become experienced at making your own probiotics at home, you'll find it's a great alternative to store-bought varieties. With a small investment of time and effort, you can enjoy the many benefits of cultured and fermented foods you prepare and enjoy as part of your diet for long-term health.

Why Ocean And Sea Vegetables?

I rarely find that any books on diet and nutrition, let alone yeast infections, focus much if any attention to this particular category of foods, the amazingly healthy sea vegetables. Just like the fermented and cultured foods, once you start to eat these foods you will notice that you can take your health to a whole new level. I'd like you to consider adding this group of vegetables into your diet slowly, just start with only one addition like hijiki, kombu or wakame and take it from there.

I first got introduced to ocean and sea vegetables when I was a naturopathic student after completing a cooking class that included Japanese cooking and got hooked right from the start, since then I have enjoyed many different types of seaweed in my diet. If you have ever eaten sushi or are familiar with miso soup which often includes pieces of seaweed, then you will already have eaten seaweed of some kind and be already familiar with these foods.

There will be no looking back once you finally adopt a diet that regularly includes ocean and sea vegetables, because you will have rounded out your diet by including some of the healthiest of foods you will find in your health-food shop.
If you adopt all of the healthy food suggestions as outlined in this first section of the book, your Candida Crusher dietary food suggestions should include foods from the following groups:

- Land-based vegetables, especially leafy greens and the colored vegetables.

- Fruits such as blueberries, avocado, kiwi, lemon and lime.

- High quality protein sources like fresh fish and lean meats.

- Free range eggs and chicken.

- Nuts, seeds like almonds, Brazil nuts, sesame and pumpkin seeds, etc.

- Alkaline grains such as quinoa, millet and buckwheat.

- Fermented and cultured foods including yogurt, kefir, kimchi, tempeh, etc.

- Sea-based vegetables, including agar, kombu, hijiki, nori and wakame.

After you have completed reading all sections of this seventh chapter, this group of foods will also include the special anti-candida foods that you will read about in section 4.

Seaweeds have been harvested for many hundreds if not thousands of years and used as a very important part of the daily diet in many traditional cultures around the world. Most people think of Asia when they think of seaweed, and countries like Japan in particular, but seaweeds were and still are an important food source for almost every country that has an ocean near it. In New Zealand, the Maori used wakame for centuries as a food source long before the white man came to its shores.

The seaweed called nori which you may be familiar with if you have tried sushi, was once only reserved for royalty only in countries like Japan and Hawaii.

I'll explain more about each kind of seaweed soon, but first, let me explain a bit about why these sea-weeds are so beneficial for your health.

The Most Mineral Rich Natural Food Source

Unlike land-based vegetables, seaweeds cannot obtain their food supply from the soil through their root systems, and they have to rely on obtaining all the nutrition they need from the ocean's water. There are almost 60 different minerals found in seaweeds, and every single mineral and trace element your body requires can be found in sea and ocean vegetables. Does your multivitamin contain this level of minerals? I doubt it.

In many Western countries, soils are becoming increasingly stressed and gradually depleted of many of our essential minerals and trace elements due to modern farming methods. This is certainly not the case with seaweeds because these mineral abundant foods contain hundreds of essential trace elements and minerals in the most assimilable forms that can nourish the cells of our bodies. Some nutritional experts in fact believe that these aquatic groups of foods are nutritionally among the densest on the planet, because they contain the highest concentration and broadest range of minerals of any currently known food. Are you starting to pay attention now, to this class of superfoods?

Perhaps you should consider adding some of these foods to your diet, especially if you want to boost your overall health and wellbeing to the highest levels and get rid of that yeast infection permanently.

Sea Vegetable Health Benefits

Sea vegetables contain an amazing array of minerals, including calcium, magnesium, potassium, iron, and an incredibly large variety of trace elements, some not anywhere else. Sea vegetables may be one of the only dietary ways left to get precious trace elements such as cobalt, copper, chromium, fluorine, iodine, manganese, molybdenum, selenium and zinc back into your diet.

These foods are also a rich source of B vitamins, vitamin C and vitamin K. In addition, sea vegetables are nature's richest source of iodine, required by your thyroid gland in particular and contain good amounts of a carbohydrate-like substance called fucans that has strong anti-inflammatory properties. Sea vegetables are particularly beneficial for those with autoimmune disease because of their immune-boosting and anti-inflammatory properties.

I like all patients with adrenal fatigue and hypothyroidism to included some sea vegetables into their diet, and because half the population has some degree of hypothyroidism, and three quarters have varying levels adrenal fatigue issues ranging from mild through to extreme, I guess it just about sums up everybody to some degree. Just like rice bran, oat bran, Jerusalem artichoke, and linseed/sunflower/almond mix (LSA), sea vegetables contain high quality prebiotic fibers and are perfect for those who are interested in re-populating their digestive system with beneficial bacteria, especially those with a yeast infection.

Health Tip:

Careful with sea vegetables if you have thyroiditis

I would caution those with Hashimoto's thyroiditis when it comes to eating sea-weeds, and to regularly have their urinary iodine levels checked. Those with autoimmune diseases of the thyroid such as Grave's disease and Hashimoto's thyroiditis are particularly sensitive to iodine and certainly don't want too much in their diet.

Here are but a few of the many health benefits you can derive from eating ocean vegetables:

- Improve the condition of hair, nails, bones, connective tissues, skin and teeth.

- Inhibit growth and reproduction of pathogenic bacteria, candida and viruses.

- Help chelate heavy metals, especially lead, mercury, arsenic and cadmium.

- Increase the diet's fiber content and encourage daily eliminations.

- Facilitate healthy thyroid function, due to the iodine content.

- Assist with adrenal fatigue, stress and burnout.

- Prebiotic qualities, feeds up the good bacteria.

- Fight the growth of cancer cells.

- Blood pressure lowering action.

- Powerful antioxidant action.

- Anti-inflammatory action.

- Reduce cholesterol levels.

- Anti-inflammatory action.

- Alkalize the blood.

Ocean Vegetables In The Kitchen

So what do you do with seaweed you may be wondering? These foods are very versatile because they can combine with just about any dish you may prepare. Seaweed is alkaline and combines easily with any vegetable, protein or grain dish. You can use them in salads or with cooked dishes and the possibilities are virtually endless. I recommend that you go to your local library or bookstore and obtain a few books about macrobiotic cooking; there you will find many different recipes relating to sea vegetables. The Internet is also an excellent source of more information.

You are unlikely to buy sea vegetables from your local supermarket, apart from nori sheets perhaps. If you want to buy seaweed I recommend that you visit your local health-food store, and the bigger stores will most likely have the best varieties. Don't forget your local Asian supermarket, they have a surprising amount of fresh, frozen and dried seaweeds on hand. Just like their land-based counterparts, the colors of sea vegetables are incredible and can range from black, green, yellow, brown and even red or purple varieties.

Try different varieties and you will soon settle of two or three and include them regularly into your diet. Most varieties of seaweed require soaking so that they can be reconstituted before use. Generally a half an hour of soaking is all that is required, and you will find that seaweed will greatly increase in size the longer you leave it soak.

Some varieties like kombu are just flat leaf, whereas other varieties like hijki are long thin strands. Varieties like wakame have inedible stems that are discarded after the leaves have been removed. Some types of seaweed like wakame or dulse do not necessarily require soaking and can be crushed easily and sprinkled onto many foods to add a salty taste and a crispy texture.

The 7 Most Common Varieties

- **Agar.** Agar is often used to make sweet or savory gelatin types of dishes. It has prebiotic properties and nourishes the digestive tract. You can buy it as a powdered form or in larger pieces of chunks. It dissolves in water and sets like jelly. (Jell-O) Some people even use agar regularly to keep them regular.

- **Arame.** Arame is fine and delicate seaweed that has a sweet taste. It cooks well with finely cut onions, carrots and zucchini. Add to egg and quiche dishes, add to salads or as a side serve to a main dish. Soak well and then chop fine, it is best when added raw in small amounts to salads, or as a more generous amount as a side with your main meal.

- **Dulse.** Dulse is my personal favorite, closely followed by hijiki and nori. It has a nice purple color and does not need soaking and has a sweet, tender flavor. Try wrapping a little piece of dulse around a Brazil nut. This seaweed can be powdered and used as a condiment or left in a chunky form and added to soups and stews. Try it, you may like this one, it is high in iron and packed with antioxidants too.

- **Hijiki.** Hijiki is also one of my favorites; it comes in black long thin strands and looks a bit like very thick black hair. I find it most agreeable when soaked for half an hour in tepid water and the cooked lightly with sesame oil and mixed in with some lightly steamed broccoli on which I have tossed a little roasted sesame seed. While it does take a little longer to cook, it is worth it because it has a great texture and tastes nice and is a rich source of many minerals, including magnesium.

- **Kombu.** Kombu is the other sea vegetable I enjoy; it is flat seaweed and an inch or two wide. Kombu makes an excellent stock and is commonly added to miso soup. Just simmer a few pieces of kombu in water for about 30 to 40 minutes and then add some miso stock and you have instant miso soup. Kombu stock is mineral rich and very nourishing. I also add a piece of kombu to the water when I boil a root vegetable like potato or sweet potato.

- **Nori.** Nori is probably one of the most popular of sea vegetables, and you may well know it as sushi. There are many ways you can enjoy nori, personally I like to roll up nori with quinoa and add salmon, avocado, cucumber, and a wide variety of other vegetables into the filling. I like roasted nori sheets and just crumble them up and add them to salads or sprinkle on top of steamed broccoli.

- **Wakame.** Wakame is delicate and can range in color from a pale green right through to a very dark green. I find that after soaking it is tastes not unlike spinach and is most agreeable as a side serve or great when added to salads.

Tips On Using Sea Vegetables In Cooking

- Always read the instruction on the pack carefully, some sea vegetables need soaking for longer than others. Some you cook with dried, like kombu, whereas others you soak and then cook, like hijiki, arame and wakame.

- Roasted sesame oil is a very nice seasoning that seems to complement the texture of many kinds of seaweed. I find that toasted sesame seeds a great match with soaked and cooked seaweed as well.

- Try mixing seaweed with carrots, onions and cucumbers to begin with, you will soon get the feel of it and begin to experiment more with this groups of foods.

- Add a two-inch piece of the flat seaweed kombu to dried beans when you are cooking them, the cooked beans will be easier to digest.

- Rinse then roast some sesame seeds with sea salt, perfect with seaweed.

- Add seaweed to casseroles, stocks or vegetable soups.

- Make miso soup and add seaweed to this.

- Try making your own sushi, you can even lightly toast the nori sheets to add extra flavor. I like making sushi with quinoa and tahini instead of rice and sweet rice wine vinegar. You'll find a recipe online.

- Add soaked seaweed to your favorite salad, toss in a little toasted sesame oil and add a few roasted sesame seeds for a real taste treat.

- Try to saute' some arame or wakame with carrot strips and onion, and again, try the sesame oil and roasted sesame seed combo, it's absolutely delicious!

- Agar agar is seaweed that sets like jello; you can make a really nice dessert with agar agar and blueberries for example. Look online for recipes on how you can incorporate this unique seaweed into your diet because it has great prebiotic properties.

- How about a sandwich with arame or dulse? Saute' one of these seaweeds and have on some toasted sourdough bread along with avocado, delicious.

Sea Vegetable Pollution Warning

Unfortunately the world's oceans are becoming increasingly polluted, and with only about ten percent of the world's population living in the Southern Hemisphere, it stands to reason that the cleanest oceans are down under. We are fortunate living in New Zealand, and have possibly the world's cleanest ocean, the Southern Ocean. Some of the world's best wakame comes from the South Island of NZ, and the flavor is quite amazing.

There has been a lot of concern amongst scientists over the past several years with regards to the high levels of pollution in the world's ocean waters. Sea vegetables readily absorb what is in the water surrounding them, including heavy metals like mercury, arsenic, lead and cadmium, and if they have been harvested in polluted waters or around large industrial cities they are likely to contain heavy metals and other potentially toxic elements. Deep-sea kelp is a safer alternative for example than wakame that may have been harvested close to the shoreline.

Some forms of seaweed have been discovered to contain high levels of arsenic, while others have been found to contain traces of mercury. Try to get a high quality product harvested in areas known to contain low levels of pollution, and make enquiries with the company if you are uncertain as to the origin of the product.

Improving Your Digestion and Bowel Function

Just about every person I see daily in my naturopathic practice has digestive problems to some degree, and I'm sure that many people who practice natural medicine reading would tend to agree. It is incredible how many people needlessly suffer with regular bouts of constipation, diarrhea, irritable bowel syndrome, bloating, nausea, and various kinds of food intolerances. Most of these problems can be avoided or corrected by eating a healthy a well-balanced diet to begin with.

If you are plagued with digestive problems, then I'd recommend you slowly start to change your habits and include more of the following into your diet: water, vegetables, probiotics and the specialized foods I talk about later in section 4 of this chapter, including garlic, ginger, coconut products and fresh herbs as well as the fermented and cultured foods and sea vegetables I have just outlined before.

Always Adopt Dietary Change Slowly

One of the most important points to emphasize with regard to diet change is to start right away yet to adopt these new habits *slowly*. All too often I have found that when I make a recommendation in the clinic to a patient then these recommendations are adopted too rapidly and almost overnight, meaning that their whole diet and lifestyle is changed literally within 24 hours. You can imagine the misery this can bring about, years of sloppy or bad eating habits changed in an instant, and the result for many can mean bad headaches, nausea, plenty of gas and bloating, more constipation or diarrhea and sometimes insomnia, headaches and fatigue. It doesn't sound like fun, does it? But it happens regularly in the clinic, so I must warn you again – begin to adopt health dietary changes slowly, preferably over a two to three week period to be on the safe side.

I know that you want to feel better fast, but slow dietary changes will mean less misery in the long term, and a greater chance that you will adopt these changes permanently. Perhaps you can remember once when you went on that health kick or exercise program some time back, you made sweeping changes to your diet overnight, or were a little too enthusiastic with exercise. Can you recall how you felt after two or three days? Need I say anymore on this topic?

Your Beneficial Bacteria
And Digestive Enzyme Levels Will Improve

Believe me, it is not difficult to improve your digestion and bowel function, it is just a matter of adopting the correct lifestyle and dietary habits, and then keeping these habits going until they become engrained enough to have become habitual in your life. Start with my following my 12 recommendations for a full twenty-one (21) days straight without a break. If you can manage to continue these habits for a full three weeks, then it is likely they will last and stay with you long enough, for at least three to four months. An important concept to understand is that when you make long-term and positive changes to your eating habits that the microorganisms in your stomach and intestines will change as well, the bad ones will reduce in number and the good ones will increase.

Your yeast infection will not like these good partners whatsoever, as it likes to rub shoulders with the bad guys, candida will also hate the fact that your body is starting to produce healthier amounts of digestive enzymes in all areas of your digestive system in your stomach, pancreas, liver and small intestine. This in itself will bring about a renewed vigor you may not have felt for years, and as your digestive health improves, which is your foundation for great health, then the superstructure you build on top of this foundation, your body's trillions of cells, will become healthier and stronger as a result. The end result is a solid structure, able to withstand just about anything that nature throws at it, and this is called good health.

12 TIPS For Improving Digestive And Bowel Function

1

Add Fermented And Cultured Foods To Your Diet. You have just read the section on fermented and cultured foods; doesn't it make sense to start including some of these you're your diet *every day*? These kinds of foods include yogurt, kefir, kombucha, tempeh, fermented coconut water, miso, soy, tempeh and no doubt there will be several other kinds fermented foods. Besides containing beneficial bacteria like lactobacillus and bifidobacterium, fermented and cultured foods provide your body with lactic acid, and lactic acid is what feeds beneficial bacteria like lactobacillus acidophilus.

A good way to begin to incorporate these foods into your diet is to include a small portion, about three to four tablespoons, of a natural yogurt into your diet each day. Beware though, as I mentioned before, not all yogurt is created equal, and some brands are laden with artificial sugars and don't even contain a shred of beneficial bacterium. Always read the label first, and if in doubt, avoid buying yogurt from your supermarket and purchase from your organic wholefood suppliers instead, these kinds of folk are often less motivated to look only at profit and are focused on providing you the consumer with foods that are actually healthy.

2

Slowly Begin Adding Soluble And Insoluble Fiber To Your Diet. It never ceases to amaze me how many patients I have seen over the years who simply don't eat much fruit at all, perhaps one piece every so often, and the vegetables they consume are either bought frozen or consumed after having being been boiled or microwaved. Fruits and vegetables contain some of the best levels of soluble and insoluble fiber you can get, be sure to read what I have written further ahead in this section on fiber in your diet. There are so many ways you can increase the amount of fiber you can take in, but once again, go easy to begin with. You've heard it all before; go low and go-slow is my motto when it comes to making any changes to your diet and digestion. It is a fact that most people eat a small amount of fiber (20 to 40 grams) when compared to people who live in the undeveloped nations (80 to 120 grams), and as a consequence they experience all the digestive problems that go hand in hand with such low-fiber diets.

2

Start by including small amounts of beans, lentils, fruits (wait until your candida improves first before including too much fruit), vegetables, raw or partially cooked are best, seeds, whole grains such as brown rice, quinoa, amaranth, millet are best, and continue to add these foods slowly over a two-week period until over half of what you eat are these kinds of foods.

So you want to eat less, lose weight, feel full and improve your bowel tone? Then eat more soluble fiber; these foods include pears, oranges, strawberries, kiwi fruit, carrots, psyllium hulls, slippery elm bark powder, lentils, rolled oats, and cucumber. Soluble fiber fills you up as it swells up in your stomach due to its ability to hold water; you feel fuller and thereby eat less.

So you want to bulk up your bowel motions, or perhaps clean out that lazy bowel? Then try including insoluble fiber into your diet. These foods include brown rice, onions, leafy green vegetables like broccoli and spinach, celery, bulgur (cracked wheat), chia seeds, various nuts and seeds and whole grains.

So you want to reduce the amount of gas and bloating you have and feed up any good bacteria you have? Then I recommend you consume a combination of fermented and cultured foods as well as foods which contain pre-biotics, basically these are beneficial sugars which feed the friendly bacteria. The pre-biotic feeds the pro-biotic, and these foods include Jerusalem artichoke, artichokes, garlic, onions, shallots, scallions, and spring onions.

3

Cut Back On Sugar And Fat In Your Diet. This is quite a simple achievement, just reduce the amounts of foods you buy and eat which contain sugars and fats. Be sure to read the labels of processed foods you buy to see how much sugar and fat they contain. It won't be difficult for you to do this if you prepare most of your own meals from meats, grain and vegetables, because you control what other ingredients then go into your meals and not some manufacturer in a factory far away. The problem with foods containing sugars and fats is that they will also contain all manner of chemicals such as artificial colors, flavors and preservatives that you may not be aware of, especially if these foods are highly processed foods. The less of these foods you consume, the better your digestion will work and the more likely that you will be able to build good levels of beneficial bacteria. This will result in an easier ability for your body to crush a yeast infection.

Drink Water.
This sounds like a simple tip but is the one health boosting tip that many never seem to be able to achieve, to drink more water. Your digestive system will work so much better when you consume ample water, and you will be quite surprised how much better you feel overall when you are more hydrated.

Your digestive system will work that much better, especially your stomach, pancreas and intestines, and although no proof exists that water actually aids digestion I have certainly noticed that those with a yeast infection who do drink water and considerably less coffee, tea or alcohol, appear to have much less bother with many different digestive problems. Remember

4

also, that when you slowly add more fiber into your diet that it really pays to drink a lot more water. The best approach in improving your digestion however, is to cut back on sugary, salty and fatty foods, increase the number of fruits and vegetables and whole grains your consume (fiber) and drink more water every day. Try this for twenty-one days and you will be delighted at the difference these simple dietary tips can make to your life.

5

Avoid Three Large Meals A Day, Eat Several Smaller Meals Instead. Did you know that one of the best-kept secrets to crushing candida permanently is to improve the ability of your digestive system to produce digestive enzymes? Many high quality candida supplements contain enzymes, and now why would that be? It's because enzymes can help to bust open the walls of yeasts, bad bacteria and other nasty bugs which may invade your digestive system. By eating smaller meals more frequently, you avoid over-loading your digestive system and because your body is better at digesting smaller quantities in one sitting you will be improving the way the digestive organs work. Can you recall I mentioned just before that your stomach is like a cement mixer, it functions best when half full and not overloaded? First you will need to figure out how much food you need to eat per meal, and then try to keep a regular schedule that your body can adjust to. This will take about two or three weeks.

6

Eat Small Amounts Of Lean Protein. Look at the palm of your hand, and if you are a meat eater, that's the size of the piece of meat you should be eating each day. Many adults eat too much meat, and the portion sizes are just too big. While protein is essential for good health, you will find that smaller amounts of lean cuts of meat are less likely to cause digestive discomfort such as heartburn, bloating or gas and will be quicker to digest. In general, high-fat meats take longer to digest than low-fat meats, so always choose meat containing less fat.

7

Chew Food Well. How could I forget to mention that it is important to chew proteins in particular more slowly and carefully than you would other foods? That way you prepare your digestive system for what's to come as chewing promotes the release of enzymes and acids in your stomach and small intestine. Make sure that you chew all foods well, but especially the high protein foods. That way you will also help to reduce them to a much smaller size and allow your digestive power to more easily render these foods to their components called amino acids which will be much more readily digested and absorbed.

8

Try 30 Minutes Exercise Every Day. Did you know that those who walk daily have a significantly better digestive health than those who don't? Are you creating "sitting disease" by being chained to your computer or iPad? Walking stimulates digestion and is one of the best things you can do to improve the tone of your small and large intestine especially, so if you are not in the habit of walking most days get started. Just get up and out of your chair and start moving, don't take the escalator, take the stair instead. Regular movement such as walking, swimming and dancing for example helps food to move through your digestive system, stimulates your metabolism and aids significantly in weight loss.

9 Alcohol And Tobacco Are Two Big Enemies Of Your Digestive System. You will never beat a yeast infection if you can't give up drinking alcohol for at least 4 months, end of story. Those who are serious about their health will know that cigarette smoking is crazy, but I'm very much surprised how many patients I have seen with yeast infections who want to continue both smoking cigarettes and drinking alcohol yet still want to beat their yeast infection. It is not likely to happen, and the day you are prepared to become disciplined and say "NO" to these destructive habits is the day your health will change. Once your yeast infection has significantly improved you should be able to drink socially again, but may soon realize that moderately heavy drinking may lead you down the path of another yeast infection.

10 Learn The Art Of Relaxation. Your digestive system is very much affected by stress, especially any acute or ongoing low-grade stress. I'll talk a lot more about the effects of stress, your digestive and immune system and candida later on in this book. When you learn to counter the effects of stress in your body you will be amazed at how much better your digestion works, in fact it is another one of those best-kept and totally understated health secrets. Stress has the ability to impair your stomach and digestion in general, and has been shown to cause weight gain, constipation, diarrhea and a lowered immune system. For example, I see many guys in my clinic who complain of heartburn or indigestion related to stress. A few methods you could use right now to reduce stress in your life is to get involved in yoga, meditation, and having regular massage.

There are many other relaxation techniques that can help you handle stress and improve digestion but I'll expand much more on them later in this book.

11 Understand Your Digestive Habits. If you have recurring digestive problems and can't get a handle on them then try to use a diary or your daily journal to write down what you eat along with any increase or reduction of digestive symptoms you experience. Sometimes it is only the simplest things in your diet and lifestyle you have to change in order to get an amazing improvement in your health. It may be the combination of a few dietary indiscretions you are consuming simultaneously, or you may be eating too late or too fast, either way, by keeping a symptom diary you will be in a much more powerful situation to truly establish any cause and effect.

12 Don't Treat Yourself, Go Your Naturopath or Doctor. OK, so you have made all the necessary changes, you are exercising regularly, learning to relax more, drinking more water, eating plenty of vegetables, lean meats, etc., but you still don't feel quite right. May I suggest that you contact your naturopath or nutritionally minded natural medicine doctor? You may need testing for food allergies or intolerances, you may have an underlying bacterial or parasite problem or there could be any one of a dozen hidden causes such as heavy metal toxicity that may need exploring in depth.

Food Reactions - Allergies And Intolerances

There are lots of people with yeast infections who are talk to me about their food allergies and intolerances, and unfortunately many people kind of get confused and think that all food reactions are food allergies, when in fact, many reactions which develop as a consequence of eating food are in fact food intolerances and not food allergies. So how do you distinguish between them both? How do you know if you are actually allergic to something, or simply can't tolerate a food? We call the latter a non-immune mediated food reaction.

A food allergy is just one type of adverse food reaction that is mediated by the immune system. An adverse food reaction may comprise any symptom following the intake of a particular food. Symptoms may be any perceptible change in how we feel and/or function. A symptom may present, for example, as a rash, achy joints, or fatigue. But first let's take a look at the different kinds of reactions which are possible after you eat a particular food, some of these reactions may be familiar to you whereas others will be unfamiliar.

Adverse Food Reactions Are Classified Into 3 Subgroups

1. **Toxic food reaction.** These reactions are commonly known as **food poisoning** and are as a result of contaminants (often bacteria) in the food. Most of us will have had a case of eating something "not quite good" or that "didn't quite agree", and this may have resulted in cramps in the stomach, vomiting, and diarrhea.

2. **Psychological or food aversion.** These food reactions are more difficult to diagnose and are generally related to **a former bad experience with a particular food**. These kinds of reactions are largely psychosomatic in nature. An example is when my younger brother burned his mouth quite severely when he was younger with a mushroom, and since then he has not been able to eat any mushrooms.

3. **Non-toxic reaction.** This group is the most common and can be divided into two groups - immune (**food allergy**) and non-immune mediated responses (**food intolerance**). I'll focus on these two groups in more depth and explain the difference between them both.

    In my experience, those who have had digestive problems for years may be more prone to toxic food reactions and others who have had an eating disorder like anorexia or bulimia in the past may have developed psychological or aversions towards certain foods. The most common category however is the non-toxic reaction group, and non-toxic food reactions seem to top the list.

A practitioner has to have a good amount of clinical experience and common sense when trying to understand a patient's presenting digestive problems, because a non-immune-mediated food reaction, a food intolerance, can often mimic an immune-mediated allergic inflammation and may occur from a particular food additive such as a color or preservative, any pharmacological compound such as antibiotics found in commercial chicken meat, or an enzymatic deficiency such as lactose intolerance or hypochlorhydria, an underactive stomach.

The Coca Pulse Test

Have you heard about a simple home test you can perform to determine whether you have a reaction to a food or drink you consume? The Coco Pulse Test will not define whether the reaction is an allergy or intolerance, but with a bit of skill it can certainly reveal any underlying and hidden reactions. You may like to try the pulse test, developed by Dr. Arthur F. Coca in the mid 1950's after working and refining his technique with many patients. Dr. Coco identified many different substances to which his patients were sensitive to, and was surprised how effective his test was at identifying the problems foods in a person's diet.

The Coco Pulse Test is based upon the premise that the stress caused by your nervous system in response to a food or drink, which you may be sensitive to, will increase your decrease your resting pulse. Dr. Coca's pulse test is a technique I have used in my clinic for over twenty years, and it must be performed strictly according to Dr. Coca's guidelines if excellent results are to be expected. This test is easy to perform, but before you start you will need to establish your baseline, i.e., what your pulse is normally like without being challenged. I use the stopwatch on my iPhone, but a wristwatch with a second hand is OK as well. Now I will explain the whole protocol in detail, and you should be able to perform it at home easily.

1. First, take your pulse fourteen (14) times per day for three con-secutive days as follows: once before rising in the morning (on waking and before getting out of bed), once before each meal, 3 times after each meal (at 30 minute intervals) and again just before going to bed.

2. Take the pulse for one minute (**an entire 60 seconds**), don't make the mistake I used to make and count the pulse for 15 sec-onds only, and then multiply by four.

3. All pulse rates should be checked with the person in a seated and relaxed position, except for the first pulse rate of the day that is checked lying down, before you get up and out of bed.

4. Make a Microsoft Excel spreadsheet and record all the results, along with what you have consumed with each meal.

5. No snacking between meals, but if you do then you will need to account for the food you consumed and what the pulse rate was before and after.

6. Make a note of the lowest and highest pulse readings over the three-day period. The difference can be between 10 to 16 beats per minute, and a significantly higher or lower pulse rate will indicate that you have consumed something to which you are allergic or sensitive to.

7. Any food that increases or decreases the pulse rate by 12 beats per minute indicates a suspected food and should be eliminated.

8. To figure out which offender is causing the problem, eliminate the suspect food for three days and test around that particular meal again.

9. Take into account that smoking and various pharmaceutical drugs like Beta blockers (blood pressure drugs) may cause false readings, so do take this into account.

10. Any pulse readings should always be performed, and will give the best results while resting quietly.

Another method I have found that works is to simply take your resting pulse each morning and evening throughout all three stages of Candida Crusher Diet. Once you start noticing an increase or decrease in your pulse of 10 to 12 beats per minute over a three-day period, you are on to something. Now you will need to work out what it is that has caused this pulse fluctuation by way of challenging your body with a food or drink you have eliminated. With a bit of trial and error you will find it.

Foods That Are Suspect Are:

- Foods you crave or have a strong desire for.

- Foods that often make you feel lousy or different in any way.

- Foods that one of your blood relatives is sensitive to.

- Key trigger foods or foods you have a strong suspicion about.

The Food Reactions Diagram

Non-toxic adverse food reactions are either immune-mediated food reactions, or food allergies are divided into IgE (immediate) and IgG (delayed) reactions, or non-immune mediated food reactions, enzyme deficiencies, food additives or pharmacological compounds. Other causes of food reactions are either toxic (food poisonings) of psychosomatic (mental/emotional) by nature.

Below is a simple diagram to put all of this into visual perspective as defined by the European Academy of Allergy and Clinical Immunology EAACI).

Thanks to EAACI for permission to use this diagram.

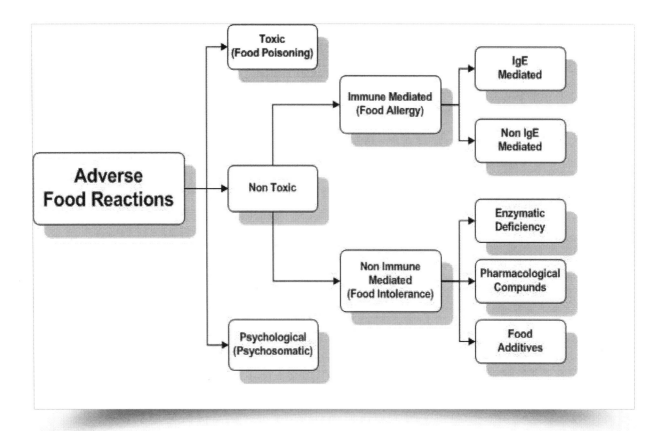

Food Allergies

A true food allergy is not as common as you may think, although much emphasis is placed on these kinds of food reactions in a clinical setting, and food intolerances are much more common in my experience. It is a lot easier for a practitioner to run a battery of tests and then to point the finger at one or several foods that will then need to be eliminated from the patient's diet. This supposedly cures the problem, but in my experience it never does. True food allergies certainly do exist, but they are more rare than most people realize, and there is always a reason for these allergies.

In some cases, the true allergy will be inherited but in many other cases it will be acquired. A true food allergy is always immune-mediated, and involves an immune reaction to a food or drink. Food allergies can be categorized into two groups, those which are more immediate (IgE responses), and those which are more delayed (IgG responses), now let's take a deeper look at both.

Immediate Food Allergies - Type 1 or IgE Response

Food allergies are either immediate or delayed. In the case of an immediate reaction, it will be quite noticeable and could take place within minutes to a few hours after ingestion of the offending substance.

The best-known and most studied form of food allergies is called a Type 1 immune reaction, or IgE mediated response. Type 1 food allergies occur in less than 5 percent of the population, and mostly in children, they are also called immediate-onset, and/or atopic food allergies. These types of allergies usually occur in the genetically predisposed individual, because one or both parents will be found to have an allergy, and the immune system begins to create a specific type of antibody called IgE (immunoglobulin IgE) in large amounts to specific foods.

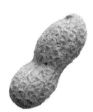 An IgE reaction occurs very much immediately after exposure to a particular allergen, which can be a food, and inhalant like dust mite or even venom like a bee sting. The early phase reaction usually occurs as little as 15 minutes after exposure to the allergen. Other types of IgE reactions may occur 4-6 hours later and persist for days with increased inflammation including symptoms such as swelling, puffiness, redness and itching. I have often heard patients tell me that they will eat a certain food, or perhaps be exposed to a certain inhaled allergen like pollen and literally within hours have a reaction ranging from itchy skin to feeling just about completely disabled.

So what happens with these immediate responses? One side of the IgE antibody will recognize and firmly bind to the allergic food. The other side of the antibody is attached to a specialized immune cell called a mast cell, packed with histamine. Ready and waiting for action, the IgE antibody now only has to patiently wait for re-exposure to particular allergens. For example, when the allergic food is eaten the next time, IgE antibodies hungrily latch onto the food. Almost instantly, histamine and other allergy-related chemicals (called chemical mediators) are released from the mast cell, bringing on various signs and symptoms rapidly.

Since this pathway occurs immediately, it is very easy to recognize a Type 1 allergy as a problem after an exposure to the irritant. This is the immunological pathway behind seasonal allergies such as hay fever. The most common test for this type of reaction is the scratch or RAST test that is performed by doctors or immune specialists. This involves scratching the skin and applying a test substance and then waiting for a wheal and flare response, often a skin reaction. The problem I find here is that this test is not always a reliable indication of an allergy, with many patients showing a "false negative" test and at times even an exaggerated positive response. The test substance may be too old to invoke a reaction or the test substance may not specific enough to the particular person and therefore does not invoke the reaction. There are simply too many reasons why this test can fail, and it does, so don't rely on it to be 100 percent positive.

There are no guarantees in this life, certainly not in immune testing so never rely one hundred percent on any antigen/antibody testing. As usual, don't get paralysis from analysis.

Type 1 Food Allergy Symptoms

The allergen and resulting symptoms are unique to the individual affected, and any symptoms can be very individual. However, many people don't have any idea that they may well have an underlying and often undetected food allergy. Once the potentially allergenic foods are digested and their protein derivatives enter into the bloodstream, some of these food nutrients or other food components are rejected by the body because a tendency develops of the antibodies and other related immune system elements are to fight back.

Not long after the response, allergy symptoms become apparent including swollen hands, itchy and swollen eyes, sensations of the lungs, and if acute even the closing of the larynx or throat. Anaphylaxis is the most alarming response (can't breathe, fast heart rate, panic) and other symptoms may include stomach cramping, diarrhea, hives, swelling, itching and various skin rashes.

Immediate Food Allergy (IgE) - Good Summary

We call these immediate allergic reactions the Type One immune reactions, and they are quite obvious. You know when you have one because your body suffers a notable and almost instant reaction, some people can die from consuming peanut, fish or crab meat. Did you know that more people die in Australia from bee stings (an IgE response) than from snakebites annually?

- Generally 1 or 2 foods are involved in causing these severe allergic symptoms. It is usually the one food that causes the strongest response.

- Even the tiniest trace amounts of food can trigger these intense allergic reactions, including anaphylaxis in which a fatal reaction can occur literally within minutes. It is not the quantity of the actual allergen, but the severity of the allergy that will dictate the response. I have known of patients to be hospitalized after only smelling fish or having the tiniest piece of peanut in their mouth.

- Allergic symptoms commonly appear 2 hours or less after consumption of offending foods, but may occur within a few minutes.

- Primarily affects the skin, airway and digestive tract manifesting in such classical allergies as asthma, rhinitis, urticaria, angioedema, eczema, vomiting, diarrhea and anaphylaxis.

- Common in children, these reactions do occur in adults although less commonly than the delayed (IgG) allergies.

- Some experts claim that addictive cravings and withdrawal symptoms are rare to nonexistent in children with IgE allergies, but this is certainly not my experience with Type 1 allergies and children.

- With the exception of infants and young children, due to single food and the immediate appearance of allergic symptoms, the offending food is commonly self-diagnosed. As a result, many patients never see a physician.

- Allergic food is food that is rarely eaten; the person has learned to avoid that food which causes them to feel not so good.

- IgE allergies are commonly permanent, fixed food allergies - but again, I have seen with some patients that no allergies are fixed or permanent. Even the most violent IgE allergic reactions in some cases become rather mild, and on a rare occasion actually disappear entirely. The immune system is very much like the weather; the only thing you can be certain of is, change.

- Frequently an IgE RAST (scratch) test can reveal a positive skin test result, but this may not reflect in a positive immune stimulus in the person's body when they are subjected to that particular food or allergen. It all depends on the experience of the person doing the testing, the conditions the test was performed under for example, and even if the patient was taking drugs such as antihistamines beforehand, or how much Vitamin C the patient took that morning. As you can see, there are simply too many variables that may cause a false negative test result, and this can all leave you quite confused.

Delayed Food Allergies - Type 3 or IgG Response

Non-IgE-mediated allergies involve antibodies other than IgE (generally IgG). Symptoms of an IgG-dependent reaction may occur hours to days following exposure to the allergen.

These are often referred to as "delayed food reactions". The IgG antibody may bind to the food antigen and form an immune complex, and these immune complexes may deposit in various tissues and trigger inflammatory reactions.

It is most unfortunate, but conventional medicine does not recognize these types of delayed immune responses.

Delayed Food Allergy (IgG) - Good Summary

Delayed food reactions are not immediate, and this can make them almost impossible to detect without sophisticated blood testing. I find it rather hard to believe that many conventional immunologists virtually ignore the IgG response, citing lack of scientific evidence as the main reason they won't test for it.

- More allergic responses typically occur here in the person suffering from an IgG food allergy, anywhere from 3 to 10 food allergens may be clinically involved, and sometimes even up to 20 foods have been reported in some cases.

- It is more rare for a person to be only allergic to one or two foods in this category.

- Unlike IgE allergies, typically larger amounts of food often in multiple feedings are commonly needed to provoke these types of allergic reactions. Reactions may not in some cases even occur after a single food challenge.

- Allergic symptoms commonly appear 2 to 24 hours after offending foods are eaten, but in my clinical experience, symptoms often appear 48 to 72 hours later.

- What makes it hard for the doctor or skin specialist to distinguish between an IgE and a IgG allergic response is that virtually any tissue, organ, or system of the human body can be affected, even the so-called classical allergic areas.

- Very common in children and adults, and well over 50 medical conditions and 200 symptoms have been reported to be provoked, worsened or caused by IgG allergic reactions to foods.

- It has been estimated that addictive cravings and withdrawal symptoms can be clinically significant in 20 to 30% of patients suffering from this type of allergy.

- Due to multiple foods and delayed onset of symptoms, the offending foods are rarely self-diagnosed. Multiple doctor visits involving different physicians are the rule, not the exception, before proper diagnosis and treatment is provided.

- Allergic foods in delayed reactions are commonly the person's favorite foods, frequently eaten, and eaten in larger amounts. It is interesting that people are often drawn to the foods their bodies need the least. This is unlike the Type 1 (IgE) response, where the person will have more of a tendency to avoid these immediately aggravating foods because they make the person feel unwell sooner. Even tiny amounts can provoke severe reactions in a Type 1 response.

- Allergy to foods is commonly reversible. Symptoms often clear following 3-6 months of avoidance and especially with repair of the person's leaky gut.

- Skin test negative, IgE RAST will be negative. This is a non-IgE antibody-mediated allergic reaction to foods.

- IgG ELISA (Type II) positive; IgG food immune complex (Type III) and/or cellular (Type IV) reactions may be involved as well.

- Sensitized lymphocytes, eosinophils, platelets, release of PAF and leukotrienes may be more prevalent.

Food Allergies - Learning What To Do

Food allergies are often inter-related with chronic illnesses such as arthritis, asthma, diabetes, yeast infections, and ADHD (Attention Deficit Hyperactivity Disorder), I have often seen changes in patient's behaviors and emotions once the chronic allergic reactions were overcome. Dealing with food allergies whether the condition is mild, moderate, or severe, must be learned. It includes learning the causes of allergic reactions, how to recognize the onset of symptoms cause by foods or inhaled allergens, the best options for preventing and fighting food allergies, and integrating ways into your lifestyle to avoid food allergies.

Major allergens may include eggs, dairy, gluten or wheat, corn, peanuts, shellfish, fish, oranges, bananas and chocolate.

The Hypo Allergenic Diet Sheet will give you good indications as to the most allergenic and least allergenic of foods. It is a handout I have used in my clinic for over fifteen years and it has helped countless patients over the years. You can print it and hang it on your refrigerator. Sufferers from food allergies can in time still eat the types of food they love, especially if they initially work on avoidance, food rotation and build up the integrity of their digestive system.

Candida Yeast Infections And Food Allergies

OK, so you have a yeast infection and suspect that you may have a food allergy. You may have been diagnosed with a food allergy or suspect you have one. After you have completed stage 1 implementation of the Candida Crusher Diet, it's time to move into stage 2, which is the Hypo Allergenic Diet.

Make sure you read this stage 2 section well and implement it; it will make a huge difference to your outcome long-term. After you have healed your digestive system and moved onto the 3rd stage, the Foods Re-Implementation Stage, you will notice that over time your health will have improved immensely and that your food allergy need not be a life sentence after all.

Food Reactions - Intolerances

Food intolerances are reasonably common, and many stem from poor digestion such as leaky gut, drugs like antibiotics and the ingestion of chemicals that have been added to foods, and even chemicals that are naturally occurring in foods such as salicylates and amines. But how do you determine the difference between food allergy and food intolerance? It is easier to test for a food allergy initially, especially if you have major food reactions, and if you do then I highly recommend that you complete a comprehensive IgE/IgG food allergy blood test. This will rule out any possibility of a food allergy.

Diagnosing A Food Intolerance

An elimination diet is probably the best way to diagnose any potential food intolerance. First of all, remove any suspected foods (start with processed or refined foods) completely removed from your diet for one to three weeks. A small amount of this food is then re-introduced and if symptoms reappear, the intolerance is confirmed. This elimination/challenge test can also be performed to diagnose a food allergy. If you suspect that there may be a risk of a severe reaction, foods should never be re-introduced without first consulting a health professional, especially in children. For some people, undertaking an elimination diet to get to the bottom of what is causing your food intolerance may prove to be a slow and rather frustrating process. Try to eliminate those food items you buy and enjoy regularly first. You may be quite surprised to discover that you have hit the jackpot. Above all, try to stick with it, because being free of food intolerance symptoms will be well worth in the long run.

As usual, there are no quick fixes when it comes to diagnosing and fixing a food intolerance; be very suspicious of anyone offering an easy answer, and if it sounds too good to be true, it usually is!

Common Food Intolerances

Almost any food can cause intolerance, but there are some types of food intolerances that occur more commonly than others. Lactose intolerance, a condition in which a person cannot digest the sugar found in dairy products, is one of the most common food intolerances. The main symptoms here will be bloating, gas and diarrhea.

I have seen several patients over the years that were not responsive to any food allergy test, when I suspected a food allergy, and only responded positively once certain food items were removed from their diet. I've found that salicylate, amine and glutamate sensitivities are more common than you may think, and that is why I have added this information into this section of the book.

Maybe you are at a loss as to why your allergy test has come back as negative, but you know you have issues with certain foods or drinks. It may well be salicylates, amines or glutamate. Be sure to avoid these foods and then challenge yourself to see if this is the case. You will find that a sensitivity to naturally occurring food chemicals may in some cases cause symptoms of intolerance, and these chemicals may include:

Salicylates, natural preservatives found in a wide variety of fruits, vegetables, nuts and spices.

Amines, produced during fermentation, aging and ripening

Glutamate, an amino acid found naturally in all protein foods.

Gluten, a protein found in wheat and certain other grains. It has been estimated that about 1 in 300 people in Western nations has gluten intolerance.

In some cases, it will be quite difficult to distinguish between food allergy and food intolerance, but in the end, does it really matter? In some cases only by careful elimination and challenge will you be able to discover the real culprits. So be patient and take your time, it is best to eliminate one food or food group at a time before moving onto the next. Now let's look at amines, salicylates and glutamate in a little more detail, we have already covered gluten intolerance elsewhere in this section of the book.

Salicylates

Salicylates are chemicals that occur naturally in many plants, acting as preservatives to delay rotting and to protect the plant against harmful bacteria and fungi. They are a type of insecticide that is designed to protect the plant from various bugs and insects, which they readily poison. Salicylates are stored in the bark, leaves, roots, and seeds of plants. They can be found naturally in some foods and its compounds are used in various products. Chemically speaking, salicylates resemble aspirin, and as such those who cannot tolerate aspirin will not be able to tolerate the high salicylate-containing foods either.

People can generally consume much larger amounts of these chemicals than insects, without causing too much irritation. Salicylates can affect some adults considerably though, and can particularly affect children, sometimes causing their behavior to be hyper, particularly so when a child already had asthma or eczema as well or an inherited immune weakness.

Many foods contain varying levels of naturally occurring salicylates. These allegedly may trigger symptoms in aspirin-sensitive patients. I have found the most common symptoms affecting adults to be coughs, nasal congestion, nasal polyps, post nasal drip, sneezing, rashes around the mouth and in children behavioral problems, especially hyperactivity. Only by carefully eliminating the suspected foods and challenging will you be able to work out the offenders.

Children And Salicylates

Research has discovered that up to a staggering 70 per cent of children with behaviour problems ranging from depression, lack of self control to aggressive and even violent behaviours, are affected to some degree by salicylates, artificial colours, flavours and preservatives, when compared to only about 40 per cent affected by amines.

What Are The Signs And Symptoms Of Salicylate Intolerance?

Common Symptoms
Can't smell
Congestion
Hyperactivity
Itchy skin
Rash or Hives
Nasal polyps
Persistent cough
Post Nasal Drip
Urgency to pass water
Bedwetting
Lack of concentration or Memory
Fatigue
Headaches
Sinusitis

Less Common Symptoms
Asthma
Breathing difficulties
Changes in skin color
Some cognitive and perceptual disorders
Stomachaches or upsets
Swelling of eyelids, face, and lips
Swelling of Hands and Feet
Wheezing.
Watery or Swollen eyes
Mouth ulcers or raw hot red rash around mouth
Anaphylaxis (rare)
Irritability
Diarrhea

Salicylate Content Of Foods

Fruits

Negligible: banana, pear (peeled)

Moderate: lemon, loquat, mango, pear (with skin), persimmon, red apple, rhubarb, tree tomato, kiwi fruit, and fresh fig.

High: avocado, grapefruit, granny smith apple, lychee, mandarin, mulberry, nectarine, peach, tangelo, watermelon, dried fig, and passion fruit.

Very high: apricot, blackberry, blackcurrant, blueberry, boysenberry, cherry, currant (dried), dates, grapes & grapevine leaves, guava, loganberry, orange, pineapple, plum, prune, raisin (dried), raspberry, redcurrant, rock melon (cantaloupe), strawberry, sultana. All dried fruits are generally too high in salicylates for consumption by sensitive persons.

Vegetables

Negligible: bamboo shoots, cabbage, celery, lettuce, potato (peeled), swede, dried beans, dried peas, brown lentils, red lentils, rice.

Low: Brussels sprouts, chives, choko, green beans, green peas, leeks, mungbean sprouts, red cabbage, shallots, potato (with skin).

Moderate: asparagus baby squash, beetroot, broccoli, cauliflower, carrot, kumara, marrow, mushroom, onion, parsnip, pumpkin, spinach, sweet corn, turnip, tomato (fresh), kohlrabi, black olive, chili (yellow & green).

High: alfalfa sprouts, broad beans, cucumber, eggplant, watercress, tomato (stewed/cooked)

Very high: capsicum, champignon, chicory, endive, gherkin, radish, tomato products (tinned, paste), zucchini, green olive, chili (red).

Nuts & Seeds

Negligible: poppy seeds.

Low: cashews.

Moderate: peanut butter, Brazil nut, coconut, hazelnuts, macadamia, peanuts, pecans, pine nuts, pistachio, sesame seeds, sunflower seeds, walnuts.

High: peanuts (with red skins on)

Very high: almonds, water chestnuts.

Amines

Amines are a type of chemical that occur naturally in many foods. Amines occur due to the breakdown of certain proteins or when they ferment as part of normal ripening or aging of the fresh food. Amines are responsible for giving food its flavor. The amine content will be normally higher in a food with a stronger, more intense flavor, so the more you keep that food, and the longer it ripens, the higher the amine content is likely to be. The best way to determine whether you have amine intolerance is by way of an elimination and challenge diet. Many patients I have seen over the years have worked out that one key food which can send them into a tailspin, and it could be red wine, chocolate of a soft cheese like Camembert.

What Are The Signs And Symptoms Of Amine Intolerance?

Here are some of the most common signs and symptoms of amine intolerance. I have discovered that the most common presentation for amine intolerance would have to be dull headaches, can't concentrate, IBS, lethargy, and nasal congestion.

Common Symptoms	Less Common Symptoms
Headache or migraine	Asthma
Inability to concentrate	Aggressive behaviour
Irritable bowel syndrome	Atopic dermatitis (eczema)
Lethargy (tiredness)	Depression
Nasal congestion	Diarrhea
	Fever
	Heart palpitations
	High blood pressure
	Insomnia (disturbed or lack of sleep)
	Lack of self-control
	Skin rash

Which Foods Are The Highest In Amines?

It is easier to avoid amines in your diet as opposed to salicylates, because the highest amounts of amines can be found in chocolate, aged cheeses, wine and many alcoholic beverages, cured, aged and smoked meats like sausage or salami, canned or smoked fish, fruits like banana, avocado, and tomato.

Remember, the amine content increases as certain fruits ripen or as the meat or fish ages, so if you are sensitive to any of these foods or drinks then my advice for you is to only consume the very freshest of produce, meats and fish.

Glutamates

Glutamic acid is a naturally occurring amino acid just like its brother glutamine, which is much more neurologically active. Glutamic acid is found in many foods, especially in gluten grains like wheat, barley rye but also in legumes like soy, peanuts, in dairy products, various nuts and seeds, meats and even in the gluten-substitute grains like amaranth, quinoa, tapioca as well as sorghum, millet, and flaxseed.

You will rarely hear of problems with glutamic acid as is considered to be safe, but certain side effects such as fatigue and headaches have occurred with a few people. Additionally, glutamic acid supplementation can have complications in those with kidney or liver disease, as well as people suffering from certain types of neurological diseases. I have only seen two or three people over the past twenty years of full-time naturopathic clinical work who needs to go have presented with glutamate sensitivity, and certainly seen many more people presenting with salicylate and amine sensitivities.

Glutamate converts into glutamine by the cells lining the intestinal tract, and glutamine is one of the principal foods of the tiny cells lining the walls of the small intestine. It is a good thing that the liver and kidneys also help to convert glutamate into glutamic acid, because gluten-based foods, soy, corn and dairy products (all glutamate foods) are also foods that have a tendency in susceptible people to destroy the integrity of the microvilli which line the walls of the small intestine.

What Are The Sign Of Glutamate Toxicity?

Severe headache or a throbbing headache, feeling of head expanding and contracting dizziness, pin-prick sensations, jaw tightness or throat tightness.

Did you know that it has been estimated that up to an incredible 30 percent of celiac patients may have glutamate sensitivity? Were you sensitive to vaccines? Some vaccines are high in glutamate, and an intolerance or reaction to a vaccine can be an indication of glutamate sensitivity. If you are very sensitive to MSG (monosodium glutamate) then you will almost certainly want to avoid HFCS (high fructose corn syrup) as well.

Dr. Jack Samuels, and expert in excito-toxins (nervous system poisons), states that all corn syrup products potentially contain high levels of MSG, because the producers do not remove it during processing, and it can concentrate to high levels in the syrup. Enzymes are added to HFCS as well, preventing any further breakdown of the protein. If you suspect that you are sensitive to glutamates, simply avoid corn, gluten products, soy and dairy products. A trial will soon reveal if glutamates are the culprit of not.

After a period of avoidance along with taking digestive enzymes and probiotics, you will have repaired the lining of the small intestine (leaky gut), otherwise you may become increasingly intolerant to glutamates and develop many more intolerances or allergies.

10 Tips On Avoiding Food Chemicals

1   Eat fresh foods that are low in the suspected chemicals. Plan your meals well in advance and eat fresh whenever you can. Remember that processing, reheating, transporting and storing foods can change the chemical content and may provoke symptoms. For a more trustworthy diet, always eat fresh.

2   Processed foods are not the best. The more processing the food has had the higher the risk that it will contain unwanted chemicals, additives, flavors, colors and many different preservatives.

3   Fresh meats are always preferred over smoked or processed meats. Eat fresh meat as soon as you purchase it; otherwise freeze it as soon as possible. In my opinion, processed meats are amongst the worst of all processed foods you can eat when it comes to your health.

4   Consume produce promptly. Fresh fruits and vegetables are best consumed within a few days of purchasing them. If you have two bell peppers, and pepper # 1 is one day old and pepper # 2 is three days old, the first pepper will have less amine in it. Eat fresh produce soon and buy every two to three days, or grow your own.

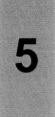

5 Avoid MSG. MSG (E621) is an amino acid commonly found in Asian foods, monosodium glutamate is an additive commonly added to foods enhance the flavor. This chemical is commonly found in Asian foods, especially Chinese foods, many snacks, chips, cookies, Campbell soups, lunchmeats, frozen dinners, and various seasonings. Studies have shown that regular consumption of MSG may result in unwanted symptoms like depression, eye damage, disorientation, headaches, and obesity. If you eat out regularly, be sure to check with the chef to make sure that there is no added MSG.

6 Avoid food dyes. Did you know that up to 90 percent of food dyes are colors that are derived from a petroleum source? Studies show that food dyes are linked to hyperactivity and disturbed behaviors in children. There are searchable databases online, and you will be able to find which synthetic dyes are used in your favorite foods.

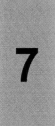

7 Avoid non-stick pans when you cook food. This may seem like a convenient way of cooking, but most non-stick cookware is made using PFOA (perfluoro octanoic acid), a toxic chemical linked to cancer and other chronic health issues. Choose stainless steel, cast iron or enameled pots and pans instead. Replace your non-stick cookware, like Teflon, with another healthier alternative. If you do continue to use non-stick cookware, be careful not to let it heat above 450°F. Throw out those non-stick pans as soon as they show signs of wear, and then go out and buy stainless or cast iron instead.

8 Avoid artificial sweeteners. Aspartame (E951), more popularly known as NutraSweet or Equal, is found in foods labeled "diet" or "sugar-free". Aspartame is now believed to be neurotoxin and carcinogenic and accounts for more reports of adverse reactions that all other food additives combined. This sweet poison is known to affect intelligence and short-term memory, and may lead to a wide variety of chronic illness including brain tumor, Parkinson's, Alzheimer's, emotional disorders like depression and anxiety attacks, dizziness, headaches, nausea, mental confusion, migraines and seizures, lymphoma, chronic fatigue, fibromyalgia, diabetes, and multiple sclerosis. You will find Aspartame in breath mints, toothpastes, chewable vitamins, ice tea, yogurt, table top sweeteners, cereals, diet foods, drink mixes, sugar-free gum, desserts, Diet Coke, sugar free soda drinks, diet drinks, Coke Zero, and jello.

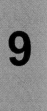

9 Avoid sodium nitrite/sodium nitrate. These chemicals are used as preservatives, flavorings and colorings. The USDA tried to ban sodium nitrite back in the 1970's, but the food manufactures won the battle as they claimed that they had no other way of preserving meat products that were packaged. This chemical is widely regarded as toxic, it is in fact carcinogenic and once it enters the bloodstream it can affect the liver and pancreas especially. You will find sodium nitrite/nitrate in smoked and preserved meats especially, such as sausages, bacon, ham, luncheon meats, corned beef, hot dogs, and canned smoked fish.

10

Avoid GMO foods. Genetically modified organisms are animals or plants that have had their DNA modified. In the United States for example, the majority of canola, corn, cotton and soybean crops have been modified genetically. The unfortunate thing is that one or more of these food items can now be found in most processed foods commercially available. The FDA has not completed sufficient safety testing on these GMO items to ensure the public that they are guaranteed 100 percent safe, especially for pregnancy women and children. Some studies have shown that consuming GMO foods increases your risk of allergy susceptibility, immune suppression, antibiotic resistance as well as increasing the risk of cancer. In light of this evidence and lack of sufficient testing, it is in your best interests to consume as little of these items as possible and to eat other foods instead.

Health Tip:

Avoid BPA

BPA is a toxic chemical used in the lining of most tin cans. Bisphenyl-A is a synthetic estrogen linked to breast cancer, reproductive problems, ADHD, obesity, other serious health problems like immune system damage. You can significantly reduce your intake of BPA by limiting your consumption of certain canned foods. The main offenders are canned foods that are acidic, salty or high in fat, because BPA is more likely to leach into these foods. Did you know that foods in cans or tins are one of your largest sources of the chemical BPA? A study has found that you can reduce your BPA intake by 60 percent in three days by avoiding packaged foods. The top ten canned foods to avoid are: Coconut Milk, Soup, Meats, Vegetables, Meals (e.g. ravioli with sauce), Juice, Fish, Beans, Meal-Replacement Drinks, and Fruits.

What To Do If You Have Been Diagnosed With A Food Intolerance

Like a food allergy, most food intolerances are dose-dependent. In some cases, large amounts of the offending food will need to be consumed before symptom become apparent, but in other instances only small amounts of foods need to be consumed. I've never seen any violent reactions in those with food intolerances like I have in those with IgE Type 1 food allergy cases however.

In some rare cases, some patients can be so violently allergic to foods like fish or peanuts that just the slightest smell of these foods can invoke the most extreme anaphylactic reactions and require the patient to be hospitalized. Look at a bee sting, for you and me it is painful and probably gone in 10 minutes, but if my son gets stung then he needs to see a doctor fast and will require a shot of adrenalin.

Those with food intolerances will probably be eating their offending foods much more regularly than those with food allergies and in larger amounts, so in many cases they will find that just be reducing the quantity of these foods there will be a significant reduction in symptoms. The amount of offending food/s tolerated is very individual, so once you have discovered what is causing your symptoms, you'll have to learn how much affects you.

Health Tip:

Take A Digestive Enzyme If You Have Any Food Reactions

A good tip when you have both food allergies and/of food intolerances is to take a digestive enzyme and a top quality probiotic, particularly as you reduce the amount of offending food/s, it will help support your digestive system significantly and you will be happy with a reduction in symptoms.

The Candida Crusher Diet

" Let your food be your medicine and medicine be your food. "
Hippocrates

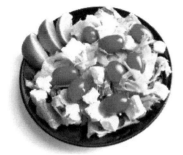

For many reasons, the mainstay of therapy for any yeast related illnesses must be directed at dietary changes. Many books and websites that specialize in candida yeast infections are product-focused, and some even call the candida diet an unachievable diet. I can tell you after treating many yeast sufferers; it is impossible to think that you will be able to cure your yeast infection permanently unless you adopt the right dietary approach long term.

The Candida Crusher Diet Is In 3 Stages.

Before you get into the Candida Crusher Diet, it pays to tidy-up your diet and lifestyle, this will pay big dividends as you go through the first few weeks of the Candida Crusher Diet.

The best results will be achieved after a person completes an initial clean up of their diet in particular, and for this reason I have devised the Big Clean Up which lasts for one week, and is ideally begun before you start on stage 1 of the Candida Crusher Diet. I'm sure that you will want to achieve the best possible results from your program, and by completing your initial Big Clean-Up you will be well on your way to achieving your goal of a permanent yeast solution with the minimal of aggravations or unnecessary yeast die-off, so commonly spoken of, so please don't skip this stage.

Don't be put off be the Candida Crusher Diet being in three-stages, after much trial and experimentation I begun to realize that the best outcomes with yeast infected patients in our clinic was when they incorporated an initial clean-up I call the Big Clean-Up, followed by an induction diet known as the MEVY Diet, and then after two to three weeks started to work on improving the integrity of their digestive system by removing any potentially reactive or allergic foods and drinks from their diet, the Low-Allergy or Hypo-Allergenic Diet, which was then followed finally by the Food Re-Introduction Diet. The duration of the Candida Crusher Diet varies from person to person, and anywhere from three to four months is on average.

Try not to skip any of the three stages for the best possible outcome, and be sure to read this section, section 1 of chapter 7 all the way through to really understand the significance of not only what foods to eat and what foods to avoid, but about diet and nutrition in general. This section is probably the most important part of this book, so be sure to follow the advice and you will almost certainly experience the same great outcomes that candida patients do who visit me in my clinic.

I wanted to make sure that you had easy access to all the contents of this book, and for this reason made an extensive contents section at the beginning of this e-book book. Each link is clickable, and hyper-linked to the information contained ahead in this comprehensive book. All you have to do is find what you are looking for in the contents and then click the link to get you to that particular information, the back-button will bring you back to the contents.

The Three Diet Stages

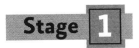

Candida Crusher Diet - Induction (The Mevy Diet) Stage

The Candida Crusher diet is in 3 stages, and each part will be covered in detail. The first stage is the Candida Diet Induction (The MEVY Diet) Stage; this stage lasts generally from two to three weeks and is best followed strictly, NO exceptions! This diet is easy to follow; you have plenty of food choices and will find it easy to do.

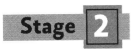

Candida Crusher - Diet Low-Allergy (Hypo-Allergenic) Stage

The second stage is the Candida Diet Low-Allergy (Hypo-Allergenic) Stage and this can last from two through to six weeks. Depending on your results in stage 1, you may not even need to go ahead with stage 2, but I would like you to do stage 2 if you are a long-standing candida sufferer, have consumed alcohol regularly for a few years or in particular have any history of taking an antibiotic (*even many years ago*), the oral contraceptive pill or any pharmaceutical drug regularly. This stage is important when it comes to healing the lining of your digestive system, especially leaky-gut, which is one of the biggest health challenges those with chronic candida face.

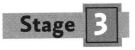

Candida Crusher Diet - Re-Implementation Stage

With the third stage it is time for Candida Diet Re-implementation Stage, this stage is mandatory like the first stage. We are now returning your diet back to normal and go about expanding the range of foods you eat, carefully testing foods to establish those which are best left alone for some time and in some cases maybe even permanently dropped off your menu. In time you should be able to eat a normal diet again, like you did before you became unwell. Do you find this hard to believe? I've seen countless people go back to foods they were told they would never eat again, in so many cases. Don't believe for one minute that you will have to avoid eating the foods you love forever, just because somebody told you so.

The Big Clean-Up

It makes sense to clean up your digestive system even before you start on the Candida Crusher Diet, even if you believe that you have a perfect diet or appear to have no digestive problems. Before you landscape your garden to perfection, doesn't it make sense to first clean up all that garbage around the garden? The first thing you do is to pick up all the rubbish, especially all that rubbish hidden in the corners and out of sight places of your garden and take it all away. Similarly, before you set about restoring your body and eradicating all that unwanted yeast overgrowth and its toxic by-products, it pays to clean up your digestive tract.

The surface area of your digestive system is huge, and not unlike a large garden. There are many places where potential yeasts, bacteria, parasites and protozoan can hide and thrive, and by sweeping out the small and large bowel in particular with a bowel purge and then a seven day cleansing diet, you will find it that much easier to tackle your Candida Crusher Program. This stage is important because it sets the foundation and will help to ease you into the Program with a lot less potential discomfort and candida die off that many people talk about.

For chronic yeast infection sufferers especially, the Big Clean-Up offers the opportunity of moving out the accumulated debris from your intestines, thereby flushing out not only the candida yeast overgrowth, but many other accumulated bugs so that Candida Crusher Program can finally deal with that ongoing infection once and for all.

When it comes to cleansing reactions of your body after commencing natural medicine treatment, I like to use the metaphor of cleaning a room. When you clean a dirty and dusty room in your house and sweep the ceiling for cobwebs, wipe down the walls and then proceed with cleaning the windows, curtains and floor you will notice that there will be dust floating in the air, you may even cough and sneeze if there is a lot of dust. You don't feel clean when you clean a dirty room, and cleaning a house properly can leave you rather dirty, have you noticed? You feel dirty and want to have a bath, because all this house cleaning has made you feel literally toxic, especially if you have left it for many years.

Cleansing your body can have you feeling rather terrible at times as well, you may sneeze and cough, develop a skin rash or fatigue, have a dull headache and potentially plenty more. Sometimes patients tell me that they are worried about "side-effects" of natural treatments, but this reaction is generally nothing more than all that dirt and grime coming to the surface of the body and causing problems.

Don't worry, these reactions are only temporary and soon clear up, and like a room you have cleaned from top to bottom, you will be delighted with the end result. Do you like a clean house? Of course you do, then tell me why are you living in a body that rarely ever gets cleaned on the inside? You take a bath daily, but what about all those organs inside, do you think that rubbish and toxins never accumulate?

Bodies, just like houses, can harbor many different and varied kinds of hidden toxins, like molds, heavy metals, pesticides, herbicides, xenoestrogens, man-made estrogen mimickers found in every day products like thin plastic cling film and countless other kinds of poisons. Sometimes these poisons can remain hidden and undetected for many years, but when you finally do detect them and remove them your health will often elevate to a whole new level, once all that dust has settled so to speak. These undetected toxins can often be the hidden source of a mystery illness, like a candida yeast infection. Yeasts like to grow in environments that are conducive to their survival, and once you change your inner environment for the better, candida will find it very difficult to gain a foothold.

A Change Is As Good As A Holiday

> *There is no true healing unless there is a change in outlook,*
> *peace of mind, and inner happiness.*
> Dr. Edward Bach

I have on many occasions witnessed that when a patient who had a chronic yeast infection moved from one house to another, or changed the country they lived in that their health improved, and in some cases the chronic yeast infection even went away entirely without any further intervention. This is a true fact, and something that used to really surprise me many years ago.

But why did this happen, and why did it take a move to bring about such a change in their health? My experience has led me to believe that it was because the person left some kind of stress behind; like work stress, a relationship stress, maybe their son, daughter, ex partner, mother in law, etc. Maybe it was a change in diet; they were deficient in a mineral or vitamin or allergic to a certain food, or perhaps a change in the air temperature or humidity.

An improvement in health can come about for many reasons, and often a change in the person's outlook by changing their residence, their occupation or their key personal relationships will bring about an improved state of health. Dr. Edward Bach (Bach Flower Essences) was a doctor many years ahead of his time, he gave a public lecture in London in the 1920's about the emotional causes of ill health and was very much scorned by the medical establishment who thought he was a fool, after all, how could emotions be a causative factor in illness, when any self-respecting doctor knew in the 20's knew that there was only one cause, and it was those nasty germs.

The upside about cleansing your body is that you will feel a lot better once this dust has finally settled, much better in fact than you have in fact for many years.

If you want a room in your house to be really clean and one that *stays* clean, you will need to clean it regularly and thoroughly, and if you want your entire house to sparkle from top to bottom then you will need to do some basic housekeeping every single day to ensure that not only the dirt doesn't build up, but that cleaning it eventually doesn't become an impossible task.

Small cleaning tasks performed regularly make a lot of sense, otherwise through procrastination a major clean up becomes overwhelming to the point that it is simply put in the too hard basket. Some people's houses, just like the inside of their bodies,

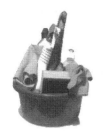 have become a real mess, and they give up even trying a simple cleansing regime causing them much embarrassment if others come to visit! You may know somebody with body odor, bad breath or a major weight problem. In some instances some people who have developed conditions such as this simply avoid social contact for embarrassment or fear of rejection and live a lonely life.

Likewise, if you drink fresh clean water every day, eat plenty of fresh, high quality organic foods and make those wise dietary and lifestyle choices your body will tend to get clean and stay clean, but don't confuse the Big Clean-Up with detoxification, I'll elaborate a lot more on detoxification in section 3 of this chapter.

Cleaning a room is certainly like cleansing your body on the inside. Dust and grime such as toxic residues may appear from those hidden recesses of the bowel, liver, kidney and lungs in particular, and deposit in the blood stream and lymphatic system.

You don't wait 30, 40 or even 50 years to clean your house, but rarely consider your body when it comes to cleansing it on the inside, so when it does finally get a clean you can and should expect some aggravations, particularly if your room has had little to no attention for several decades. Doesn't this make sense to you? It doesn't to the medical profession, who never talk about cleansing or detoxification. They claim that there is "no scientific proof" that cleansing is necessary, and that the kidneys and liver are perfectly capable of keeping the body clean. I suppose those self-cleaning ovens and dishwashers are perfectly capable as well, the fact is that we always seem to need to call the repair guy for these amazing "self-cleaning" appliances because they clog up at the least opportune moments.

The Big Clean-Up gives you the opportunity to step-down from the diet and lifestyle you were leading, including dietary and lifestyle habits that may have contributed towards the development of your yeast infection. If you are serious about beating a yeast infection then it makes sense not to skip this important cleansing step, and the longer you have had yeast issues the more reason you will need to complete it.

If you have been unwell for a number of years and can relate strongly to many of the signs and symptoms of a candida yeast infection in chapter 3, then my recommendations are for you to complete both Phase 1 (the colon cleanse) and Phase 2 (the seven day cleansing diet) and as outlined below, both of these cleansing regimes are part of the Big Clean-Up.

The Big Cleanse Is NOT Designed To Be A Detox Program

But why you ask should you clean up your digestive system, isn't that what the Candida Crusher Program is about itself? The Big Cleanse is designed to be just that, a quick cleanse, and not a detox, I'll be talking a lot more about detoxification further on in section 3 of chapter 7.

A thorough detox is not unlike reconditioning your entire house from top to bottom, you will be working on much more than just a superficial level.

Detoxification is more like completing a major renovation on your house rather than giving it a spring clean, because now you are looking at a much more heavy-duty cleansing approach which may lead to re-decorating, re-painting, and more. The first good detox you do will be like your first big renovation, after you have completed several renovations they will become much easier and with potentially a lot less aggravation because you will have removed plenty of deep seated grime that has built up over the course of many years.

Sweat Equity

Have you ever completed a major renovation on a house before? I can tell you; once you come out at the other end you realize that you overlooked several things, and that with your next renovation there would be things you would do differently. This is because there is nothing like experiencing something for real and working through all those problems that seem to arise. It is called sweat equity, and you always seem to learn best by the mistakes you make the first time round.

Would I do things differently the next time? You bet I would, and the same goes for your first cleanse, after you have completed one or two of these one-week cleanses you will begin to realize how easy they are and what to look out for the next time around. You get to know the pitfalls and traps, and just like completing small renovations which eventually give you the courage and experience to complete a major renovation, the Big Clean-Up will give you the confidence in time to complete a three or four-week detoxification program. Be patient, it will all happen in time, and you are best to wait until you have recovered from your yeast infection. You have plenty of time in the future to complete an intensive detoxification and cleansing regime but for now just concentrate on a one-week cleanse before you start on the diet.

When I recommend a detox program, I generally recommend a certain diet and a series of specialized herbal or nutritional supplement treatments to be used at the same time such as digestive enzymes, liver and kidney herbal medicines, certain probiotics and special bowel cleansing products. A detox for some people will imply the cleansing of heavy metals or chemicals, and I'll outline this kind of protocol in section 3 later in this chapter, in Understanding Cleansing and Detox. As you may be aware, a good detox is well out of the scope of the Big Clean-Up, which is just a bowel purge followed by a seven day cleansing diet and is a prelude to your Candida Crusher Program.

4 Reasons To Do The Big Clean Up

Poor diet – By neglecting to sufficiently feed our lawns, shrubs, trees and flowers, we end up with a poor garden, not unlike somebody suffering with malnutrition. Many who are about to undertake the Candida Crusher Program rely on a diet that contains nutrient depleted vegetables, grains, fruits as well as meats containing antibiotics and hormones. This type of diet provides an inadequate amount of essential nutrients for the body's countless metabolic processes, including internal cleansing.

These dietary habits, and the fact that many of us eat a limited variety of foods, consume alcohol and caffeine-containing beverages, can result in the internal congestion of our organs of elimination, in particular the small and large bowel. Even you have been adopting a "perfect" diet for some time but have a yeast infection which you have had for a long time, you will benefit from the Big Clean-Up.

Poor absorption rates – By sweeping the paths, mowing the lawns and weeding the garden you will find that the fertilizer you apply will be that much more effective. (An under-active stomach) We can get better crops, bigger flowers and truly enjoy the fruits of our labor. The other major advantage of this initial big cleanse is that the probiotics, anti-fungal foods, supplements and herbs which I recommend during the Candida Crusher Program will work that much better. The more efficiently your digestive system works, the more efficient will be your body's ability to digest foods, herbs and supplements, absorb nutrients into cells and excrete wastes.

Poor bowel functioning – By neglecting to prune the shrubs and trees, neglecting to weed the garden beds and letting the garbage pile up we end up with a garden that becomes a real eyesore. It also becomes a haven for pests and vermin, just like a person's bowel that has been neglected for many years. Some gardens have become so neglected that they may even have oil poured onto the soil, and that can mean that the garden is so seriously affected that nothing will grow there for years. This to me is like one of those gardens where you will find a dumped car body, some beer bottles thrown over the fence as well as ice cream wrappers and cigarette butts around the place. Not unlike bowel cancer, it takes years for bowel cancer to develop and the signs and symptoms have been there for many years and either ignored or accepted as a normal part of that person's life, symptoms like bloating, gas, constipation and many other digestive issues. Just because there is no pain it doesn't mean there is nothing wrong, and that's why so many people are quite surprised when the diagnosis finally comes: "But doctor, I didn't feel a thing". Some people live with a dysfunctional bowel for many years and never expect it to eventually turn into cancer. About 80 percent of people I see in my candida clinic have issues with their bowel functioning, and if you skip the occasional bowel motion or have difficulties passing daily motions easily, then you would be foolish to skip this Big Clean-Up. During the big cleanse your bowel is cleansed and purged to eliminate undesirable bowel matter and bowel plaques and helps to make your whole intestinal tract clean. This process eliminates places where yeasts, bacteria and parasites like to hide and thrive. You will not only eliminate sludge and plaques but also accumulated toxins, helping you to prevent the re-absorption of toxins when we do a proper detoxification program well down the track by allowing a clear and unhindered passage of toxic wastes to be excreted. The benefits of this initial cleanse go way beyond treating your yeast infection, and you will discover that regular bowel clean ups can help increase your energy levels, improve your mood and concentration, and help significantly with weight loss.

Poor immune system functioning – A neglected garden over time becomes a sick garden and each year the weeds become more vigorous than the year previous. The lawn, once beautiful, has now become a large tract of weeds that will take a lot of hard work to restore to its former beauty.

Some gardens in fact are all weeds and the birds and other pests just keep on spreading weed seeds until it becomes a difficult task to remedy (ulcerative colitis, leukemia, Non-Hodgkin's lymphoma, etc.) This is not unlike your immune system, and if neglected can take quite a few years to bring it back to its original and powerful state. Healthy gardens are not only beautiful and a joy to behold, they require only a few hours of work each week to maintain them.

Another concern I have with people launching straight into the MEVY Diet or stage 1 diet without cleansing their digestive tract is that they may have developed potential intolerances or allergies to some of the most commonly eaten foods like cow's milk, wheat and gluten containing products, eggs, soy, oranges, peanuts, and even banana. And how often do you hear of somebody with a yeast infection suffering from allergies, hay fever, asthma, or sinusitis? Most people I see with a chronic yeast infection have a compromised immune system, and a bowel cleanse makes digestive restoration down the track that much easier, particularly if the person has leaky gut syndrome.

I have outlined below a straightforward and very effective cleansing option below, which is a bowel purge followed by a simple cleansing diet with the option of a juice fast, and followed by a more powerful colon cleanse we call a colonic. Before you begin however, there are a few things that you need to consider:

Please Read This Before You Start Your Big Clean-Up

Before you start on the Big Clean-Up, it makes sense to eliminate any potential causes of your yeast infection. What is the point in cleaning up your digestive system if you don't address any likely causes of your yeast infection? Have you read chapter 2, the causes of a yeast infection? If not then I'd recommend you go back to chapter 2 right now, because now is time to address any likely causes, let's get rid of them once and for all. Why do you think I call the Candida Crusher Program the permanent yeast solution? If you tackle the cause and clean up the problem you have right now then you solve any future recurrence, simple as that, it can be permanently resolved.

You May Feel Worse Before You Feel Much Better

You may want to read "Aggravations and how to deal with them" previously in chapter 7. If you are quite toxic, for example, and have never completed a cleanse or detoxification program previously, or if you have had a candida yeast infection for some time then you may experience what we call "die off", you would do well to read "How people think they get well" and "How people actually get well", you will find these articles also previously in chapter 7. These articles were written to explain the healing process and they will make a lot of sense to you when you are going through or have been through the up and down process of healing from a yeast infection. Sometimes all you will need to do to reduce any aggravations is to ease up a little, drink plenty of water, rest up, take a nice long shower, bath or nice relaxing sauna and have plenty of Vitamin C.

The Big Clean-Up is in Two Phases

There is no single way which is the right way when it comes to a bowel cleanse, I have tried many and varied methods with patients over the years and will mention the main techniques which I tend to use now.

It really depends on what you want to achieve and the time you have to be able to do this cleanse. You can still complete the Big Clean-Up, even if you work full-time. For example, start your bowel flush on a Saturday and by the time Monday comes around, you will have enough experience with a bowel purge product to have enough confidence in its use, and to know how much to take.

There is no reason why you shouldn't be able to complete the Seven Day Diet while you are working, others may want to complete the Seven Day Diet during their holidays or whenever they have a quiet time at work. It makes sense to start the initial cleanse while you are working, after all, the four-month Candida Crusher Diet will be undertaken when you are working, unless you plan on going on a four to six month holiday.

I have seen many people start with the Bowel Purge (Phase 1) and then go on to complete the seven day cleansing diet (Phase 2) before they embark on the Candida Crusher Program, and this is the best option and the one I now recommend. Alternatively, you may want to complete the Bowel Purge and then simply go into a predominantly juice-based approach for five or seven days as a Phase 2 option, more on this later.

Phase 1 – The Bowel Purge

There are many different ways you can achieve this phase, but I recommend you use either a good quality Vitamin C powder or a product that was especially made to gently cleanse the bowel, Colozone.

I tend to use a dietary supplement called Colozone for a colon flush; it is a great product and works time and again. Colozone is a dietary supplement made of magnesium oxide and magnesium hydroxide; it was made specifically to gently release oxygen in the digestive tract for the purpose of cleansing the bowel. Colozone releases oxygen in the intestines for rapid and thorough, yet gentle cleansing, creating a clean and healthful internal environment and enhancing nutrient uptake. It provides much needed oxygen for proper digestion and cleanses the digestive membranes to allow better uptake of nutrients. Colozone is a high-tech solution to bowel cleansing and was developed by NASA to obtain the maximum possible oxygen release in the digestive tract.

Once the digestive tract is free of unwanted wastes, the oxygen liberated is free to be assimilated through the walls of the intestines and colon providing needed metabolic oxygen. This is a great way to begin the Candida Crusher Program and is the method of bowel cleansing I now recommend. The Big Clean-Up should be considered in any health-cleansing regime, and by cleaning the digestive tract before starting out on a candida diet most healing crises or detox reactions can be reduced significantly or even avoided.

A bowel purge can dramatically enhance the effectiveness of regimes like the Candida Crusher Program and should be seriously considered by those who want the best results. You can read all about how to take Colozone on the side of the pack or make enquiries through your supplier.

Phase 2 – The Seven-Day Cleansing Diet

There are two options available to you in the Phase 2 stage. You can either do the Seven Day Cleansing Diet, or the juicing phase. I'd recommend that if you have little to no experience that you stick with the seven-day diet option, but incorporate some juices into this diet. If you have some skills with eating very healthy, have adopted a healthy diet the past several weeks including salads, steamed and raw vegetables and have a well functioning bowel, then you could go for the Phase 2 juicing option, and you can read more about this in a moment. Try this seven day cleanse once per year for best effect, but do the Bowel Purge first to give yourself a good foundation *before* you do the diet. This cleanse is best performed is spring or summer but can be completed at any time of the year if you want to do the Candida Crusher Diet. Why spring or summer you ask? Because there is an abundance of fresh produce at this time of the year, especially fresh vegetables, berries and herbs, and you will be inclined to drink plenty more water at this warmer time of the year too.

During this seven-day period, you can eat all you want but the selection of food is quite important. It is highly recommended that no alcohol or caffeine be consumed during this cleanse. It is best that you start to reduce coffee or tea consumption a week or two before attempting this detox, and start making some changes for the better, like drinking more water and less tea and coffee. You will also notice that I recommend you have very little in the way of fruits, except for avocado or berries, and no starchy vegetables. This is because they contain sugars, which may aggravate an underlying yeast infection. A fresh juice each day is OK however, but stay with green apple, carrot, celery and beet and dilute with water, because straight vegetable juice can be a bit too strong, especially when you just start out with juice. There will be some people with candida who can tolerate certain fresh vegetable juices with The Seven-Day cleanse, more on juicing later. It is important to note that juice has very little protein and virtually no fat so by itself it is not really a complete food, therefore you should ideally be using juices in addition to your regular meals and not in place of them or you may feel tired, washed out and rather depleted. Unless you are undergoing a juice fast or a particular detoxification program it is probably unwise to use juicing as a meal replacement. Ideally, juices can be consumed with your meals, a small amount in that case, between meals or as a snack.

The Seven Day Cleanse will increase your sense of health and wellbeing and will help pave the way for the Candida Crusher Program to follow, believe me, it is THE way to go and will make your program to follow that much easier.

Your diet for the week does not have to be boring! We have found the following foods the best to have during this cleansing period. You will feel better as your body releases more and more accumulated matter, clearing digestion and restoring vigor and energy, especially if you follow-up with the Candida Crusher Diet, the stage 1 MEVY Diet, which is not unlike this seven day diet.

For many, a well performed bowel cleanse is a completely invigorating and rejuvenating process for the whole body and mind, particularly when combine with two or three saunas during this period, some dry skin brushing, perhaps followed by colonic irrigation. It is particularly important to drink plenty of water and rest up. When it comes to food, keep any cooking fresh and simple, get a cookbook from your bookstore or library and you will find plenty of options using the foods listed below.

Why A Seven-Day Diet?

This brief diet plan can be used as often as you like, but I would suggest doing it once a year, at the very least. If you follow this week long eating plan correctly, it will clean your body of impurities and can give you a feeling of wellbeing you may not have experienced for many years. Here are a few reasons why you should do this short cleansing diet:

Weight-Loss Benefits - After only a week, some people may begin to feel considerably lighter, many by five pounds, quite a few others by ten pounds, and I have even seen one or two lose as much as an amazing twenty pounds! While weight-loss results may vary from one person to another, most will lose some weight on this cleanse. Now you are thinking, how is it possible to lose this much weight in such a short period of time? It's because those whom are overweight lose a lot of accumulated fluid at first, not fat, and the fluid comes off fast, especially if you don't cheat on this diet!

Energy and Vitality Benefits - Most who undertake the Seven-Day Diet will have almost certainly noticed an abundance of energy and vitality by the end of the week. As your digestive system becomes cleansed on the inside and you take out alcohol and caffeine, the healthy food choices you have made begin to make a real difference to your health. The many cells of your body can finally utilize nutrients such as vitamins and minerals, amino acids, carbohydrates and fatty acids much more efficiently as they are taken up more readily in your stomach, small and large intestine and you start to feel great as a result. What you will probably also notice is that you will feel a positive difference in both your physical as well as your emotional and psychological disposition.

Is My Yeast Infection Gone? – Quite a few patients have asked me this question over the years. Unfortunately your yeast infection has not gone, it is still there and all you have done is cleaned up your digestive system a little. You will have reduced the yeast population by a small amount, but you simply cannot eradicate a chronic yeast infection in a mere seven days, and anybody who tells you that is incorrect and misleading you. It takes time and commitment to eradicate a candida overgrowth, and by initially taking this seven-day step you have begun your journey. Most people should count on a four-month yeast eradication program if they are serious about a permanent yeast solution.

From One Week Up To One Month - Some people may want to continue this one-week eating plan for a fortnight and some for even up to a month before they embark on the Candida Crusher Diet, especially if your diet and lifestyle have not been the best for some time, then extend this Seven-Day Diet for an extra week or two and don't be in a hurry to commence the Candida Crusher Diet. The more junk food, alcohol, and caffeine you have consumed, the more time you may want to take with this initial cleansing approach.

Get the foundation right before you start the Candida Crusher Diet in earnest, you will be glad you did, because you'll experience a lot less aggravation, trust me on this one! On the other hand, there will be others with a chronic yeast infection who have been living a healthier and cleaner lifestyle and diet for some time already, they will be content to do bowel purge then the seven-day cleanse before starting on the Candida Diet. These are the folks who don't experience major aggravations unless they push themselves really hard with the dietary supplements.

Bowel-Cleansing Additions - The Seven-Day Diet is not unlike the 1st stage of the Candida Crusher Diet, the MEVY Diet, except it is more cleansing in its approach in that we discourage any red meats and encourage white meats and even more vegetables and cleansing foods. The main reason why the Seven-Day Diet is different is that you incorporate extra bowel-cleansing foods and drinks into this cleanse, over and above what you would do while on the Candida Crusher Diet. You can read about these in a moment.

The Seven-Day Diet

20% Of Your Diet ✓
Foods to have: Fresh Fish, (no tinned, smoked fish or shellfish), Free Range Eggs & Free Range Chicken (avoid commercial poultry, get certified free range), Amaranth, Beans, Grains (whole); i.e., Barley, Oats, Lentils, Rye, Quinoa, Extra-Virgin Olive Oil, Flaxseed Oil, Unsalted Butter, Nuts (Almond, Brazil, Walnut, Hazelnut), Rice (Brown is best), Sourdough Bread, Wheat Germ and Kelp.

80% Of Your Diet ✓✓✓✓
Foods to have: Artichokes, Asparagus, Avocados, Green Beans, All Berries, Brazil Nuts, Broccoli, Brussels Sprouts, Cabbage, Capsicum, Carrots, Cauliflower, Celery, Cherries, Cucumbers, Eggplant, Endive, Herbs for seasoning (i.e. Basil, Oregano, Thyme, Coriander), Lemon, Lettuce, Mustard Greens, Okra, Parsley, Peppermint, Plain Popcorn, Pumpkin Seeds, Radishes, Rice milk, Sesame Seeds, Sunflower Seeds, Sorrel, Spinach, Tahini, Tomatoes (fresh), Turnips, Water Cress.

Some Particularly Good Bowel Cleansing Foods & Drinks: Alfalfa Sprouts, Almonds, Aloe Vera Juice (20mls twice daily in water or juice) Artichoke, Barley Grass or a Green Powder (1 heaped tsp./day in juice or water), Beetroot, Buckwheat, Broccoli, Brown Rice, Cabbage, Capsicum, Chives, Garlic (eat 2 fresh cloves daily), Ginger (eat some fresh grated ginger every day), Herbal tea, Millet, Onions (includes: Leeks, Red & Brown Onions & Shallots), LSA Mix – have 1 – 2 tablespoons per day on foods (linseeds, sunflower seeds and almonds ground up), Parsley, Pure Water, Turmeric Powder ($\frac{1}{2}$-1 tsp./day). Eat bitter foods: Lemon, Capers, Endive, Rocket, Organic Cider Vinegar (Bragg's). Herbs, the best are Rosemary, Thyme, Sage, Marjoram, Oregano and Parsley. Fresh is the best. Use spices like Cloves, Cinnamon, Pepper and Nutmeg to help wipe out any bad bacteria in your digestive system & to add flavor and interest. Each morning, have one large glass of water with the juice of ½ - 1 Lemon – then follow with a glass of water to which you have added ½ - 1 tsp. of Vitamin C Powder.

Drink: Dandelion Root Coffee, and also plenty of freshly filtered, bottled or mineral water (non-sparkling), organic herbal teas e.g. Chamomile, Dill, Lemongrass, Lemon Balm, Nettle, Peppermint, etc. For an excellent cleanse, drink Vegetable Juice daily. Drink at least 1 glass of a blend of Carrot; Green Apple, Celery and Beetroot juice daily, mix together, as this is excellent for cleansing the bowel, liver, and kidneys and for purifying the blood. Dilute with 50% water and have half a glass to one glass twice daily between meals.

Better To Avoid: Bananas, Chocolate, Processed Cereals, Commercial Bread Toppings like Marmalade, Jam, Peanut Butter and Chocolate Spreads, etc., Fruit Juice (with added sugar), Soda or Energy Drinks, Gravies, Jellies, Candy or Sweets, Peanuts, Pistachios, Meat Pies, Pastries, Shellfish, Sugar (white or brown, any), ALL Dairy products such as Milk, Ice Cream, Sweetened Yoghurt (Natural Yogurt is best), Cream, all Cheeses, Margarine, Wheat based Breads, Pasta or other Wheat Flour products e.g. Breads, Cakes, Bagels, Donuts or Biscuits, Cookies. Red Meats, Pork, Lamb, Venison, Take Away, Pizza, Burger Take-Out Foods like McDonalds, Milk Shakes, Chicken Nuggets, etc.; in fact, any foods that contain a high element of sugar, salt or fat.

Don't eat out for the Big Clean-Up; it is best to prepare all your own food at home. Don't deep fry foods in fats or oils but steam, grill or simmer foods, this will be easier on your digestion. Use Olive Oil primarily in cooking.

It is best that you avoid all fresh and dried fruits for seven days (except Avocado and Berries) as well as starchy vegetables such as sweet potatoes, potatoes, yams, corn, all winter squash, beets, peas and parsnips. They all contain sugars and by stopping them now you will find it a lot easier, and by doing so you will find the MEVY Diet of the Candida Crusher Program easy if you follow this seven day cleansing diet beforehand. Just follow the above dietary approach for 7 to 10 days and do it strictly.

The main thing is to avoid all fast or take-out foods, eat fresh and if at all possible, eat organic produce. You can cleanse your bowel most effectively by just cutting out the garbage foods from your diet and focusing on steamed vegetables, high quality proteins (lean meats) and drinking plenty of good quality water, it's as simple as that. Although you can achieve a good result without requiring colon cleanse (option 2), colonic irrigation in conjunction with this Seven-Day Diet will give you a fantastic foundation to begin you Candida Crusher Diet.

5 Cleansing Recipes For Your Big Clean Up

1 The Potassium Broth

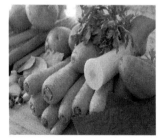

Potassium Broth is a kind of soup made from vegetables (root vegetables in particular), which are rich in many minerals, including potassium, calcium and magnesium. This beverage is an excellent rejuvenator and tonic for those who want to cleanse and alkalize their body. Potassium broth is excellent for those who are interested in detoxification or for those who have recently had surgery or suffered with an extended chronic illness.

It is also a good choice for a woman who has recently had a child and who wants to give herself a good boost. Be sure to use the freshest vegetables you can, and preferably home grown or organic. If you want to boost Potassium Broth then add a few tablespoons of liquid whey (Molkosan) during the cooling stage, whey will assist digestion and absorption of the copious amounts of potassium and the many other minerals present in this broth. You can read more about Molkosan, the amazing Swiss whey tonic under the section on Fermented and Cultured Foods previously in this Chapter.

The Potassium Broth Recipe

- 3-4 potatoes, peeled and diced

- 1 small onion, diced

- 3 stalks of fresh grown celery, thinly sliced

- 2 fresh grown carrots, thinly sliced

- A small bunch of fresh parsley

- 1 large handful of chopped greens such as kale, chard, or leek

- Liquid whey

Place ingredients in 3 quarts (about 3 liters) of good quality clean water. Bring to boil and gently simmer for 20 minutes, strain the liquid and discard the vegetables. If you'd like to spice it up a little, throw in some cayenne pepper. You should drink 2-3 bowls of this vegetable broth each day to replace depleted minerals. Use organic vegetables whenever possible.

You might be wondering, "If root vegetables such as potatoes and carrots and are on the Candida Foods To Avoid list in the Candida Crusher Diet, then why are they in the Potassium Broth you recommend?" Good question and it shows me you are observant, you are only taking this broth for a seven-day period, and because the broth has simmered for some time and has whey added to it, I have found that it doesn't cause any problems whatsoever with aggravating an existing yeast infection.

Have you made more Potassium Broth than you can consume in a few days? This dish freezes well, so freeze what you will not use in three to four days.

2 Lemon –A Most Alkalizing Drink

Now here is a great morning drink that has an amazingly alkalizing effect on your body. It takes a little getting used to but if you want to blitz a bacterial or a yeast infection and prepare yourself for a good cleanse then I can highly recommend this amazingly effective morning drink.

It not only alkalizes your body totally, and especially your digestive system that houses candida, it makes peroxide inside your body, which encourages apoptosis, the death of rogue cells or cells which may turn cancerous, and is a super powerful anti-oxidant boost. This drink has a particularly powerful effect on your liver and gallbladder and is an amazingly effective liver cleanser and regenerator, especially if you are like me and consume plenty of olive oil in your diet. After all, lemon juice and olive oil are the two main features of a liver & gallbladder flush.

Bacteria and yeasts thrive in an acid environment, and by taking this drink regularly before breakfast you are discouraging dysbiosis and encouraging your body eradicate yeasts and bad bacteria. Lemon juice has no effect on beneficial bacteria.

The Alkalizing Drink Recipe

Try juicing 3 – 4 whole lemons and drinking the juice straight, preferably with little or no water. I told you it takes a little getting used to! Rinse your mouth with a little water after and swallow. Caution with straight lemon juice in your mouth, some may notice that their tooth enamel may be sensitive to the effects of citric acid, so be sure to rinse with clean water after and swallow.

3 Dandelion Coffee & Tea

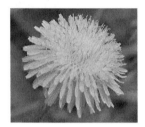

Have you ever tried dandelion coffee from roasted 2-year-old dandelion roots, or dandelion tea, dried leaves of 2-year-old dandelion plants? Dandelions are a great source of iron, vitamin A, calcium as well as potassium. Dandelion root coffee is good for your liver, whereas dandelion tea made from the leaves will have more of an action on your kidneys. These beverages eliminate bodily toxins through your liver and kidneys and are an excellent adjunct with your Big Clean Up.

The Dandelion Drink Recipe

Take 6 tablespoons of 2-year-old dried dandelion roots and 6 tablespoons of 2-year-old dried dandelion leaves in 4 cups of purified, boiling water. Leave the brew with the lid on in a stainless steel, ceramic or glass teapot. Avoid aluminum. If you are after a more kidney cleansing effect, try 12 tablespoons of fresh dandelion leaves and allow brewing for ten minutes. If you are after a more liver tonifying effect, have the dried root. You can grow dandelions readily in your garden or buy these items dried from your health-food store.

4 Creamy Coconut Drink

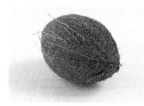

You can read more about the virtues of coconut and candida later in this book, but suffice to say this is an excellent cleansing, satisfying as well as a very tasty drink for those who are interested in beating candida. Coconut contains caprylic acid that has a prominent anti-fungal action. Be sure not to add any form of sugar to the following drink, just add some pure vanilla extract or some real vanilla bean and you will be most impressed by the flavor and fragrance of this wonderful beverage. Have one drink each day; you can have this drink throughout both the Big Clean-Up as well as the entire Candida Crusher Program. Once you get used to the wonderful flavor of coconut drink it is hard to beat. By the way, avoid coconut milk in a can or tetra pack, it may contain Bisphenyl-a, as your retailer for a BPA free coconut milk, there will be one.

Creamy Coconut Drink Recipes

Home Made Coconut Cream Recipe

You can either buy coconut cream from the grocery or health-food store, or you can save pennies by making your own. All you need to do is to mix organic shredded dried coconut with pure luke-warm water and blend it well, simple as that.

I have found that a ratio or one part coconut to three or four parts water works best. The best way and the way to liberate most of the oil from the shredded coconut is to add one cup of boiling water to four parts of shredded coconut and blend immediately until creamy, then strain through a fine mesh strainer or a fine colander. This creamy milk will store in your refrigerator for several days, but I doubt it will last that long! And again, try adding vanilla bean to this recipe.

B Hot Coconut Drink Recipe

Now that you have some coconut cream, all you need to do is to add one cup to a small saucepan, add ¼ - ½ teaspoon vanilla extract (or better still, add half a dried vanilla bean) and bring to a high temperature, stirring well for a few minutes. Take off the heat, pour into a mug and enjoy. This is a great drink to have before you go to sleep.

Water

Yes, plain old water, not exactly a recipe, but certainly a recipe for disaster if you don't drink water during cleansing or detox. Have you ever tried to clean a house or a car without water? The reason why I added this here is to remind you to drink! Most people I see in my practice are dehydrated, and if you are dehydrated and expect to get the most out of your Big Clean-Up, and also from the Candida Crusher Program then you are kidding yourself.

Water makes up well over half of your body weight; every system in your body relies on water. Water is responsible for giving you beautiful, supple skin and regular bowel motions and is particularly important in helping to remove and flush out toxins and carry those all important nutrients to the countless cells of your body, needless to say - water is critical for good health. Daily you will lose an incredible ten to twelve cups of the stuff through perspiration, breathing, and urine as well as by way of bowel motions. While food and drinks do account for a lot of water we need, we invariably end up with a shortfall so it is most important that you drink more, and you need more especially if you expect to clean your body up.

Great Health Tip:

Great Health Tip

Drink a glass soon after you wake up, because you always wake-up dehydrated, and also before each meal. Avoid distilled water; it is essentially dead water that is devoid of oxygen making it a most unnatural way of drinking water. Stick with water bottled, preferably in glass, or get a reverse osmosis water purifier. Avoid drinking water containing fluoride or chlorine if you can, filtered water is always better.

Fiber For Cleansing

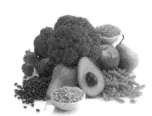

Fiber is a great idea when it comes to cleansing your digestive system, but some people tend to think that fiber is only good for those with constipation. Fiber performs many beneficial actions once inside your digestive tract, for example it combines with bile acids, and dead bacteria and other waste that enables a good bowel motion to be formed which in turn allows the easy passage of wastes from the digestive system. Fiber also slows digestion down a little and allows better control of the appetite, which allows you to be able to maintain your weight better. But wait, there's more, those who eat plenty of fiber are less likely to develop a whole host of chronic diseases like cancer, heart disease and diabetes.

Fiber and Candida

Although fiber does not eliminate candida-related health problems directly, dietary changes certainly have been linked with reduced symptoms, according to the University of Maryland Medical Center in America. And this is why I think it is smart for you to stop thinking only about killing candida and rather about re-populating your digestive system with friendly bacteria. The killing method is almost always encouraged by dietary supplement companies who may tell you that you will be unable to conquer your yeast infection by diet primarily, but the truth is you can, but it is difficult and drawn out process and therefore I have always found it best to recommend a few high quality supplements to speed up the process and ensure a more effective, complete and thorough eradication of candida. But in saying that, nothing takes place of a diet high in nutrients and fiber, nothing. Always remember that food is your medicine and medicine is your food. A great diet in addition to great supplements will win hands down, particularly with the right lifestyle changes.

A diet which is high in added sugars often lacks fiber, vitamins and minerals, and by following a diet high in fiber it will invariably lead not only to an increased fiber intake which will be good for your digestive system in many ways, it will also ensure by default that you get a good boost of vitamins and minerals which are often found in these high fiber foods, and that will certainly boost your wellness, especially if you eat organic or high quality fresh produce.

Furthermore, fiber allows a better balance of beneficial bacteria in your digestive tract and tends to put the squeeze on candida species, reducing their numbers. Fiber is important to re-establish a healthy bowel function, and could hold the key between success and failure if you are serious about improving your digestive health and finally ridding your body of that yeast infection you have had for years. There are several options when it comes to having more fiber in your diet, you can have high fiber foods and also include a few high fiber supplements in your diet.

Great Health Tip:

Introduce fiber gradually into your diet, you will have less gas

If you introduce fiber into your diet too quickly, you may well experience a lot more gas and possibly bloating. By introducing fiber slowly into your diet you allow the beneficial bacteria to grow in direct proportion, they crowd out the bad bugs and reduce your ability to produce gas. Make sure you drink lots of water; because plenty of water in your digestive system moves things around a lot easier, and without the liquid your stool becomes a stronger bind in the colon. Do the eyeball test, pay attention to what you flush and if it formed much too hard, e.g. it is quite difficult to evacuate or very hard, then increase your fiber intake gradually. Still having lots of gas? Then try a good probiotic containing Lactobacillus acidophilus and take one capsule with each meal. That should put an end to the gas within a week, no more embarrassment.

Avoid Commercial High-Fiber Powdered Products

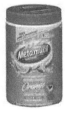

If you want to take a powdered supplement, my recommendations are to stay away from commercial high-fiber powdered products; many include the addition of artificial sugars, colors and preservatives and some are made by drug companies. On the Metamucil Smooth Powder pack it states: "Sucrose, Psyllium Husk Powder". Great, so you buy a product to add fiber to your diet, and the main ingredient is… sugar?

Other commercial psyllium powders contain aspartame, an artificial sugar. Be sure to read labels before you buy any commercial product and see for yourself and if it contains any sugar, put it back.

Do the sensible thing and get yourself some slippery elm bark powder, the pinker the color, the higher quality the grade, and try also some psyllium hulls. Any good health food shop will be able to help you with a top quality natural fiber supplement.

Psyllium is very effective, but can be a bit hard on the intestines for those who suffer from leaky gut syndrome. Another alternative is to try acacia powder or pure apple fiber. Flax seed meal is good too, and you may like to try the LSA mix you will read about further on.

Soluble and Insoluble Fiber

What is the difference? Soluble fiber dissolves in water and insoluble fiber does not. They both have their merits, but let's examine both these types of fibers in more detail and see what benefits they have to offer you.

Soluble fiber attracts water and forms a gel, which slows down digestion. Soluble fiber delays the emptying of your stomach and makes you feel full, which helps control your appetite and therefore your weight. Slower stomach emptying may also positively affect your blood sugar level and have a beneficial effect on insulin sensitivity, which may help control diabetes. Soluble fiber can also help lower LDL, the bad cholesterol, by interfering with its absorption and maximizing excretion of bad cholesterol.

Sources of soluble fiber: oatmeal, oat cereal, lentils, apples, oranges, pears, oat bran, strawberries, nuts, flaxseeds, beans, dried peas, blueberries, psyllium, slippery elm bark powder, cucumbers, celery, and carrots.

Insoluble fiber is considered a digestive-healthy fiber because it has a laxative effect and adds bulk to the diet, helping prevent constipation. These fibers do not dissolve in water, so they pass through the gastrointestinal tract relatively intact, and speed up the passage of food and waste through your gut. Insoluble fibers are mainly found in whole grains and vegetables, especially the leafy greens.

Sources of insoluble fiber: whole wheat, whole grains, wheat bran, corn bran, seeds, nuts, barley, couscous, brown rice, bulgur, zucchini, celery, broccoli, cabbage, onions, tomatoes, carrots, cucumbers, green beans, dark leafy vegetables, raisins, grapes, fruit, and root vegetable skins.

How Much Fiber Do I Need?

It is a fact that most of us adults in Western countries get only about 15 grams of fiber per day in their diet. Experts agree that around 25 to 30 grams per day is a good amount for most adult females, and males require more at around 30 to 35 grams. I'll bet you won't be consuming this amount right now, and if you start eating the way I recommend with the Seven Day Diet you will most certainly be increasing your intake of fiber.

Don't be too concerned about what type of fiber you eat, soluble or insoluble unless you are looking to improve a specific health problem like lowering your cholesterol. Soluble fiber will help lower cholesterol levels. Just focus your attention on a diet rich in vegetables, fruits, (remembering to avoid the sweet fruits initially), whole grains, legumes, seeds and nuts. Eating a diet like this will provide your body with a wide range of both soluble as well as insoluble fibers.

The High-Fiber Cleansing Drink

Here is a great drink you can have once a day on the Seven Day Cleansing Diet, I highly recommend this drink that is best consumed in the morning before breakfast. Try the psyllium hulls, but if you have food allergies, leaky gut syndrome or irritable bowel syndrome then you may want to try a tablespoon of slippery elm bark powder instead.

- 1 large glass of water (about 300mls)

- 1 tablespoon of soluble fiber slippery elm bark powder or psyllium hulls.

- 1 tablespoon of bentonite clay (or take 4 – 5 capsules).

Bentonite Clay For Cleansing

A question I have heard numerous times is why should I drink clay?

Bentonite clay is a powerful cleanser because it grabs toxins in the bowel and helps to pull them out. When bentonite clay absorbs water and swells up and is stretched open like a highly porous sponge. In fact, according to the *Canadian Journal of Microbiology*, bentonite clay can even absorb pathogenic viruses, as well as herbicides and even pesticides. Toxins are drawn into these spaces through electrical attraction and are bound to it. Due to bentonite clay's highly charged microscopic crystal formation, some experts even believe that it contains an electromagnetic energy capable of improving cell repair time. Bentonite clay is completely safe when taken internally because the body does not absorb it. Clay has been gaining popularity in many countries around the world because of its ability to bind to, absorb and then rid the body of many different kinds of toxin; therefore it is perfect for our Seven Day Cleanse.

Bentonite clay doesn't mix that well with water, be sure to stir the psyllium and clay mixture very well in water for several seconds and then drink before it settles. For the best results, drink a second glass of water immediately after. The combination of the clay and the soluble fiber (psyllium or slippery elm bark powder) will help to bind to toxins in the digestive system and move the waste out of the colon. There is no reason why you couldn't continue to take this High Fiber Cleansing drink well into your Candida Crusher Program, especially if it benefits your bowel function and you feel better for it.

High Fiber Supplement – LSA Mix

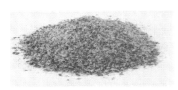

Have you tried LSA mix? LSA *(Linseed-Sunflower-Almond)* is a seed-meal supplement often recommended by the natural health fraternity, and easy to make at home, don't buy it – make you own. This food supplement is an excellent source of essential omega 3 oils, protein-building amino acids, minerals, vitamins, and fiber. LSA is not only a good choice for those on the Seven Day Cleansing Diet; it can be used throughout the Candida Crusher Program.

You can sprinkle LSA over breakfast cereals, desserts, salads, or any dish to pump up the wholesomeness. Health food shops often sell it, but they charge a premium over the raw ingredients and it may not be as fresh as you think! Here's how to make your own:

LSA Ingredients

1.   Kitchen blender

2.   1 cup raw linseed (flax seed)

3.   2/3 cup raw sunflower seeds (hulled)

4.   1/3 cup raw almonds (shelled)

5.   An airtight storage container

Great Health Tip:

Edible Bean De-Gasification

Beans are a great source of dietary fiber, but the unfortunate thing is that they sure can make you pass a lot of wind. How many times have you eaten chickpeas, navy or pinto beans or any other type of beans and had a problem with wind? Well, here is an effective solution and one that I've tried myself, it works and is a great idea.

I heard this great tip a while ago when I was at a health seminar in Seattle, it is called "edible bean de-gasification" No kidding! When soaking beans before cooking, add 2-3 drops SSKI, (super saturated potassium iodide) and allow soaking for at least one hour. (SSKI inhibits the amylase inhibitor in beans, allowing better digestion and less gas. (Thanks go to Richard Kunin, M.D, USA.)

You should be able to buy SSKI from your chemist or find an online supplier.

Another tip I heard from a vegetarian patient who eats beans every day is to soak beans and then drain and freeze them for several hours before cooking. You will find that this too has an effect of reducing the amount of gas your bowel seems to produce after you have eaten cooked beans.

Cleaning Up With Fruit and Vegetables Juices

As I mentioned earlier, there are two ways you can do Phase 2 of the Big Clean up, you can either do:

1) **The Bowel Purge and then the Seven Day Cleansing Diet**

   Or

2) **The Bowel Purge and then the Juice Diet.**

Who Should Do The Seven Day Cleansing Diet?

But why should you have the choice of either these two programs, why make it difficult by offering different choices? Because some who attempt the Big Clean-Up will have less experience than others when it comes to eating healthy, they may want to improve their health after drinking coffee, alcohol and maybe even smoking.

For those folks I'd recommend option 1 - Phase 1 (the Bowel Purge) and then Phase 2 (the Seven Day Cleansing Diet).

Who Should Do The Juice Diet?

Other readers will have already begun to clean up their act so to speak, may have taken dietary supplements and/or herbal medicines for some time. They may have previous experience with a naturopathic doctor, a detox program, a weight loss program or feel a lot more confident generally in tackling a different approach, and for those I'd recommend the second option: the Bowel Purge, followed by the Juice Diet. You have already read about the Seven-Day Diet previously, now I'd like to explain about option 2 that involves the juicing cleanse.

If you are serious about the Big Clean-Up and want to tackle the juicing cleanse, then first let's establish one thing, bowel function. The Bowel Purge is especially relevant if you have a history of a problem bowel with regular bouts of constipation, maybe a history of antibiotics or have relied on fiber products or even laxatives on/off over the years. But even if you consider your bowel to be in good shape, the Bowel Purge will pave the way for further cleansing.

Why Juicing?

> *When you're green inside, you're clean inside.*
> Dr. Bernard Jensen

After having worked with many candida patients I am absolutely convinced that juicing can be one of the most successful nutritional options, it can give yeast infected patients a radiant, energetic life, and truly optimal digestive function leading to excellent health.

Juicing may not agree with some people with yeast infections, but with others it will be fine, so it may be a case of trial and error for you.

I'm not there to assist you with your particular case so I'd recommend you give it a try, particularly as you improve. Here are some of the main reasons why juicing is so good:

1. Juicing is so good because all those valuable and sensitive micronutrients locked in your fresh foods become damaged and even destroyed when you heat up foods, and juicing every day ensures you lose virtually none of these nutrients. As soon as you heat up food and process it in any way you begin to alter the shape and chemical composition.

2. You may well have heard that we all need to eat between five to eight servings of fruit and vegetables daily if we want to maintain optimal health, and what easier way to achieve this than by juicing. Daily juicing is the easiest way to guarantee than you will take in your daily quota.

3. Nutrients are more easily absorbed from juices as opposed to eating them cooked. Many people reading this will have an impaired digestive system, and consuming vegetable and fruit juices allows your body to more easily access all those critical minerals, trace elements and other nutritional factors.

4. You eat a larger variety of vegetables and fruits by juicing them. It is a fact that most of us tend to eat the same vegetables and fruits, by juicing you eat a much larger selection and therefore increase your chances of getting all those important nutrients you wouldn't otherwise consume. Eating the same vegetables and fruits violates the principle of food rotation and increases your chance of developing an allergy or intolerance to a certain food.

Keep an open mind and don't think that juicing is not for you because you have a yeast infection, or because you have been told or read online that you should strictly avoid all fruits and limit many vegetable juices because the yeast will thrive of the sugars in juices. Can you imagine what the cells of your body experience once you start to drink fresh juice every day?

You will be absolutely amazed at the difference it can make to any underlying chronic health complaint you may well have had forever, regardless of whether it is diabetes, heart disease, high blood pressure or a chronic candida yeast infection.

Great Health Tip:

Avoid 100 percent fruit juices because most contain too much sugar.

When some folks here of the word "juice", they immediately think of a glass of fresh sweet orange or grape juice. These juices are full of sugar and contain little to no fiber generally. Some people switch soda drinks for orange juice and believe they are doing themselves a healthy favor, when in fact they have swapped one sweet drink for another. Consider mixing vegetable juice (80%) with fruit juice (20%) for a healthier drink.

Faster Uptake by Your Bloodstream

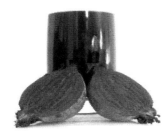

When you drink fresh vegetable and fruit juices you are greatly reducing the digestive process that normally occur when you consume whole food. The vitamins, minerals, antioxidants and enzymes of fresh juice are easily transported across the intestine walls into the bloodstream, where they become available for use by the body.

Need to Improve Energy Levels, Reduce Aging, Lose Weight?

Fresh vegetable and fruit juices have been proven to contribute to overall good health. People who juice regularly have more energy and stamina, and improved immune function, which will mean fewer colds. Juicing has also been shown to have a positive effect on cardiovascular health, blood pressure, and the aging process itself. It can also be very important in any weight loss program.

Is A Typical Western Diet Dangerous To Your Health?

Most people who eat the typical diet are consuming too many overcooked and processed foods that are high in fat, calories, sugar and salt. In addition, these foods contain food additives, preservatives, and artificial colors and flavors. Fresh juices are a way for you to get the good nutrition you need without the calories, fat, or additives. Natural juices are certainly far more healthful that the liquids we often consume, like soft drinks, coffee, tea or alcoholic beverages.

Even bottled, canned, or concentrated juices cannot match the nutrient value of freshly prepared juices. Most canned or bottled juices have been pasteurized which destroys many of the nutrients in juices. Often preservatives and artificial colors are added.

Great Health Tip:

Don't throw away that fiber!

Only one cup of freshly juiced carrots contains the nutrients in found in an amazing four cups of raw, chopped carrots. Did you know that two cups of mixed vegetable juice gives your body the same amount of live enzymes, vitamins, and minerals that are available in two large vegetable salads? Not only are the same amounts of nutrients available, they are available in a form that is much more easily digested and assimilated. If you drink juice you then have to get your fiber elsewhere so why not blend everything together – the juice and extracted pulp and eat whole foods like nature intended?

The problem I have with vegetable juicing is that many people who juice, throw the valuable fiber away. They just drink the juice and don't consume the fiber, and that doesn't make sense to me.

But why have the fiber AND juice? Here are 4 good reasons:

1 **Your blood sugar will be more stable.** If you drink straight juice then the sugars get into the bloodstream too quickly, rapidly raising your blood sugar and causing other problems the body has to then deal with, such as high insulin and cortisol. It can be counter-productive and do more damage than good. The fiber allows the nutrients to enter the blood stream at the right amount, just like nature intended because it created the juice and fiber at the same time. Juicing may even cause your blood sugar to rise rapidly like drinking soda. This is especially the case if you drink carrot juice made from those fancy new hybrid carrots or apples, bred to taste sweeter. Yes, many fruits and vegetables are hybridized to contain more sugar for increased consumption with their unnaturally high sugar content. I believe the real reason many love to drink carrot; apple or orange juice is because they are in fact satisfying their craving for sugar. They may be in the erroneous belief that giving up that chocolate bar for a glass of carrot juice is a healthy choice, when in fact they are just trading sugars to feed their addiction. Whole foods slow down the digestive process as well as the assimilation of vital nutrients that helps to prevent low blood sugar. Diabetics for example should avoid juices with no fiber, and will feel much better when they include fiber in their diets.

2 **Fiber is your intestinal broom.** The second reason is that all that pulp or fiber inside the fruits and vegetables you juice acts like an intestinal broom inside your digestive tract. And this fiber is a critical part of the whole digestive process. Without the fiber, the system slows down and can even come to a grinding halt causing constipation. Fiber is also essential for many other reasons; for example, beneficial bacteria require fiber to thrive.

3 **Whole foods are best consumed.** It makes sense to eat whole foods, because this is exactly what nature intended us to eat. Whole foods like fruits and vegetables contain water, minerals, vitamins, and many other phytonutrients in addition to plenty of fiber.

4 **Juices containing fiber satisfy you for longer.** When you drink juices containing fiber, you will find that they satisfy your appetite longer than juices containing no fiber. This can result in an improved appetite and reduction in foods consumed that will lead to improved weight control.

Drink The Juice
Of Vegetables And Fruits You Actually Enjoy Eating

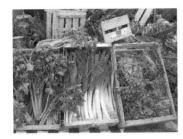

When I first started juicing I read a few books that were written by people who were juicing fanatics. I started to experiment with many different types of fruit and vegetable juices and in different combinations. I now tell patients to juice the vegetables they actually like to eat, and with experience they can start to juice the vegetables they don't generally like to eat, and these are often the stronger tasting or bitter vegetables.

You will generally keep eating and drinking things you like the most, and tend to avoid those things you like the least, but it is the things you like the least that your body seems to need the most. The bitter vegetables stimulate your digestion and are required by most people; especially those with yeast infections, and people with rampant and chronic yeast infections most always favor the sweeter foods. Sweeter juices can promote the proliferation of yeasts in the body, but only when drunk in excess.

Remember to listen to your body, and if you start to feel nauseous or your stomach starts to make all kinds of sounds after you have had your juice then you may have taken a vegetable or fruit in that you shouldn't have. Before you decide that it's not for you, try diluting the juice with water and try different juice combinations. Experience will soon tell you what suits your taste as well as your digestion and what doesn't, and with experimentation you will discover over time that you will soon work out what suits and what doesn't in terms of your yeast infection.

For example, drinking too much alcohol will soon make you realize that are going to feel pretty bad, and intelligent drinkers will know their limits. Intelligent folk who juice regularly will soon work out what kind of juices they can tolerate, how much juice they can drink and when and what the best juices for them are. Unlike alcohol, vegetable and fruit juices are actually *good* for you and never let anyone tell you that juices make a yeast infection worse unless you drink straight orange juice or other high sugar containing fruit juices on a regular basis.

Are You Are New To Juicing?

Some of you who are reading the Candida Crusher will have never juiced before, others may have tried it in the past and not continued on, and yet others juice daily. If you are a newbie, then I'd highly recommend starting out with these vegetables that are not as nutrient dense as others, but they are the easiest to digest and tolerate:

Category 1 Juices

- Celery

- Carrot

- Fennel (if you like an aniseed taste)

- Cucumber

- Granny Smith Green Apple

- Tomato

You don't need to blend them all together, try each one on its own to get a feel for the taste, and then combine and see what you like. When you first start out you may want to initially dilute your juices with up to 50 percent of filtered water. Some candida patients can tolerate pineapple juice and find it an excellent fruit juice to combine with vegetables, others I know simply cannot tolerate pineapple. It's all about trial and error.

It won't be long before you will want to experiment more with other vegetables, when you gain a little experience with category 1, try these:

Category 2 Juices

- Lettuce (red, green, romaine, etc.)

- Endive

- Spinach

- Rocket (and other salad greens)

- Bok choy, Chinese vegetables

- Peppers

- Beets

- Coriander

- Kiwi Fruit

Are you ready to take the plunge and go all out when it comes to juicing? These are very nutrient dense choices and considered some of the healthiest vegetables and many of these choices are a wise addition to your juices for those with a yeast infection. You can of course try them as a beginner, but my suggestion is to start with category 1 choices first, move to category 2 and then move on to these choices, category 3.

With increasing experience you will want to go for these juices, they can be blended in with the others suggested above. The strongest tasting juices generally confer the most health benefits. They contain an extensive amount of phytonutrients and enzymes and will be a great step in the right direction as far as great health is concerned. Be warned, category 3 juices are not for the faint hearted, they taste strong and are best taken once you have a little experience with the other two categories.

Category 3 Juices

- Broccoli, Cauliflower, Brussels sprouts, Collards

- Leeks, Garlic, Onions and Shallots

- Radish

How Can I Make My Juice Taste Better?

Occasionally somebody asks me how they can make juice taste better, I've heard the odd person over time complain that juices taste unpalatable. This need not be so! As you gain more experience with juices, it will become apparent that this becomes much less of an issue, trust me. Here are a few things you can do to improve the flavor and palatability, however:

- Lemon or lime juice. Citrus juices add a fresh taste to your juice, and in some cases they will stop juices from becoming brown. I like to juice a small lemon or lime whole, and include the rind as well as the seeds.

- Berries. You'd be surprised how nice juice tastes with the addition of a few berries; you can add them fresh or frozen.

- Pineapple. If you can tolerate fresh pineapple you are lucky, I know that many with candida can and find that juicing is great because of it. This tasty fruit can add a whole new dimension to your juicing regime, experiment!

- Ginger. Add a little grated fresh ginger to your juice, it will give a little zing to your juice and I have found that ginger can go in just about every juice combination. Only by experimentation will you be able to discover what works for you and what doesn't.

- Vanilla. Try adding a few drops of natural, organic vanilla extract. This stuff is heaven and can transform a bitter, and seemingly unpalatable drink into bliss.

- Icecubes. These add texture and drop the temperature of the drink, sometimes just by adding two or three ice cubes you change the whole experience, try it.

Green Vegetables

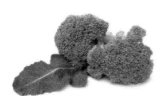

Green vegetables are important sources of potent phytochemicals that can have a major impact on your health; they are an excellent choice for those with a yeast infection looking for an instant way of gaining many valuable minerals, trace elements and many other important plant based chemicals not stored in your body.

Most of this benefit will be gained when consuming organically grown vegetables, because conventionally grown vegetables have often been raised with artificial fertilizers and pesticides. The great health benefit derived from green juices includes the fact that they are a great source of potassium, magnesium, bioflavonoids, iron and calcium and chlorophyll. In fact, green leafy vegetables dedicate much of their energy to maximizing the production of chlorophyll. Chlorophyll is a great blood purifier and is therefore of great benefit for those undertaking the Big Clean-Up.

Red Vegetables

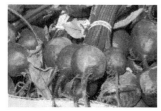

Benefits of beet juice are that it is a strong blood builder and purifier. This is due to the fact that beets optimize the utilization of your oxygen stimulating red blood cells. Beet juice in moderation is good for those with chronic candida, and the leaves are just as good if not better than the beet itself.

Are you congested, have high cholesterol or have a stomach ulcer? Then be sure to add a tiny amount of red hot pepper to your juice. Be careful! They can really add zing to your juice, so be sure to start with a tiny amount and feel free to experiment. The health benefits of cayenne pepper include its pain-reducing effects, its cardiovascular benefits, ability to help prevent ulcers and its effectiveness in opening congested nasal passages.

Some red vegetables and fruits like the humble tomato are good source of phytochemicals such as lycopene that is a powerful antioxidant with anti-cancer properties.

Juices Contain Little Protein

I started to notice some time ago in my clinic that the patients who were placed on juice fasts felt great for the first few days but them became tired by the end of the first week. After ten to fourteen days they felt really washed out and went back into normal eating, including various proteins like eggs, fish and chicken and plenty of carbohydrate or energy-producing foods like bread and potatoes.

Many on the juice fasts lost weight; in fact for some it was quite a dramatic weight loss with results that were quite astounding. It is very important for you to know that juices contain very little in the way of protein and virtually no fat so they are not really a complete food, if you want to do nothing but juice for a week or two this is fine, but be sure to add a good quality protein powder containing either brown rice or yellow pea protein. Both of these protein choices are low in allergic potential, unlike whey (cow's milk) protein powders that may contain copious amounts of sugars. Just take a scoop or two a day of protein powder can make all the difference, and add this to water or to the juice you like best when you are on the juice fast and your energy won't suffer.

Health Tip:

Caution With Fruit Juices Initially With a Yeast Infection

Do you have a chronic yeast infection and crave sugar or sweet things? Maybe you have diabetes, are overweight or obese or have high blood pressure or high cholesterol (high triglycerides in particular). Then I'd advise caution with high fructose containing fruits, the very sweet fruits, and it is best to limit these fruits until you normalize your condition. Yeast infections, especially when chronic, can initially aggravate with fresh fruit juices, but in my experience if you persist with an 80% vegetable juice and 20% fruit juice blend you should be fine after a few days. Providing you only take in vegetable and fruit juices, and avoid all other solid foods containing any form of sugar for up to a week. Yes, it is possible to have juice if you have a yeast infection, just make the right choices and experiment. Stop if you feel worse or an aggravation of your symptoms, you may need to experiment with different combinations until you've worked out what best suits your needs.

You are always safe with lemon and lime however, and these two fruits are a good addition to any vegetable juice that is bitter, as these citrus fruits are great at masking any strongly bitter flavors of some of the more beneficial deep leafy greens.

As you improve, you should be able to include more fruits in your diet over time and as usual – experiment to see what works best for you.

Preferably Use Organic Fruits And Vegetables – Or Grow Your Own

When you juice, be aware that if you buy fruits and vegetables from your local supermarket that you may be consuming a hefty dose of unwanted chemicals.

You are most probably aware that commercially grown fruits and vegetables contain chemical residues of herbicides and pesticides. Whenever possible, be sure to buy organic fruits and vegetables which contain no chemicals, or grow your own. Here is a list of the fruits vegetables that are the ones most likely to contain pesticides according to the Environmental Protection Association:

1. Celery

2. Pears

3. Spinach

4. Kale

5. Collard Greens

6. Lettuce

7. Carrots

8. Cucumber (not as bad if you peel the skin)

Drink Now Or Drink Later?

I find that juicing takes a lot of time, don't you? First you have to obtain the vegetables and fruits, wash them, juice them and then comes the clean up. Like me, you are probably thinking "Can I juice once a day and drink some now and some later?" Not really, some folks recommend that you cover the juice well, or fill the container to the top (to exclude oxygen), whereas other people tell you to get a vacuum pump and suck out the air from the container, thus reducing the amount of oxygen in contact with the freshly made juice. Why bother? Just make it and have a fresh juice once a day, you make it and then drink it and then clean up. That way you won't be compromising the quality of the juice and its over and done with!

Most people juice in the morning, but if that does not work out well for your schedule, please feel free to choose whatever meal works best for your lifestyle.

Which Juicer Should I Buy?

There are three main types of juicers, I own all three options and can tell you that the last option, the Vitamix, is the only you will want to seriously consider if you are really into good health and want the best. Let me explain the three different types and you can make up your own mind.

Talk to people who own these types of juicers and they will be quick to tell you that one of the most important things to consider is how long it takes to clean.

The Centrifugal Juicer.

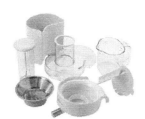

I call these juicers "screamers" because that is what they do, they scream when you use them. These juicers operate at a very high speed and can make a lot of noise. The centrifugal juicer cuts up the fruit or vegetable with a flat cutting blade.

It then spins the produce at a really high speed (anywhere from 3,000 up to an incredible 14,000 RPM) to separate the juice from the pulp. Although this style of juicer can juice most types of fruits and vegetables, it unintentionally heats the juice from friction and exposes the juice to significant amounts of air to cause oxidation, both of which causes large amounts of vitamin loss in the juice and greatly shortens the juice's shelf life. Besides, it takes ages to strip it down and clean it and all that engine speed is going to guarantee that it probably won't last too long.

Can you really be bothered spending all that time in the kitchen cleaning your juicer after you have made juice? I have my screamer still from years ago buried somewhere in the back of a kitchen cupboard, complete with a box full of parts. I must get around to putting it on EBay one of these days.

The Masticating Juicer

The masticating juicer is a better choice in my opinion rather than the screamer, especially if you want a quieter and more robust juicer that will last for years and produce a good quality juice. A masticating juicer uses a single auger to compact and crush the chopped up fruit and vegetables before squeezing out its juice along a static screen while the pulp is expelled through a separate outlet. Unlike centrifugal juicers, masticating juicers can juice wheat grass and other leafy greens and herbs like parsley.

The drawback is that this type of juicer tends to be more expensive than a centrifugal juicer and slower, but it is certainly more efficient and produces higher yields of juice. The juice also tends to be more nutritious and has a longer shelf life because the juice has not been exposed to as much heat or air as the centrifugal juicer. But once again, be prepared to strip it down and clean it after you juice, but the good news is that it doesn't contain quite as many parts as the screamer.

I have used the Champion juicer for a several years and found it to be excellent. Masticating juicers can be single or twin gear, but the principle is still the same. I like mine for carrot or wheat grass juice but only use it infrequently these days because I bought the Vitamix. I think I'll keep the Champion, so it's not up for sale.

The Vitamix Blender

The Vitamix is my personal choice and the juicer I now recommend, it is in fact a super blender. After having used several different types of juicers and blenders over the years I now just use the Vitamix, simply because it produces a high quality juice in seconds and takes seconds to clean! I love it because it is fast, juices anything and is extremely tough and will most probably outlast me. If an appliance is easy to use and quick to clean you tend to use it every day, and a glass of fresh juice daily is one of the best ways to build good health on any health program.

I have a Vitamix, the Champion masticating juicer and a Panasonic centrifugal juicer which is gathering dust. We use our Vitamix on a daily basis and the Champion juicer occasionally, I do like to use this juicer for wheatgrass juice at times. The clean up with most kinds of juicers is the big deterrent for me. And you end up wasting so much fruit and vegetables. We love our Vitamix for so many reasons, it can also make so much more than a juicer as it makes batters, dressings, soups, smoothies, ice cream, bread dough, perfect nut butters, excellent nut milks, creams, shakes, Frappuccino thingies, etc. But best of all, it is super easy and quick to clean. The Vitamix blending container is really tough and made of a special type of indestructible plastic, when I bought mine, the salesman even jumped on it with all his weight to demonstrate how tough this appliance really is.

At the top of the container is a lid to prevent ingredients from escaping during operation, and at the bottom is the high quality blade assembly. The container rests upon a base that contains an extremely powerful and very long lasting motor for turning the blade assembly that has several variable speed controls.

This baby is even capable of milling grains into flour and crushing ice cubes into slush in seconds without assistance. The biggest drawback with this superb machine is the hefty price tag, but I do believe in the saying that the quality long remains after the price is forgotten because the Vitamix truly is the Rolls Royce of the juicers and blenders.

Because it only takes a minute to make the juice without generating heat unless you let it run for ages, the Vitamix is more efficient and does produces a higher yield without waste, and the result is a top quality juice. When I make juices, I just cut an apple in four and leave the skins, stalk and seeds intact, thrown in a roughly chopped carrot, a stalk of celery (broken into three or four pieces) and hit go for 30 seconds - done. I drink the lot including the pulp, which incorporates ground up seeds, skins and even the stalk as well as the skin of the celery and carrot.
If you are serious about juicing and can afford the very best, get a Vitamix or otherwise settle for the Champion or Omega masticating juicer.

If you own one of these long enough you will probably end up buying the Vitamix down the track like many do. I'd recommend that you bypass the centrifugal juicer, unless you want to spend time with some form of hearing protection when you operate these screamers and then spend ages stripping it down and cleaning it, in comparison to how much time you will spend drinking the actual juice.

Juice Recipes

Why not add a healthy green drink each day as part of your cleansing regime? This is just another way to incorporate fresh fruit & vegetables into your diet. The best thing about raw vegetable and fruit juice is that these foods are packed full of many essential vitamins and minerals, enzymes and amino acids that are all critical in maintaining excellent health. Here are some of my favorite recipes:

Clean and Green

Carrots	4
Celery	2 Stalks
Parsley	1 Handful
Spinach	4 Leaves

CBS

Carrots	3
Beet	1/2
Spinach	3 Leaves

Carrot Cleaner

Carrots	3
Beet	1/2
Cucumber	1/2

Candida Crusher Drink # 1

Oregano fresh	Small bunch
Garlic	2 cloves
Green apple	1
Lemon	1

Candida Crusher Drink # 2

Coconut Milk	200 ml
Aniseed	½ tsp.
Ice Cubes	6

Candida Crusher Drink # 3

Grapefruit seed extract	5 drops
Colloidal silver	1 tsp.
Coconut milk	250mls

The Yeast Killer Caution – Strong!

Grapefruit juice	1 cup
Garlic	2 cloves
Oregano oil	1 capsule
Colloidal silver	1 tsp.
Grapefruit seed extract	5 drops

Colonic Irrigation

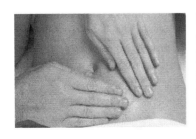

Have you ever had a colonic? Many people swear by them, and I regularly refer patients to a colon therapist. I'd like you to keep an open mind when it comes to this form of therapy and try to understand the benefits you can get from this amazing treatment. Colonic therapy is something a lot of people would never consider as a treatment and it is certainly not a therapy supported by mainstream medicine. But it is important to remember that mainstream medical doctors regularly prescribe antibiotics and do not believe in the concept of a candida yeast infection either. Colonic therapy is a very valid form of therapy and if you go to a professional person you need not be embarrassed either. I know of several colonic clinics in both Australia and New Zealand that have been treating patients for many years with excellent results, especially those who have had chronic digestive issues for many years.

Why Colonic Irrigation With Candida?

Having a colonic makes sense if you have been suffering with a yeast infection, especially a chronic one. Colonic irrigation is a great way to get the most out of your Big Clean-Up; it will assist in loosening and removing any unwanted and hardened fecal matter from your large intestine. This treatment will ensure that there are virtually no places for the yeast to hide in your large bowel, and give your digestive system a clean foundation. If you are considering colonic irrigation, then a colonic cleanse is best attempted now before you start on the Candida Crusher Diet. I have seen less noticeably less aggravations during the candida treatment phase in those who have a colonic at the start compared to those who didn't.

What Am I Likely To Expect With Colonic Treatment?

Your colonic therapist is a person who is experienced in this area. Be sure to enquire how much experience he or she has had, and it is important to enquire which professional colon therapist association your therapist belongs to.

A treatment session lasts anywhere from 30 - 45 minutes, and the patient initially will have a nice relaxing abdominal massage in the lower stomach area. This helps to loosen any bowel plaques or accumulated matter that the colonic irrigation treatment will help to expel from the body. After the massage, your therapist will insert a small disposable tube into the rectum through which warm water is passed into the colon. You may find the first treatment a little strange, but you soon get used to it. The water is expelled after, along with any loosened matter. The best way to find a therapist is to ask your local health food shop, or go online or look in the yellow pages. I recommend anywhere from one, two or even three treatments during your cleansing week, but your therapist will best be able to guide you on the frequency of treatment.

How Can I Make My Big Clean-Up More Effective?

Even though the Big Clean-Up is designed to be only of short duration, there certainly are a few good tips I can recommend with regard to getting the most out of your cleansing program. Although not mandatory by any means, it is a good idea to have a liver, gallbladder and kidney flush added as well, you could read more about cleansing in section 3 of this chapter, Understanding Cleansing and Detoxification.

Follow These Tips
To Get The Most Out Of Your Preparatory Cleanse.

- Do the Bowel Purge using Colozone or Vitamin C powder first.

- Stay well hydrated; drink plenty of clean fresh water.

- Avoid all alcohol, caffeinated tea and coffee. Don't even think about it!

- Eat fresh and raw, partially raw or steamed vegetables.

- Buy organic produce and poultry if at all possible.

- Fresh fish and free-range eggs are OK, but no red or other meats.

- Drink the High Fiber Cleansing Drink each day, in the morning is best.

- Get plenty of rest and sleep.

- Try to complete this cleanse when you are not very busy.

- You will benefit a lot from regular relaxation and meditation.

- Complete this cleanse over a seven-day period if your diet and lifestyle have been really good up until this point.

- Complete this cleanse over a two-week period or even longer if you have been drinking alcohol most days, having several cups of coffee or tea or know that your diet and lifestyle have not been the best up until now.

- You are ready to begin the Candida Crusher Diet after this cleanse.

- Consider Colonic Irrigation if you have had a chronic bowel problem.

- Consider liver, gallbladder and kidney cleansing if you have undertaken the two-week or longer option. (See section 3 of this chapter)

STAGE 1

The Induction Diet Stage (The MEVY Diet)

" When you are tough on yourself, life is going to be infinitely easier on you "
Zig Ziglar

This first stage is the induction, and requires effort; there is no doubt about it. It requires complete elimination of refined carbohydrates; all alcohol, all sugary foods and yeast containing foods and this restriction should be maintained for two to three weeks.

The whole idea of this first phase is to limit your eating which disallows exposure to the refined carbohydrates, alcohol and junk foods in general and to eliminate the yeast containing foods as well, because these foods provide direct nourishment for the stimulation of yeast growth and development. Candida and bad bacteria prefer an environment of refined sugars and any convenience or processed foods that tend to be high in sugars or yeasts. The best initial diet approach in my opinion is the MEVY diet, and acronym for Meat, Eggs, Vegetables and Yogurt.

The Candida Crusher diet induction phase is not unlike the Dr. Aitkin's Diet Induction phase that also lasts two weeks, it is high in protein and low in carbohydrates (breads, flour products, etc.).

Have you completed the Big Clean-Up? You will find that by having done so, the MEVY Diet stage will be easier and your outcome will be better as well, because you have laid a foundation for your digestive system upon which to build good health.

5 Good Reasons to Enforce the MEVY Dietary Change

1 Previously Poor Diet. An incorrect diet will have been one of the major reasons you got into trouble with yeast in the first place. Now you have a golden opportunity to have a diet makeover. Remember, not only will your yeast infection go away, your health will become better than it has in years.

2 Weight Loss. Many people with yeast infections carry a bit too much weight. While this certainly won't be the case in every situation, I've found that only about 15 to 20 percent of people I see with chronic yeast infections do not need to lose any weight, and this leaves us with about 80% who certainly could do with losing from anywhere from one to fifty pounds. By being tough on your diet, your weight will come off and by keeping on track with my dietary suggestions and lifestyle habits you will keep it off, for good.

3 Don't Forget your Immune System's Involvement. Until your immune system is strong enough to handle the insults of your current diet, foods that challenge your immune system, stimulating possible food allergies, in addition to the foods that stimulate growth of candida, the sweet foods, carbs, yeast containing foods and drinks, must be eliminated. Many people with a yeast infection tend to forget the immune system's involvement, and the MEVY Diet will lead into stage 2 of the Candida Crusher Diet, the Low-Allergy Diet, for this very reason.

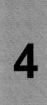

4 Eat Foods That Build Health. The foods you eat while on the MEVY Diet are the foods that will assist in nourishing and rebuilding your body rather than just killing your yeast infection. This is an important point, because if you want to get well and remain staying well you will need to rebuild healthy cells and repair the body's systems such as the digestive and immune system, systems that will be in a state of dysfunction. Your ability to eliminate the symptoms which have been plaguing you ages such as bloating, gas, sinus, itchy skin, vaginal itching, toe nail fungus, nasal congestion, brain fog and other troubles depends on how well your body's cells can rebuild these key areas. Do you want outstanding health as you age? Of course you do, and a healthy, nutritious and balanced diet is one of the best ways you can achieve this objective.

5 Yeast - It's All About Balance. It is important to remember that you want to get the yeast in your body in balance with the other beneficial bacteria in your body, both good and bad. You will never escape from yeast or eliminate it altogether from the mouth, vagina, around the foreskin, rectum, intestines and other body areas anymore than you will never eliminate every criminal in this world. Whenever an opportunity arises, there will be some people who will be ready to offend and commit crimes, it is the same with a yeast infection, and candida is always ready to commit an offence if you let it. There will always be good versus bad; it is about balance and harmony, and if you don't let candida have the opportunity then the balance will swing in your favor. Of all the therapies recommended to you to fight yeast infection, following an appropriate eating plan most probably assists with rebalancing the best.

The MEVY Diet

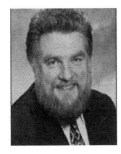

The **M.E.V.Y.** Diet (**M**eat, **E**ggs, **V**egetables and **Y**ogurt) for those with yeast infections is not a new concept; in fact you will find this diet in the book called "The Yeast Syndrome" (Bantam Books 1986) by Dr. John Trowbridge and Dr. Morton Walker. This is one of my favorite yeast infection books; it is excellent although a little heavy reading for some. The lengthy food charts tend to make the yeast infection dietary approach confusing and complicated. In my experience, unless a diet is kept as simple as possible it will be difficult to follow for many.

Dr. Trowbridge once said that the majority of people he has seen over the many years exhibit minor symptoms of a candida yeast infection, while almost thirty percent of those living in Western developed nations population are severely affected, and that was way back in the 1980's. My experience spanning of treating yeast infections certainly supports his assertion. Dr. Trowbridge has also said that candida is a precursor for almost every chronic degenerative disease because of its connection to cause harm to virtually every single body system, now you can see why it is important to tackle this all too common problem.

I prefer the simple and short-term approach to the MEVY diet, and while this diet is OK if you follow very strictly for 3 to 4 weeks, it fails as a complete nutritional program and does not supply your body with a sufficient amount of nutritional factors in a sufficient balance. It is best to adopt the MEVY diet in its strictest form for the first two weeks especially, then to loosen up a little for the next two to three weeks as you implement the low-allergy stage (stage 2) of the Candida Crusher Diet. Some may soon tire of being ultra-strict, but dietary discipline is a good thing, and as you begin to experience the cause and effect of the foods you have been eating and have been omitting, you will most probably want to stay reasonably strict for some time. I have found that others have no problems in enforcing a strict dietary protocol for themselves and remain on the MEVY diet for many months until they really improve.

It is really up to you to decide how long you want to stay on this dietary approach, but either way, let me assure you of one thing, the MEVY Diet works, and it works very well for those who adhere to it for some time, albeit in a modified fashion after enforcing it strictly for a week or two. I have trialed and experimented with many candida diets over the years and always seem to come back to the MEVY Diet for the simple reason that it works so well, time and again.

The MEVY diet is just a term for a low-carbohydrate diet, and was recommended in a time that was well before the low-carb diet craze. But unlike many other diets low in carbohydrates, Dr. Aitkin's Diet for example, the MEVY Diet isn't recommended primarily as a weight loss diet, although you will most certainly lose weight on the MEVY Diet if you have weight to lose, particularly if you follow it well. Instead, this particular restricted dietary modification will suppress and starve a candida yeast infection.

The MEVY diet brings the intestinal flora back into balance, and in my experience if you adhere to this diet you will discover that not only will your yeast infection and weight problem disappear over time, you will discover that your overall health will improve to a remarkably high level as a consequence. The Candida Crusher Program was not designed with the sole aim of ridding your body of candida; it is about getting your healthy life back.

While on this initial MEVY induction diet, you're allowed to eat all meats, eggs, most all vegetables (except initially the high starch vegetables like potatoes, carrots, pumpkin, sweet potato, peas, corn and beets) and plain, natural acidophilus yogurt. Eliminate foods and beverages made from grains or yeasts such as cereals, pasta, conventionally leavened breads (containing yeasts and sugars), pastries, chips and alcohol. I must emphasize, do avoid breads containing yeasts and sugars that are the leavened breads, although I have found that sourdough bread is OK. You also avoid all dairy foods, except natural unsweetened acidophilus yogurt.

No fruits, no forms sugars or vinegar (unless naturally fermented vinegar like Bragg's) are allowed. And that's it, a simple diet yet highly effective and as you can see, there are plenty of foods you can eat so you really don't have to starve. You are fine to have the fermented and cultured foods, as well as the sea vegetables of course.

MEVY Diet Effects

The idea behind this diet is that sugars and starches encourage the overgrowth of candida albicans in the intestinal tract. Remember that the Candida Crusher MEVY Implementation Diet is strictly a therapy employed *against* feeding candida and a usually will not be continued for more than three or four weeks at the very most. In some cases I have found patients to continue this phase for a month or two but then soon want to move on as they stabilize and improve. Most people find that two to three weeks is sufficient with stage 1, they've simply had enough at the end of this stage. Others I know continue this diet on for several months but in a slightly modified version, they simply add a few of the items that they originally avoided. So how do you know when you have had enough of the MEVY Diet, when can you stop? You stop when you don't seem to be improving anymore, that's when.

Remember, these are recommendations only. No diet is fixed or absolute by any means, it can be adapted entirely to suit your needs. But in saying that, I'd like you to follow this stage one MEVY Diet approach strictly for at least two weeks as a bare minimum, but preferably for three weeks initially for best results. Don't forget to take the Candida Crusher supplement recommendations; you'll be glad you did.

Stage One MEVY Diet Summary

1. **Avoid all junk food** (white sugar, white flour, soda drinks, take-out foods).

2. **Include liberal amounts of fresh, unprocessed and nutritious food** from a wide variety of sources. Shop at Farmer's Markets and your local butcher and produce store rather than buying all your food from the supermarket.

3. **Avoid all sugars and sugar containing foods** such as candy, chocolate, honey, molasses, and maple syrup.

4. **Avoid most fresh fruits and fruit juices** from 2 to 4 weeks and definitely no dried fruits of any kind! If you feel significantly better on a "no or low" fruit approach, you may want to continue this. You are allowed a few fruits, see below.

5. **Try not to eat the same foods every day**, rotate your foods if possible.

6. **Feature low carbohydrate vegetables, seafood, lean meats, and eggs and natural acidophilus yogurt** (try sauerkraut, kefir or Kim chi if you are allergic or can't handle real yogurt). Try to incorporate some **fermented and cultured foods** as well as the **sea vegetables** into your diet.

7. **Stage 1 MEVY Diet is one of the most important parts of your diet** along with the Big Clean-Up, because they form the foundation. The MEVY Diet is the induction, so try to factor it around a time when you can take it a little easy and are not working very hard.

8. **Be prepared in case you aggravate**, I find it best to ease somebody into this phase especially if they have been drinking lots of coffee, tea and alcohol right up until they want to commit to the Candida Crusher Program. And for that reason I recommend they complete the Big Clean-Up.

Try my "warm turkey" approach, because going cold turkey can be tough and distressing for many; it makes sense therefore to make reductions in your consumption of caffeinated drinks and alcohol well before you start on the MEVY induction phase. Start a few weeks before you get serious with stage 1 by gradually cutting back on alcohol and caffeine and you will sail a lot smoother through these potentially rough seas.

9. Multivitamin, take one with each meal, **digestive enzymes** – take one with each meal. You can read a lot more about the Candida Crusher dietary supplements in section 4 of this chapter.

10. Did you get constipated on this MEVY Diet? Try eating less meat, no more than 500 grams red meat in a week, and more vegetables. Pay attention to the fiber information in this chapter.

11. Stay on the MEVY Diet strictly for the first two weeks then allow yourself some starchy carbohydrates and maybe even a little fruit, depending on your level of improvement. Keep on the MEVY approach as you move into stage 2, the Low-Allergy Candida Diet phase.

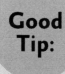

Good Tip:

The "Warm Turkey" Approach

Slow down certain foods & drinks before you cut them out
Everybody has heard about going "Cold Turkey", but who has ever heard about going "Warm Turkey"? It's a concept I came up with a couple of years ago with a patient who had problems coming off coffee. Does it not make sense to gradually reduce alcohol and caffeine and sugars in particular before you decide to cut them out of your diet? Of course it does, and you can do this over a two-week period before you start on the stage 1 MEVY diet approach. Do you drink 3 cups of coffee a day, or a few glasses of wine or a few beers daily? Then reduce over two weeks and then consider the stage 1 Candida Crusher Induction Diet. This approach will dramatically lessen any potential aggravations you may experience, which in turn will increase your compliance, enabling you to stick to the diet long-term. The more alcohol, caffeinated beverages or sugar you consume, the more gradual your reduction should be if you want to avoid any major aggravation. Try warm turkey, cold turkey is Yuk!

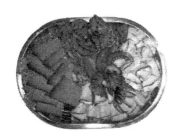

M.E.V.Y – Meat

You can eat all the meat you want on this diet, but within reason of course. Animal protein has no effect on a yeast infection, but eating too much red meat especially can cause digestive disturbances such as constipation and encourage putrefactive dysbiosis, so eat no more than 500 grams in a week.

This means that you will encourage too many bad bacteria as a result of too much meat in your diet, and it is therefore important that you eat plenty of vegetables in addition to meat, and make sure you take the digestive enzymes and probiotics in addition.

Meat Choices

Chicken, Turkey, Beef, lean cuts, Veal, Pork, Lamb, Venison, Shrimp, Crab, Crayfish, Abalone, Tuna, Salmon, Mackerel, Cod, Sardines, Eggs, other fresh or frozen fish.

Watch Out For Commercially Raised Poultry

You know by now to avoid as much as possible the broad spectrum anti-biotics and immunosuppressant drugs like cortisone, prednisone and inhaled steroids, birth control or hormone replacement therapy pills whenever possible.

Today's powerful antibiotics are able to suppress good micro flora and cause candida overgrowth in just a few days. But wait, in all Western developed countries, and probably your country if you live in a developed nation, we are feeding millions of chickens per year low-doses of antibiotic every day of their lives. Chicken feed can also include Roxarsone, an antimicrobial drug that also promotes growth but unfortunately contains arsenic. You may be interested in reading this Wikipedia page to become enlightened about commercial poultry production: http://en.wikipedia.org/wiki/Poultry_farming

A politician in New Zealand discovered that there were several strains of antibiotic resistant bacteria in 2002 in the very first chicken that was tested. Do you eat supermarket chicken? Chances are that you will also be consuming antibiotics in a low dose, and it doesn't take a genius to work out that long-term low dose antibiotics is the same as short term high dose.

The solution is to look for clean, preferably free-range chicken and eggs and avoid the well-known commercial brands that almost always contain traces of antibiotics. Some of these companies are clever, and while they promote themselves as "our chicken contains no growth hormones"; they do contain traces of antibiotic residues, arsenic and probably other toxins. How else can you keep thousands of birds healthy when you stuff them in cages, keep them in the dark and give them a totally unnatural lifestyle? You may recall when people were kept in inhumane conditions like this in German concentration camps during the Second World War, millions died of infectious diseases.

It is preferable to eat organic poultry and all meat whenever possible, and this includes beef, lamb and pork. Venison and ocean fish are probably your best protein choices because they haven't been tampered with. Your grandparents probably kept a few chickens and grew their own vegetables; remember how expensive chicken used to be? Now that chicken is cheap and plentiful and commercially produced just like farmed pink salmon is today, you will need to be aware of the potential for these proteins to be of rather dubious quality.

There will always be farmers who cut corners to make bigger profits by using cheaper feed and more chemicals to control pests and diseases. Just look next time how much fat is finely laced through the chicken breast and then imagine what chemicals are lurking in that meat, and particularly the fat, because that is where most of the drugs and chemicals go in an animal's body. Just look next time how brightly orange-colored the salmon is and wonder what chemical they used to achieve this bright yet artificial orange coloration.

Eat Organic Grass-Fed Beef

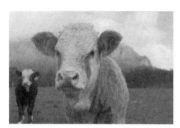

Studies have shown that the longer you feed cattle grains instead of fresh grass, the greater the fatty acid imbalance is likely to be. Unfortunately, many cattle in the USA are fed for 200 days or more on grain. We are most fortunate in New Zealand that all our sheep and beef are grass fed and our animal proteins are generally of a high quality.

I do believe that grass-fed beef and sheep are available in America but at a premium price. Bison is available as a grass-fed animal protein and may be an option. Real beef, sheep and bison that has been raised naturally without hormones and not having been fed antibiotics has added benefits to your health.

Grass-fed animal protein is loaded with many natural minerals and vitamins, and in addition is a great source of CLA (conjugated linoleic acid), which is a fat that reduces the risk of cancer, obesity, diabetes, and a number of immune disorders.

Caution With Fish

Fish, while generally a leaner food choice than beef, is very much promoted as an excellent clean protein that is a rich source of the omega-3 fats. One of the biggest problems with fish is the contamination with mercury; nearly all fish caught today are contaminated with mercury. The situation is so bad in many parts of America that even the conservative US government is warning pregnant women to avoid eating fish. Avoid canned tuna; apparently albacore tuna is lower in mercury than yellow fin or blue fin.

Once again, we are more fortunate in New Zealand and still have plenty of clean oceans and plenty of clean fish, particularly in the Southern Ocean; one of the few oceans remaining that is still relatively clean in comparison to the Northern Hemisphere where ninety percent of the world's population lives. Eat younger fish, they have shown to be much less contaminated that older fish and certainly avoid fish like shark, swordfish, grouper, and tuna if you can, the older and larger the fish, the more likelihood that it will be contaminated with heavy metals like mercury. A good idea is to get a Hair Analysis once every few years to determine whether you have a problem with heavy metals in your body.

Eat No More Than 500 Grams Of Red Meat A Week

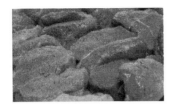 When Dr. William Crook and Dr. Trowbridge wrote their landmark candida books back in the 1980's, little attention was paid to red meats and cancer. Today this is different however; we know the link between those who eat lots of red meat and an increased risk of bowel cancer in particular.

My recommendations are for you to reduce the amount of red meat you eat, and to consume more white meats like free-range chicken and also nuts, seeds and free-range eggs for protein sources.

In 2007, the World Cancer Research Fund recommended a limit of 500g (1.1lb) of red meat per week. Since 2012, health experts in England have been advising that consumers should reduce their daily red meat intake to 70 grams (2.5 ounces) a day, or 500 grams (1.1lb) per week in the light of evidence emerging of the link between bowel cancer and red meat consumption. I still see a few yeast infection websites still recommending those with candida to eat 8 ounces of meat a day, that is 225 grams of meat a day or 1568 grams of read meat a week.

Did you know that a third of the adult population in your country, if you live in a Western developed country like America, Australia, NZ and Europe, consumes more than 100g (3.5oz) of red meat per day? This includes beef, pork and lamb. Current advice regarding red meat consumption, from 1998, suggests that 90g (3.2oz) a day was a healthy amount, and that people were only required to cut back on the amount red meat they consume if they were eating more than 140g (5oz) every day.

Whether you agree or not, there are established links between red meat and cancer, and with bowel cancer rates sky-rocketing in Western countries I think this advice is sound, limit your portion size and do not eat red meat every day. I prefer to go for quality and not quantity, and once a month enjoy a nice juicy medium-rare steak with all the trimmings at my favorite restaurant.

In 2005, a European study found those who regularly ate 160g (5.6oz) of red meat a day increased their risk of bowel cancer by an amazing thirty percent. In 2011, Sir Liam Donaldson, (Chief Medical Officer for England) said cutting consumption of all meats by 30 per cent would prevent 18,000 premature deaths a year in England.

High consumption of not only red but also processed meat in particular has also been linked to many other types of cancers, including breast, bladder, stomach and other digestive organs such as pancreas.

Naturally, the meat industry fiercely defends the role of red meat in a balanced diet, and claims that there is "no evidence" that the consumption of meat has any link with cancer whatsoever. A 38 year-old male who happened to control a large meat export business in New Zealand, came to see me after his diagnosis of bowel cancer. His breakfast consisted of lamb chops; he enjoyed sausages for lunch with bread and had steak most nights for dinner. He left my rooms furious after I mentioned that there might be the possibility of a connection with eating meat three times a day for several years and cancer. Unfortunately he didn't make 40 and left a wife and two children behind.

Similarly, drug companies would also like you to believe that their toxic wares are entirely safe for human consumption with no concerns for side effects. It's your life and the decisions you make today will have a direct impact on your health tomorrow, the ball is in your court. I am not here to patronize you or to tell you what to do, I'd like you to put the time into researching like I have and come to your own conclusions. Once you do, I'll bet that you cut your meat consumption by half at least.

Processed and Smoked Meats

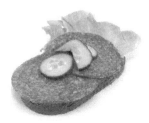

Controversially, the 2005 European study I mentioned just previously has said that children should never consume ham, sausages and bacon, the processed meats. When on the Candida Crusher Diet, it is best to avoid all processed meats from the supermarket, and this includes pickled and smoked meats and smoked fish including sausages, hot dogs, corned beef, pastrami and pickled tongue. Keep away from the delicatessen section of your supermarket.

Good Tip:

Avoid smoked meats

Smoked meats may increase your risk of cancer

Eating smoked meats may place you at a higher risk of developing certain cancers. Smoking adds flavor to the meat, but it also acts as a preservative. The problem with smoked meats is that smoking meat increases your exposure to a known carcinogen called PAH, otherwise known as polycyclic aromatic hydrocarbons. These potentially cancer causing chemicals are formed when animal fat from the meat comes in contact with the heat source thereby creating smoke, and this is how the PAH chemicals are then transferred to the meat. A 2010 study published in the journal *Circulation* also found that eating smoked meats may also increase your risk of heart disease. It was discovered that eating fresh red meats had a lower risk than smoked meats.

Reference: "Circulation"; Red and Processed Meat Consumption and Risk of Incident Coronary Heart Disease, Stroke, and Diabetes Mellitus; Renata Micha, et al.; May 2010

There are many theories as to why red meats may increase your cancer risk, and it is not the scope of this book to elaborate on them. Suffice to say, please do reduce your intake of red meats and processed meats. Eat more certified free-range eggs and chicken and when you do eat meat just reduce the portion size, it is easy as that. Focus on a large vegetable content of your diet and keep your meat intake down, there is no need to have a large steak every day as part of your diet.

Nuts And Seeds – High Protein Yet No Meat

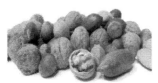 Although not meats, nuts and seeds are significant sources of protein. Caution is advised, tree nuts can be quite allergenic for some. Don't overdo it here, and avoid roasted or salted nuts and choose fresh whenever possible.

Careful of rancid nuts, be sure to select fresh nuts only. You may like to try pumpkin and sesame seeds, they are great lightly roasted and make a perfect condiment or snack. Peanuts are not nuts but legumes, and like soybeans can be highly allergenic and should be avoided by those who are proven to be allergic to them. Fermented soy products like miso or tempeh are generally OK, and I have found them quite well tolerated, even by many people who have shown to have soy allergies.

Best nut and seed choices: almonds, Brazil nuts, cashews, hazelnuts, macadamia, walnuts, and sunflower, pumpkin or sesame seeds. Nuts and seeds make excellent snacks or garnishes for salads and vegetable dishes.

M.E.V.Y - Eggs
Eat Organic Free-Range Poultry And Eggs

We keep our own chickens because we know exactly what we feed them, organically grown grains, like corn and wheat, as well as vegetables we grow ourselves, they also get plenty of kitchen scraps.

Chickens that eat organically raised vegetables along with plenty or worms, insects and lots of fresh green grass, provide superior eggs rich in fatty acids including omega 3. I always get the most positive comments from those who we regularly give eggs to, as they are used to buying the supermarket variety.

Unlike red meats and processed meats, eating organic free-range eggs daily has not been linked with an increase in cancer. In fact the opposite applies, those who eat high quality proteins like fresh and unfarmed fish and high quality eggs have lower rates of all cancers, when compared to those who eat a predominantly land based animal protein diet such as beef, pork and sheep.

Eggs Are OK, But Only If You Are Not Allergic To Them

Dr. William Crook recommended eggs as part of his overall diet plan, and so did Dr. Trowbridge. Some candida patients I have seen over the years have an egg allergy, and if you are allergic to eggs then you will obviously want to avoid eggs. Interesting, I have certainly seen egg allergies over the years, but I've never come across a person with a chicken meat allergy. Egg allergies do exist, but they are certainly not as common as dairy allergies so in most cases you should be able to tolerate eggs. Eggs are a fantastic source of protein and contain all the essential amino acids, they make an excellent breakfast and I highly recommend that you eat eggs several times a week. Given the extent of the candida dietary restrictions, being able to eat eggs is a big step towards superior nutrition; so do try to get them into your diet regularly. And be sure to only buy free range, or keep your own birds, they make the most wonderful pets.

M.E.V.Y – Vegetables
Vegetables

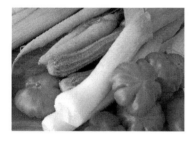

Most of the vegetables I recommend contain lots of fiber and are rich in phytonutrients and are relatively low in starchy carbohydrates. It is best to buy them from a local Farmer's Market or your local greengrocer rather than a supermarket. Better still, grow some of your own vegetables. I like patients to eat at least 3 to 6 servings of vegetables each day, and preferably to rotate so that they and don't get caught eating the same ones each and every day. There are many ways you can eat vegetables, did you read the section I have written previously on vegetables in this chapter for more information on how to prepare your vegetables and of the various ways you can add them to your meals?

Fresh organic produce is the best if you can afford it, otherwise try to grow some of these vegetables yourself, growing vegetables is not difficult and most rewarding. The following vegetables can be fresh or frozen and you can eat them cooked or raw: All fresh and dried herbs, asparagus, artichoke, bean sprouts, beets, beet greens, bok choy, broccoli, Brussels sprouts, cabbage (1 cup/day), capsicum (bell pepper), cauliflower, carrots, celery, cucumber, eggplant, endive, garlic, ginger, horseradish, kale, spinach, mescalun salad mix, mustard greens, garlic, lettuce, leeks, okra, onions, parsley, radishes, radicchio, salad greens, sprouts, string beans, seaweed, tomato, turnips, watercress and zucchini.

Fruits

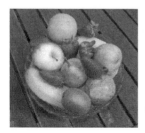

It is very important that you minimize fruit, so do your best to avoid most fruits in the first few weeks. Fresh fruit is often recommended by many practitioners as being OK, but it is certainly not when you start out on the Candida Crusher Diet. Remember, we want to reduce the candida food supply, and fruit contains plenty of sugar, especially fructose, a nice and easy food if you have a yeast overgrowth. I do recommend the following fruits, but if you notice any reactions on any of the following fruits then do avoid them, naturally.

Avocado, blueberries, coconut, green apples, strawberries - limit 6 per day, lime or lemon are always OK, they are in fact highly alkaline and a good cleanser. Some people can tolerate pears and pineapple, and experimentation will soon tell you if you can or can't. The less fruit you eat, the better, at least initially.

Beverages

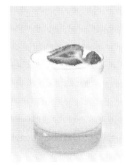

It goes without reason that alcohol gets the red light on my program, and this is non-negotiable as far as I'm concerned. Those with a chronic yeast infection will have no issues here and those that want to continue a daily drink that do have a yeast infection have wasted their money by buying the Candida Crusher book. This book is for those who want to win their fight against a yeast infection, not for those into denial.

Drink water and non-sweetened herb teas. Don't get caught out with alcohol, soda drinks and caffeinated beverages, stick with water. I prefer patients to avoid caffeine but have no problems with patients consuming one good coffee or cup of tea daily without sugar or milk during the entire Candida Crusher Program. Best to have your one coffee in the morning. Look for herbal teas with an anti-fungal activity like Pau d'arco, which I will talk a lot more later on. I'm developing an amazing herbal tea blend just for those with yeast infections, you will hear all about it when I release this product hopefully a bit later in 2013.

M.E.V.Y – Yogurt

Yogurt is a most beneficial cultured dairy food, and most people with a yeast infection will be able to eat a small amount every single day. I'm not going to talk a lot about yogurt here, as I have already given you an extensive rundown on this excellent cultured food. Do try to make your own yogurt, and avoid buying yogurt from your supermarket if you can avoid it, as many will be flavored and even contain artificial sugars. You can buy a natural yogurt from your supermarket, but you will need to carefully read labels! I have always found it best to buy this food from my local health-food shop, and you are almost certain to have a good one close by. Use a premium organic yogurt as your starter culture, and make your own delicious and creamy yogurt in your own home. I've written extensively about yogurt in this section, you may want to go back and read this information.

Foods You Should Eat With Caution for the First Month
The High Carbohydrate Starchy Vegetables

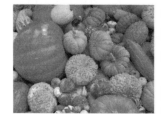
With all cases of chronic yeast infection I prefer the patient to avoid the starchy vegetables for the first several weeks, especially if they crave or love eating them.

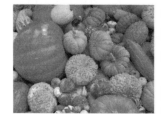
I found that when I made strict dietary restrictions, particularly refined carbohydrates like yeast containing breads, muesli bars, take-out, chocolate, cookies, potato chips, corn chips, etc., then the patient would start to consume plenty of potato, (like fries or potato chips) pumpkin, corn and sweet potato in addition to meats and green vegetables.

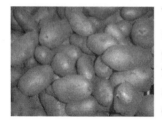
The fact is that most of the starchy carbohydrates offer little nutrition, especially in comparison to carbohydrates from deep green leafy vegetables. Why is it that many of us like to eat fries, those tasty deep-fried potatoes smothered in salt when we have sides or choose a take-out meal? It is because they contain lots of sugars, they satisfy us and hit the spot when it comes to a food craving. Deep fried potato chips are refined carbohydrates and they can help to feed the bad bugs in your digestive system, not unlike bread.

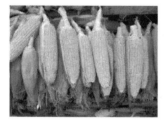
These starchy carbohydrate-containing vegetables can be broken down much more rapidly to form a convenient food for a yeast infection, more so than other carbohydrates such as spinach, broccoli and beans. Do you love pumpkin soup? Perhaps you are a fan of boiled, fried or mashed potato or fries? Maybe you like a few cobs of corn smothered with butter? If you want to recover from your yeast infection, and especially if you can relate to craving these kinds of vegetables then is best that you stick with other low carbohydrate vegetables, especially the green leafy variety for several weeks. This will ensure that you are doing everything you can to reduce that food supply of candida.

Passing a lot of gas and feeling bloated? Have you tried to cut out those starchy vegetables and sugars? You will have a lot less gas I absolutely guarantee it.
Carrots should be OK, but I have noticed that eating them aggravates some patients. If you have a problem with carrots then try eating them raw, steamed, stir fried or boiled, one of these ways is sure to be OK with your digestive system if the way you are currently consuming them is not.

Health Tip:

Do you want to lose weight?

Many patients I see are overweight, and all too many patients with yeast infections in particular are carrying too much weight. The MEVY diet will certainly cause you to lose weight, and it is not unlike the initial induction phase of the Dr. Aitkin's High Protein/Low Carb Diet. But following the MEVY diet you will lose weight rapidly if you want to, especially if you increase your activity levels and walk daily.

By cutting out the refined carbs (sugar, cookies, ice cream, and many junk foods), the breads containing yeast and now the starchy carbohydrate vegetables, you can understand how the weight will come off. The MEVY approach will not only get rid of your yeast infection, but your expanding waistline as well. By staying off the starchy vegetables, the refined carbs and breads you will be blown away at how much weight you can lose.

Carbo-hydrates do just what they say; they are a carbo that will "hydrate" your body and puff up your butt and thighs or other body parts like your upper back or arms. This is why you will urinate plenty once you kick the carbo habit and lose that puffed up weight rapidly, at least for the first two to three weeks. You are losing all that puffy fluid from your body.

Be sure to drink enough water and eat sufficient fiber to keep those bowels going or you may find yourself a little constipated. Some people I have seen have lost amazing amounts of weight (150 pounds or more) on the MEVY diet approach, and many have kept if off because they kept up with their good eating practices. If you go back and eat and live how you used to, you just may find that your weight will probably come back again, and all this yo-yo type diet approach will make it almost certainly impossible to shift in the years ahead.

The Main Starchy Offenders

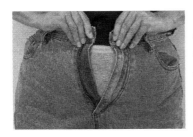

It is particularly important that you avoid these foods initially, especially if you have a lot of digestive problems like bloating, gas, burping or suffer regularly from indigestion, food allergies or food sensitivities. Remember that these starchy vegetables can cause aggravations if you have plenty of bad bacteria in your digestive system.

Best to avoid this group for several weeks, or even several months, if you have had a major bowel or severe yeast related problems for many years; but if your problems with yeast are quite minor or of a recent origin then you are probably OK if you are sensible about this food group. There are many diet books that are just starting to come out which focus on the low or no starch diets, and they make this recommendation for a good reason.

There may be one starchy vegetable in particular that you love; it could be said to be your favorite. A lady once told me she is a potato girl and enjoys potatoes cooked in variety of ways, whereas another lady told me that she adores pumpkin in any cooked in any way, in soup, baked and even in pumpkin scones. What is your favorite? Is it fries, sweet corn or maybe baked parsnip? Identify with it and avoid it, it could make all the difference.

Starchy High-Carb Vegetables

The main vegetables to be avoided when reducing carbohydrates to cut off the candida food supply are the starchier and sweeter vegetables:

- Peas
- Lima Beans
- Broad Beans
- Dried Beans
- Winter Squash (acorn and butternut)
- Sweet Chestnuts and Water Chestnuts
- Parsnips
- Potatoes in all forms
- Sweet Potatoes
- Corn, Sweet Corn or Maize
- Plantains
- Pumpkin, all vaieties

Health Tip:

Eat more complex carbohydrates - you will have better bowel flora

If you want to promote good health with a yeast infection, I always stress not to go indefinitely on a low-carbohydrate diet. It is important (but not commonly known) that a diet rich in complex carbohydrates, especially vegetables, is one of the best ways to promote healthy normal bowel flora with a candida yeast infection, leaky gut and many immune dysfunctions.

I like to see patients become wise about their carbohydrate choices on the Candida Crusher Program, and recommend they cut out many carbohydrates initially (especially sugar containing foods, the refined carbs) and then carefully phase them back in as they improve.

Eat Low-Carb Vegetables

This list is roughly arranged from lowest to highest carbohydrate counts, but all are non-starchy and generally low in carbohydrates. These are the best vegetables to eat when you have a yeast infection, remember, avoid the starchy carbohydrates for at least two to three weeks or longer if need be. Some patients I have seen avoid the high starch carbohydrates until well down the track whereas others reintroduce them much earlier. It all depends on your recovery, how much you miss them or were addicted to eating them, and how they affect you when you do reintroduce them eventually.

- Asparagus

- Artichokes

- Bok Choy

- Bamboo Shoots

- Broccoli

- Brussels Sprouts

- Cabbage (or sauerkraut)

- Carrots

- Cauliflower

- Celery

- Celery Root (Celeriac)

- Cucumbers (fresh)

- Eggplant

- Fennel

- Green Beans and Wax Beans

- Greens – lettuce, spinach, chard, etc.

- Hearty greens - collards, mustard greens, kale, etc.

- Herbs - parsley, cilantro, basil, rosemary, thyme, etc.

- Lettuce – all varieties, Cos lettuce is good

- Leeks

- Okra

- Onions

- Peppers (red, green & colored bell peppers)

- Radicchio and endive count as greens

- Radishes

- Rutabagas

- Scallions or green onions

- Sea Vegetables (nori, kombu, wakame, etc.)

- Snow Peas, snap peas, pea pods

- Sprouts (bean sprouts, alfalfa, etc.)

- Spaghetti Squash

- Tomatoes

- Tomatillos

- Turnips

- Zucchini (courgette)

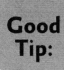

Good Tip:

Eat Bell Peppers
Do You Miss Sweet Foods On Your Candida Diet?

Many people appear to miss sweet fruits not long after they start the candida diet. I have found that sweet peppers (bell peppers or capsicums) are a great substitute, and once you get used to the sweet taste of red bell peppers you won't be missing those sweet oranges again. Try a red bell pepper; make sure you wash them well as a fungicide may have been used on them if you buy the commercial ones. They taste great roasted, stir-fried or just raw and are perfectly fine to eat if you have a yeast infection.

Whole Grains

It is a common misconception that people with yeast infections should go on a "no grain and 100 percent gluten free diet". I am not an advocate of this, you will most certainly need to avoid gluten if you are a celiac or have a gluten allergy, but not everybody with a yeast infection necessarily has a gluten allergy, I can assure you. Gluten is often to blame when a person has a chronic ongoing digestive problem, but try blaming the poor bacteria and levels of candida yeast in the digestive tract before you go pointing the finger at gluten. You are OK to eat wheat and gluten products in most cases, providing you eat bread for example made from just whole meal flour, salt and water, bread which contains no yeast or sugar. Have you tried to make the sourdough bread yet?
I see no problems, unless the person has a known allergy, with consuming barley, millet, oats, rice or wheat.

Breads, Biscuits, Cakes and Muffins

All breads, biscuits and muffins should be made with baking powder or baking soda as a leavening agent. Again, we don't want any commercially prepared products containing sugars or yeast. Best to make and bake your own. Be particularly careful with this category of foods, and if your yeast infection is severe, chronic or has been of a long duration, then you will need to avoid most all cookies, muffins, breads, scones and baked or flour-based products for some time until you improve to a high level.

Dairy

Natural yogurt (100% sugar free, natural and sour yogurt), buttermilk, butter. Pure butter is OK as well, and you will probably have no problem with hard cheeses or sour cream. Some will, some won't and again, experimentation is best. The main offender is cow's milk; I have found it to be the most allergenic of all dairy products.

Stocking Up On Foods – Your Pantry

The essential ingredients in this diet are the fresh foods; fresh vegetables, eggs and meat are essential. Also, fresh yeast free-breads and cereals are also excellent – unless you are allergic or intolerant. Shop as frequently as possible and try to have the freshest foods on hands for up to three days at a time is best.

Make certain that there is no mold or mildew on your fresh foods, and be especially careful with your vegetable crisper that you clean it out at least weekly. Plan your meals ahead, that way you will be able to select the foods you need and never fall short. Make sure you buy any ingredients you have not previously had and keep them in stock.

It is best that you make your own cottage cheese and yogurt but if this is not possible buy only small quantities. Make sure your selection of perishables is fresh, by checking the expiry dates.

Great Tip:

Shop Smarter And Take Note Of Expiration Dates

Here is a good trick my Jewish mother taught me, when selecting perishables from your supermarket, always select the products which are placed right at the very back and not the very front of the shelf of the refrigerated section. You will find that the difference in expiry dates can vary from one day right up to one week. The container right at the back was placed there more recently, and the shopkeeper wants you to buy the product at the very front, with the shortest expiry date, and the least fresh. How is that for a clever tip.

It is best not to leave any half-opened containers in your refrigerator or pantry. Buy small quantities of fresh produce, dairy products, vegetables, meats, eggs, grains, nuts and seeds and replenish stores frequently. As you will be shopping rather frequently for fresh produce, you will be able to produce exciting meals within minutes.

Here is an example of minute meals:

- Soup and pita bread

- Brown rice and stir fried vegetables

- Meat and salad

- Pancakes topped with home-made sour cream

The Deep Freezer

A clever thing to do is to think ahead with your meals, and this is particularly important if you are a busy person. When you start the diet, set aside some time to make standard meals you consume regularly which are suitable for our purposes, or make up recipes and then go on to create your recipe book. A good idea is to store pre-made meals or foods in your deep freezer well ahead. Be sure to clearly label the date of freezing and what the food actually is. This is very smart, because you will always have some food on hand in case on any emergency or if the unexpected arrival of guests such as family or friends catches you out. There will also be days when you just can't be bothered to cook and just want something quick and easy, am I right?

Here is an example of foods to freeze:

- Soups

- Pancakes

- Cooked rice

- Whole meal pitta or sourdough bread

- Casserole

- Cooked chicken of beef

Foods You Should AVOID

> *When diet is wrong medicine is of no use.*
> *When diet is correct medicine is of no need.*
> *Ayurvedic medicine quotation*

Candida loves carbohydrate and yeast rich food, but we are talking mainly refined carbohydrates, the simple sugars. It is important to repeat myself here; it is considered important in the beginning to also avoid any foods that contain or have the potential to contain fermented products like molds or fungi. And that means cheap commercial vinegars, alcohols, yeast extract spreads, mushrooms, melons and soft cheeses, etc.

Once the yeast is controlled, there is no reason to keep a strict prohibition however, but the return of your symptoms like abdominal bloating, gas, etc., after eating one of your offending foods will tell you that it is time to return for a period to the offending food avoidance strategy.

ALL Sugar and Sugar Containing Foods

Sugar and other quick-acting carbohydrates including sucrose, high-glucose corn syrup, fructose, high fructose corn syrup, maltose, lactose (cow's milk), glycogen, glucose, mannitol, sorbitol, galactose. Also avoid honey, molasses, maple syrup, maple sugar, and date sugar.

Packaged Foods

Canned, bottled, boxed and other packaged and processed foods usually contain refined sugar products and other hidden ingredients. For example, you will find many small pieces of dried fruits in packaged cereals and muesli.

Breads, Pastries And Other Bakery Goods, Milk And Cheeses

While you don't have to strictly avoid wheat products such as breads, flat breads are ok, made with flour, water and salt only, it is better to avoid wheat, rye, barley, spelt and even oats, all gluten containing grains, for a while until your digestion and immune system improves. If you have been unwell with a chronic yeast infection for many years, only a careful elimination and challenge will let you know if wheat based breads and grain based foods are working either for or against your health. You will soon know with a careful elimination and challenge. You can always try the Pulse test we have spoken about previously.

In my experience, you will improve rapidly if you do decide to eliminate wheat in chronic cases. If you must eat wheat, then eat mountain bread or flat breads made with only flour, water and salt, that way you avoid the yeast.

Alternatively, use a sour dough technique to make bread. Hard cheese is usually fine, but do bear in mind that any cheese has the potential to go moldy. Especially avoid moldy cheeses such as Camembert, Brie and Blue Vein.

Aren't they great though with a glass of wine and some crackers? See, you have plenty to look forward to when you recover!

ALL Alcoholic Beverages

Wine, beer, whiskey, brandy, gin, rum, vodka and other fermented liquors and beverages such as cider and ginger beer. Alcohol is an absolute no-go zone, and if you can't stop drinking until you are really well then the Candida Crusher Program is NOT for you! There is no "safe" alcohol, one website with plenty of yeast infection information surprises me by stating that gin and vodka are OK, but wine, beer and other spirits are not. Is it any wonder folks get confused when reading information online?

Condiments, Sauces And Vinegar Containing Foods

This is a very much and completely over looked area, because most people who have a yeast infection tend to narrowly focus on the sugar and yeast containing foods. Did you know that this group has the potential to contain even more yeasts, molds and unhealthy bacteria than all the other groups put together? If I went to your refrigerator right now, how many jars would I find that have been residing there for weeks or even months? You would be surprised how often you have bought a jar of some sauce and forgot about it for ages. Do you check expiration dates on bottles foods in your refrigerator? I'll bet you don't.

Sauces And Condiments To Avoid For A Few Months:

Barbecue sauce (sugar containing)

Bottled olives (supermarket)

Chili sauce (sugar containing)

Mustard sauce (sugar containing)

Tomato sauce (sugar containing)

Hoi sin sauce (sugar containing)

Horseradish sauce

HP Sauce (sugar containing)

Mayonnaise (sugar containing)

Oyster sauce (sugar containing)

Pickles (sugar containing)

Pickled vegetables (sugar containing)

Relishes (sugar containing)

Sauerkraut (sugar containing)

Salad dressings (sugar containing)

Shrimp sauce (sugar containing)

Soy sauces

Steak sauce (sugar containing)

Mincemeat (sugar containing)

Tamari

Worcestershire sauce

White vinegar

Avoid ALL kinds of vinegar-containing foods such as mayonnaise and salad dressing especially those fat-free dressings that are high in sugars and these sugars are often artificial as well.

Freshly squeezed lemon juice may be used as a substitute for vinegar in salad dressings prepared with extra virgin olive oil. You can use vinegar providing is has been naturally fermented, like Bragg's Vinegar. Most people who treat yeast infections will tell you to avoid all vinegar strictly, this is not right in my experience.

I have found that most all patients with a yeast infection can tolerate an organic and naturally fermented vinegar that has not been pasteurized.

Malt Products

Malted milk drinks like Milo, Ovaltine, Horlicks, and cereals. (Malt is sprouted grain that is kiln-dried and used in the preparation of many processed foods and beverages.)

Edible Fungi

All types of mushrooms, champignons and truffles.

Melons

Watermelon, honeydew melon and especially cantaloupe (rock melon). Melons are particularly high in sugars and molds.

Coffee and Tea

Regular filtered coffee, instant coffee and tea, stop green tea, especially the first two weeks. This is tough, but if you were a slave to caffeine you would do well to slowly come down off your caffeine addiction, reduce to one cup per day. Remember, we are looking at improving your overall health to the highest level possible, and caffeine certainly does not play any beneficial role here. I do allow one cup of coffee a day on the Candida Crusher Diet for those caffeine addicted souls who tell me that they would simply die if they didn't have their morning cup. Have one coffee a day, but skip on the sugar and milk if you can! Try stevia, it's nice in coffee if you need a sweetner.

Believe me; you will not miss your several cups of coffee or tea once you start to eliminate these beverages from your diet. You will feel much better once your body is used to generating energy naturally and has become less reliant of caffeine to fuel it.

Fruit Juices and Sodas

Fruit juices are a big trap for many who believe that a glass of orange juice is a great way to start the day. You will need to avoid canned, bottled or frozen juices, including orange juice, grape juice, apple juice, pineapple juice and any other fruit juices.

Tomato juice should be fine – providing it is sugar free. All soda, carbonated and energy drinks are to be avoided entirely. About a year ago I started to experiment with a few patients with grapefruit juice, to which they added 5 drops of GSE (grapefruit seed extract) and I found it to be a great success. You may want to try this option, providing there is no added sugar in the juice.

Dried and Candied Fruits

Many people I have seen with yeast infections just love dried fruits, and routinely snack on them. Avoid them, as they are loaded with sugar. Apricots, dates, figs, pineapple, prunes, raisins, currants, dried apples, dried bananas, dried paw paw, etc.

Leftover Foods

Here is a problem I see with many who present with yeast infections in my clinic, they eat for lunch what they had leftover from dinner the day previously. Don't make the mistake of cooking food for dinner, and then placing it in the refrigerator after covering it with plastic-film, or placing it in a container with a lid ready for reheating the next day. Molds grow in leftover refrigerated food.

Freezing is much better as soon as the food cools down, then heat to a high temperature to kill any molds, spores or bacteria. You are better off cooking just enough for your meal, and prepare fresh meals each day. This takes a little more time but you will ensure that the foods you do eat has no molds or spores on it which has developed overnight.

The MEVY Quick Check List Of What To Eat

1. Eat meats, seafood, vegetables and eggs. **The MEVY diet – M**eats, **E**ggs, **V**egetables and **Y**ogurt for the first two to three weeks.

2. **Eat no more than 500gr red meats a week**. Eat more eggs, chicken, nuts/seeds and fish.

3. **Avoid starchy vegetables for the first two weeks** (potato, pumpkin, peas, corn, squash, beans)

4. **Feature complex yet low carbohydrate vegetables** like leafy greens, spinach, celery, green beans, broccoli, cauliflower, etc.

5. **Eat the allium family of vegetables** – onions, spring onions, and garlic.

6. **Avoid most fruits initially** (except allowed) for two to three weeks, the longer the better)

7. **Fermented and cultured foods** are excellent and highly encouraged. Try to eat some regularly throughout the MEVY Diet and beyond. Try sauerkraut, kim chi, yogurt or kefir, and fermented tofu like tempeh.

8. **Sea vegetables** are one of the world's best super foods, try to incorporate some into your diet regularly.

9. **Butter (real butter)** and shop bought or home-made (traditional sour) yogurt is OK. Hard cheese and sour cream *may* be OK, experiment.

10. **Include liberal amounts of nutritious food from a wide variety of sources**.

11. **Drink water, herb teas and especially Pau d'arco herbal tea**. I'll speak a lot more on the virtues of the amazing herb Pau d'arco later in this chapter, in section 4.

STAGE 1

Quick List Of What To Avoid

1. Avoid ALL white sugar, white flour, soda drinks and take-away foods.

2. Worst foods & drinks – Most all junk & take-away foods, high sugar or yeast (risen bread) foods, alcohol, soda/fizzy drinks. In my experience what you crave the most is what you need to avoid the most.

3. Avoid ALL chocolate, honey, molasses, and maple syrup.

4. Avoid ALL fruits and fruit juices for the first 2-4 weeks, and definitely no dried fruits of any kind, not even in muesli or packaged cereals.

5. Try not to eat exactly the same foods every day, rotate your meats and vegetables

6. If you have severe candida, or have suffered with yeast related bowel problems for years, then avoid the high carbohydrate vegetables: sweet corn, peas, snow peas, squash, pumpkin, lima beans, white potatoes, sweet potato and carrot may be ok, experiment for the first two or three weeks.

7. If you have food allergies or react to foods then follow the Stage 2 Low-Allergy Diet for three weeks in addition straight up, no need then to wait until you begin the second stage of the diet. Avoid dairy products (cow's milk, all cheese, ice cream and cream. Butter and real yogurt are OK.

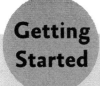

Getting Started

Making Your Candida Diet Work

1. Have you started to get rid of the foods from your refrigerator and pantry that you should avoid in stage 1? Go out and buy a vegetable steamer and re-organize your cooking space, clear that clutter.

2. Have you gone shopping yet and bought the foods that you should be consuming? Have you bought the right grains, nuts and seeds, oils, spices, fresh garlic, organic apple cider vinegar, coconut products and Pau d'arco tea? You have thrown out all that junk including all those old jars out of your fridge, haven't you?

3. Have you started to make a shopping list? Hang a shopping list on your fridge, plan your meals and buy what you need ahead of time. Buy small amounts of fresh fruit and vegetables 2 to 3 times weekly.

4. Have you tested yourself with the various candida home tests yet, which you can find in chapter 3? Are you tracking your test results yet with the Candida Test Tracker? See chapter 3.

5. Have you completed the online yeast infection survey yet on yeastinfection.org?

6. Have you started to fill out your Candida Symptom Tracker yet? It is important to test and measure if you are to find out what works and what doesn't for you. You will find an explanation of the Candida Symptom Tracker in chapter 3. Keep going if you improve, stop – assess and change what needs changing if you don't improve. Easy.

7. Are you prepared for the inevitable ups and downs you are likely to face in this first stage? Keep telling yourself that you are going to beat this thing once and for all and that it will be well worth your efforts in the long run. You want a permanent yeast solution, and that's why you bought this book.

Dietary Supplements During The Stage 1 MEVY Diet

Along with these dietary changes, you will get optimal results from your Candida Crusher Program if you take a few highly specialized dietary supplements. While nutritional supplementation is not absolutely necessary, it does play a crucial role in recovering from a yeast infection. The supplements I recommend will not only speed-up your recovery, but in many cases they will be found necessary for a complete and deep-seated recovery from the dysbiosis (bowel overgrowth of poor bacteria), leaky gut, fatigue and brain fog, food allergies and many other chronic health problems associated with a chronic yeast infection.

The Candida Crusher supplements I have chosen have been specifically selected based on my experiences in working with many patients with chronic yeast infections for their cleansing, healing and deeply restorative effects, and I will explain the significance of these formulations in section 4 of this chapter, because it is important for you to understand why these supplements have been included as part of your Candida Crusher Program, and the necessity of taking them regularly.

The supplements I recommend in the first stage of the Candida Crusher Program are the **Candida Crusher Formula,** the **Candida Crusher Multi**, the **Candida Crusher Digestive Enzyme** and the **Candida Crusher Probiotic**.

Here's why you need to take these dietary supplements during stage 1:

1

The Candida Crusher Formula is one of the most effective yeast infection inhibition and eradication products you will find; it is made of the finest raw ingredients and from ingredients that have proven to be the best at eradicating and killing candida. This unique formula will be released in 2013. Stay tuned to yeastinfection.org and candidacrusher.com

Good advice is to wait about a week or two into the MEVY Diet before you start taking the Candida Crusher Formula; this is to prevent any potential die-off or aggravations from occurring. For those with a serious yeast infection, start at the rate of one dose per day initially and slowly build up the dosage. Most people with a candida overgrowth will be able to tolerate between two to three doses per day without too much problem, but do wait a week or two the Candida Crusher Formula after you have started the MEVY Diet before you begin supplementation with, just to be on the safe side, particularly if you are sensitive, aggravate or feel weak when you first start the treatment plan. This is a powerful product and will most certainly crush your yeast infection!

2

The Candida Crusher Multi is intended to help combat any potential nutritional deficiencies while you are on the Candida Crusher Program. It was designed with the candida patient in mind and contains the most bioavailable nutrients available. This is an excellent product and will ensure you don't run into any deficiencies throughout the different stages of the Candida Crusher Program. You generally take one with each meal; three a day is the optimal dose.

The Candida Crusher Digestive Enzyme is intended to assist in the proper digestion of foods because it will help to boost the production of digestive enzymes; this will help to improve your digestion (stomach, pancreas, small intestine and liver/gallbladder) tremendously and help improve bowel function. I found the digestive enzyme to be particularly important for the first two to three weeks of the diet because the protein intake will be increased and the refined carbohydrate intake decreased, including fruits. This can often lead to a sluggish bowel and an increased load placed on the stomach and small intestine. You will discover that the better the process of absorption, digestion and elimination work in your body, the sooner you will overcome your yeast infection and with the least discomfort and aggravation.

The candida Crusher Probiotic, this formula has been incorporated into the digestive Enzyme product. Probiotics are important supplement to aid in the recolonization of friendly bacteria.

You can read all about special anti-candida foods, supplements and herbal medicines in section 4 of this chapter, chapter 7.

Consider Stopping
Your Current Supplement Regime For 4 – 6 Months

Have you been taking up to a dozen or more dietary supplements until now to fight your yeast infection? You may be taking a few, several or even a large amount of dietary supplements like a Vitamin B Complex, Vitamin D, Vitamin E, Calcium or Cal/Mag, Zinc, urinary formula, liver detox formula, etc.; etc.

In section 4 you can read about some people who take up to two-dozen or more supplements daily when they have a yeast infection. There is no real need to take so many products on the Candida Crusher Program, trust me. I routinely take patients off many different types of products whilst they on the Candida Crusher Program, and have done so for many years. Incredibly, not one patient has died or even become ill due to a deficiency of any vitamin or dietary supplement that I have come across whilst on my program.

I'd like you to think carefully about taking all those different dietary supplements you may be taking currently while you are on the program. How long have you been taking them for? In many instances, there is no need to continue with so many dietary supplements at this stage. Just take one top-quality candida formula the Candida Crusher Formula, along with the Multi-Vitamin and Mineral formula like the Candida Crusher Multi, a digestive enzyme like the Candida Crusher Digestive Enzyme and probiotic like the Candida Crusher Probiotic for now.

Taking several dozen dietary supplements each day is no guarantee of yeast eradication, it is the combination of diet, lifestyle and carefully balanced and highly targeted supplementation that will give you the results you are looking for, a permanent yeast solution.

The more supplements you take, the more you will confuse your treatment and we will not know what is happening and what is working and what is not working if you continue to take all manner of vitamins and minerals. Remember, you can always go back taking all your supplements after you have completed your Candida Crusher Program, so just put them in a box and store them in a cool dark place.

STAGE 2

The Low-Allergy Foods Stage

Now that you have completed the first two to three weeks on the stage one MEVY induction diet, it is time to clean up the diet a bit more by eliminating the foods that potentially challenge your immune system. As you go into Stage 2, be sure you adhere to the principles as outlined in the MEVY Diet, but after two or three weeks on Stage 1 you may loosen up a little depending on your level of improvement.

This is the low-allergy diet stage and is especially useful for those who have suffered with a yeast infection or any chronic digestive problem for some time. It is particularly beneficial to do this stage if you have been on a course of antibiotics or take any pharmaceutical drug regularly. Still drinking occasional alcohol? Then you simply must complete this stage or you will not recover entirely, and this has been my experience after helping many thousands of yeast-infected patients back to health.

You can skip this allergy-avoidance stage and I have no doubt that many will, but your recovery will probably only be partial, especially if your yeast infection is chronic or you can relate to the list of the several reasons I have described ahead. This list contains the main reasons why you may want to include the avoidance of potentially allergenic foods as part of your Candida Crusher Diet.

Once you have completed between two to three weeks on Stage 1 MEVY Diet, you should be starting to feel better, it is time to withdraw any potentially allergenic foods from your diet. With Stage 2, it is time to follow the Hypo-Allergenic Diet (also known as the Low-Allergy Diet), this is because certain foods have an increased tendency to create allergenic responses, and most patients I have seen with chronic yeast-related problems have various issues with their small intestine including leaky-gut syndrome, parasites, dysbiosis as well as their yeast over growth.

If you have a mild case of yeast infection, like a mild case of toenail fungus or a very mild bowel problem, then you may not need to complete Stage 2 at all. The longer you have suffered or the more resistant your yeast infection is to treatment, the more likely you will benefit from Stage 2, and the longer you may need to implement this stage before your digestive system has turned the corner and repaired itself.

Good Reasons To Enforce The Low-Allergy Diet Stage

- o   Those with a history of eczema, asthma, hay fever or allergy.

- o   Those who have candida yeast infection and have tried many different treatments with only partial success.

- o   Anybody who has taken an antibiotic, especially if you have had several courses of an antibiotic.

- o   Anybody long-term on any prescribed pharmaceutical drug.

- o   Any chronic (more than 12 months) case of candida yeast infection.

- o   Those who have had a history of poor diet or alcohol consumption.

- o   Those with a yeast infection who are shift-workers, nurses, taxi or truck drivers or any occupation with unusual or long hours.

- o   Those who have irritable bowel syndrome or any bowel or digestive complaint which is resistant to treatment.

- o   Those who are celiac or have inflammatory bowel syndrome (ulcerative colitis and Crohn's disease) .

- o   Those who feel better when they avoid dairy foods, gluten, or any particular food group.

- o   Those with an auto-immune illness (like rheumatoid arthritis, asthma, Hashimoto's thyroiditis, grave's disease, multiple sclerosis, or any one of the sixty auto-immune illnesses).

- o   Those who have had a chronic case of vaginal thrush (vaginitis).

Most people who have a yeast infection will be able to relate to one or several of these points, and for this reason they should complete the Stage 2 Low-Allergy Diet component of the Candida Crusher Diet.

The Low Allergy Diet (The Hypo-Allergenic Diet)

Food allergies and food sensitivities are common with candida. The things you crave are frequently what the yeast itself craves. Try to identify any possible allergies or sensitivities and weed them out. This can help a lot and will allow you to recover much faster than if you skip this step. In particular, steer clear of milk products, oranges, bananas, peanuts, and all foods to which you suspect you might be allergic or sensitive to. Reducing the workload on your immune system enables your system to harness sufficient energy to kill candida. I have found this to be a key but often a very overlooked factor to a complete recovery.

It is important to bear in mind that the Hypo-Allergenic Diet sheet does not take into account the fact you may be a celiac, or be sensitive to dietary salicylates, amines, colors, flavorings or certain kinds of preservatives. You will need to bear this in mind, and need to further consult with your practitioner on these matters. You may also have food intolerances, which also may need to be addressed. These can come about due to poor digestive enzyme levels or many other factors. I intend to expand considerably on the topic of food intolerances and sensitivities in the second edition of the Candida Crusher. The immune system is the one that finishes off the job, but only if it has the energy to do so.

Eating foods that have a high allergy potential (cow's milk, bananas, peanut butter, oranges – see the list) or typical yeast promoting foods (like bread and alcohol, chocolate, etc.) tires out your immune system since it is forced to shadow box any antibodies it has built up that mimic candida.

It is my belief that the only way you are going to get fantastic results and permanent results once and for all is to get serious with your diet and lifestyle, and by avoiding all the potentially allergenic foods until your immune system improves significantly, that way you will get results much faster than by any other method you will try.

I've always told patients if they are looking for a good doctor, then I'm looking for a good patient. In fact, the greater the patient's compliance, the better the results and the faster he or she will achieve them. That's how your reputation grows as a practitioner, with results. The more you put in, the more you get out, and that's how it is with any endeavor in your life.

Ahead you will find the Low-Allergenic Diet I have been using in the clinic for many years now. The trick is to avoid foods in BOLD until your digestive and immune system improves considerably. You will notice that once you remove the key offending foods that symptoms improve, and if you re-introduce too soon then you will aggravate.

Be sure to read what I have written previously on allergies, especially about IgE (immediate) and IgG (delayed) allergies. Immediate allergies are the allergies usually caused by foods such as cow's milk, bananas or for example strawberries. However, quite violent IgE food allergies are caused in particular to foods like peanuts, eggs, shellfish or fish. Most people with these types of allergies know they have an obvious allergy to a particular food they eat, or in some cases only have to breathe around the food, and bingo, the allergic response is produced.

The foods you see in bold below in the Low-Allergenic Candida Diet are the ones most likely implicated in immediate food allergy responses. If you are confused and want to know the difference between an allergy and intolerance, something many people get confused with, just go back and read what I have written previously in this chapter about the difference between allergies and intolerances, it will all make sense.

The foods in the column on the right in the Low-Allergy Candida Diet are the ones I would like to see you avoid for two to three weeks, and if you may want to avoid them for a longer time because you will feel great. There are three categories of foods in the right column:

- **Bold listed foods**
- *Italics and underlined foods*
- Plain font listed foods

In Stage 2, the Low-Allergy Diet Stage, be sure to avoid those foods listed in bold first for two weeks. If you are severely affected and have known food allergies or strongly react to foods in your diet, then I would suggest that you avoid for two weeks in addition any foods in the right column that are in italics and underlined.

It should not be necessary for you to avoid all the foods in plain font in the right column, I have listed them here as foods which may have a tendency to creating immune reactions, so the more severe or extreme your case, the better it is for you to eat less, but do not necessarily avoid altogether, the foods listed in the right column. It certainly is in your best interest to eat foods more in the left column, as these are the foods least likely to create any unwanted immune reactions, especially if you have a case of leaky-gut syndrome involving lots of bloating, gas, constipation or diarrhea.

You will notice that included in this list are all raised breads (baked breads containing yeast) all soft cheeses, wine, beer and spirits and vinegar, chocolate, peanuts, and sweets (candy). In this category I would also place bananas and oranges, pineapple and mandarins as well as dried fruits, but limes and lemons are fine.

Don't kid yourself that one small piece of chocolate occasionally is OK. This is not the way to tackle the beast called yeast, just say "NO" and learn to discipline your discipline. You will feel fantastic in time and the healthier you get, the stronger your self esteem and resolve to never go there again. I have seen this in many yeast-infected patients over the years; many of the worst cases eventually become the best advocates for living a naturally healthy lifestyle. After all, I was one of these cases, remember?

Drink Water And Lemon Juice

During Stage 2 the body will need to adjust to cleanse the toxins that are released by a yeast overgrowth and this is achieved by drinking plenty of water. I like patients to drink water when they get up, before meals, in the afternoon and early evening. In addition, tepid to warm water with a small squeeze of fresh lemon is a great detoxifying agent, and lemon is a fruit that is permissible during the Candida Crusher diet.

Eat More Anti-Fungal Foods

During Stage 2, I recommend that you increase your intake of vegetables including salads and especially those key foods with anti fungal properties that inhibit the growth of candida albicans. You will be able to read about these in more detail in section 4 in this chapter, Understanding Special Foods, Herbs and Supplements.

Ensure that there are sufficient levels of protein in the diet, by increasing the amount of fish and poultry in the diet. It is recommended by some experts that red meat be avoided during the first 4 weeks of this diet as it can place further strain on an already weakened digestive system. The MEVY Diet can be a bit protein top-heavy for those who are not used to eating lots of proteins and vegetables like this, I an assure you, this diet is excellent for those with a chronic yeast infection. You will need to keep those bowels going, and that's why selecting the right amount of vegetable fiber along with plenty of fresh water and lemon juice makes sense.

When your bowels work better, you will eliminate plenty of toxins and bad bacteria from your bowel. And what animal protein should you choose? That's really up to you, I personally like fresh fish and free range egg with a bit of organic grass-fed beef and lamb. You will need to decide what is right for you, you may even wish to go vegetarian, and in that case there are plenty of choices as well.

Leaky Gut Syndrome Is Very Common With Candida Sufferers

I guess LGS sums up most of the candida patient population to some degree. In my experience, people with long-standing candida albicans often have food allergies or food intolerances and this may result from problems which have occurred to the lining of the small intestine called "leaky gut", you can read a lot more about what constitutes leaky gut in section 2 further on in this chapter.

Leaky gut goes hand in hand with a yeast infection, and is often one of the main underlying causes of most all food allergies I see in patients in my clinic. Subsequently to developing a leaky gut, a person's immune defense may become increasingly weakened. Leaky gut is a particularly common occurrence in those with a history of antibiotic therapy or other prescribed or non-prescribed pharmaceutical drugs, which is not uncommon in those with a history of candida, and at the risk of sounding like a broken CD player that keeps jumping onto the same track, if you have had *any* antibiotic treatment in the past then you should certainly NOT skip Stage 2, the Low-Allergy Diet stage.

But why don't we take these potentially allergenic foods out at the beginning you ask, why do it now? That's a very good question, and the answer is that we don't want to compound any potential aggravations you have as you simultaneously eliminate all sugars, refined carbohydrates and the yeast containing foods along with more problems caused by the withdrawal of any potential allergenic foods. A person may develop an aggravation as they commence the program, especially in the first few weeks. By making the diet even more restrictive I have found that the candida diet becomes just too much to cope with in many cases, and it certainly can be called the "impossible diet" if too many restrictions are placed at the onset.

It is a person's best interest to make any food withdrawals staggered and in increments over a period of time. I have trialed various dietary approaches over the past several years and have found this multi-stage approach to work the best with the large majority of candida patients I have worked with. You are welcome to go ahead and try your candida program by making lots of exclusions right up front, but do expect aggravations, especially if you have had a chronic candida problem many years duration. Believe me, the best approach is to stagger your food withdrawals, just like the best approach is to carefully and to systematically re-introduce the potentially aggravating foods as you recover.

Staggered Withdrawal – A Clever Approach

Stage 2 is a clever approach in the clinic, and I started to realize the value of this second stage approach several years ago, and it works really well. Most books on candida I have studied never mention the value of staggering the withdrawal of initially the refined foods, junk, alcohol and breads (yeasts) and THEN to implement the Low-Allergy Diet, they just ignored this step and went from Stage one to Stage three – the re-introduction. While it is true that many of the potentially allergenic foods are removed in Stage 1, little to no attention is paid in my experience to the Stage 2 Low-Allergy Diet approach by most health-care practitioners, and those with candida are frequently allowed to continue consuming cow's milk, commercial breads and even peanuts throughout the treatment. You will find that these are the patients who improve to a degree, but never feel really good or have experienced significant improvements right across the board. Recovering from a yeast infection means recovering your immune and digestive systems, it involves what you eat, how you eat it and how you live your life. It takes time and a commitment to improving these aspects, and that is why the biggest part of this book is by far devoted to diet and nutrition and lifestyle.

Stage 2 of the candida diet is not compulsory by any means, but you will find that if you follow this part of diet in the sequence I have outlined, you will get the very best results – I guarantee it. Your digestion will improve faster and you will halve the amount of time it takes for your digestive system to beat this thing for good once and for all. And besides, it has taught you one important thing – discipline, and that's not a bad thing when it comes to making the right dietary choices.

Tailor Your Withdrawal And Food Re-Introduction To Suit Yourself

Do you have a bad case of candida and have tried many different dietary approaches all to no avail? Here's what you can do before you start on the Candida Crusher Diet. I'd like you to carefully write down all the foods you currently eat in a long list, all the foods. This includes all the grains, proteins, fruits, vegetables, spices, everything. Now do the same for all the drinks/beverages.
Take your time and be very thorough, not missing out a single thing. Put this list away for a week then come back to it, adding what you may have overlooked previously. Now, try this: with your pen, mark each food or drink with a score. Place 3 next to the food you enjoy the most, number 2 next to the food you enjoy and a 1 next to the food you find OK. What we are trying to establish is the foods you are drawn to the most and those you are drawn to the least. If you make your lists in columns you will have an easier overview of the food and drink items and their respective scores.

As far as the forbidden and allergic foods are concerned, the foods you withdraw more slowly (and for longer periods of time) are the category 3 foods, followed by category 2 and then category 1. The foods you introduce first are the category 1 foods, followed by 2 and then 3. By following this principle you are the least likely to incur any major dietary aggravations, because you have intelligently withdrawn and challenged you body with the key foods your body has a particular affinity with. This affinity will be specific to you and is as unique and individual as you are.

Key Benefits Of The Low-Allergy Stage 2 Diet

- Less chance of any major aggravations

- More chance of identifying any key allergenic foods, clearing up any underlying food allergies that may have plagued you for years.

- An easier approach than stopping potentially allergenic foods, sweet foods, alcohol and yeast containing foods all at once.

- Longer lasting results because there is more time to heal the leaky gut

- You become more disciplined and learn to control your diet more long-term

- You will find an improvement not just in physical health, but in your emotional and psychological health as well. Why do you think they call the gut the second brain? When a person heals their digestive system on a deeper level, they heal their entire wellbeing.

3 Reasons Why Your Tolerance To Foods Will Improve Over Time

I have found in most all cases those who have previously found themselves to be intolerant, and some cases even reacted violently to certain of these foods, could over a period of time re-introduce those foods without a problem. Why is this so? There are several reasons for this, but here are what I believe are the three main reasons for this to occur:

1. **Your digestive system becomes renewed** over the course of the Candida Crusher Diet. As your beneficial bacterial and digestive enzyme levels improve, you will digest foods better, absorb foods better and even excrete the wastes better. Less bloating, flatus, nausea, etc.

2. **Your immune system improves and becomes less reactive to potentially allergenic foods.** Newly restored, your tolerance increases over time and even disappears in many cases. People who thought they were gluten intolerant for example can now eat bread again without any real problems. Less bloating, gas, itchy skin, hot or cold sweats, fatigue and more.

3. **Your yeast population and bowel flora become more balanced,** and once your intestinal flora once again becomes healthy and normal your reactions will become much improved to the point where most all foods become tolerable. Less brain fog, more energy, less bloating, flatus, etc.

The Low-Allergy Candida Crusher Diet

The low-Allergy Candida Crusher Diet sheet does not take into account the fact you may be a coeliac, or be sensitive to dietary salicylates, amines, colors, flavorings or preservatives. You will need to bear this in mind, and need to further consult with your practitioner on these matters. You may also have food intolerances, which also may need to be addressed. These can come about due to poor digestive enzyme levels, etc.

FOOD GROUPS	🙂 FOODS WHICH ARE OK *Foods which don't generally cause immune reactions*	🙁 FOODS SUSPECT OR NOT OK *Foods which may cause immune reactions*
Meat, Fish, Chicken, Legumes, Eggs	Chicken, turkey and venison. All Legumes dried peas, lentils. You should be OK with most fish, unless you know you have fish allergies.	*Red Meats*, *Lamb*, Pork, Cold Cuts, Sausages, Corned Beef or Canned Meats, *Eggs (white & yolk)* or Egg substitutes. *Soy products*. Processed Meats in general. *Fish and shellfish*
Dairy Products	Milk Substitutes (*caution* with soy) Almond or nut milks, Rice milk, Oat milk. Stop all ice cream, including "soy" ice cream.	**Milk, Cheese, Cottage Cheese, Yoghurt, Ice Cream, Cream, Non-Dairy Cream.**
Starch	Sweet potato, Arrowroot, Tapioca, Rice, Buckwheat, Millet, Amaranth, Quinoa, All Gluten-Free products.	*All Gluten containing products* including Pasta, All *Corn* & Corn Containing Products.
Breads and Cereals	Any flat (yeast free) bread made from Rice, Quinoa, Amaranth, Buckwheat, Millet, Potato Flour, Tapioca, Arrowroot, All must be (certified) 100% Gluten-free based products.	Any bread (containing sugars and yeast) made from *Wheat*, Oats, Kamut, *Spelt*, *Rye*, *Barley*, and even any '*Gluten-Free*' containing grained breads.
Vegetables	All Vegetables, preferably organic, freshly grown, (pref. not frozen). Garlic, onions, etc.	Creamed or made with prohibited ingredients.
Fruits	Blueberries, coconut and avocado are the three best fruits when you have a yeast infection. Green apples are generally OK.	Fruit drinks, Cocktails, **Oranges**, **Banana**, *Pineapple*, Strawberries, all dried fruits preserved with sulphites. (Like the glazed apricots). Avoid all dried fruits.
Soups	Clear, vegetable based broth, Homemade vegetarian. It is best to avoid packet or tinned soups, make your own from scratch using fresh vegetables & meats.	**Canned or Creamed soups**. Avoid soups with glutinous flours & grains
Drinks	Stay with filtered or pure water and unsweetened herbal teas. Pau d'arco tea, works well. Lemon juice in water, grapefruit juice to which you add 5 drops of grapefruit seed extract per 250 mls.	**Milk** or **milk-based drinks**, **dairy** based products, avoid alcoholic drinks, soda and energy drinks, diet drinks and most citrus drinks, **Orange Juice**.

Oils and Fats	Cold pressed oils, preferably in dark amber bottles; best oils are linseed, olive, and sesame, sunflower, walnut, pumpkin and grape seed oils. Oregano oil. Coconut	Margarines, shortening/lard, butter, vegetable oil blends, salad dressings, spreads (sugars), deep-fried foods.
Nuts and Seeds	Almonds, brazil and hazelnuts, walnuts, pecans, pumpkin, sesame, sunflower, squash seeds, nut/seed butters made with allowed ingredients, watch those sugars.	**Peanuts**, pistachios, cashew nuts, **peanut butter**, hazelnut spread (sugar)
Sweeteners & Treats	Brown rice syrup, fruit sweeteners. Xylitol or Stevia are acceptable, in very small amounts.	*White or brown sugar, caster, icing, Demerara, soft brown and all types of sugar, honey, molasses, maple & corn syrup, fructose, glucose, malt, dextrose.* **Chocolate** *Avoid candies & sweets as well*

Dietary Supplements During The Stage 2 Low Allergy Diet

The supplements I recommend in the second stage of the Candida Crusher Program are the **Candida Crusher Formula,** the **Candida Crusher Multi,** the **Candida Crusher Digestive Enzyme** and the **Candida Crusher Probiotic** and we introduce in the second stage the **Candida Crusher Omega 3**.

Here's why you need to take these dietary supplements during stage 2:

1   The Candida Crusher Formula. This product is maintained throughout the three stages of the Candida Crusher Program and beyond until you are yeast-free. You will have been on the MEVY Diet for several weeks now and have already introduced this powerful product into your supplementation regime. It is time to step-up the dosage if you can and to get out of your comfort zone, if you were taking 3 each day try 4 or 5. There is nothing wrong with increasing the dosage, but do it carefully and controlled. Great improvements can come about at times just by making slow increases; you will reduce the candida population steadily and surely this way. Stay on the Candida Crusher Formula during Stage 2, as you start to reduce any potential allergenic foods from your diet. We want to keep any advancing yeast, parasite of bacterial populations at bay so if you can, increase the dose and be sure to take this product seven days a week. As your diet continues to change, there will be subtle changes in the micro-flora of your digestive system and we don't want the yeast to take advantage of any opportunities.

2   The Candida Crusher Multi is intended to help combat any potential nutritional deficiencies while you are on the Candida Crusher Program. This product is also maintained throughout the Candida Crusher program and beyond, until you feel really well. This Stage 2 low-allergy diet includes the removal of certain foods, which may be challenging your immune system, but it also potentially includes the removal of several sources of important nutrients from your diet and you are therefore wise to supplement with the Candida Crusher Multi. Take one dose three to four times daily with meals or snacks. Some will need more, some will need less.

3   The Candida Crusher Digestive Enzyme is one of the most important supplements you can take during this second stage. This unique enzymatic formula will ensure a more complete and efficient digestive process, allowing the more complete breakdown of foods thereby reducing the risk of increasing any allergenic potential of the foods remaining in your diet after you have removed the most likely allergy culprits. Take with each meal, and more with a protein rich diet. You may want to try the "stomach tolerance method" outlined in section 4 of chapter 7. In addition, this formula will assist in reducing any inflammation in your digestive system and along with the probiotic help to heal the lining of the digestive system.

4 **The Candida Crusher Probiotic.** You will want to continue with this product throughout the Candida Crusher Program, just like the other two products already mentioned. Most people do fine on dosing twice daily with a probiotic, and don't need to take it three to four times daily like most other supplements.

This product is a good immune-booster and anti-inflammatory as well, which are two great actions to have in your digestive system when you are eliminating potential allergy causing foods. With acute digestive problems you can dose more frequently, however.

5 **The Candida Crusher Omega 3** is a product we are introducing into the program during stage 2. But why not take it earlier you ask? Well you can, but I prefer that you take fewer products during the initial month or so and place more focus on your diet and lifestyle. Many people who begin the Candida Crusher Program will be already taking dietary supplements and may be taking an Omega 3 already, which is OK to. The reason why I like you to take the Candida Crusher Omega 3 supplement now during this second stage and for the rest on the treatment, is to reduce any potential inflammation as we are particularly interested in healing the lining of the small intestine (leaky gut) and want to counter and inflammation in stage 2. In addition, Omega 3 has been shown to boost the immune response and this is an important action we are looking for during this second stage. Be sure to take one capsule twice daily with meals.

Don't forget, you can read all about special anti-candida foods, supplements and herbal medicines in section 4 of this chapter, chapter 7.

The Diet Re-Introduction Stage

People always ask me this question: "How long do I have to stay off these foods for?" Once you have started to feel really good, which does take time, then it's time to move to Stage 3, the Diet Re-Introduction Stage.

This stage is very important, and if properly implemented can provide the solid foundation for your future digestive health. Always remember that a healthy and balanced digestive system will keep you from having a candida yeast overgrowth again in the future.

The rate of recovery varies from person to person; some folks can re-introduce foods more rapidly than others. It is best that you slowly re-introduce foods into your diet because if you introduce foods too quickly you may find that you may quickly revert back to a candida yeast infection once again. Your long-term candida dietary approach is explained in this section as well. You need never have a candida yeast infection again if you follow this long-term dietary approach carefully.

There is no point in eradicating a yeast infection only to find that a year or two later it is back again. Once your health is fully restored in time, the Stage 3 long-term dietary approach is very important because it will most likely provide you with your own weapon against falling victim to a major candida yeast infection all over again.

The duration of Stage 3 depends entirely on your rate of recovery, and I sometimes find that men and children recover quicker than female patients.

This could be partly due to the fact that many women with a yeast infection affecting their digestive system have a vaginal infection as well. While this may seem a bit generalized, it is just my experience after treating many patients. But this is certainly not true in all cases; some men I have treated just don't seem to recover as fast as others and pediatric cases can be more resistant to recovery if the child is constantly sick and getting antibiotics.

Your favorite foods can and should be re-introduced one at a time, don't be in a big hurry to reintroduce too quickly and especially too many foods at once, this is a very common mistake you can make and most patients I have seen who seem to relapse, or those who almost get well but then quickly crash yet again fall into this category.

You have come this far and have started to feel great one again and now you could potentially blow the whole thing due to impatience.

Remember earlier on in the introduction to this chapter, we spoke about your recovery in terms of fantasyland and the reality check? The reality is that you can and possibly will aggravate when you reintroduce certain foods or drinks in Stage 3, but this does not mean that you are back to square one, it just means that you have to back off a little and slow down. Just remove that offending food or drink, and once more your symptoms should subside and when you are starting to feel a lot better, it is time to re-introduce that food back into your diet once again.

Not Certain If You Have Cleared Your Yeast Infection?

Those who have initially completed the online survey (candida questionnaire) and then the Candida Symptom Tracker along with the Candida Test Tracker will have a much clearer picture of which direction they will be heading in. They will know if they are improving, standing still or going backwards as far as treatment is concerned.

You may wish to complete the candida questionnaire again, and if all is well with your health you should be getting quite a different outcome to the questionnaire than when you first started. You can complete the test online at www.yeastinfection.org, which I recommend, as this will give you a score and is just a matter of going through the screens and clicking away.

Your energy levels should be up, your head clear, no more brain fog or dizziness, and you should be able to eat most foods without any major aggravations. If you have not improved as much as you would have liked, then I recommend you stay with Stage 1 and Stage 2 of the Candida Crusher Diet for a few more weeks and keep taking the Candida Crusher products. Each case of a yeast infection is different, with some patients respond more rapidly than others so there is no set time limit on each stage.

Start by re-introducing those foods that contain the least amount of sugar and yeast. As mentioned earlier, the foods you avoid initially are those that are the highest in sugars, and the chart below for example will give you an insight in to the highest and lowest sugar containing fruits. If you are very serious about your recovery, then please be committed and prepared to make long-term changes to your diet!

Fruit Re-Introduction

I always find that the two big areas people feel deprived of once they start the Candida Crusher Dietary Program are fruit and breads, containing sugars and yeasts. For those who have recovered from a yeast infection, they may enjoy the following fruit treats. As I have mentioned previously, it is best that you avoid eating very sweet fruits until you feel much better, especially better in your digestive system.

Once you feel a significant improvement, and you have already added kiwi fruit, green apple, pears, berries and maybe even pineapple back into your diet, there is no reason why you shouldn't be able to introduce other sweeter fruits back into your diet. It is advisable however not to eat too much of the sweet fruits in one day and not every single day either. Be sensible, you are recovering from a yeast infection and yeast loves sugar to feed on, whether it is in the form of sweets, fruit or alcohol.

The safest way to begin reintroducing fruit into your diet is to start with a small bowl of fresh natural acidophilus yogurt and add a few blueberries, kiwi or a few slices or freshly peeled orange or mandarin. From there you may want to progress to a fruit smoothie, but hold on the ice cream please, too much sugar! Fresh fruit smoothies taste fabulous when made with yogurt and ice cubes, then add some berries, pear, pineapple or orange.

Feel free to experiment and work out the combination that suits your taste, the variations are endless.

- **Frozen fruit smoothies** are hard to beat for a treat and my absolute favorite would have to be this recipe: about three large mangos, just cut the pulp away from the seed, and include the juice of three large juicy oranges, blend and enjoy!

- **Try making a fresh fruit salad** made with banana, passion fruit, green apple, lemon juice, orange and pineapple. The passion fruit will give this salad a truly exotic flavor.

- **Fresh creamy yogurt with frozen blue berries.** I blend this in my Vitamix with a few ice cubes.

I generally allow berries in the candida diet right at the beginning, as they are low in sugar, especially blueberries. It pays to first re-introduce foods in the left column, those fruits that tend to be lower in sugar than fruits found in the right column. Introduce the low, then moderate and then the fruits that are high in sugar (fresh). Always introduce dried fruits way down the track, once you are feeling great and then use a lot of caution here, many people simply overdo the dried fruits and eat too much. You may find it interesting to see avocado in the low-sugar fruit list, many people think that avocado is a vegetable when technically it is a fruit and is OK to eat when you have a yeast infection.

Fruits Low In Sugars

- Avocado
- Blueberries
- Blackberries
- Cranberries
- Lemon & lime
- Raspberries
- Strawberries
- Rhubarb (don't add sugar)
- Green apple

Fruits Moderate In Sugars

- Cantaloupe (rock melon)
- Guavas
- Honeydew Melon
- Apples (some mod. & some high)
- Melon
- Nectarines
- Papaya
- Peach
- Watermelon

Fruits High In Sugars

- Apricots
- Banana
- Cherries
- Dates
- Figs
- Grapefruit
- Grapes
- Kiwifruit
- Oranges
- Pears
- Pineapple
- Plums
- Pomegranates
- Mangoes
- Prunes
- Raisins
- Tangerines

Now that you have completed the hard work of defeating your yeast infection, don't blow it by reintroducing foods too quickly! Start slowly and add back one food at a time. This has the added benefit that you will easily be able to pick out any food allergies as you go. You can start by adding back some fruits; particularly those with lower sugar content like green apples and berries. Fruits which are considerably higher in sugar, like oranges, grapes and bananas should still be avoided until you are really sure that things are OK, trust me, don't blow it at this stage, you may be excited and think things are just great until you go to a wedding, a diner party, etc.

Most candida patients will be able to add complex starchy vegetables back into their diet soon enough, but some won't and will find that if they add sweet potato, yams, pumpkin and other starchy foods like beans back into their diet too rapidly, they will suffer with gas and bloating. It's all trial and error really, what will suit you won't necessarily suit another. I prefer to use the cautious approach when it comes to re-introduction. It took you some time to start feeling better, don't blow it by being impatient, let's get it right this time and beat this thing, once and for all!

Good Health Tip:

How To Re-Introduce Bananas Into Your Diet After A Yeast Infection

Everybody loves bananas, they are such a convenient snack and so tasty. Besides being packed full of nutrition, bananas are a good source of pre-biotics and are a good addition into your healthy diet, but I do advise caution here and feel it is better upon re-introduction to initially eat them when they are partially green/yellow and don't wait until they are very ripe and very yellow or over ripe with some brown discoloration. The reason for this is that as they ripen they become sweeter, and the starch which is very high when bananas are green, converts to fruit sugars, especially by the time they are spotted brown.

If you eat one or two bananas each day that are ripe or over-ripe too prematurely, you may quickly find that you run the risk of lots of gas and bloating, and may be potentially setting yourself up for developing that yeast infection all over again. Eat a banana once or twice a week to start, and eat them partially green and yellow, that way you should be able to avoid most aggravations.

Vegetable Re-Introduction

Vegetable re-introduction is no big deal, the main thing to bear in mind is that with chronic cases of yeast infection it is really in your best interests if you avoid the starchy (usually root) vegetables for the first few weeks and the bring them slowly back into the diet.

As I have mentioned earlier, some folks will tend to eat more of the sweet starchy carbohydrates as a substitute for the sugar they have removed from the diet. Do you crave pumpkin or potato? It may be the sugar you are looking for, and the stronger the craving for a starchy vegetable the more likely you will be having a problem with it in your diet.

A good tip is that upon re-introduction of the starchy root vegetables, to be aware of these two issues, and if it has become a real problem then ease up a little.

Gas & bloating – introduce more slowly and in smaller amounts, try a different cooking method. You are taking the Candida Crusher Digestive Enzyme and the Candida Crusher Probiotic, aren't you?

Bowel motion issues – constipation or diarrhea, reduce portion sizes, try a different method of cooking. You are taking the Candida Crusher Digestive Enzyme and the Candida Crusher Probiotic, aren't you?

Follow The MEVY Stage 1 Diet If Any Major Stress Is Coming Up

For example, if at any time in the future should you need to take an antibiotic; it is wise to follow the Stage 1 anti-candida implementation phase again for a few weeks, whilst taking the probiotic.

And although the susceptibility to candida infection may remain high for a number of years into your future, it can reoccur literally at any time if the conditions are right and the right formula for its re-growth are there. For this reason I'd like you to be very aware of your body and its vulnerabilities. You certainly don't have to wait for all the symptoms to re-appear.

For example, if you have a stressful event coming up like a wedding, a large family occasion, the birth of a child, exams or perhaps a job interview – then do something about it before you begin to feel unwell. Follow Stage 1 of my dietary approach and you will have no problems at all and will most probably avert any aggravations from occurring. Many people beginning a candida diet believe they must stay on a restrictive diet forever; this is certainly not my experience. While the final phase of the diet is intended to be a long-term maintenance plan, candida dieters will typically re-introduce most foods and avoid only the ones that exacerbate their symptoms. Most people will continue on with some form of reduction in their consumption of dairy products, breads, sugary sweets and soft drinks but most return to eating fruits and high carbohydrate foods. In general, fresh fruits and vegetables, high-quality proteins, whole grains and unprocessed foods are the best way to keep any future yeast overgrowth in check.

Benefits Of Re-Introduction

One of the biggest benefits of following Stages 1 and 2 of the Candida Crusher Diet in an immediate sense is that it helps to regulate your gastrointestinal system and reduces many problematic symptoms such as gas, cramping, pain, constipation, diarrhea and bloating. Many people who have followed the Candida Crusher dietary approach feel more energetic and considerably less fatigued, and many lose weight along the way and for these reasons quite a few patients have remained on variations of the stage 1 and 2 eating approach for months, and some even for many years.

And why would you change if you feel so good on a particular eating regime? Well, many do want to go back and enjoy those foods they used to like a long time ago, and this may include bread, alcohol and the occasional treat like chocolate or cookies. But common sense prevails, and any intelligent person should understand that a steady slide down to a poor diet and sloppy lifestyle might bring a yeast infection back once more with a vengeance. But it would also increase the person's chance of any one of a hundred other chronic health conditions too.

> *If we are creating ourselves all the time, then it is never too late to begin creating the bodies we want instead of the ones we mistakenly assume we are stuck with.*
> Deepak Chopra

Good Tip:

When do I know I'm better and can stop treatment?

If your yeast infection symptoms are changing for the better, change nothing but continue on with the treatment until there is no more improvement.
If you continue to improve, stay with what you are doing – it is obviously working for you.

No more improvement but still not well? You need to make changes until you notice improvement again. Is nothing changing, or are you still feeling bad? Then you may need to change *everything you are doing and start over*. If nothing is changing you may need to change everything!

Be sure to read section 5 at the end of this chapter, particularly the end of section 5. I will give you plenty of solutions about what to do if all else fails and you just can't seem to get right, in spite of all your best intentions.

The 3 Golden Rules of Re-Introduction

After a period of time ranging from 6 to 12 weeks there are many foods that may gradually be re-introduced back into your diet, although this will depend greatly of course on the progress you have made in reducing symptoms.

Golden Rule # 1

With your food and drink re-introduction, examine the foods you liked to eat before you started on the Candida Crusher Program, when you were at the peak of your dysfunction. It makes sense that if you go back to the pattern of eating and living the way you used to, that you may well end up with a yeast infection all over again. You need to change is your candida needs to go for good!

Golden Rule # 2

If your yeast infections symptoms are getting better (some symptoms may be getting better, some are not) then keep on with treatment, I have absolutely no doubt in my mind when I state that a general lack of perseverance is the number one reason why most people will fail to recover 100 percent from a yeast infection. In fact, it's the number one reason they fail to accomplish many great things in their life.

Golden Rule # 3

If you are not improving at all, in spite of following my Candida Crusher Program including the dietary, lifestyle and supplementation advice to the letter, then you may well have an "obstacle to cure". You can read all about these obstacles in section 5 of this chapter.

Dietary Supplementation During Stage 3

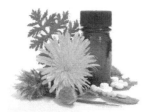 The supplements I recommend in the third stage of the Candida Crusher Program are the **Candida Crusher Formula,** the **Candida Crusher Multi**, the **Candida Crusher Digestive Enzyme** and the **Candida Crusher Probiotic** and the **Candida Crusher Omega 3**.

Here's why you need to take these dietary supplements during stage 3:

1 The Candida Crusher Formula. This product is maintained throughout the three stages of the Candida Crusher Program and beyond until you are yeast-free. Now that you are re-introducing foods back into your diet in stage 3, there is the potential danger that you may slowly slip back into your old dietary habits, be careful! The Candida Crusher Formula when taken at a lower dosage of one or two a day for several months after you complete the program will ensure you don't get a re-occurrence of your yeast infection.

If for example, you did start to eat some of those offending foods you once did which contributed to your yeast infection, at least with this product you are reducing your risk of a full-blown regrowth. If you do stop this product, keep it handy so that you can take it whenever you feel that the problem resurfaces, because the recurrence rate for a yeast infection (especially if you've had a chronic infection in the past) is considerably high. So, unless you are behaving yourself, the risk can be high of a recurrence.

2 The Candida Crusher Multi is intended to help combat any potential nutritional deficiencies while you are on the Candida Crusher Program. This product is also maintained throughout the Candida Crusher program and beyond, until you feel really well. As you go back onto your regular diet, this product can be maintained for as long as you need a multivitamin and mineral dietary supplement. You can stay on one, two or three daily, depending on how much support you need, and how good your diet is.

3 The Candida Crusher Digestive Enzyme is a very good product to take during stage 3, because you are changing your diet once again and along with that there will be a shift in your intestinal pH and micro-flora population. Whenever there is dietary change like this, there is a potential for bloating, gas, and bowel function (and bowel motion) changes. Stick with two or three doses daily. Have you tried the Stomach Tolerance Method yet, as outlined in section 4 of chapter 7? You may be quite surprised to see how much enzymatic support you really need.

4 The Candida Crusher Probiotic. This is the last product you finish off with. In my experience, most patients I've seen with yeast infections never seem to take enough probiotics and never for long enough to really benefit from them. The rule of thumb in my clinic is for every week you have been on an antibiotic; you take a

4 probiotic for 2 months. If you are going back into eating commercial (not certified free-range) chicken, stay on the Candida Crusher Probiotic indefinitely. Stay on the probiotic for at least three to four months after you complete the Candida Crusher Program, and even longer if you continue with a little alcohol or diet with refined, processed or take-out foods.

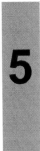

5 The Candida Crusher Omega 3. You may be well aware of the multiple health benefits you can get from a high quality Omega 3. The Candida Crusher Omega 3 has been made from the finest raw materials and will help you in many ways to contribute to your health and wellbeing. I have been personally taking Omega 3 daily for over thirty years and will continue to do so, along with my multi vitamin and mineral. The Omega 3 and Multi Vitamin when taken daily form a cheap health-insurance policy against the premature development of many chronic and degenerative diseases of modern civilization like heart disease, cancer and diabetes.

The third and last reminder, you can read all about special anti-candida foods, supplements and herbal medicines in section 4 of this chapter, chapter 7.

Frequently Asked Candida Crusher Dietary Questions (FAQS)

When Can I Have Fruit Again?

I always find that one of the first food groups that the patient will want to re-introduce is fruit. Some experts believe that fruit has such amazing health benefits that it is believed that they outweigh the potential problems that more fruit sugars in the diet may cause. It is important that fruit is re-introduced slowly, particularly if you have been eating plenty of fruit in your diet previously, and by plenty I mean 3 or 4 pieces of fruit or more daily. I believe that fruit should only make up a small proportion of the diet and not be a major focus. You will need to be particularly careful with the re-introduction of fruit juices back into your diet. It is interesting to note that some folks with a yeast infection keep eating fruit right throughout their candida program; they just eliminate sweets and yeast containing foods and still get a great result. This is for the minority of yeast sufferers however; I can assure you that in most cases this is not the case and that a careful elimination of all fruits (except avocado and berries, lemon, lime, kiwi fruit and Granny Smith apple, will be found to be most beneficial in the early stages of the candida diet.

How Long Does Stage Three Last?

There are no rules with the food re-introduction stage, and each case is different. It is important that you understand that because nobody knows how you are feeling, you will need to be the judge of how you complete the food re-introduction. Only you are best to gauge when you are ready to take on a new food, so don't be afraid of trying a new food or taking your time when you do re-introduce. If you feel bad at any time, re-assess what went wrong and make changes, just revert back to what did work for you previously and hang in there a little longer. By taking your time and not being in a hurry, you will develop a higher level of patience, a factor that is critical in your recovery and re-introduction stage.

The third and final stage has no real end stage, some patients I have seen have successfully re-introduced foods back into their diet and are leading normal lives again within four months of commencing the Candida Crusher Program, whereas others are still having issues a year down the track. Some people find that they feel fine after a period of a few weeks of food re-introduction, only to discover that their previously major symptom begins to aggravate once more (although not as bad a previously experienced).

This will typically be caused due to the fact that they felt increasingly better, and with this renewed level of health and vitality they began to enjoy life to its fullest once again, and this possibly included favourite "likes" such as alcohol, sweets, ice cream, breads, staying up late, pharmaceutical drugs, too much stress, etc., which caused them to crash. Not an uncommon scenario, and one I have seen one hundred times or more. It would have been the combination of these several contributing factors put together that reached a point where their digestive system once again supported a level of yeast and bad bacteria that brought those symptoms to the foreground previously. Back to the drawing board in that case I say.

Should I Continue With The Multi, Digestive Enzymes And Probiotics?

Many patients I see believe that you only need to take dietary supplements like the multi, digestive enzymes, probiotics, Omega 3, etc.; when you feel unwell, and once you feel better then you can discontinue them. It is not uncommon for me to recommend a product to a person who will take that supplement for a month or so and then stop taking it, because "it didn't work". I'll speak a lot more on dietary supplements and herbal medicines in general with regard to yeast infections in section 4 of this chapter.

It makes a lot of sense for you to continue on with the multivitamin, digestive enzymes and probiotics for several months, even the entire next year. I like a patient to get well and stay well and continue that way for at least three to six months after they have beaten candida before they decide that supplements are not that necessary any more.

How Quickly Should You Re-Introduce Foods?

This is where many people run into problems, they either re-introduce too many foods at the same time or re-introduce certain foods and drinks prematurely, before they have improved to the point where they can tolerate those foods and drinks that they previously had difficulties with. Now that you have done all the hard work by eliminating the offending foods and allergenic foods, don't blow it be re-introducing foods too quickly! The trick is to be patient and introduce one food at a time, and over a three-day period. For example, when you first re-introduce fruit, add a piece of fruit for three days and then try another piece for the next three days in addition to the first, etc. Introduce your favorite fruit last, and try not to eat anymore than two to three pieces of fresh fruit per day until you are really well and even beyond.

Which Foods Should You Reintroduce First And Which Foods Should You Reintroduce Last?

A good question and one I often get asked. As I mentioned previously, I believe the smartest approach here is to re-introduce the foods you love and crave the very last, because these are the foods and drinks your immune system has most likely become the most sensitive to, simply because it has been exposed to these foods and drinks the most. There is a reason why you wanted these foods in the first place, especially if these were sweet, sugary or yeast containing foods. And now you are telling me that you want to re-introduce them right away? You must be crazy in that case!

Some patients who are overcoming a yeast infection often tell me they want alcohol back in their lives, or chocolate, bread, ice cream or another food that potentially may plunge them head-on into a yeast infection yet again. If you are really serious about crushing your candida permanently, and I take it you are or you probably wouldn't be reading the Candida Crusher, then reintroducing an offending food should be the last thing on your mind. Why is it that we as humans can tend to be a bit like moths drawn to the flame? How many times in the past did you have a hangover or indigestion yet weeks later you found yourself with a glass in your hand or eating too much or the wrong kind of food?

How Long Will It Take Until I'm Eating My Normal Diet Again?

It is very important to understand that there is no fixed time period when it comes to eating your normal diet again. Some patients I have seen are re-introducing foods back into their diets that they previously could not tolerate, within 3 months. Others are not so fortunate, and find that they are still having issues with foods after 6 months. Some candida patients I have seen over the years have struggled for decades with their diet re-introduction unfortunately, but these folks are certainly a minority. Please don't expect a quick and easy solution if you have been chronically unwell for many years. There are many factors that may account for how long it will take before you are eating the foods you love again, and some of these factors include:

- How successful you have been at eradicating your yeast infection.

- How successful you have been at re-introducing beneficial bacteria.

- How well and committed you have been in sticking to the 3 Stages of the Candida Crusher Diet.

- How successful you have been in understanding that to eradicate your yeast infection does not solely mean taking supplements and eating healthier, but that it involves making changes to your lifestyle as well. See sections 2 and 5 of chapter 7 in particular.

- How successful you have been in attending to any causes of your yeast infection.

- If you have ben experiencing a local complaint like jock itch, vaginal thrush or toe nail fungus, it all depends how well you have treated the local complaint in addition to following the Candida Crusher Dietary Program. Local complaints need local treatment either daily or very regularly, in conjunction with my lifestyle and diet advice if a permanent yeast infection result is to be expected.

At the risk of repeating myself time and again, the foods you need to re-introduce last are obviously the foods that have caused you the most aggravations, and for most people these foods include the white refined carbohydrates, alcohol and the sugary processed foods.

I want you to go into these three candida dietary stages with your eyes wide open and to not have totally unrealistic expectations. If you follow the Candida Crusher Program earnestly like many have, and you are honest with yourself then you will get results, it is as simple as that, and the more you apply yourself, the sooner those results will seem to appear to happen.

When Can I Drink Alcohol Again?

I knew you would ask this question sooner or later! It really depends on your level of improvement, but as I have stated a few times already in the Candida Crusher, alcohol is probably the strongest item you can take into your diet in terms of affecting your digestive system and aggravating any underlying yeast infection. You are best to wait for a considerable length of time before you do re-introduce alcohol, from 3 to 6 months, but many who will be reading this will most probably drink socially or very occasionally whilst on the C.C. Program anyway, let's face it!

I do see the occasional patient who complains of little to no improvement in spite of a perfect diet and lifestyle. I wonder if this person may be taking in a little too much alcohol if they do happen to be drinking? It is important to remember that self-delusion is the worst kind of delusion there is.

To answer this question, I would say that it is best you wait long enough until you feel really good, and then start very slowly with alcohol and be sure to also include plenty of water, fruit & vegetable juices and herbal teas into your diet in addition. Is wine better than beer, or are spirits better then cider? It does not really matter, alcohol is alcohol and its effects are similar in the body. It is all about dosage and frequency of dosage that counts, and if you want to drink regularly once you have recovered, be sure to have several days during the week in which you drink no alcohol, this will allow your body, especially your digestive system, to recover. This will ensure that you are much less likely to develop any re-establishment of your yeast infection, and will give you enough time to work out if alcohol is a causative factor and to what degree with your yeast infection.

Final Words

Always Think About Healing That Leaky Gut

You should be able to eat an increasing amount of foods as you digestive system heals. It is very important that you fully understand this concept. What we have done initially, when you think about it, is to remove those food items that contributed to the yeast overgrowth, and then we removed food items against which you may have, unbeknown to you, experienced allergies towards.

The foods that are re-introduced first were the least of the reactant foods because your immune system will have had the time to recover, after this you should be able to handle the re-introduction of the increasingly provocative foods. As a result, you should be less symptomatic, even if you are eating food items to which you formerly had been allergic or reacted to. This principle is one of the major foundations on which the Candida Crusher diet is based.

As you are able to tolerate foods that you previously couldn't, you leaky gut is showing signs of recovery. As your leaky gut heals, your immune system improves and your reactions decrease and eventually your signs and symptoms disappear, trust me, this will all happen in good time.

Repetition Is The Best Way To Learn

If you have read this chapter all the way through, you will have found that I have repeated myself on several occasions. This was done to serve a purpose, to drive the point home. Repetition is the way to learn and if you pick up of the key repetitive messages in the Candida Crusher, then I believe that you are well on your way to yeast infection recovery. And that is why I wrote this book, and I thank you again for investing in the Candida Crusher.

Don't forget to read the rest of this book; Candida Crusher was intended to be a manual that offers you a holistic mind and body approach to overcoming your yeast infection.

Here's to your health!

Eric Bakker ND

SECTION 2

Candida Crusher Immunity –
Understanding Immunity, Metabolites And Stress

> *An investment in knowledge always pays the best interest*
> *Benjamin Franklin*

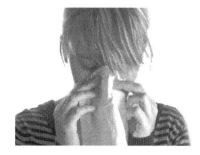

When it comes to the immune system, most people are only familiar with terms such as infections and allergies. Many people I have seen are not even aware that stress can play a fundamental role in the development and maintenance of their yeast infection. This is an important section of the Candida Crusher, because you are about to learn that stress can and does take its toll on your immune system, reducing your resistance and increasing your susceptibility of a yeast infection.

Once you understand the stress/candida connection and know that you can do something about it, you will be in a better position to be able to fully recover from your yeast infection. This chapter is one of the key areas of the Candida Crusher, and often one of the forgotten aspects of yeast infection recovery. Your immune system is greatly influenced by your stress levels, and a powerful immune system can help you recover rapidly and permanently from a yeast infection. Once you learn about the stress/candida connection and work on balancing your autonomic nervous system, (more on this in section 5 of this chapter) you will be amazed and delighted at how quick your body can recover from a fungal overgrowth that may have been plaguing you for years.

This information will be especially helpful for those with candida who get better but don't seem to fully recover; they only partially recover and then seem to slowly get worse again. They have followed a strict diet, take supplements and exercise regularly. They get enough sleep but still can't seem to get on top of their yeast infection. Have they looked at the influence of stress in their lives?

First let's explore the topic of immunity and candida a little further and take a look at the interplay between candida metabolites and your immune system in particular. A metabolite is just a fancy term for any products of metabolic change, i.e., what your immune system does to candida and also to any chemicals that candida produces, like waste products.

In this section of the book I will also explain what I call health busters and health builders and then elaborate on the relationship between adrenal fatigue, stress and yeast infections. I'll finish this section on what you can help to beat a yeast infection by boosting your immune system and beating stress, one of the biggest, most misunderstood and hidden causes of chronic ill health today.

Metabolites, Mycotoxins, Immunity And Yeast Infections

Mycotoxin means fungus poison in Latin, and is a toxic secondary metabolite produced by organisms of the fungi kingdom, commonly known as molds. The term mycotoxin is usually reserved for the toxic chemical by-products produced by fungi, and one mold species may produce many different mycotoxins, and the same mycotoxin may be produced by several species.

Many people are probably unaware of the effects of the yeast cells on the immune system. Yeast cells are quite complicated and have many thousands of complex reactions both within their own cells as well as with the many millions of cells in their surrounding environment. Just like all other living things, yeast cells need food to live and to multiply, as well as having the ability to produce wastes.

When yeast is living in your digestive system and in other areas of your body, mycotoxins are released from yeast cells which can then circulate throughout different areas of your body, for example in the circulatory system such as the blood and blood vessels, as well as throughout your digestive system, the stomach, small and large intestines, liver, pancreas, etc., in particular, but they can also travel through the blood-brain barrier and create problems in the brain and affect the way you think and feel.

Several of these individual metabolite components have been identified over time as being toxic to your immune system, causing reactions including a chronic low-grade state of inflammation. And it is these chemical reactions that can literally exhaust your immune system and wreak havoc on your brain, digestive, hormone, musculoskeletal and nervous systems.

Acetaldehyde

In 1986, Dr. Orion Truss wrote about acetaldehyde, a chemical that at toxic levels can make its way into the brain from candida. The consumption of sugar ensures that candida produces acetaldehyde in the digestive tract by way sugar fermentation. Anyone with a yeast overgrowth who also drinks beer, wine, spirits or liqueurs not only produces acetaldehyde from alcohol itself, but also delivers more sugar for the yeast production of acetaldehyde, creating a double-barreled dose. Acetaldehyde produced in the gut eventually reaches more parts of the body and even into the brain, flooding the system and increasing the risk for damage*.

*Truss CO. Metabolic Abnormalities in Patients with Chronic Candidiasis: The Acetaldehyde Hypothesis. J Orthomolecular Psychiatry. 1984; 13(2): 66-93.

Gliotoxin

A gliotoxin is a mycotoxin produced by several species of fungi, including pathogens of humans such as *Aspergillus*, and also candida.

A study* published in 2010 revealed that candida could produce a substance called a gliotoxin (GT), an immunosuppressive toxin. It is now believed that GT's immune-suppressing activity contributes to the survival of candida albicans in the blood stream during infections. In addition to GT's immunosuppressive properties, this mycotoxin may also suppress and cause apoptosis (cell death) in certain types of cells of the immune system, including neutrophils, eosinophils, granulocytes, and macrophages.

This explains why this parasite can be so hard to eradicate by so many people's immune systems. GT has also been discovered to have antithrombotic properties, which means that it prevents the formation of clots and thins blood, allowing it to travel more freely through the bloodstream and giving it the ability to be able to access areas of the body where it couldn't normally go. GTs also explain brain fog and the severe and debilitating feelings many people feel when they are on the candida program.

*Thrombosis and Haemostasis. 2010 Aug;104(2):270-8. doi: 10.1160/TH09-11-0769. Epub 2010 Apr 29. Bertling A, Niemann S, Uekötter A, Fegeler W, Lass-Flörl C, von Eiff C, Kehrel BE. Department of Anesthesiology and Intensive Care, Experimental and Clinical Haemostasis, University of Muenster, Muenster, Germany.

In addition, yeasts continually die as well as multiply causing yet even more chemicals to be produced and circulated throughout your system, and some of these chemicals other than aldehyde have also been identified as being toxic to the brain, capable of causing various behavioral disturbances. Is it any wonder that a yeast infection can leave you feeling so lousy?

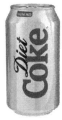

A chronic yeast sufferer may consume large amounts of foods or drinks which are continually causing a large amount of these toxic metabolites to be formed in their body, and these foods may include alcohol, soda or cola drinks, breads, fries, confectionery, dried and fresh fruits, chocolate, refined carbohydrates, and sugar. It is surprising how many people drink diet drinks, in the belief that they are entirely harmless.

A hidden problem surfaces when there is a large amount of toxic metabolites like gliotoxin and mannan present in the body, with more being continually produced along with the large amount of yeast and bad bacteria already present. The big problem arises however when these formed toxic metabolites begin to challenge the immune system, along with the candida itself.

If your diet is high in the foods that candida love, the foods and drinks I have clearly outlined in the first section of this chapter, then you may well be producing far too many yeasts themselves in addition to their metabolites, thereby challenging your immune system on a continual basis, twenty four hours a day.

Sometimes the sheer volume of these toxic metabolites in combination with very poor levels of beneficial bacteria may be even too large for your immune system to cope with, because your body may already be having to deal with numerous hidden food allergies, bad bacteria and parasites, leaky gut syndrome and low-grade inflammation present elsewhere in your body. Now you can understand how a chronic yeast infection can affect you at any time of the day, and in any one of a hundred or more ways!

Mannan

Mannan is a glycoprotein found in the cell wall of candida, and it is released by candida in response to an infection around it, usually in the digestive system. This is different from gliotoxin, which is an actual toxin released by candida itself which spreads toxins directly in its surroundings. A study* has shown that tiny mannan fragments are liberated in the digestive tract and then get absorbed slowly into the bloodstream. These tiny proteins then stimulate an immune response and go on to cause suppression of the immune system, and it is this response then renders the immune system less capable of fighting a yeast infection. This explains in part why some people just don't seem to recover that well or constantly relapse with candida yeast infections.

Here's what typically happens, a person takes one or several courses of an antibiotic for an infection which kills the infection, but also kills many beneficial bacteria in the digestive tract. That you already know, but then candida gets the upper hand and begins to slowly proliferate as an opportunistic organism. That you probably know too, but what you may not know is that this proliferation of yeast cells in the digestive system then slowly release mannan proteins continually which drip feed into the blood stream. Even after the yeast is cleared or brought under control eventually by anti-fungal supplements, foods or drugs, mannan will continue to circulate for some time, sometimes many months or even a year in chronic cases in my experience, until these miniscule proteins are finally cleared. The unfortunate thing with mannan protein is that it can take a very long time before it is finally broken down and eradicated from your body, and this explains why your digestion may appear OK, your thrush may be under control but you still feel lousy, tired and miserable. Brain fog can still be there for some time, so you will need to be patient! Now you know some of these reasons.

Recurring and persistent yeast infections of the mucus membranes, especially involving the vagina and the entire digestive system, have been linked with a poor and ineffective response of white blood cells called T-lymphocytes, and guess which part of the immune system are affected most by gliotoxin and mannan? You guessed it, the T-lymphocytes. We call this the cell-mediated immune response, and shortly I'll tell you a bit more about this, and how you can significantly boost this part of your immune system.

There are lots of scientific papers I have researched that have clearly linked candida yeast infections and immune suppression, and candida-produced agents like gliotoxin and mannan often cause this kind of suppression. This may give you an indication why yeast infections can be so hard to clear in some people's bodies, because it is not just a matter of killing the yeast, it is a matter of stopping the foods which allow candida to produce these toxic metabolites, assisting in the removal of candida in addition to their metabolites as well as boosting your immune function.

*Clinical Microbiology Review 1991 January; 4(1): 1–19. Candida mannan: chemistry, suppression of cell-mediated immunity, and mechanisms of action. R D Nelson, N Shibata, R P Podzorski, and M J Herron

Reducing Metabolites And Boosting Immune Function

I have discovered that patients who only partially recover and who remain feeling unwell for some time appear to have very low, low or borderline SIgA levels as well. You can read a lot more about SIgA (antibodies) in chapter 3 under comprehensive digestive stool analysis testing.

It would certainly pay to increase your SIgA levels, that way your immune system will get a significant boost and may help to pull you out of a sustained aggravation you are going through, the SIgA antibodies form part of your immune system's humoral response. This part of the immune system fights the enemy at a distance, unlike the cell-mediated response that fights the enemy close up. You will find that with higher SIgA levels you will be able to tolerate foods more easily, which you previously were having aggravations from in many potential ways.

With a reduction in candida metabolites through boosting the cell-mediated immune response, you will find that your brain fog, fatigue, feeling unreal, stoned or spaced out will be reduced much more quickly. By boosting both aspects of immunity (cell and humoral responses), you will begin to feel better than you have for a long time, possibly even several years. This is one of the key secrets I've discovered to a deep-seated recovery from chronic yeast infections that I have not seen mentioned elsewhere.

The best way to work on the immune system if you want to get rid of your yeast infection is to boost both the cell and humoral mediated responses, the two main branches of your immune system. This is a bit like renewing your troops on the frontline, more white blood killer cells, the cell mediated response, and giving them better weapons with a higher accuracy and more killing power, boosting the humoral-mediated response.

Your Immune System And Candida

I'm not going to give you any big or lengthy explanations of how your immune system works, I'll keep that for a future edition of Candida Crusher, but what you need to know is basically this, that your immune system works on yeast infections in two main ways.

1 The Cell-Mediated Immune Response – consider this hand-to-hand combat. This group is like the marines who are sent in first to do the dirty work; they are tough and get the job done, their mortality rate is higher. The white blood cells are killing on contact and eradicate yeasts, bacteria and other pathogens directly. The cell-mediated response can be boosted significantly by taking selenium, zinc, Coenzyme Q10, beta-carotene, vitamins B6 and B12 and vitamin E and the herbal medicines ashwagandha, astragalus, cat's claw, mistletoe, Siberian ginseng and ligustrum. The most specific probiotic for enhancing the production of the cell-mediated T-helper cells is Bifidobacterium lactis. Omega 3 fish oils are also a very good idea, as they reduce any inflammatory response and boost many aspects of your immune system function.

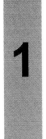

1 The other point I'd like to make it to ensure that you have sufficient cortisol production by your adrenal glands, as cortisol has a significant effect on your lymphocytes, so be sure to get a salivary cortisol test completed with the assistance of your health-care professional. As I have mentioned elsewhere in the Candida Crusher, adrenal fatigue treatment is one of my best-kept secrets when it comes to recovery of impossible cases of candida yeast infections. Both the cell and humoral mediated responses are significantly boosted with strong adrenal function.

2 The Humoral-Mediated Immune Response – consider this part of your immune system, it is fighting the enemy at a distance. These guys are the snipers squads and the artillery; they either can't see the enemy or can kill them from miles away. In this case, white blood cells produce antibodies that travel widely throughout the bloodstream and can kill yeasts, bacteria and pathogens anywhere the bloodstream will take them.

The humoral response is responsible for your body's SIgA production. Go to chapter 3, Diagnosing, Identifying and Testing For Candida yeast Infections and then read The Best Nutritional Way To Increase SIgA, you will find it under the information on comprehensive digestive stool analysis testing.

Different Yeast Presentations In The Clinic

Candida can and often does affect your digestive system primarily, but it can also affect just about any other system of your body. The candida and toxic metabolites can travel anywhere your circulation will take them, they can even affect a person's brain functioning. In chapter 2 you may have read about the study published in *Lancet*, which revealed that when a candida albicans sample was swallowed it could be cultured literally within a few hours from a person's blood and urine samples.

Imagine if candida had stayed long enough in the body to be able to produce the toxic metabolites as well. These metabolites can and will travel throughout the body and even into the brain and create all kinds of neurological symptoms.

Here are but a few of the many different presentations of yeast-infected patients I see in my clinic, to illustrate in what ways candida and its toxic metabolites can affect the body's immune system in various ways.

The 7 Different Patients
With Yeast Infections Commonly Seen

1 **Digestive problems.** High level of candida and metabolites in their digestive system and low levels in their systemic circulation. These cases are common, they are the patients who are tired and may well have fatigue, and their digestive complaints may be strong affecting the quality of their life. I don't generally find many mental, emotional or neurological symptoms here. They will have leaky gut syndrome becoming increasingly chronic over time without proper treatment. As the gut becomes more permeable, they develop increasingly more allergies and risk metabolites and associated neurological symptoms like brain fog and mental fatigue affecting the rest of the body.

2 **Chronic digestive problems.** Low or average levels of beneficial bacteria, high levels of candida and metabolites and high levels of bad bacteria and parasites in the digestive system, some degree of candida and metabolites in their circulation, high or low levels. Expect digestive pain, chronic bowel or digestive complaints, possibly nausea, gas, bloating and irritable bowel syndrome. These are the patients who often present with multiple food allergies and may have lost a lot of weight. These can be quite reactive or sensitive to many foods and dietary supplements. They respond slowly but surely over time and need to be patient. I work primarily on their digestive system for a long time, up to two years in severe cases, and especially with the Candida Crusher Formula. You can read a lot more about the Candida Crusher formulations in section 4 of chapter 7.

3 **Peripheral problems.** Candida and toxic metabolites in their digestive system but much higher levels of gliotoxin and mannan in their systemic circulation and organs or body systems peripheral to the digestive system. These are the patients with ongoing chronic low-level digestive problems, multiple food allergies that may cause major reactions, possibly food intolerances and a significantly chronic leaky gut. These patients are often tired and can feel literally wasted; some complain of brain fog, others may have varying levels of depression or anxiety and many will suffer from severe adrenal fatigue. These are the patients who tick literally every symptom box on the case-talking form. Some have recurrent vaginal thrush; others may have bladder or prostate irritation. Some will have problems with their muscles or joints. With a particularly high systemic load of candida and toxic metabolites some can even feel spaced-out to the point where they can find it difficult to even function on a day-to-day basis. These are the impossible cases and don't often get the right treatment, they will generally be prescribed antidepressants and told to see a psychiatrist by their doctor, and they may have visited a dozen or more practitioners.

4 **Vaginal yeast infection.** A recurring vaginal yeast infection yet little or no digestive or systemic yeast issues. These are the women who may have had a history of taking the Pill and/or antibiotics and may have used applicators and fluconazole initially but gave up on medical treatment years ago. They recover well on the Candida Crusher Program but need to address their digestive system

4 health and need to be tough on their diet as well as concentrate on continual local treatments for several months. Some of these women may have had a problem here for twenty years or more. Women with vaginal thrush and strong digestive complaints need the same treatment, balancing local treatments but with an even stronger emphasis on their diet, nutrition, and lifestyle. They need to be particularly careful about personal hygiene as well.

5 **Chronic and Severe Candidiasis.** Multiple areas of concern such as toenail fungus, vaginal thrush, bowel issues, brain fog, depression and irritability can sometimes all be seen in the same person. These people are a combination of category 2 and 3 I have just described, they have serious gut yeast infection issues and systemic metabolite issues. These patients can be very immune-compromised and will need to pay particular attention to the Low-Allergy Diet section on the Candida Crusher Diet. They are best to stay with the Candida Crusher Diet principles for some time while they heal their digestive system. I like them to take the five key Candida Crusher dietary supplements daily (section 4 chapter 7) and work on all the local areas of concern while paying particular attention to their leaky gut. Sometimes they come into the clinic on half a dozen drugs, including antidepressants, sleeping pills, antibiotics, antihistamines and steroid creams. They often benefit from fresh garlic; grapefruit seed extract and by using tea tree oil on their problem areas twice daily. These can quite possibly be the most challenging cases to work with and can take two years or more to heal.

6 **Minor skin or nail yeast infection.** Skin yeast infections and hardly any other candida issues. I routinely see cases of patients who only come into the clinic with tinea or toenail fungus, or only with jock itch, for example. Careful questioning will most always reveal some degree of underlying digestive issue, their small intestine will be leaky but only to a very mild or mild degree. These are often the people who are oblivious to any underlying health issues and drink alcohol regularly and may have a very average or even poor diet. They are best to follow the Candida Crusher principles and avoid especially the one or two key trigger foods or drinks they know they like. They recover well and generally in three to four months.

7 **Chronic skin or nail yeast infections.** These cases often present with major digestive and genito-urinary issues, like recurrent urinary tract infections and vaginal thrush along with tinea or toenail fungus. These patients will generally be older and may well have used antibiotics, creams or other drugs for years to little avail. These cases have some of the most compromised immune systems of all and the serious cases can take three years or more to heal. The skin will be the last thing to improve, as the body needs to heal from the inside out. The gut will be quite leaky indeed and the patient will need to strictly follow the diet plan for a long time. I expect to see various aggravations, as the body will need to throw out toxic drug residues locked inside organs from years of suppressive drug taking. Compliance increases as the thrush and UTIs begin to clear, but decreases as the aggravations occur. These are the cases that nobody wants to treat, and if this person only came to the clinic when he or she was a category 6 it would have been so much easier!

As you can see, there are potentially as many different yeast infection scenarios as there are people, and each case will be slightly different from another, but there will be common threads tying them together. I have learned much of my knowledge by carefully taking the patient's case in addition to comprehensive stool testing. With stool testing you can work out if the yeast infection is predominantly in the person's digestive system or not, what levels of bacteria, good and bad, as well as if there are any parasites present. You can also see if there is any inflammation present and how their digestion is coping under the load.

The stool test will also reveal an immune marker (sIgA) which can reveal if they are reactive to their diet and to what extent, and further specialized testing such as the lactulose/mannitol test will reveal if they have leaky gut and how significant it is. So you see, there are ways of working out what is happening to the patient and how their immune system is affecting them. This information is priceless and can help you the patient significantly. You can read a more about functional medicine testing in chapter 3, and especially a lot more about sIgA, an important gut immune marker.

While the toxic candida metabolites can affect just about all cells of all organs and systems of a person's body thereby causing just about any symptoms, candida albicans will often tend to initially have more of a direct impact on the digestive system causing gastrointestinal symptoms, and from there it will spread to different parts of the body.

I am especially on the lookout for and mental, emotional or visual disturbances. This will tell me that we are potentially dealing with toxic metabolites, and I expect the small intestine to be especially permeable in such cases. I look to see if the patient has more peripheral symptoms like brain fog, numbness & tingling, feeling unreal or spaced out. With any presenting neurological symptoms, you can figure out to what degree the candida and toxic metabolites have moved the person's digestive system into their circulation, other organs and even into their brain.

To cope, some people under continual stress unfortunately drink alcohol, raising their immune response further. An even further assault can occur to their immune system when they take drugs like antibiotics, anti-histamines, sleeping tablets or a blood-pressure drug, for example. Likewise, the immune system may be challenged by molds which may come from living or working in a moldy environment, or from ingesting foods containing molds or spores, such as those foods placed in the refrigerator which were cooked the day before. Did it ever occur to you that these air or food-borne yeast spores can become trapped in your respiratory or digestive system and challenge your immune system further?

How Candida Metabolites Invade Your Body

In a healthy and strong body, the respiratory or circulatory system can trap these microscopic spores and the immune system can then effectively deal with them, and likewise, a health and strong digestive system will be minimally affected by candida. Digestive acids and enzymes along with healthy levels of beneficial bacteria ensure that candida metabolites are effectively dealt with.

But in a weak and immune compromised body, the candida spores can invade your immune system situated in the lungs and small intestine, where the yeast can readily change to its mycelial form, the vegetative part of a fungus consisting of a mass of branching threadlike filaments, which literally burrows into the lung or intestinal lining where this infestation irritates and effects the lining so much so that it eventually loses its ability to act as an effective barrier, allowing the candida metabolites to pass directly into the bloodstream. Once inside, these toxic metabolites are ready to circulate and create havoc throughout both the body and brain wherever your blood travels.

Now you can understand why a yeast infection can become a systemic problem and affect literally the entire person, from their emotional and psychological wellbeing creating a cotton wool feeling, feeling drunk or spaced-out, depression and anxiety, right down to their toenails, creating athlete's foot.

Poor diets, especially those high in the simple carbohydrates and immune-challenging foods and poor environments, moldy environments, can compromise your immune system because they can significantly boost the production of these immune-challenging toxic candida metabolites. This kind of diet and lifestyle also provides inadequate supply of minerals and vitamins so desperately required by your body to maintain and repair, sustain and nourish the entire system, thereby encouraging flare-ups or multiplication of the candida related problems.

After learning about the immune system's critical involvement, you should now be able to have a better understanding as to why it is critical for you to follow the Low-Allergy Diet stage as part of your yeast infection recovery, and to make not only digestive rejuvenation a focus of your program, but immune rejuvenation as well.

Health Builders And Health Busters

I have always been big on trying to identify the cause of a person's yeast infection, because if I can understand what caused their yeast infection in the first place then I can probably help that person turn things around and get rid of it. It sounds simple in theory doesn't it? But it isn't always that easy to uncover one or several of the causes of a yeast infection, a person may have had their yeast infection for twenty, thirty or even for fifty years and in such cases it may even become an almost impossible task to determine how this mess all started.

One thing is for certain, there were one or several causes, and that cause was a stress to the body which either occurred on an emotional, mental or physical plane or a combination of one or more of these factors. This stress, a health buster, created a shift to the left of the stress pyramid I have drawn (see diagram), and when that shift occurred the patient became increasingly susceptible, and as their resistance dropped they increased their susceptibility for a bacterial, viral or fungal infection.

Many people who develop a yeast infection do so because their immune resistance becomes compromised and their susceptibility towards a yeast infection increases. If you look at the diagram below you will see a line with susceptibility on the one side, and

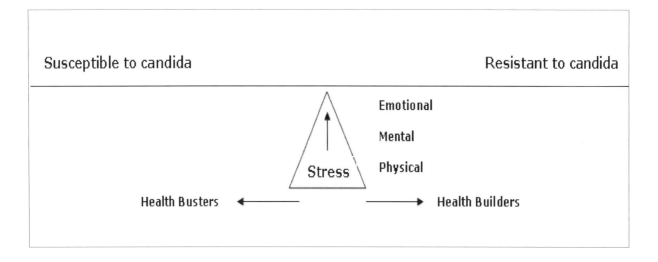

resistance on the other. In the middle you will see a pyramid with the word stress in it, and to the right you will see the words emotional, mental and physical.

But what does this mean, and what has stress got to do with getting and keeping a yeast infection? To answer these questions we need to take a closer look at how diet and lifestyle affect immunity and increase your susceptibility of contracting a yeast infection.

Likewise, if a person decides on health building activities, their resistance will increase and their susceptibility will drop. Like any infection, candida yeast infections occur for a reason; you develop them because you became more susceptible to them due to various health busting activities.

Candida Health Busters

Candida health busters are often the exciting and maintaining causes of yeast infections. These causes break down the body's resistance and affect the immune system either directly or indirectly by causing problems with the HPA (stress) axis, which I will explain shortly. The cause of a yeast infection may occur as a stand-alone occurrence, such as taking an antibiotic, but will occur more commonly due to a combination or accumulation of these causes or triggers.

- **Mental and Emotional** – anger, hatred, jealousy, envy, greed, anxiety, depression, other negative attitudes and beliefs, work related stress, financial pressures, fears and phobias, marital or relationship stress, unemployment stress, study/mental over-exertion, death of a loved one, prison term, birth of a child, divorce, lack of relaxation, constantly driving yourself, trying to be perfect.

- **Physical** – Smoking, alcohol, caffeine, junk foods, poor eating habits and a general lack of good food, sugar and white flour products, yeasty and moldy foods, toxins, chemical toxicity, heavy metal toxicity, over-exertion or over-training, antibiotics (a big cause), prescription and non-prescription pharmaceutical drugs (antibiotics, the Pill, etc.), adrenal fatigue and thyroid imbalances (common), no exercise, damp or moldy living conditions, infections (acute and chronic), root canal therapy, mercury amalgam fillings. EMF (mobile phones, radiation, microwaves, etc.). Physical causes also include environmental causes like wearing nylon underclothing (increasing the risk of jock itch or vaginal thrush), wearing socks and shoes for too long (toe nail fungus), and having hands wet for too long (fingernail fungus). Over-breathing can be a cause of many different health problems; many people hyperventilate due to stress.

People And Relationships Are Some Of Our Biggest Stresses

Some of the biggest stresses we face involve other people, and most people can relate to the fact that there is one person they know in general, like a son, ex-partner, employer, husband, employee, mother-in-law or daughter-in-law, etc.; that is causing them stress right now, ranging from very mild and occasionally to severe and extreme.

The emotional stresses are the ones you will notice which are on top and close to the line I have drawn near the pyramid.

Most people consider the physical stresses to be the most toxic (like chemicals, heavy metals, etc.) whereas in fact it is the constant low-grade emotional stresses that cause us the most harm in my opinion. They continue on and sit in the background of our mind, sometimes for years or even decades and slowly wear down the ability of our body to help us recover from stressful events. These kinds of stresses are hidden from view, virtually un-diagnosable and accepted as being a normal part of our lives, unlike parasites, mercury, mold or microwaves, etc.

As our HPA (hypothalamic-pituitary-adrenal) axis becomes increasingly compromised, our immune system becomes incrementally compromised as well, and this is often how we become increasingly allergic or hypersensitive to foods and substances in our environment, we develop less resistance to many different types of infectious diseases like urinary tract infections, skin infections, respiratory infections, etc., we have an increased tendency to developing any one of the eighty auto-immune diseases like ulcerative colitis, Crohn's disease, rheumatoid arthritis, Grave's disease, etc.; and finally we can even be prone to developing one of the many different types of cancer.

It the accumulation of the many and varied different types of stresses which tips the balance, however. And if we can recognize stress for what it is and deal with these different stresses in our lives, whether they are emotional, mental or physical, than we will be in a much better position to avoiding falling victim to a yeast infection because our resistance will be high and our susceptibility will remain low. As you will soon discover, continual low-grade stress causes a strain particularly on our adrenal glands, and once these powerful little glands become compromised our susceptibility to virtually any immune problem increases significantly. Be sure to read section 5 of chapter 7, Understanding the Health Lifestyle, because in this part of the book I explain much more about stress and what you can do about it.

Candida Health Builders

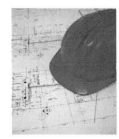

These are the health-building activities that reduce your risk of a yeast infection and increase your resistance to developing or maintaining one. The following activities boost your health and especially your immune health. With an increased resistance comes a lowered susceptibility, and this is good news for you. The good thing is that you can do plenty to get rid of your yeast infection if you want to, just be aware of the health busting activities and finally deal with them while at the same time increasing your health-building activities.

- **Mental and Emotional** – happiness, laughter, not trying to be perfect, learning to say no to people, not over committing yourself, daily relaxation, lettings things go and not dwelling on unpleasant thoughts or unpleasant people, regular meditation or prayer, consciously slowing down your mind and thought processes and your life!, effective time management.

- **Physical** – not smoking, avoidance of alcohol and caffeine, eating a healthy, balanced diet, consuming plenty of fresh organic foods, avoiding sugar, alcohol, junk and white flour, eating at regular times and never skipping meals, regular detoxification of chemicals, heavy metals, etc., daily exercise, regular dental check-ups, caution with mobile phone and microwave use, avoidance of mercury fillings and avoidance of root canal therapy, relying on natural medicines and not pharmaceutical drugs, getting plenty of sleep and rest as well as unstructured time. Taking a vacation regularly.

The end result will be that your immune system will not only be considerably more capable of dealing with your yeast infection than by relying on dietary supplements and diet alone, this form of focused activity on your behalf will also keep your level of immunity at an all-time high, thereby reducing your risk of any future recurrence of many problems like food allergies, many different types of inflammatory disease, dysbiosis and leaky gut, bacterial and viral infections and a host of other immune-related health problems.

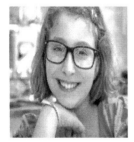

With a healthy HPA stress axis you will find that you will have lots more energy, improved sleep, better control of your cognition, including clarity of thoughts and memory, less chance of mood swings including anxiety and depression, quicker wound healing or recovery from any stressful events, being more productive, and having a state of wellness that is truly priceless. True health really is the greatest of all wealth, and you can't buy this health with all the money in China.

All the money on the entire planet could not give you the state of wellbeing that a balanced stress axis could. A healthy and balanced stress mechanism may even save you from developing one of the big three, namely cancer, heart disease and diabetes.

Most all books and articles I have read on yeast infections unfortunately don't drive home the importance of connection between stress, immunity and a yeast infection, and that's exactly what I'd like to explain to you right now.

If you can master but one thing when it comes to beating a yeast infection, master the ability to understand the relationship between your immune system and a yeast infection, but more particularly, the relationship between your adrenal glands and a yeast infection.

Did you know that about 90 percent of all visits to the doctor are stress related? Many of these visits are regarding conditions such as insomnia, headaches, digestive problems, I have routinely found in the clinic that the tendency is there for an immune weakness to be expressed in a highly individual manner, and it may be expressed with the patient's inherited or familial weaknesses, for example if the patient has a family history of heart disease, arthritis or asthma, the individual weakness is much more likely to be expressed in these key areas. The weakest link for some genetically may be their heart, for others their lungs, and yet for others it could well be their joints. Stress has the amazing ability to expose these weak links of the chain and bring them to the foreground. If the person is of a nervous or a sensitive type, the dysfunction, their individual signs and symptoms, may be expressed in the nervous system, digestive system or other system most susceptible to that person, especially when stress is factored into the equation.

After having specialized in stress for the past six years in my clinic and treated many patients who suffer from adrenal and thyroid issues, I would like to believe that I could give some good advice in this area. You will find that stress affects your immune system in several ways profoundly, and once you learn about the connection you will be in a better position to avoid the common pitfalls that so many succumb to.

There are many other reasons naturally for an immune dysfunction to be expressed in a person, for example with toxicity. The ability of your body to cope with or be affected by the toxic effects of any foreign matter such as heavy metals, chemicals, etc.; is dependent on your immune system's ability to cope with that foreign material and is influenced by many factors.

3 Most Important Factors Affecting Your Immune System:

1 Your Nutritional Status

In order to function optimally, your immune system is like any other system in your body. It needs adequate nutrition to operate at peak efficiency and must be supplied with a whole range of nutrients, particularly the vitamins C, D and E as well as the key immune minerals magnesium, zinc, copper, iodine, iron and selenium. A deficiency in any one or several of these important nutritional contingent factors can significantly increase your risk of a yeast infection. Poor nutritional status can come about from a deficiency due to a poor dietary intake or a poor ability of the digestive system to digest and absorb these vital nutrients.

2 How Stress Affects You.

Stress is one of the most universal underlying causes of many infections, including yeast infections. Whenever your body is exposed to any kind of stress, whether it is an emotional stress such as for example grief, anger, anxiety, or a physical stress such as an injury, toxicity or infection, many chemical changes occur in your body, which in turn may have a significant effect on your immune system.

Your Toxic and Allergenic Load.

3 Your toxic and allergenic load is the total quantity of potentially toxic and allergenic substances that have entered your body, and it is this load that your immune system has to deal with. There are different ways for your body to receive both toxic and allergenic materials and they can be absorbed and incorporated into your body in many different ways.

Toxins Are A Forgotten Cause Of Immune Dysfunction

Toxins and allergens include substances you breathe in, such as pollen, bacteria or mold spores, dust and various chemicals such as pollutants (car fumes, heavy metals, etc.) or by way of additives to the foods you eat (colors, flavors, preservatives, etc.) Toxicity also commonly occurs due to pharmaceutical drugs, and many people with a yeast infection today will have taken an antibiotic or the oral contraceptive pill in the past, besides headache pills, sleeping pills, antidepressants, or any one of a dozen other commonly doctor-prescribed or self-prescribed over the counter drugs.

There are also the naturally occurring toxins such as the bacteria, viruses and molds that will be found in our foods or environment. Other ways you may become toxic or allergic or develop parasitic infections is by coming into contact with animals, do you have any pets or live on a farm?

Some patients I have seen in my rooms over the years work in potentially toxic occupations like mechanics, printers, dry cleaners, truck drivers, painters, plumbers, tanners, welders, sheet metal workers, gardeners, dentists, factory workers and many other occupations which all potentially place their workforce in toxic environments.

Many of these chemicals can increase your incidence of an abnormal immune response, including the production of immune modifying substances produced to cope with any potentially underlying toxic onslaught. When an increasing toxic or allergenic load overwhelms your immune system, it is unable to resist a yeast invasion and as your resistance breaks down you are increasingly likely to develop a chronic yeast infection.

The best way to deal with toxins is to regularly undergo detoxification, and you can read all about this in section 3 of chapter 7, Understanding Cleansing and Detox.

It is important to consider boosting your immune defenses, because it is the sole responsibility of your immensely powerful immune system to hunt down, identify and destroy any allergic or toxic substances before they have a chance of wreaking internal damage. Without an adequate defense mechanism you are leaving your body wide open to a myriad of different health complaints directly related to poor immunity, including a chronic yeast infection.

Adrenal Fatigue, Immunity And Yeast Infections

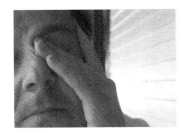 Not long after my clinic began to specialize in treating patients with chronic yeast infections, I began noticing that many of these patients also suffered from a common condition known as adrenal fatigue. Those with strong adrenal gland function did not appear to be bothered as much with yeast infections in comparison to those who had weak adrenal gland function.

But after having treated several thousand patients with adrenal fatigue, I have come to realize that those with chronic yeast infections can actually develop adrenal fatigue as a consequence.

There are many complex immune mechanisms involved in the interplay between a yeast infection and the adrenal glands, but suffice to say, there certainly is a correlation between them both. By treating adrenal fatigue and a yeast infection simultaneously, the patient tends to recover *much faster* than by treating either as a stand-alone condition. Unfortunately, in the worst case scenario, neither condition is treated because both a yeast infection and adrenal fatigue were not recognized as distinct syndromes, or because the practitioner just treated the patient's many presenting symptoms with either drugs or a combination of drugs and dietary supplements.

If a practitioner wants to achieve optimal results with their patient with a chronic yeast infection, they would do well to employ complementary adrenal support to maximize their patient's chances of a full recovery. Ideally this will be achieved both from a dietary and lifestyle intervention perspective, as well as including highly specialized adrenal nutritional support to maximize their patient's outcome.

An adrenal treatment plan may not be necessary at the onset of yeast infection treatment, but at some stage during the patient's recovery phase he or she is going to benefit from adrenal treatment, particularly if she has been unwell for a considerable period of time. When a person feels unwell with a yeast infection for a very long time, and I've seen some suffer for 20, 30 years or even longer, then this person may begin to develop anxiety and/or depression which becomes an additional stress adding to the severity and duration of their yeast infection and adrenal fatigue. This is especially so with a sensitive patient who is not taken seriously, something I have witnessed time and again over the years.

It has been known for some time that those with adrenal fatigue are more prone to developing a yeast infection; it is however rarely acknowledged that a chronic yeast infection can actually be the cause of adrenal fatigue in certain cases. One of the main reasons is because a chronic yeast infection can cause chronic over-activation of the adrenal glands, and this occurs due to a continual up-regulation of the powerful hormone cortisol, which has several important immune modulating properties when it comes to fighting a yeast infection.

It was discovered some time ago that high levels of cortisol suppress various aspects of immune function, especially SIgA levels, the prime antibody found in all the mucosal surfaces which defends the body from an overgrowth of yeast and bad bacteria. If you want to finally crush a candida yeast infection permanently, you will want to make certain that you have a viable and supremely powerful immune system, and one of the best ways of achieving this is to have your adrenals working for and not against you.

What Is Adrenal Fatigue?

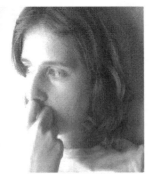

Adrenal fatigue is a very common condition most practitioners will see almost daily in their practice, but first let's take a look at what adrenal fatigue actually is, what the cause of this well know condition is and how yeast infections and adrenal fatigue can be linked.

The adrenal glands are small glands that sit on top of your kidneys, they are glands that produce almost fifty hormones and are critical in helping you recover from any stressful event.

Adrenal Fatigue is any decrease in the ability of the adrenal glands to carry out their normal functions. This happens when your body is overwhelmed, and particularly when stress over-extends the capacity of your body to compensate and fully recover from any stressful events. Consequently, the adrenal glands become increasingly depleted and fatigued and are unable to continue responding adequately to further stress.

Adrenal Fatigue is a collection of signs and symptoms, known as a syndrome that results when the adrenal glands function below their necessary level. Although adrenal fatigue is commonly associated with intense or prolonged stress, it can also arise during or after acute or chronic infections, especially respiratory infections such as influenza, bronchitis or pneumonia, but also a yeast infection. Many factors can reduce adrenal function, and it is often an accumulation of triggers over a period of time that is responsible for this syndrome. As the name suggests, the main symptom is fatigue, a kind of fatigue that is not relieved by sleep, but adrenal fatigue is not a readily identifiable or diagnosable entity like a low iron count or Vitamin B12 in the blood, which is typically viewed by the medical profession as the cardinal sign of fatigue.

The Adrenal Fatigue syndrome has been known by many other names throughout the past century, such as non-Addison's hypo-adrenia, neurasthenia, adrenal neurasthenia, adrenal apathy and more recently as having a nervous breakdown. Although both adrenal fatigue and yeast infections affect the lives of many millions of people around the world daily, conventional medicine does not yet recognize these health complaints as distinct conditions.

Japanese Recognize Adrenal Fatigue As An Illness

After Dr. James Wilson, the adrenal fatigue expert, spoke to over 3,000 doctors on adrenal fatigue in Japan after the tsunami and Fukushima nuclear power plant meltdown in 2011, the Japanese government declared adrenal fatigue as an illness in its own right. The World Health Organization has also recently recognized adrenal fatigue as a separate illness, yet conventional medical science in the Western world still cites "lack of evidence" as the main reason they believe this syndrome simply doesn't exist. I certainly have seen plenty of evidence in my clinic, after having treated several thousand patients with adrenal fatigue since I began to specialize in this syndrome since 2006, and the results have been spectacular.

Adrenal Fatigue Can Wreak Serious Havoc With Your Life.

In the more serious cases, the activity of the adrenal glands is so diminished that you may have difficulty even getting out of bed for more than a few hours per day. With each increment of reduction in adrenal function, every organ and system in your body is more profoundly affected. Changes occur in your carbohydrate, protein and fat metabolism, fluid and electrolyte balance, heart and cardiovascular system, and even your sex-drive.

Many other alterations take place at the biochemical and cellular levels in response to and to compensate for the decrease in adrenal hormones that occurs with adrenal fatigue. Your body does its best to make up for under-functioning adrenal glands, but it does so at a price.

Just like with a yeast infection, you may look and act relatively normal with adrenal fatigue and may not even have any obvious signs of physical illness, yet you continue to live with a general sense of unwellness, tiredness or gray feelings.

People suffering from adrenal fatigue often use coffee, tea and other stimulants to get going in the morning and to prop themselves up during the day. Younger people may rely on caffeinated or energy drinks. Some adults may rely on the regular even daily use of alcohol in the late afternoon or evening to unwind.

Others may take medications such as sleeping pills, anti-depressants or rely habitually on paracetamol (acetaminophen) for tension headaches that may be caused by stress. Those with adrenal fatigue may crave salty foods such as potato chips, olives, pretzels, etc., because sodium will become more easily excreted as the adrenal gland's energy becomes increasingly depleted. This occurs to the adrenal gland's reduction in the output of a hormone called aldosterone that assists in the body's regulation of sodium and potassium levels. This is why many with adrenal fatigue complain of vagueness, weakness, dizziness, feeling like blacking out and low blood pressure.

Have you suffered from stress, and more importantly, can you recognize any of the following signs and symptoms? Many people tell me that they are not stressed and that stress does not figure in their lives, but if you have a pulse and you are breathing then you will suffer with stress at some point in your life because you are a living human being!

Warning Signs and Symptoms of Stress

Cognitive Symptoms

- Memory problems
- Indecisiveness
- Inability to concentrate
- Trouble thinking clearly
- Poor judgment
- Seeing only the negative
- Anxious or racing thoughts

Physical Symptoms

- Headaches, backaches, neck aches
- Muscle tension and stiffness
- Diarrhea or constipation
- Nausea, dizziness
- Insomnia
- Chest pain, rapid heartbeat
- Weight gain or loss
- Skin breakouts (hives, eczema)

Emotional Symptoms

- Constant worrying
- Loss of objectivity
- Fearful anticipation
- Moodiness
- Agitation
- Restlessness
- Short temper
- Irritability, impatience
- Inability to relax
- Feeling tense and on edge
- Feeling overwhelmed
- Sense of loneliness and isolation
- Depression or general unhappiness

Behavioural Symptoms

- Loss of sex drive
- Frequent colds
- Eating more or less
- Sleeping too much or too little
- Isolating yourself from others
- Procrastination, neglecting responsibilities
- Using alcohol, cigarettes, or drugs to relax
- Nervous habits (e.g. nail biting, pacing)
- Teeth grinding or jaw clenching
- Overdoing activities (e.g. exercising, shopping)
- Overreacting to unexpected problems
- Picking fights or arguments with others

Are You At Risk Of Adrenal Fatigue?

If you can recognize several of these signs and symptoms of stress, then you may be at a greater risk of developing adrenal fatigue. Here is a list of those who are most at risk of developing adrenal fatigue, see if you are in this group and if you are, can you relate to the conditions I just mentioned?

- People who are highly ambitious or competitive with themselves and others, all work and little play.

- Perfectionist people who set impossibly high standards for themselves and then fail to achieve them.

- Professional sports person with a grueling training schedule. I have seen several patients over the years that have competed at the highest levels with severe adrenal fatigue.

- People who are constantly on-the-go and rarely give themselves permission to truly relax.

- People addicted to computers, laptop, iPad, mobile phones, or watching too much TV. Those who feel compelled to check emails very frequently or are addicted to social media like Facebook, Twitter, etc.

- Full-time university students, PhD candidates, especially students who have to work through their studies to support themselves financially.

- Single parents with little downtime, or parents with children with autism or behavioral syndromes.

- Career or working mothers trying to juggle work and children.

- People in unhappy personal or professional relationships.

- Unhappy employees in stressful working conditions.

- Shift-workers, air-traffic controllers, flour millers, factory workers, truck drivers, police officers, miners, pilots, nurses, doctors, etc.; those working irregular or long hours needing to adjust their sleep & work patterns regularly.

- Adults caring for their sick or elderly parents or sick children while trying to juggle their busy lifestyle.

- Self-employed people in start-up companies, financial stress, huge mortgages, etc.

- Drug or alcohol abuse.

Testing For Adrenal Fatigue

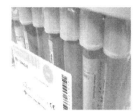 Did you know that testing for Adrenal Fatigue could be conducted by a simple saliva test? The Cortisol Salivary Test is an excellent way for you to determine your levels of the stress hormone cortisol; it provides an evaluation of how cortisol levels differ throughout the day. Speak to your health-care professional about this test.

Here is a simple test you can do right now, take the Adrenal Fatigue Home Test:

- Low risk: If you can answer yes to 3 or more of the following questions, you may be at risk of developing adrenal fatigue.

- Medium risk: If you can answer 5 or more of these questions, your risk is certainly greater than if you can only answer one or two questions. Take a look at the manifestations of adrenal fatigue below, if you have any of these, see your health-care professional.

- High risk: If you can answer 7 or more correctly, you probably have adrenal fatigue right NOW. See you health-care professional soon!

1. Do you have difficulty getting up in the morning; do you like to stay in bed an extra half an hour before you get up?

2. Could you easily sleep in?

3. Do you still feel tired and fatigued even after sleep?

4. Are you not really fully awake until after 9.00am?

5. Do you have an energy drop between 2 to 5pm?

6. Do you feel better after your evening meal and get a "second-wind? Later in the evening from 10-11pm?

7. Is it common for you to stay up to 1 am or beyond?

8. Do you feel less enjoyment or happiness in life and constant lethargy?

9. Does everything seem like a chore?

10. Do you feel fuzzy mentally and often lose track of thought, short-term memory concerns?

11. Have you been diagnosed with depression, panic attacks, or anxiety?

12. Have you got a poor sex drive or no libido?

13. Do you feel anxious about things that never previously bothered you?

14. Are you more irritable with your partner, children or co-workers lately?

15. Is it taking you longer to recover from an illness, injury or trauma (i.e. the cough you got two months ago is still lingering on)?

16. Do you suffer recurrent colds, flu, sore throats, skin infections, etc.?

17. Have you been prescribed antibiotics several times in the past few years?

18. Do you have recurrent asthma, hay fever, pneumonia or bronchitis?

19. Have you suffered increased PMS, i.e. bloating, tiredness, irritability, craving chocolate?

20. You have suffered with menopause, i.e. hot flashes, vaginal dryness, irritability, accelerated ageing, etc.?

21. Do you get feelings of vagueness, dizziness or feeling like you might blackout yet no cause can be found?

22. Do you "need" two or three cups of coffee or strong tea daily?

For a much more comprehensive explanation of how stress and Adrenal Fatigue affect your health and what you can do to recover and protect yourself see Dr. James Wilson's book, Adrenal Fatigue: The 21st Century Stress Syndrome. I have known Dr. Wilson for several years and consider him to be one of my mentors in my continuing education of natural medicine.

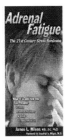 Once adrenal fatigue sets in, you may become susceptible to a long list of health complaints including respiratory infections, asthma, allergies, candida yeast infections, chronic fatigue syndrome, fibromyalgia, and a host of other immune disorders. Here are some of the more common conditions we see in those with adrenal fatigue. They are all potential manifestations of adrenal fatigue:

Manifestations Of Adrenal Fatigue:

- Alcoholism

- Allergies

- Anxiety, anger (short-fuse), irritability, depression

- Arthritic pain

- Asthma

- Adult-onset diabetes - Type 2 Diabetes

- Auto-immune disorders (rheumatoid arthritis, lupus, ulcerative colitis, many more)

- Confusion, poor concentration, and memory recall

- Chronic fatigue syndrome

- Common to stay up to 1.00 am or beyond.

- Cravings for salt or sweet foods

- Decreased immune response - recurrent coughs, colds, flu

- Difficulty during menopause (the adrenals take over the role of the ovaries after menopause) especially with hot flushes, anxiety and mood swings.

- Dysbiosis

- Everything seems like a chore.

- Fatigue in spite of sufficient sleep. Trouble getting up in the morning, likes to sleep in that extra half an hour.

- Feeling fuzzy mentally.

- Fibromyalgia

- Food allergies

- Frequent respiratory infections

- Hypoglycemia - erratic or abnormal blood sugar levels (very common)

- Increased fears, anxiety, and depression

- Insomnia

- Libido issues

- Premenstrual tension

- Post viral syndromes (history of glandular fever is common)

- Reliance on stimulants such as coffee, tea, energy drinks

- Reliance on alcohol to "unwind"

- Reliance on sleeping pills, anti-depressants, and a host of other pharmaceutical medications related to stress-induced diseases.

- Thyroid problems, many hypothyroid patients have adrenal fatigue

- Tired in the afternoon especially between 2.00pm – 5.00pm

- Weight gain

- Yeast infection

Adrenally Fatigued Yeast Infection Patients Aggravate More Easily

A problem I used to encounter in my early days of treating those with chronic yeast infections who were adrenally depleted is that those patients with major adrenal fatigue were not able to readily handle treatment aggravations or die-off (Herxheimer reactions) without having severe reactions. Their bodies were simply not able to cope with any kinds of aggravations, apart from trivial or very minimal, and these were the patients less likely to return for a return visit.

Immune resistance certainly declines as adrenal function goes down; this increases the chance of an aggravation when yeast infection treatment is commenced. This is something I had to learn by making many mistakes with patients in the early days, and it is a mistake I don't want you to make! Either find a practitioner who knows how to recognize and treat adrenal fatigue or become enlightened yourself by buying Dr. Wilson's Adrenal Fatigue book, then you can make up your own mind and request treatment when you recognize this all-too-common syndrome in yourself.

I have learned and don't tend to have these kinds of violent reactions with chronic candida patients anymore, and if you carefully follow my recommendations as outlined in the Candida Crusher, you won't either. But I want you to seriously consider whether you have adrenal fatigue or not, and if you can relate strongly to this part of the Candida Crusher book, then please speak with a practitioner who is familiar with Dr. James Wilson's Adrenal Fatigue protocol, you will be glad you did.

The Adrenal-Cortisol Connection And Yeast Infections

Once the adrenal glands become compromised due to stress, their ability to function optimally is impaired, and as cortisol output is decreased so is the adrenals ability to optimize the immune system.

One of the most important hormones made by your adrenal gland is cortisol, a powerful steroid hormone that performs many different functions in your body. According to Dr. James Wilson, the world authority in adrenal fatigue, all of your body's cells have a requirement for cortisol apart from your nails and your hair, but the cells which have possibly the highest affinity for cortisol are your white blood cells, your immune cells. In the initial stages of stress, the alarm phase, your body's cortisol levels will tend to be elevated, but as your adrenal glands become increasingly depleted due to long-term low-grade stress, the resistance phase of stress, cortisol levels eventually become depleted, and eventually they may even hit low levels, the exhaustion phase of stress.

One of the common symptoms we find in those with adrenal fatigue is recurring immune problems and poor recovery from minor infections. Those with adrenal fatigue also tend to have more problems with leaky gut syndrome, food allergies and all manner of digestive and bowel problems. Unfortunately, the doctor's answer to many of these common stress-related complaints is a prescription for antibiotics, and this may lead to or further exacerbate any underlying yeast infection.

An All Too Common Scenario

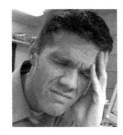 A common scenario I have seen in my practice time and again is that a person suffers from recurring stress and may develop a symptom such as headache, insomnia, constipation, recurring cough and cold, a skin infection or a recurring urinary tract infection. According to the doctor, it was a bacterium that was the cause of their unwellness, and this will naturally mean that a prescription for an antibiotic is called for. The patient may develop a digestive problem including a yeast infection or vaginal thrush requiring more antibiotics and so this drug merry-go-round continues.

Case History # 19
Anne, 56 years

Anne is an accountant who came to me complaining of having had vaginal thrush "for ever". She mentioned that she first noticed this most annoying problem when she was in her mid-twenties after she came back from England to New Zealand to live and work. About ten years ago she started to develop constipation and this later turned into irritable bowel syndrome about six years ago. She has had two marriages, and her second marriage was about to come to an end.

Anne has led quite a stressful life, her first husband committed suicide when she was in her mid thirties, leaving her with two young children. Her son found if difficult going and didn't really adapt to a stepfather coming into his life, which caused additional stress. Anne went through a period of several years of financial hardship with her second partner who turned out to be less than supportive. Anne is a particularly sensitive woman, and has had to rely on sleeping tablets and regular headache medications as well. I soon realized that she was adrenally fatigued and in fact was severely affected; as she has had to juggle two jobs, raise her children literally by herself and cope with the pressures of dysfunctional relationship. She took it very hard when her mother died two years ago and still has not resolved her grief.

Anne's diet has become very restricted since her doctor diagnosed irritable bowel syndrome, and she has noticed that many of even the most common foods were now causing digestive upsets, making it very challenging for her to enjoy eating out or even socializing with friends. That's when she decided to visit my rooms. The condition she most wants to conquer however is that annoying thrush, but feels that nothing can be done because her case is hopeless and her doctor has long given up.

I worked with Anne for several months and initially treated her adrenal fatigue and at the same time placed her on the Candida Crusher Program. I asked Anne to do a salivary cortisol test that revealed a very low morning cortisol level, indicative of severe adrenal fatigue. Likewise, a stool test revealed that she had yeast in all three stool samples, from samples taken on three concurrent days.

After following my two-stage thrush eliminating protocol (in this book) it took almost four months to get rid of her thrush, but it has now gone entirely. As her adrenal energy improved I noticed some remarkable changes in Anne, she finally plucked up the courage to leave her second husband and now happily living alone with daughter and her two cats. Slowly but surely, Anne began to tolerate an increasing amount of foods that she had been unable to eat for many years. She also started to gain weight and looks much healthier today than she did a few years ago (her weight hit rock-bottom at 84 pounds but is now a healthy 120 pounds at 5' 7").

These are the chronic cases that are often discarded by many practitioners or simply placed in the too hard basket. It is much easier to spend five or ten minutes with the patient and to shuffle their drugs or supplements around when they return for a follow-up visit than it is to deal with causes of their chronic health problems. Such chronic patients end up more and more unwell as their yeast infection and adrenal fatigue slowly but surely become increasingly chronic as the years roll by. What started out as a feeling of occasionally being unwell eventually gets to the stage where the person's occupation and livelihood are threatened and their lifestyle becomes more and more compromised, by the time they come to me they sometimes have been on a government sickness hand-out and are stone broke from years of paying out for these ineffective and generally useless treatments.

In my experience, if the patient does not improve, the whole case needs to be re-taken and the root causes finally addressed, and if you dig deep enough you will often find yeast or bacterial overgrowth in their digestive tract along with a pattern of adrenal fatigue from many years of dysfunction.

What Is Leaky Gut Syndrome?

Leaky gut syndrome describes a condition of altered or damaged small bowel lining, caused by antibiotics, toxins, poor diet, parasites, a yeast infection or stress which can lead to increased permeability of the gut wall to toxins, microbes, undigested food, waste or larger than normal macromolecules.

It has been estimated that around 60% of your immune system is located in your small intestine, and incredibly, a high percentage of this activity is concentrated in the first three inches (75ml) of your duodenum. In a normal healthy person, the small bowel behaves like a colander or a sieve, allowing only the breakdown of the very finest molecules of digestion into your bloodstream. A healthy membrane of the small intestine allows only very small nutrients and fats, proteins and starches which are all broken down to extremely small particles to enter into the bloodstream, while the larger molecules and many different types of toxic compounds are kept out.

When the small intestine is affected by LGS however, this process does not occur. Tiny food particles by-pass the cells which normally absorb them and slip in between tiny intra-cellular spaces which have been created by the LGS and challenge the immune system on the other side. Now let's examine this in a little more detail.

Yeast Infection And Leaky Gut Syndrome

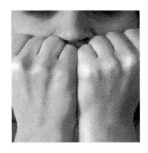 Leaky gut syndrome (LGS) is one of those non-descriptive syndromes, which like candida yeast infections and adrenal fatigue simply does not exist according to Western medicine. I once heard someone say that some doctors have a tendency to be down on things they are not up on. The fact of the matter is leaky gut syndrome is a very real and valid functional complaint from which millions suffer around the world on a daily basis. LGS has ample scientific evidence supporting its existence, and there are a variety of scientific papers in a wide variety of medical journals written by medical researchers from many parts of the world regarding this functional digestive complaint.

Because LGS is a disturbance affecting a person's core, their small intestine, leaky gut issues may well be implicated and play a role in a wide range of chronic diseases including heart disease, auto-immune diseases, depression and chronic fatigue syndrome. It is important to understand that LGS is actually a symptom of something else, and like all health complaints there are specific causes.

To effectively treat LGS, the underlying cause must first be identified and treated, as well as the gut damage that occurs in this syndrome. Many yeast infection patients suffer with LGS, and it is one of the prime reasons they develop food allergies. Just as in adrenal fatigue, candida can cause LGS, and LGS can also increase one's susceptibility to a yeast infection. You need to be aware of these syndromes because your health-care provider may not, so be educated enough to know what is going on in your body, then you will be in a better position to understand your starting point of treatment and monitor the progress of your yeast infection as time goes by.

Microvilli

In your intestinal tract, there reside small microvilli, microscopic finger-like projections that come off the lining of the intestinal tract with hair-like cell membrane extensions called the brush border. Microvilli serve as the major point of absorption of nutrients. A thin layer of mucous forms on this brush border in which beneficial bacteria thrive, and once this layer becomes compromised, the friendly bacteria reduce in number and the bad guys including candida species have an easy time or colonizing the brush border. This brush border is also home to SIgA, the major antibodies find in your digestive system. I go into great detail about SIgA in chapter 3 under comprehensive stool testing.

Antibiotics in particular can really wreck this brush border, causing severe damage, now you can understand who taking an antibiotic is not such a good idea and can easily lead to a yeast overgrowth in your digestive system.

Specific nutrients like glucose, amino acids and electrolytes are carried through these microvilli and into the cells via active transport, and there are even specific carrier molecules to take the nutrients across the cell membrane border. Active transport is the movement of a substance across a cell membrane against its concentration gradient from low to high concentration.

Leaky gut syndrome causes the intestinal lining to become inflamed and the microvilli then become damaged or altered, active transport does not occur effectively and even the cells themselves that transport nutrients into the bloodstream suffer as a consequence. These damaged microvilli then cannot go on to produce the necessary enzymes and secretions that are essential for a healthy digestion and the absorption of nutrients.

Because LGS impairs the body's ability to move nutrients from the digestive system into the bloodstream and eventually to all the cells of the body, it is not hard to see the consequences, poor absorption and an impaired uptake of vital nutrients. The outcome eventually is fatigue and a host of other chronic complaints over time. These cells lining the microvilli together form a strong, sturdy and almost impenetrable structure, preventing those larger molecules from passing through. When an area becomes inflamed, this weakens the structure of the allowing those larger molecules to escape through.

These larger molecules provoke an immune system response that in turn stimulates the production of antibodies. Antibodies themselves are highly specific proteins that are utilized by the immune system to locate and attack foreign objects to fight off the molecules, as they are perceived as antigens, and antigens are substances that are capable of triggering the production of antibodies. These antigen-antibody complex structures move around in the bloodstream to distant sites, provoking inflammatory reactions far away from the digestive system.

Leaky Gut Syndrome May Affect Your Liver In Time

A healthy immune system has the ability to control many toxic substances but as it becomes overloaded, toxins can affect the liver resulting in an overburdened liver. The liver is the largest organ in the body, and plays a critical role in detoxification as well as having many hundreds of other functions including:

- Producing bile containing bile acids, which aid digestion. Bile is stored in the gallbladder.

- Filtering out toxins, such as drugs, alcohol and environmental toxins.

- Breaking foods down after a meal to be converted to glucose to regulate blood sugar levels.

- Storing excess glucose as glycogen.

- Helping to break down many different toxins and assist in excreting them.

- Converting ammonia to urea and removing damaged red blood cells.

As LGS progresses, it can overwhelm the liver in time causing it to become flooded with additional toxins diminishing its ability to function normally. One of the liver's main roles is to detoxify the body and help keep the bloodstream clear; it was designed to neutralize chemical substances. When the liver cannot cope with an increasing level of toxins, it will begin to expel these toxins back into the bloodstream. The circulatory system will then over time begin to store these toxins into various parts of the body, including other organs, the connective tissues and even the muscles where they are stored to prevent major organ damage. The immune system will recognize these toxins as foreign and may begin to mount an inflammatory response, tying up valuable immune resources. Regular detoxification will rejuvenate the liver and is an important part of keeping your immune system in fine form.

The Immune System Becomes Activated

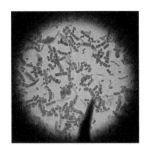 As the intestinal lining of the small bowel becomes damaged over time, substances larger than particle size such as undigested food particles, disease causing bacteria, yeasts, and potentially toxic molecules can pass through these weakened and leaky cell membranes. These molecules enter the bloodstream, triggering the production of antibodies and cytokines, which are protein molecules released by the immune system to cause a reaction in other cells, to fight the antigens. The cytokines alert the white blood cells, the lymphocytes, to fight the particles that have escaped through the intestinal lining. These cytokines along with other cells produced by an over-alert immune system start to cause allergic reactions and inflammation throughout the body.

The result can be low-grade pain in the bowel and a generally uncomfortable sensation in the lower part of the abdomen. The bowel motions become altered; there may be constipation or diarrhea, bloating, gas or various other sensations experienced. Have you noticed a little pain from time to time in your lower abdomen? It may be LGS, especially if you have plenty of gas and bloating and crave carbohydrate and especially the sweet foods like chocolate, cookies, ice cream or candy.

A healthy small intestine is normally coated with the thin layer of mucus I described earlier to keep out foreign substances as well as to facilitate the growth of friendly bacteria. LGS slowly develops as this mucus layer becomes weakened and the good and bad bacteria as well as yeasts, which usually reside in the intestine, will begin to inhabit other parts of the body as well. This is called bacterial translocation, and it happens as a consequence due to the intestinal permeability. Is it any wonder that candida can become a systemic problem?

It Takes Time To Heal LGS

To sum LGS up, your intestine develops microscopically tiny leakages allowing substances that would normally be digested to enter your bloodstream. These substances and toxins are slowly passed to the liver to deal with, but in time it simply cannot cope with this increasingly and overwhelming load of toxins and will attempt to store them in the body tissues. The liver eventually becomes overworked as the intestinal lining gets consistently weaker over time, and more and more toxins and undigested food progressively enter into the bloodstream. Your immune system sends out an increasing amount of antibodies to fight these foreign substances and in doing that toxic chemicals are produced that attack the body tissues causing allergic reactions and pain and inflammation throughout the body.

There are several ways to remedy a permeable bowel, but you will need patience and the right approach to cure LGS. You are well on the way by following the Candida Crusher Diet, especially if you take a quality probiotic a few times a day for a three to six month period non-stop. Be sure to avoid all sugars and refined foods and most importantly, do not take an antibiotic anymore unless it is absolutely necessary.

Without a firm diagnosis of an underlying bowel condition, a doctor's hands are often tied due to a lack of evidence. Diet are lifestyle factors certainly do play a significant role in leaky gut, but a visit to your gastroenterologist for a colonoscopy and perhaps an endoscopy is a good idea to initially rule out any pathology (disease) with any chronic digestive complaint. Lifestyle modification, especially stress reduction, is now seen by most holistic doctors as being one of the most important factors in LGS recovery, particularly when no underlying condition has been identified. I will speak a lot more about the importance of lifestyle in the fifth section of this chapter.

Boosting Glandular Function

It is important to write about an area on what used to be an important part of conventional medical practice that many may not be familiar with. Glandular therapy is certainly a very interesting topic and well worth paying attention to, as it is one of the very few natural medicine treatments that has emerged with a pedigree backed by amazing medical credentials. I recommend you get an understanding about glandular therapy and consider if is right for you.

By boosting your body's flagging glandular function, you may be in a better position to take your immune system to a whole new level and beat your yeast infection that much more quickly and easily. It is important to remember that boosting glandular function is but one piece of the yeast infection puzzle though, and never forget that to successfully eradicate a yeast infection it will take a whole lot more than to just pop a few extra pills a day, you will need to look at the whole picture.

What Is Glandular Therapy?

Glandular therapy today is a treatment that uses the freeze-dried glands of various animals, it is a therapy that has been used for many hundreds of years in medicine, in fact; one might say even thousands of years. Hippocrates wrote extensively on the topic of animal glands in healing, and in biblical days it was known the testes of an ass (donkey) when boiled in milk provided an excellent boost to a feeble old man. It wasn't until the early 19th century however that conventional physicians started to take this form of nutritional therapy seriously.

Doctors discovered that desiccated pancreas helped those with "sugar-disease", now known as diabetes. In the mid 1800's to mid 1950's, physicians knew of the amazing benefits conferred by giving dried thyroid gland extract to those exhibiting signs and symptoms of hypothyroidism. Thyroid glandular extracts were considered standard treatment for hypothyroidism, and doctors successfully prescribed bovine thyroid gland extract to hundreds of thousands of patients in the USA alone. Other enlightened doctors worked out that one of the best treatments for those with Addison's disease (adrenal insufficiency) was to give the patient a bovine adrenal gland extract. Upjohn, a well-known drug company, was in fact manufacturing adrenal glandular extracts right up until the late 1950's in America.

What killed the glandular industry is of no surprise, the pharmaceutical industry. Although pharmacy started before the Second World War, it wasn't really until after the late 1950's that scientists started to artificially synthesize hormones which they claimed worked better and more consistently than glandular extracts. The truth of the matter is that instead of farming animals, they could now artificially synthesize a chemical drug in a laboratory cheaply and efficiently, and then go on to patent this chemical, thus assuring exclusivity and huge profits for many years to come.

Doctors who prescribed Synthroid (synthetic thyroid hormone) instead on Armor, a well proven and highly effective thyroid gland extract were seen as modern, scientific and progressive. Powerful and side-effect ridden synthetic steroids such as prednisolone were starting to replace adrenal cortex extracts and over time doctors even stopped prescribing ovarian extracts to women with waning estrogen levels in favor of a drug called Premarin, a hormone extract derived from the urine of pregnant mares, kept in the cruelest of conditions.

Glandular extract therapy which was once successfully prescribed in medical practice for over one hundred years by thousands of doctors to countless patients, has now became discredited by mainstream medicine, and the doctors who dare to prescribe these "outdated" therapies today often ridiculed by their more enlightened colleagues. But the good news is that there has been a revival and a big interest in glandular therapies in both America, Europe and in many other countries.

Glandular animal sources have generally been cow (bovine), pig (porcine), or sheep (ovine), with many glandular extracts now coming on the market in the USA from New Zealand, my country of residence, one of the only countries left in the world that is certified BSE free.

3 Ways In Which A Glandular Extract Works

As glandular extracts are most always hormone-free, I'd like to discribe to you the pathways by which these kinds of products works'. There are three main ways in which a glandular extract may work inside your body.

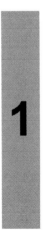

By way of active components: You don't need to be an eminent scientist to understand the logic behind glandular therapy, the gland of an animal will be reasonably close in its nutritional composition to that of a human being, and contain most of the necessary nutrients for healthy glandular function. Eating meat supplies us with ample protein, which in turn forms an important building block (amino acids, protein) for our own muscles. It is believed that glands and organs in animals and humans contain similar biochemical substances, as their functions are very similar. This is particularly true with the porcine glandular products I prefer to use from different companies. For example, a pig's digestive system produces enzymes very similar to humans, with digestive enzyme products containing porcine derived pancreatin being very popular. Pig

1 tissue contains several enzymes found in other living organisms like the human body. Two of these enzymes for example are: (1) Aldose reductase, an enzyme required for sugar breakdown, and (2) Steroid 17 -20 lyase, an enzyme for both producing steroidal hormones and for the subsequent detoxification of those hormones from the body. Thus we can deduce that the effect of using the respective biochemical compounds extracted from animals may be one of substituting an exogenous (external) source to make up for the endogenous (internal) deficiency.

2 By way of associated nutritional factors: Glandular tissues are metabolically amongst some of the most active tissues of an animal or human being. They are very dense and are most are rich in nutrients including vitamins, minerals, amino acids, fatty acids, polypeptides, nucleic acids (RNA & DNA), enzymes, and many other miscellaneous nutritional contingent factors. Glandular therapy can supply these essential nutritional needs in a highly efficient manner. This is simple really, adrenal cell extracts (or those made from hypothalamus, pituitary, gonads, etc.) are not meant to be "replacement hormones" like giving estrogen, DHEA, melatonin or progesterone as some people think, but instead provide a person's body with the essential endocrine nutrient building blocks contained in a highly specific hormonal nutrient dense form and proportion which are analogous to the human body. Most glandular dietary supplements have been made and processed in a special ways to remove all traces of hormones. Floating the raw and freshly extracted glands in a solution of alcohol and water prior to freeze-drying is one such way, as hormones are soluble in alcohol and effectively removed from the glandular tissue that way.

3 By way of an adaptogenic effect: An adaptogenic substance (like a food, herb, vitamin, glandular, etc.) is any substance that increases the body's resistance or adaptation to any physical, environmental, emotional or biological stressor and helps promote normal healthy functioning. Glandular-based food supplements contain a myriad of different tiny polypeptides, minute protein-like substances that have highly specific messenger activity and directly act on target tissues. Many hormone-like substances found in the glandular tissues, even at almost undetectable concentrations, still have potent tissue-specific activities. For example, a polypeptide material present in one tissue can have powerful and selective effects in encouraging another tissue at a different site in the body to produce hormonal materials that then may affect a final target tissue and change its physiological function. In addition, glandular extracts help cells eliminate cellular waste and speed up and revitalize their restorative functions allowing the body to metabolize for example powerful adrenalin and nor-adrenalin more effectively.

Reference: * J. Bland PhD, "Glandular-Based Supplements: Helping to Separate Fact from Fiction," Bellevue-Redmond Medical Laboratory, Department of Chemistry, University of Puget Sound, Tacoma, WA, 1980, pp. 20-21.

Thymus Versus Adrenal Gland Extracts

Your thymus gland is located under your breastbone, centrally, and close to your thyroid gland. It reaches its maximum size during early childhood and plays a large role in immune function, particularly with the developing child. The thymus is responsible for the production of T-lymphocytes, as well as the production of various hormones that are particularly important in the developing child in the years ahead. This could be partly so because there is an interplay between the thymus gland and the thyroid gland, two hormone producing glands in very close proximity to one another. Important research in 1986 discovered that the thyroid plays a significant role in modulating the activity of the thymus gland. *(J. Clin. Endocrinol. Metab. 62:474–478 1986)*

Unlike other important hormone producing glands in your body, with age, the thymus gland is the only gland which is actually replaced by fat and connective tissue, so why would there be a direct link between it's atrophy (shrinking) with age and a yeast infection, when the vast majority of adults with normally small thymus glands have in fact no yeast infection?

In my clinical experience, the adrenal glands are the most important glands to boost before you even start to look at other glands such as the thymus when it comes to those who have a chronic yeast infection. Whilst the thymus is an important gland due to its link with the production of white blood cells, notably T-lymphocytes, it is a gland more relevant to the infant's immune system rather than an adult's immune system that has been affected with a yeast infection. Although I have experimented with thymus gland extracts with yeast infected patients over the years (and in some cases did certainly notice a good level of improvement), I simply haven't found the same consistent level of amazing recovery in those suffering from a yeast infection when taking thymus gland extracts compared to those taking adrenal gland extracts, particularly when the patient took a porcine extract as opposed to bovine.

Thymus glandular extracts are generally sourced from calves. Bovine thymus extracts can be found in capsules and tablets as a dietary supplement. The best porcine adrenal nutritional supplements are those that also contain hypothalamus, pituitary and gonad in addition to cortex of the adrenal gland.

It makes more sense to me to begin with an adrenal gland extract for several reasons. For example, a top quality adrenal glandular supplement is composed of several glands including the adrenal cortex, hypothalamus, pituitary and gonad, rather than just the thymus gland. It incorporates the most important glands involved in the HPA axis, the hypo-pituitary-adrenal axis, which is the main system set up by the body to counter any stressful event, and a chronic yeast infection certainly is a stressful event.

The thymus gland extracts works primarily by inducing a higher output of white blood cells (lymphocytes), and have no effect on the body's stress regulation mechanisms, and there is a lot more to overcoming a yeast infection than just boosting white blood cells. This to me is typical of a medical approach to candida treatment, let's boost a person's immune system but forget about the fact that they may have been suffering from the stress of having a yeast related health complaint, sometimes lasting on/off for years.

HPA treatment makes more sense; you are supporting an entire system, and not just certain specific cells.

By balancing the body's underlying stress-axis, you are doing the person the world of good, but even more so if you help them understand the importance of improving their diet and lifestyle which will keep their HPA axis in fine form for many years to come.

Thyroid Glandular Extracts

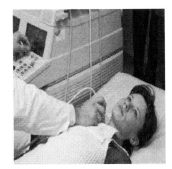

Can a yeast infection cause hypothyroidism? According to Dr. William Crook *(The Yeast Connection and the Woman, 1995)* it can. I have certainly noticed a connection between them both, and have seen countless female patients who have both a yeast infection and suffer from hypothyroidism. But whether a yeast infection causes hypothyroidism, or the other way around is something I wouldn't really know, but I certainly have noticed some type of connection in many women.

This may be co-incidental when you think about it, because many experts believe that as many as 40 to 50 percent of the female population will suffer with hypothyroidism to some degree, and it is highly likely that the percentages will be equally as high when it comes to yeast infection in women. I certainly do believe that any autoimmune condition, like Hashimoto's thyroiditis, can make a person more susceptible to a bacterial, viral or fungal infection.

Dr. Orion Truss, M.D., one of the first doctors to recognize that candida yeast infections actually caused ill health in humans stated the following "When tests are done on oestrogen levels, thyroid hormone levels, or other hormone levels and in people suffering from the symptoms of candida overgrowth, the hormones are there in the bloodstream, but they are not activating any response." Dr. Truss believed that certain toxins produced by a yeast infection in some way reduce the body's tissues from responding normally to hormones. He was probably referring to the toxic yeast metabolites, something not really studied in depth in the days of Dr. Truss. These toxins may also directly affect the functioning of the glands themselves, such as the thyroid gland.

There certainly is a large concern amongst natural health-care professionals that conventional medicine is paying little attention to the growing hypothyroid epidemic. It has even been estimated in the USA alone that as many as 60 percent of more of the entire population suffers from hypothyroidism to some degree. Dr. E. Chester Ridgway, (Chief Endocrinologist, University of Colorado), believes this figure to be as high as a staggering 70 percent. Many of the symptoms of candida in fact mirror those of hypothyroidism, such as constipation, brain fog and poor concentration, lack of focus, and cold hands and feet. Yet the blood tests all come back within normal range when it comes to the thyroid hormones.

What I have noticed with some patients is that when they started the Candida Crusher Program, within three to four months many of their hypothyroid signs and symptoms were gone, completely gone.

I'm not for one moment saying that all hypothyroid patients respond to yeast infection treatment, but some certainly do, and some magnificently. Once I started noticing this, I would include a thyroid glandular and the results are amazing to say the least. If you have a yeast infection and can relate to hypothyroidism, seek the advice of a health-care professional with experience in glandular therapy, you may benefit from Armour therapy. I would prefer you seek this treatment before a medical doctor decides to place you on Synthroid, a synthetic thyroid hormone replacement drug.

Fibromyalgia And Yeast Infections

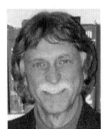
In other cases I have seen fibromyalgia patients with yeast infections experience similar improvements not just with their yeast infection, but with the pain in their muscles and joints as well. This makes me believe that by clearing the yeast from the body, some chemical must be reduced which is preventing the thyroid hormones from working effectively. If you suspect that you have fibromyalgia and a yeast infection then read Dr. John Lowe's book: The Metabolic Treatment of Fibromyalgia) and visit your health-care professional who is well versed with Dr. Lowe's pioneering work.

I worked in a medical clinic a number of years ago and used to prescribe Synthroid (T4), T3 (the active thyroid hormone), combinations of T4/T3 and also whole thyroid glandular similar to Armour. The best results I have obtained, and still do, are when I treat the patient's underlying adrenal fatigue first, present in over 80 percent of hypothyroid cases, before going onto treat their hypothyroidism. I like to use a whole thyroid glandular extract, whist at the same time addressing their yeast infection.

Do you have hypothyroidism and a yeast infection? Then both will need to be treated simultaneously, but in addition to taking a whole thyroid extract, you may initially benefit from adrenal glandular rather than thyroid glandular treatment, depending on whether your thyroid gland or adrenal glands have greater needs at the time. Either way, I certainly don't recommend you treat yourself if you have a complex set of conditions such as hypothyroidism, adrenal fatigue and a yeast infection, see your naturopathic doctor and get treatment accordingly.

Relaxation - 12 Ways To Achieve Bliss In Your Life

Relaxation is outstanding for overall health, not just for the prevention and recovery of a yeast infection. Although there are many forms of relaxation, I recommend T'ai Chi, meditation and yoga. These three techniques in particular appear to be the most beneficial because they have such a profound effect on helping a person balance their HPA axis and relax.

The concept and mechanism for how relaxation protects our stress mechanism is simple: When we relax, we elicit the relaxation response, which is opposite to the stress (fight or flight) response. Once a state of deep relaxation is achieved, for example by deep breathing and relaxing, our heart rate and blood pressure fall, (largely due to stimulation of the vagus nerve and parasympathetic nervous system), our immune system is boosted, and our circulation and digestive systems improve. Countless studies have shown the beneficial physiologic effects of relaxation therapy. In a recent study published in the American Journal of Hypertension, researchers showed that patients taught basic meditation techniques had significant decreases in blood pressure. And all they basically did was to relax and slow their breathing rates down!

With regards to a compromised immune function, which increases your susceptibility to a yeast infection, many health-care professionals believe that it can be of psychosomatic origin, especially stress and emotional conflict in nature. Improper lifestyle, faulty diet and negative thinking all play an important role in triggering many kinds of chronic disease. Our thoughts, feelings and emotions affect our body and mind to a huge extent. Any yeast infection treatment that does not take into account the powerful mind/body connection is not holistic and very much medical-focused by default in my opinion. I recommend you bypass these kinds of treatments and look more towards adopting a holistic approach that encompasses the mind and body.

Here are but a few of the many ways you can relax more around the house. Relaxing your mind and body regularly will go a long way to rebuilding those tired and worn-out adrenal glands. This in turn will ensure your adrenal and especially your immune reserves are fully topped up. Most people I see with yeast infections, especially those of a chronic nature, could well do with learning how to relax a lot more.

1

Take an afternoon nap.
I'm convinced that regular and frequent afternoon naps of short duration are the key to a long and happy life. The best time to lie down is between 2.00pm – 4.00pm, this is when your adrenal energy will tend to be at its lowest point of the day. That might not be possible in the real world, but taking a twenty peaceful minute (TPM) session in the weekend is something you can do right now.

2

Listen to your tired and stressed-out body.
Do you actually listen to your body every day? Do you down tools and put those activity lists away when you get tired or become unwell? Maybe you are one of those people who just keep on going until the wheels fall off like many do. Learn to recognize your own unique and individual energy patterns and ride these waves of energy and fatigue, and when your ocean is flat resign yourself to going home and relaxing a little until the weather (your energy levels) conditions change. In time, as you become more observant, you can master this and will be able to work out your work/life balance.

3

Spend time with your pet.
Many studies have show that spending time with a pet like your cat or dog is relaxing, fun, and can even lower your stress levels. Apart from the sheer joy your pet can bring to you, consider this:

- The increased cardiovascular activity promotes healthy heart and lungs, and all that walking and quick-start/quick-stop motion not only builds muscles, but it also sharpens your "fast-twitch" muscles, which in turn influences reaction time. Cardiovascular fitness is an important part of learning how to relax, because a fit body is a body that can relax more easily and sleep deeper.

- By learning how to increase your co-ordination and in addition learning how to relax those muscles you will be well on your way to achieving a more balanced musculoskeletal/nervous system which is exactly what I want you to have if you are to master stress in your life.

- Furthermore, for years now studies have shown that simply stroking an animal can help to lower your blood pressure. But if you have a dog, you know the best reason of all to play together, time spent with a pet like a cat or a dog you love is always time well spent. Pets give us unconditional love.

4 Learn the art of being still – turn everything OFF.

I firmly believe that in this age of rapid technological change, learning how to be still and calm without noise is one of the most valuable assets of building an abundant state of health.

- For some reason, we have become accustomed to continual levels noise and technological interferences in our lives. First, decide regularly to turn everything OFF – phone, TV, computer, and ALL electronic devices. Some folks tell me that they watch TV to relax with murder programs, hyped-up talent shows or cooking shows with constant people eliminations, etc. How can this stuff be considered relaxation when you get stressed-out watching this barrage of continual hyper-stimulation?

- Don't believe me? Then please check your pulse before and during this stimulation and you will see that this is not relaxation at all. What about mindlessly surfing Google, social media, checking emails hourly, all these interactions prevent your mind from, *stillness*.

- Are you addicted to technology? Did you know that people aged between 18 to 35 years of age now spend almost 20 percent of their entire day online?

- Spend at least one hour a day in stillness; focus on the most important things in your life, your health & wellbeing, your family/loved ones and friends and your healthy and happy future.

5 Practice regular slow nasal breathing - everyday.

I discovered some time ago with the help of a practitioner friend that one of the most powerful ways I could relieve tension and bring a deep sense of peace into my life was by way of breathing- relaxation techniques. A Certified Buteyko Practitioner, and has taught me to slow my rate of breathing down and to breathe in and out through my nose only.

- Once you understand the correct breathing technique, working with your breath is a most highly effective and convenient method of relaxation and stress-release and in addition a powerful parasympathetic stimulator.

- The incredible thing is that while breathing is essential to life, and we cannot exist without breathing, most of us do not know how to breathe correctly and actually over-breathe.

- The scope of this book is not such that I can elaborate on the Buteyko Breathing Technique, all I can say is check it out online for yourself, and see a certified Buteyko practitioner in your area for a few lessons and you may well be as impressed as I was, especially once you start to see results yourself.

- Never strain yourself when practicing any breathing or relaxation techniques (or anything else for that matter). Your breath is your best friend, so always remember to go slow and gentle.

6 Make an appointment to see Dr. Hug.

Are you a person who has minimal contact with those around you? Once you relax more (and laugh more!) you will find it easier to hug those you care about more. Hugging those you care about, or even your close friends, makes you and them feel good and connected to each other. Try it, you might just like it!

- Hug your friends, family members and especially your partner. Hugging more often not only increases happiness but also makes us happier.

- Hugs are a great way to express affection and show that you care about a person and that you support that person through good times and through bad times. Hold a hug for a moment before letting go.

- Did you know that a hug is not only one of the most powerful ways to communicate that you care for another person, but that hugs can improve the other person's mood? This in turn will improve your relationship with that person, break down tension and anxiety and allow you to relax more.

- Avoid hugging the person too tightly, and probably the best way to judge how tightly or loosely to hug someone is to let the person you're hugging indicate what he or she wants by how hard they hold and squeeze you. If they are soft and gentle, then by all means be soft and gentle back; but on the contrary, if they like more pressure and squeeze tightly, then hug back same way!

- Don't hold a hug for too long, and the more you hug the better you get.

- I have a practitioner friend here in New Zealand who wears a badge with "Dr. Hug" on it, how awesome is that. I've seen Roger hug complete strangers with a smile on his face that makes me think he has been a friend for years. Roger is one of the most relaxed guys I've known. Maybe I could book you an appointment with Roger?

7 Have a regular massage.

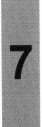

Many years ago in the earliest years of my professional work I was a massage practitioner and had a massage clinic that I worked in for several years. I noticed that some people would come in once per week for a regular massage, and the reason why they kept coming back was for stress relief. Were you aware of the amazing health benefits that a simple regular massage can have on your health and wellbeing? There are many different kinds of massage that can help to relieve tension from throughout your body. Relieving this muscular tension also releases mental, emotional and physical stress from your body. Massages are also beneficial in that they help to remove toxins from your body by relaxing muscles, joints and facilitate the circulation of blood and lymph (immune) fluids throughout your body.

- Try different massage techniques to determine which one is best suited for you. You may find reflexology (foot massage) or Swedish massage (body) to be more beneficial. Consider making massage a regular part of your regular relaxation and bliss plan.

- Swedish massage – Is often done with oils to allow a smooth experience. Essential oils may be used, and you may want a full body experience or just a focus on say legs or upper body/neck & shoulders. Swedish massage involves many different kinds of movements including plucking, pulling, stroking and stretching.

- Aromatherapy massage – This will generally be a Swedish massage utilizing a combination of various carrier oils along with essential oils such as lavender which I find relaxing, sandalwood is my favorite, and a few drops of ylang ylang is sheer bliss. There are hundreds of essential oils available and an aromatherapist will know what to use.

- Hot stone massage – Absolute magic! This form of massage uses warmed volcanic stones that are strategically placed on various muscle points to help you relax deeply. This form of massage is often used before another form of massage is begun, such as Swedish massage. This is an excellent technique for those tired, sore and tight shoulders after a day in the office. Just do it!

- Shiatsu - Shiatsu involves elements of oriental diagnosis, abdominal massage, pressure application to various parts of the body using fingers, thumbs, knees and elbows, and gentle stretches and joint articulation. A wonderful a complete body experience.

- Hugs - If you're not really into massage then do consider hugs! Touch and pressure is a big part of the success of massage; the same is true of hugs. So share a hug with someone. It will relieve stress and lift your spirits and in time as you become more relaxed will find that receiving a massage is an easy transition from receiving a hug.

 Smile and laugh more.
Learning to smile is easy; remember that smiling is the first regular step you will need to learn if you want to learn how to laugh more.

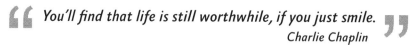
> *You'll find that life is still worthwhile, if you just smile.*
> *Charlie Chaplin*

- It's easy to smile, but do try to make your smile look natural and sincere, not strained or phony. You are trying to maintain a pleasant, happy mood, and not look half crazy! You will find it amazing that even a small, hardly noticeable to you, smile can improve the mood of those around you.

- Practice smiling when you are away from people, and make a habit of smiling frequently for no plain reason. Watch how your mood changes instantly.

- A great way to learn to smile right on cue is to think of something that gives you a lot of joy, it may be you partner or child, it maybe your car or house, it may even be you pet. Think of your favorite holiday location or the face of a very dear friend.

- Breathe-in slowly and deeply before you smile, this will help to reduce stress and dispel and tension in your body and make your smile seem a lot more natural.

- Carry a visual reminder - I have a little card that says, "Remember to Smile" with a smiley face on it. And it works! Whenever I see it, it is a good prompt. You can place a little note on your mobile phone cover or send an email to yourself or others to smile. By reminding yourself and others you know, you will be well on your way to regularly reminding yourself and others of the benefits of this simple technique.

- Turn smiling into laughing – Begin by smiling and look for things that are just plain crazy that make you laugh every day. Laughing is smiling on a roll, and if you read jokes, watch funny movies and associate with funny people regularly you will find it very easy to laugh a lot, and very easily.

9 **Engage in regular activities or hobbies that relax you find relaxing.** What are some of your favorite hobbies? Do you like playing a musical instrument, doing crosswords, cooking or baking, or gardening? The trick is to find an activity that you really enjoy and to do it regularly.

Better still; join a club of people who likewise enjoy doing the same thing. That way you will be mixing with folks who like doing what you do. This will most certainly reduce your stress and anxiety levels.

- Hobbies can be anything from simply reading a favourite book, to scuba diving with all the latest high-tech gear!

- Personally I find that oil painting is one of my favourite hobbies and now I find it one of my most relaxing activities. Have you tried sketching, water or oil painting or any other form of visual arts? Sculpting or making objects from clay (pottery) is also something many people enjoy.

- Find something you enjoy and "just do it!" as the slogan goes. It's important to find time for relaxing activities, and when you do, you will find that an enjoyable activity can be one of the best forms stress management plan for getting through life.

- Photography or filmmaking is something that many people are now getting into because of digital technology. It has never been easier (or cheaper) to have a hobby along these technical lines.

- Playing a musical instrument. How do you know unless you try it? Learning to play a musical instrument may open up a whole new world for you, and unless you give it a go you may never know what you have been missing!

10 Learn time management and how to prioritize your tasks.

- Keep a time check on yourself. Regularly throughout your day, keep an eye on what you are doing. Are you surfing the Internet again? Are you wasting your time doing something trivial because you took your eye off your important task at hand? It is truly amazing how quickly and easily we get distracted when we are working. Get back on track! Keep an eye on yourself daily and beat distractions!

- Prioritize your tasks. By setting priority levels for different tasks you need to complete each day you will get a lot more done, and more importantly, in the order of their importance. Relatively unimportant and trivial tasks can consume a lot of your day and waste a lot of your precious time, focus on the here and now and what's important and what can wait until tomorrow.

- Say "NO" to any additional work. Consider what is realistic and what is not, don't be afraid to simply say "No thank you, I'm too busy at present". Learning to say "NO" is one of the most important ways not to become overloaded by others, liberate yourself and become a little more assertive.

- Plan every day. Do you plan every day at work? By carefully planning your day it can help you accomplish a lot more and you will feel a lot more in control of your life. Do you write a to-do list and put the most important tasks at the top? Personally I find it important to keep to a schedule of all my daily activities, thereby minimizing any conflicts and any of those last minute jobs.

- Break big jobs into little jobs. Do you sometimes look at a big job ahead and find it all too difficult? Just break the job down into little steps and complete one step at a time before going onto the next step, that way you will have even the biggest job completed over a period of time. The biggest journey always begins with a single step.

- The ten-minute rule. Try this, it works for me. Is there a particular job you really have to do but you keep putting it off, procrastinating? Then just consider doing this job for a maximum of ten minutes, and no more in any one day. What you will find after a few days that you will keep on going longer than ten minutes one day and actually complete the job. Try this simple technique, it really does work.

- The art of delegation. Can you pass on any work to somebody else? Learning to effectively delegate is an important part of time management, because there is only so much you can possibly do yourself. By getting others to do more trivial and less important jobs, you will be putting out a lot less fires and save yourself a lot more time, time you could be relaxing.

- Too tired to work? Are you getting enough sleep? It is important that you get plenty of sleep otherwise you won't be able to complete tasks at your highest level when your energy levels are at their peak, generally from when you get up until about 11.00 am.

- Take a time-management course. This will not be money wasted, I can assure you. Generally your work place will be able to offer you such a course at no charge to you, otherwise find your local college or community centre that can offer you a course in effective time-management. It will be money well spent.

Chill to music.

There are many studies exploring the concept of music as a relaxation technique to help pain, sleeplessness and anxiety. Try different forms of music and see the difference it makes to your mood and energy levels, music can transform you amazingly fast and take you on a journey.

- Music as therapy is widely supported by many medical professionals, and many use it in everyday practice to create their own sense of bliss. It is great to listen to relaxing music or use other distractions so your brain shifts the focus away from any stress in your life.

- Music therapy is an excellent and safe addition to other measures such as massage or exercise, there is nothing quite like a great massage, essential oils and nice and soothing music.

- Different moods require different kinds of music tempo. You may find that when you are in an upbeat mood and you are exercising that you will want music with a higher tempo or beat (80 – 100 beats per minute) than other times such as when you are relaxing with a book or lying by the pool (50 – 60 beats per minute) Feel free to experiment with different forms of music and list these playlists accordingly such as "chill", "tempo", "party", "sleep", etc. There is a lot of research behind the tempo of music (how many beats per minute) and its effect on your heart (and stress) rate.

- Listen to music in your car. Easy going and relaxing music can make you a more easy going and relaxed driver, especially if you live and work in a big and busy city with lots of traffic.

Take a long and relaxing bath.

Have you tried to relax in a nice hot bath? A favorite way for many people around the world to relax is to indulge in a bath ritual.

- Taking a bath or spa bath or Jacuzzi, etc., is a habit that can lend deep relaxation and many therapeutic benefits to your body all year round. In ancient times, various herbal baths were used to help those who sick, while mineral baths were used for cleansing, purification and detoxification.

- Many health-care professionals today do recognize that a bath can help you relax and reduce stress levels, important in disease prevention.

- Bathing stimulates the circulation of blood and calms your muscular and nervous systems.

- Bathing can helps relieve many common aches and pains and strains associated with many common conditions such as arthritis, menstrual cramps, tension headaches, various inflammations, haemorrhoids, muscle pains, cramps and spasms.

- Insomnia - If you have any difficulty in sleeping, try taking a bath right before bedtime and be sure to add ten drops of lavender essential oil.

- Candles – Be sure to light a few scented candles and place them around your bath for a most wonderful experience. All you need now is some beautiful music.

Your 12-Step Stress-Relief And Immune Boosting Plan

" God heals but the doctor takes the fee "
Benjamin Franklin

1 Find the stress leaks in your life and plug them up. The first thing to do is to admit that stress certainly does play a role in your life, it occurs in everyone's life. I am amazed how many people who won't even admit they have stress in their lives, *any* kind of stress. Ask yourself why and how you are letting stress get to you and what you can do to mitigate the responses stress is having in your life (and more importantly on your health) right now. Examine any tension (hot) spots in your body regularly, like the sides of your jaw, neck, upper back, shoulders and lower back. Are you slowing down when you walk, talk and eat?

2 Reduce stress in your life right NOW. One of the most important points you will learn if you study psychology is that there are three things that you can do when you are in a difficult or stressful situation

1. You can *change the situation*

2. You can *change yourself* to fit or adapt to the situation.

3. You can *leave the situation.*

Remember that stresses are additive and cumulative. Removing or neutralizing your largest source of stress can make a very significant difference to your overall health and wellbeing. Most of the time, if you take care of the big stresses, the smaller ones will take care of themselves. Your body has a natural ability to handle stress and remain healthy. It is only when the stresses are overwhelming in quantity, duration or intensity that the systems like your immune system in your body start to break down.

3 Next, minimize any unnecessary stress in your life right now. What is one of the biggest things causing you stress right now? Maybe you are a worrier? Do you panic over your weight, your job, or your health or the health of your family or friends? Try concentrating on resolving the problem rather than on

3 focusing on it by completing small action steps a few times each day until you have resolved the issue, this will give you a sense of empowerment and lead you on to the resolution of bigger stresses in your life. It is easier for you to concentrate for shorter than longer periods of time initially, with experience you will be much more able to tackle the biggest stress in your life.

4 Reverse negative stress by walking each day. One of the best stress busting exercises is to simply go for a five to ten minute walk each day. Walking would have to be one of the easiest and cheapest ways to reduce the impact of stress in your life. Did you know that just by walking for twenty minutes a day three times a week, you could lower your cholesterol levels by a staggering 15 percent? Walking has a particularly favorable effect on balancing many of your body's hormones, especially your stress hormones adrenalin and cortisol and has proven to be a great stress disruptor which helps you think about other things apart from what your mind generally focuses on. Try it; you will be surprised just how uplifting a brisk walk can be, especially when your mood is low.

5 Look at your diet, each and every day. Did you know that foods could have an effect on the way your body will react to a stressful event in your life? Your body can react to a diet high in sugars and refined foods (white flour, white sugar, soda drinks, processed foods, etc.) the same way it will react when you worry about your mortgage payments, your waistline or your job security.

6 The art of relaxation, are you getting enough? It is important to balance work and play, make sure you take time out to relax every day and ensure you get plenty of sleep. Since studying stress and adrenal fatigue, I now recommend that all my patients have a quiet period of at least 15 to 20 minutes of afternoon relaxation to help powerfully build up their adrenal and immune health. Can't manage every day? Then start by doing this on the weekends and at least one day during the week. Some folk manage this well in their offices, others in their cars, if you improvise you will find a way to have this afternoon chill-out session which can be a great aid in boosting your ability to withstand stress to a much higher degree.

7 Reducing stress and anxiety through self-observation. You may be surprised to know just how quickly you run to the phone, eat your meals, take a shower, drive your car, buy your groceries, or engage in any one of a hundred other regular activities. Have you ever given yourself permission to *slow down a little?* Too many patients I see lead hurried and worried lives, and have become obsessed at completing one task before launching into several other without ever coming up for air. Pretend you are watching over your own shoulder and see how you next respond to any demand placed on you, this may come as a surprise to you. Relax when you walk to that phone, eat more slowly and chew each mouthful many more times than you normally would. Allow plenty of time to get to those meetings and arrive five minutes early and not ten minutes late, apologizing to everyone. By all means have a task list, but prioritize your tasks and be sure to place relaxation sessions, spending times with loved ones and walking on those lists – as priorities.

8 Look at increasing the parasympathetic dominators in your life. In Section 5 of this chapter I will expand greatly on some very important information with regards to your nervous system's regulation of your immune system, digestive system, and in fact most all of your body's functionality. It sounds more complicated than it is, but I'm certain that I can explain this concept to you quite easily. If you can grasp the message here and balance your autonomic nervous system (your sympathetic or "stressed out" and parasympathetic or "chilled out" nervous system) then you will be light years ahead over others who think they can beat a yeast infection with diet and supplements alone. This information alone is worth the price you paid for this book, and in fact it will be priceless if you put it into practice. By incorporating some information I'm going to discuss in detail in section 5, The Power of your Parasympathetic Nervous System, you will be delighted with how your body will not only rapidly crush your candida once and for all, but improve your overall health and wellbeing to a remarkably high level. And all of this because it is most capable of getting your health back on track in the first place, after all, your body was designed to heal itself.

9 Do you have adrenal fatigue? Have you completed the self-help questionnaire and read the section above relating to adrenal fatigue? Can you relate to adrenal fatigue? If the answer is a resounding "YES", then you need help! Contact your practitioner and see if he or she is familiar with Dr. Wilson's Adrenal Fatigue Program. By rebuilding your tired and worn out adrenals you will have a much better chance of beating the beast called yeast. Perhaps you have only partially recovered when you treated your yeast infection, but not fully? Maybe you are constantly relapsing, getting well, and then sick again? All too often, a practitioner will treat just the yeast infection by way of diet and supplements, this is my experience, but overlook the fact that their patient has suffered from many stressful events in their life, including their chronic yeast infection, a BIG stress in its own right.

10 Learn the links. I would like to mention how important it is to remember the link between your yeast infection, immune system, and more particularly how stress and poor adrenal function can dramatically hinder your full recovery. Knowledge only becomes power when it is applied knowledge; so apply your understanding of the level of your adrenal health right now and how it relates to your yeast infection. Get treatment if appropriate and be amazed at the power of your immune system.

11 Boosting glandular function. Don't forget that you may need to boost your glandular function, but be sure to get expert advice before you proceed. If you can recognize adrenal fatigue and/or hypothyroidism and in addition you have a yeast infection, I would not recommend home-treatments when it comes to glandular therapy (unless you are a qualified doctor) but rather seek out the experience of a health-care professional who has worked with glandular medicines, that way you are bound to get the best possible and least expensive results in the long run.

12 Learn the art of relaxation. Relax and slow down each day until it becomes an ingrained habit. Stressful and anxious people are much more prone to immune system problems, and will find it more easy to fall victim to a yeast infection.

SECTION 2

Candida Crusher Cleansing – Understanding Cleansing and Detoxification

Why Detoxification If You Have A Yeast Infection?

> *The primary cause of disease is not germs.*
> *Disease is caused by a toxemia that results in cellular impairment and breakdown,*
> *thus paving the way for the multiplication and onslaught of germs.*
> Dr Henry Bieler, M.D.

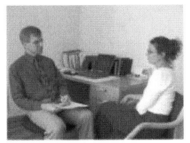

Regardless of how you feel, whether you feel OK or ill, regardless of the cause of your ill health, regular detoxification will help to free up your body's resources and improve all of its functions. My clinic has been working with detoxification programs for over twenty years which have resulted in dramatic health improvements for many patients, some who have experienced years of chronic ill health. Many people living in the Western developed nations will have some degree of intestinal dysbosis, an imbalance of the beneficial and not so beneficial flora. Detoxification facilitates the release of toxins from the liver, kidneys and throughout the body, reducing the level of pathogenic micro-organisms as well as enhancing digestion. By improving the way your body releases many and various toxic compounds you will not only assist in the prevention of many chronic degenerative disease, you will improve the way your body operates on all levels and allow healing and repair to occur more efficiently and rapidly.

There are a lot of misconceptions when it comes to detox and a yeast infection. Is detox about cleansing diets, saunas and enemas? You will gain a lot more from your Candida Crusher program if you detox correctly for several reasons:

1. Your body produces various chemicals and toxins when it comes to yeast infection, both candida as well as the immune system create these chemicals independently which your body needs to clear.

2. The candida MEVY Diet will help you liberate toxins as you invariably lose weight. Many different kinds of toxins are stored in fat tissues of your body, and as your weight is shed (even small amounts), these toxins are liberated into your blood stream entering your liver and kidneys in particular. Detoxification will to reduce the symptoms like itchy skin, bad breath, headaches, fatigue and body odour, which invariably accompany these toxic releases.

3. If you do happen to go through die-off (a Herxheimer reaction) as the yeast cells are dying, toxins will be released into the blood stream that also need clearing.

4. A good 3-step detoxification program as outlined ahead paves the way for excellent digestive health following the recovery from your yeast infection.

5. In my experience, those who detox once per year dramatically reduce their chances of developing a recurrence of their yeast infection.

What is a Toxin?

A toxin is any substance that is poisonous or hazardous to the processes that maintain life, in other words, anything that interferes with the millions of reactions that occur throughout our body and mind every few seconds.

A detoxification program will improve you health, wellbeing and decrease chances of future illness and disease. It may well be the single most effective action you can take to improve your health, wellness, and prevent illness. Dramatic results can be seen in a relatively short time, yet the benefits are felt long-term.

Environmental Toxicity

In the past 50 years, our environment has become increasingly more polluted. This has resulted in a greater human toxic burden than ever before in history. Unfortunately, over 70,000 registered toxic chemicals have been introduced into our (once) pristine environment. So, no matter where we are, or where we live, we all have some degree of toxic exposure. Add to this the use of alcohol, tobacco, caffeine, prescription, non-prescription, and illicit drugs, and you can easily see that this has created a most challenging task for our bodies to get rid of these substances. Your liver carries the greatest burden of detoxifying foreign substances, as well as substances like hormones which your body creates. You can help your liver do its job by providing your body with enough protein and nutrients and herbs involved in liver function, and by regular detoxification.

So, if we are exposed to toxic substances or if we make unwise dietary and lifestyle choices, we can build up many potentially toxic substances in our bodies. Allergies and exposure to toxins in foods, water, and the environment are being increasingly recognised as major contributing factors in many health problems. The Candida Crusher Detoxification Program is designed to allow your entire digestive system, including your stomach, pancreas, small and large intestine, as well as your liver and gallbladder to function optimally.

Daily Exposure: It Happens To Us All

Every day we are exposed to a vast number of toxic substances that we may not even be aware of - in the foods we eat, the air we breathe, the water we drink and the materials with which we surround ourselves (our clothing, building materials, household chemicals and goods, etc). In addition, the bodily functions of digestion and elimination, physical activity, combating disease and infection, and dealing with stress, produce a large number of toxic by-products. Allergic and sensitivity reactions also produce toxins. Your car probably gets serviced more regularly than your body. Does it therefore not make sense to cleanse your body internally, at least once per year?

Introduction To The 3-Stage
Candida Crusher Detox Method

My recommendations are for you not to commence detoxification until you have successfully eradicated candida. How will you know? In most all cases you will feel much better, and most if not all of your symptoms will be gone. This can take anywhere from 3 weeks right up until 6 months, so please be patient. The detox can be undertaken at anytime of the candida program, but you will gain the most benefit if you wait. Your digestive system will be functioning a lot better with candida eradication and so will our bowel, and this way you will get the most from your detox.

That is not to say that I don't support a cleanse, and the Big Clean-Up which lasts for about a week is a good thing to do before you start on the Candida Crusher Diet, as it will help pave the way and improve your bowel tone. I consider a cleanse somewhat different to a detoxification program though, a detox when doen properly will dig deeper than a cleanse and help liberate toxins stored deep inside many of the body's organs, whereas a cleanse will clear out the bowel essentially.

The following program is specifically designed to cleanse the digestive system on a deeper level including the liver and kidneys, it will help to rebalance the disturbed intestinal bacteria, restore poor digestion, prevent allergic exposure and repair the leaky gut.

To start, I most sincerely recommend you do the 7-day Big Clean-Up. But wait you tell me, "Eric, my bowels are perfectly fine, I'm passing one to two motions daily and refuse to accept that my bowels need a clean!" Sorry, you must do this stage, only then can I guarantee that this detox will really work. Remember the Big Clean-Up? Those rooms need a vacuum, the walls need dusting down, etc. Just do it!

Only after completing Stage 1 would I recommend that you commence with Stage 2 of the detox, or the deep (liver) cleansing phase.

Accumulated matter in your digestive system can create havoc, and when your system is invaded by minute toxic particles, and your body is out of balance, many factors combined contribute to the release of toxins from the gut into the body, potentially causing systemic inflammation. This dysfunction of the intestinal wall and consequent toxic invasion is associated with many chronic diseases, and the digestive repair program addresses the actual causes of these health-destroying influences.

I've worked with the following detoxification program, modified it and tried to perfect it over the years with myself as well as many clients. You will need to make adjustments to dosages of any recommended supplements and foods as you go through the program. It certainly works well, as many patients can testify who have gone through the 3-stage detox programs in our clinic.

The detox I recommend is comprehensive and is designed to help you achieve optimal health, wellbeing and longevity by way of aiding in the repair and regeneration of the trillions of cells which make up your body. It is perfect for you to attempt and to complete this detox after you have cleared you body of a yeast infection or alternatively feel that your level of yeast infection is in balance or under control. Attempting to do this detox while you are chronically sick with a major yeast infection is something I would certainly NOT recommend, or you may end up with a rather severe aggravation!

By completing this cleanse annually, you will optimize your body's function, allowing you to reach a new level of health. Digestive problems are unquestionably one of the most common health problems we see in our clinics as naturopaths, and many patients come into my practice suffering from digestive complaints such as bloating, constipation, diarrhea, gas, reflux and heartburn. Many take pharmaceutical drugs like antacids, laxatives, ulcer drugs, anti-diarrhoea preparations, etc, all which simply mask the symptoms and don't resolve any underlying problems. Armed with the information in the Cadida Crusher, and undergoing regular detoxification, you can solve many problems yourself before they really set in to become a major health crisis. And guess what? You will never need to suffer with a yeast infection ever again if you follow a regular detox, eat well, and follow the advice offerd in the lifestyle section of this chapter.

Experience and clinical observation of detoxifying many patients has shown me that for optimal results, the program is best followed in the recommended sequence for the most effective detoxification to take place. For instance, if toxins secreted by the liver were secreted into the small intestine that had not been restored to correct function, they would be reabsorbed through the leaky gut to cause more damage. Or, if the bowel is detoxified but not repaired adequately, then the "leaks" will still allow unwanted substances from the digestive system to enter the body. And thidly, if the detox is attempted but the bowels are not working very well, you will re-absorb the liberated toxins and may feel quite unwell with fatigue, brain fog and can aggravate in many different potential ways.

Just follow the recommendations because many patients with and without a yeast infection who have been through this program can testify to the amazing outcome achieved as a result of their detox.

Some Important And Handy Detox Hints And Tips:

- *Do not over-eat on a detox*! Eat less, not more, eat more slowly and concentrate on smaller portion sizes. Use smaller dinner plates, that way they will look rather full when you place a smaller portion on them, a good trick.

- Try not to eat late at night or within 2 hours of going to bed.

- Drink plenty of good quality water each and every day.

- Always chew your foods slowly and *thoroughly* before swallowing.

- Don't read anything or watch TV when you eat, *relax* and *enjoy* your foods.

- With very high levels of toxins, we generally recommend that you go easy at first, try slowly detoxing over a 2 – 4 month period for best results. It takes about that time to rest & restore your digestive function.

- Did you get a headache or hung-over feeling within the first three days of the detox? Then reduce the dosages of supplements, take it easy and prolong your detox. You will have significantly fewer aggravations and feel much better in the long run.

- For optimal results, I recommend sauna therapy; one or two saunas are generally enough per week.

- Do you want your liver to be in top shape? Then cut out all alcohol for two months entirely whilst you adopt this dietary approach. I will simply not believe you if you tell me you feel no different; you will feel fabulous and probably re-think how much you were drinking previously. I have witnessed this with countless patients over the years, many of which were only drinking one or two glasses per evening. Try it and see for yourself!

- Dry skin brushing is a most beneficial practice. Do this each day before you have a bath or shower. You will love the results.

- Water at the rate of 30 – 35mls per kg of your bodyweight is your daily target to drink.

- Visit a well-stocked health food shop for special foods and do visit the Farmer's type Markets for great organic produce.

- For an additional boost (particularly if you have poor immunity and suffer from stress) have a second glass of water after your lemon juice drink in the morning, add 1 heaping teaspoon of high-quality Vitamin C powder.

- Do you have a bowel that needs a push? Linseed & sunflower & almond (LSA) (best ground and sprinkled on salads, cereals or other foods – 2 Tablespoons a day), ground psyllium hulls (mix with water and drink, then another glass of water, they absorb water and clean the intestine) and Aloe Vera juice (add to water or fresh fruit juice), handy for restoring bowel function, clears junk out of the bowel – stay on this regularly for 3 months for the best effect.

Living A Cleaner Lifestyle – The 5 Essentials

To make the most of your detoxification program, it is essential to reduce or avoid as many toxins as possible, so that your body can truly have a chance to cleanse and repair itself. For most people, the main toxicity will be food, and we will discuss the appropriate detox (and beyond ideally) diet. The next biggest source is their lifestyle. We have listed below some essential and optional steps that you can take to give your body a fresh start. Here are some 'essentials'.

1. Exercise

Our bodies were designed for regular physical activity. We have a heart and circulatory system which pumps blood, oxygen, waste and nutrients around the body. But did you know that you also have a second circulatory system, called the lymphatic system? Unfortunately, this system doesn't rely on a pump, it relies on the big muscles in your legs and arms to pump the toxins out of the body. You should aim for at least 30-40 minutes per week (such as brisk walking or swimming) plus strengthening exercises such as weights, yoga or pilates. A well toned lymphatic system is one of the keys to well functioning immune system, and one of the main reasons why fit people don't get sick as often as couch potatoes.

2. Avoidance of alcohol and tobacco

The two most harmful drugs in our society are tobacco (3rd cause of death in many countries) and alcohol (5th cause of death in most countries). Do you use either of them regularly? then try to make a concerted effort to stop them, at least during detoxification. Can you imagine what a difference it would make to your health and your pocket if you were to stop both these poisons altogether!

3. Pure water

By now you are getting the message, one of the easiest things you can do to really get your system detoxifying is to drink lots of pure water. A good rule of thumb is that if your urine is not almost clear, then you will need to drink more. Drinking tea, coffee, alcohol, and soda drinks does NOT count when it comes to drinking water. Most of these beverages are loaded with sugar, caffeine or a host of other chemicals.

4. Detoxify your Environment

Your home and work place can be major sources of toxins. Try to eliminate or minimise your use of the following:

- Cleaning products, use natural cleansers like vinegar, baking soda, etc.

- Antiperspirants containing aluminium hydroxide.

- Pesticides, herbicides, weedicides, and all sprays generally.

- Petrochemicals, solvents, hair sprays, hair dyes.

- Pollution from cars and factories.

- Moulds, dusts, and animal furs if you are sensitive.

5. Avoid Toxic Emotions and Stressful situations

Try to avoid being around negative, energy draining people. Choose to be positive, optimistic and focused on improving your most important asset: your health. Get help from others if you have a major stress in your life. Practice relaxation techniques like Tai Chi, yoga or meditation.

Identifying The Chemicals And Toxins In Your Life

It is very important to remember that candida is not something you will beat just by changing your diet and taking a few dietary supplements. There are many other considerations to bear in mind and I'll explain a few. Just as foods that contain sugars, molds and fungi are considered undesirable, you will find in many circumstances that symptoms will in many cases be worse in humid and damp environments that are somewhat conducive of mould and fungal spores being present in the atmosphere.

Be aware of your lifestyle and environment, you may be surprised if you carefully analyse your life to find that there are potentially several sources where chemicals and toxins can enter your life. You may be interested in reading a brief description of my own case history to illustrate what I mean about a moldy environment. You will be able to read more about how serious mold is in section 5 of this chapter, "Understanding the Healthy Lifestyle".

Case History # 20
Eric Bakker, Male 25 yrs. of age (in 1986)

You may like to hear my own personal story of the yeast infection I used to have when I was in my mid twenties. I used to live by myself in a small house in an area in Brisbane (Australia) that was prone to flooding, it was cheap rent and I was working at the time in a flour-mill.

One week I would work the day shift, the next week the afternoon shift and the following week I'd work the midnight shift. I started to feel increasingly stressed and tired and one winter developed a bad cough that got worse to the point where I took an antibiotic. My little house was cold and damp and I even had to bail water out of my bedroom after it rained heavily. The walls were covered in a thin moist film that I later discovered was mold. My diet at the time was not the best; I was craving sweet foods, take-out and lots of bread. My bowels were either blocked up or I was experiencing diarrhoea and lots of gas. I felt terrible and my health was going down hill fast. My skin started to get itchy and I had developed a bad case of athlete's foot and jock itch.

To give you the background to all this, a few years prior, I had thirteen amalgam fillings replaced over a period of two weeks in 1983, but started to notice that my health was beginning to deteriorate and by early 1985 I was feeling increasingly anxious, had developed a skin rash, athletes foot and several other manifestations of a candida yeast infection, all unbeknown to me at the time, including strong sweet cravings.

I had issues with my girlfriend who thought I was a hypochondriac, because my health had deteriorated to the point where I had to seek medical help, and the doctor was of little help because all the test results all came back normal and he wanted me to see a psychiatrist. I knew I wasn't going crazy, I knew that there was something undermining my health but couldn't put a finger on it, until I later read The Yeast Connection by Dr. William Crook and then The Missing Diagnosis by Dr. Orion Truss.

My girlfriend at the time started to doubt me and told me that all my problems were in my head, a view strongly supported by her mother and that I needed to "wake up to myself", see a shrink and take an antidepressant. I decided to end that unsupportive relationship and move out of our flat and had a garage sale a few weekends later to downsize. A naturopath was looking through some of my gear at the garage sale and asked me why

I had such dark circles under my eyes. I told her about my health and the first thing she told me was to get a hair analysis done to determine the mercury levels, because she thought that having all these mercury fillings replaced may have some bearing on how I was feeling, and how the methyl mercury (released from the new fillings) may have been one of the contributing factors in the development of my yeast infection.

I went to see her and showed her Dr. Crook's book, "The Yeast Connection". What she said made a lot of sense, and I started getting treatment for my yeast infection. Unfortunately what she didn't do was carefully walk me through the various procedures of mercury detoxification and candida eradication and I had a seriously strong Herxheimer reaction ("die off") and got to one of the lowest points in my life, even contemplating suicide at one point, something I would never wish on anybody. I trust that there will be people with a significant yeast infection who can perhaps relate to my story. My whole world had come crashing down around me – I had no girlfriend, my girlfriend's mother and even my own mother thought I was nuts, I was unemployed and felt absolutely terrible. *How much worse could it get?*

After many hours of reading and study, it took over one year before I got my life back, and I did so through a careful diet regime of steamed vegetables, lean proteins, plenty of relaxation and a change of residence. In the early to mid eighties, health-care professionals did not see candida yeast infections as a problem, so you were basically left to sort out your own mess, or take an anti-depressant.

My health went to a whole new level and when I was 26, I met my new partner who encouraged me to study naturopathy. Not long after I graduated I began to specialize in yeast infections and read every single book on the topic, which was before the Internet. My health today at 53 years of age is excellent, I detox annually in the spring and undergo a one-week cleanse each fall. My weight is ideal and so is my blood pressure and I've never felt better.

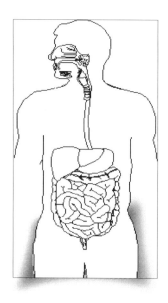

The Candida Crusher Detox Program In 3 Easy Steps

1. Purge — Clear toxic accumulations, dysbiotic bacteria fungal or parasitic infestation from the bowel. the bowel cleanse.

2. Cleanse — Release toxic accumulations from the liver and rest of the body. the deep cleanse phase. The digestive reair.

3. Feed — Repair and regenerate the digestive system, liver and kidneys to promote and maintain an optimal clearance of toxic accumulation. Rejuvenate the digestive bacterial population.

The Candida Crusher Detoxification Diet

In conjunction with the detoxification program, you will find that the best results will be obtained if you follow a healthy and cleansing diet. Often, with our busy schedules, we don't spend enough time planning nutritious meals, instead, we rely more on a on-the-run approach. These foods can have a tendency to be higher in fats, sugars, unhealthy food additives, and are generally lower in nutritional value. The candida diet approach is generally suitable for your detox, as it is designed to decrease your toxic burden by providing your body with foods that generally do not cause any allergies or food intolerances and are generally more free of preservatives, pesticides, hormones, antibiotics, and other potentially toxic elements.

Your detoxification diet should be flexible, and suit your lifestyle and personal requirements. Above all, by adopting the candida diet and detoxification program together, you will make the most of your body's ability to cleanse itself by not only reducing the toxic load coming in through your diet, but by way of facilitating toxic excretion and candida eradication all at the same time, which is a clever approach. You may even end up adopting a higher quality diet long term and avoid having any major fungal problem in the future. Common sense.

Do you remember the Big Clean-Up that you completed prior to the MEVY Diet? The following diet is similar; you can follow the 7-day Big Clean-Up diet or follow this diet. Remember, this detox is what you do after you have recovered from your yeast infection, OR you have improved significantly and feel you can cope OK. For the best results, your diet is best adjusted while you are on this cleanse. The most important things to reduce greatly or better still, eliminate, are dairy products, red meat, take-away foods, alcohol, coffee, tea, and chocolate. We are aiming for as natural a food intake as possible. Fresh is always the best.

Vegetables: sweet potato, carrots, spinach, pumpkin, citrus fruits, broccoli, strawberries, tomatoes, melons, potato, beans, capsicums, Brussels sprouts, cabbage, vegetable broths, soups, salads, stir fry, onions, garlic, spring onions, lettuce, cucumber, all sprouts. Aim for the brightly colored vegetables. Have the juice of 1/2—1 lemon each day in a glass of water, or as part of a salad dressing.

Meats: White meats, preferably: fish and chicken, venison and minimal red meat. Try to avoid lamb, pork products, and anything from the processed meat section. Eggs are fine, free range is best. Keep your protein intake up; your liver needs proteins in the form of amino acids to adequately detoxify many substances. This will also stop you snacking on the carb foods like breads, biscuits, sweets and crackers. You may even lose more weight, what a bonus.

Grains: All whole grains, rolled oats, rye, barley, buckwheat, linseed meal, millet. Wholemeal bread (two slices per day maximum), wholemeal pasta, brown rice, white rice.

Snacks: Rice & corn crackers, sushi rolls, popcorn, organic dried fruit and nuts (in moderation), (almonds & Brazil nuts are the best), sunflower and sesame seeds, almond, soy or rice milks. Fresh fruits are generally fine. Avoid peanuts, cashew and pistachio nuts on the detox.

Drinks: Herbal tea, diluted pure fruit juices, mineral water, or just plenty of filtered pure water would be optimal. Reduce or better still avoid all caffeinated drinks, such as tea and coffee (you may need to gradually cut back on caffeine to avoid withdrawal symptoms). Avoid soda drinks, energy or diet drinks.

Eliminate alcohol: This includes all beer, wine, spirits and alcohol containing products. Get real, how can your body detox when you consume any alcohol?

Reduce dairy products: Including milk, cream, cheese, cottage cheese, yoghurt, butter, Stop eating ice cream and frozen yoghurt. Have olive oil, flaxseed oil, and cold-pressed vegetable oils like sunflower or grape seed instead.

Eliminate fatty meat, fried, deep-fried foods and take-away: Avoid fast or take-away meals such as fish and chips, pizza, hamburgers, etc. Eat freshly prepared, home-cooked meals; try to avoid leftover foods from the refrigerator. Some take-away Thai or kebabs may be acceptable on occasion.

STAGE 1

Purge – Bowel Cleanse (7 days)

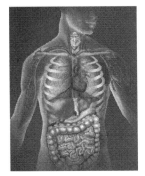

The bowel is cleansed and purged to eliminate undesirable bowel matter and bowel plaques and make your entire intestinal tract clean. Any good detoxification-cleansing program should always begin by removing any unwanted waste from your large intestine in particular. It is not a good idea to attempt to remove wastes from your liver, circulation and lymphatic system without first cleansing your bowel, the terminal part of your food processing (digestive) system. You may develop quite a strong aggravation by cleansing your body with a bowel that is not really working properly, as wastes can become recycled through the body and affect you in different ways, and I have certainly seen patients in these situations who call or email me complaining of feeling sick, nauseous, dull headaches, skin rashes, sore joints, and a host of other complaints. Just like a hangover from too much alcohol, most of these episodes are entirely avoidable.

Like anything else in this life, it is the preparation that is the key with a good detox, and if you take time and prepare your body for cleansing you can save yourself (literally) from a really nasty headache! I can remember many years ago when I first started to do regular cleansing on myself and enthusiastically took a strong liver herbal formula without paying any attention to my sluggish bowel, boy did I pay the price. Within two days I felt very unwell and extremely hung-over, I spent a whole day in and out of the bathroom and felt like a fool because I knew exactly what was going on. There is nothing quite like personal experience, is there?

Bowel cleansing can be a simple procedure for someone who has a relatively healthy digestive tract, but for somebody else with a very unhealthy digestive system it can be a major and drawn-out procedure lasting many weeks or even many months. So how do you define if your bowel is healthy or unhealthy?

Here are a few clues that will reveal that your bowel may not be healthy:

- Regular daily consumption of alcohol, coffee and tea.

- History of taking an antibiotic or taking any drugs regularly.

- Poor diet, junk food diet, eating irregularly, skipping meals.

- Not eating much fruit and vegetables.

- Eating predominantly processed or refined (supermarket) foods.

- Living or working in a high-stress environment, e.g.; shift-workers.

- Noticing that your bowel motions are not regular, you may skip a day here or there.

- Reliance on aids, laxatives or various products to help your bowel along.

- Sedentary lifestyle, little to no exercise.

- Those in a wheelchair, mobility scooter, use a rolovator or who are infirm or recovering from illness, injury or any trauma.

If you are a person who has a bowel motion once per five to seven days then you will need to take particular care when completing the 3-stage detox program, as it is good practice not to attempt a detox unless your bowel is working daily or every second day at the very least. I regularly see patients who have bowel motions every second day, and they are OK to attempt this 3 stage detox, especially if they focus on more water, fibre and plenty of relaxation.

While I have seen some chronically unwell patients over the years with major yeast infections who will probably need to work on the health of their digestive system for rest of their life, for the majority of those with a yeast infection, this will certainly not be the case, and a 7 day bowel cleanse is all is that will be required as a prelude to effective liver detoxification. The important process of cleansing and healing your bowel should not be viewed as a separate process from detoxification, and if you want to achieve the best possible cleansing outcome then this is a step you will not want to forgo. Your liver flush, bacterial & parasite cleanse and subsequent bowel repair will be that much easier and effective once a bowel cleanse is first undertaken.

It is important that you adopt the correct cleansing diet as outlined, even more so if you bowel is unhealthy. The more pharmaceutical drugs (especially antibiotics) you have taken over the years the longer it can take to clean your bowel up. The same goes for those who have lived a junk-food lifestyle for several years, it takes time to cleanse and heal that digestive tract.

You provide the necessary nutrients & herbs that allow the bowel purge process to take place efficiently, and the two products you will require are:

1. **Colozone (or magnesium sulphate powder)**

2. **Vitamin C Powder**

This is somewhat similar to the Bowel Purge you do before the Big Clean-Up (see Section 1 of this chapter, you can read about Colozone), except this is a more prolonged and thorough bowel purge, and here is why this purge is important:

- The bowel purge process eliminates places for bacteria, yeasts and parasites to hide.

- The bowel purge eliminates accumulated toxins, sludge and plaques in your bowel.

- The bowel purge will help to prevent re-absorption of toxins when you are undertaking the liver cleansing phase by allowing a clear unhindered passage of toxic waste to be excreted.

- The Vitamin C powder will help to improve the health of the cells lining your digestive tract.

Colozone *(or a similar magnesium oxide or sulphate powdered product)*

Take 1 level teaspoon in a glass of water before bedtime for 7 nights. This is a gentle and effective bowel-cleanse, and your stools will turn loose and watery. Sometimes you may feel and hear your tummy (intestines) rumbling or gurgling. Don't worry; this is quite a normal process; just reduce the dosage of Colozone if you are concerned.

Bowel Cleanse Tips:

- Just as a precaution, try not to pass early morning wind from your bowel unless you are sitting on the toilet.

- It is important to consume lots of water (1.5—2 liters) each day.

- Reduce amount of Colozone if experiencing any digestive discomfort.

- Be sure to eat light on these 7 days, stick with vegetables, rice, white meats, eggs, and decrease your portion sizes. I prefer not to eat any red meats (pork, beef and lamb) on these 7 bowel-cleansing days.

- Include lemon juice (the juice of ½ lemon in some water) in your diet, this will aid in your stomach's ability to increase output of digestive enzymes. This in turn will increase your tummy's ability to break foods down better, improving absorption, and health.

Precautions:

- Do not take Colozone or magnesium sulphate if you are pregnant, or if there is bleeding from the bowel, or if you have kidney infection or disease.

- Do not take Colozone if you have ulcerative colitis or Crohn's disease (inflammatory bowel disease). If in doubt with any of the above, please contact your health-care professional.

Vitamin C Powder

Try to buy a vitamin C powder that contains zinc, vitamin E and perhaps a few more anti-oxidants. Avoid straight ascorbic acid or sodium ascorbate as it may irritate the digestive system with prolonged use. Take 1 level teaspoon in the morning after Colozone, when you are taking Colozone for the above-mentioned 7 days.

- Designed to support your liver and intestines with Vitamin C and antioxidants, ensuring an effective bowel flush.

- If you are on the Oral Contraceptive Pill, consult your practitioner.

STAGE 2

Cleanse – Liver Detoxification (14 Days)

Your liver is now much more responsive to releasing deeper-seated toxins which have accumulated over time.

You may be thinking: "But shouldn't this second stage be about the removal of unfriendly bacteria, yeasts and parasites that may be living in my digestive tract, why is it about the cleansing of my liver?" Wait, we are going to tackle this in Stage 3, the digestive repair stage.

Be sure to read section 4 in this chapter, section 4 deals with special foods, supplements and herbs that tackle bacteria, yeasts and parasites. Do the parasite/bacteria/yeast cleanse as part of your detox once you get to Stage 3.

The liver is your cleanser and filter of the bloodstream and is of vital importance. It is the largest organ in your body and has a tremendous volume of blood flowing through it continually. It is around 8 - 9 inches in diameter, 5 – 6 inches in height and 3 – 4 inches in depth and weighs between 42 to 56 ounces. Here are but a few of the many hundreds of functions your liver performs inside your body:

- The liver is responsible for the production of bile that it stores in the gallbladder. Bile is released when required for the emulsification and digestion of fats.

- The liver stores glucose (blood sugar) in the form of glycogen that is converted back to glucose again when the body requires it for energy.

- The liver plays a very important role in the metabolism of protein and fats. In addition, the liver stores the fat-soluble vitamins A, D, K, as well as vitamin B12 and folic acid and synthesizes blood-clotting factors.

- The liver is your main detoxifying organ, breaking down or transforming substances like hormones, alcohol, chemicals, ammonia, various toxins and metabolic wastes, and pharmaceutical drugs so that they can be excreted through the bile or urine. The liver is good at removing chemicals which are foreign to your body are also known as "xenobiotic" chemicals.

- The liver is designed to remove an incredible amount of toxic matter such as dead bacterial and yeast cells, microorganisms, and all sorts of chemicals, drugs and various debris from your bloodstream.

- The liver contains many special cells known as Kupffer cells that ingest and break down toxic matter.

A Good Liver Cleanse Can Be A Person's Turning Point

Because your liver is responsible for such a wide range of functions that affect many of your body's systems, when your liver function becomes compromised the various signs and symptoms can be many and varied, and may include problems like digestive disorders, skin issues right through to memory and concentration problems, anger and emotional irritability. Stage 2 deep liver cleansing will help to restore and rejuvenate a tired and overworked liver, regardless whether the cause has been alcohol, pharmaceutical drugs, environmental poisons, illness or poor diet.

It never ceases to amaze me how much positive feedback I get from people who have undertaken a good liver detox for the first time, they are simply blown-away at their level of improvement that in turn encourages the shedding of poor and unhealthy habits in favour on adopting new habits, I have witnessed that a good liver cleanse can be a real turning point in a person's life.

Now you can understand why it is important to keep your body's main filter clean. When you do an oil change as part of your automobile's maintenance schedule, you ask the mechanic to change the oil filter. You cannot change the liver, but you can schedule regular maintenance yourself and undergo liver detoxification at least once per year. You will be amazed and delighted at the difference it makes after you have cleaned your liver up.

5 Reasons Why You Need A Liver Cleanse

Improved Mental Focus, Clarity And Moods

1

You only have to ask somebody who drinks regularly to ask what their level of mental clarity and focus is and you will soon work out that alcohol (a potent liver toxin) and healthy cognition certainly do not mix! A healthy liver gives a person a powerful ability to think with clarity and to concentrate. The liver converts ammonia, a by-product from protein digestion, into a less harmful substance known as urea. An impaired or sluggish liver will not convert ammonia sufficiently into urea, and when ammonia reaches the brain it affects the brain's ability to function optimally. This is one good reason why you will benefit from optimizing your liver's function, to allow it to metabolize chemicals like ammonia and other by-products from your digestion, not even taking into account the self-ingested toxins like pharmaceutical drugs, environmental toxins and alcohol which your liver has to deal with as well.

Those who have a great liver function are more inclined to be in a positive and upbeat mood. People with sad livers are more prone to anger, tension and anxiety, just go to your local bar on a Friday or Saturday night and watch those who drink to excess, they invariably are more prone to irritability, bad moods and anger management problems.

In Chinese medicine, the liver is certainly an organ that is connected with the emotion anger. Anything that produces a toxic liver, according to Chinese medicine, leads to anger problems and to people who have problems controlling or letting go of their anger. Obviously, the more toxic and destructive the habits like alcohol and drugs, and the longer these habits are done, the worse this angry situation and flow-on effects will become. A clean and healthy liver will make the owner feel more relaxed and at ease with their life.

Improved Digestion And Fat-Burning

I can remember having a conversation a few years back with Dr. Sandra Cabot (the Australian "liver doctor" who wrote The Liver Cleansing Diet) who mentioned that if people only knew what role the liver played in weight-loss that they would certainly pay much more attention to regular liver-cleansing. Did you know that your liver is your body's main fat burning mechanism? Your liver's role in the metabolism of proteins and fats makes it one of your most important digestive organs.

2

Your liver produces up to one pint (600mls) of bile each day that it stores in your gallbladder. Bile is one way for your body to get rid of worn-out red blood cells and other unwanted chemicals like redundant hormone residues. Bile helps to break down dietary fats and is also important for the correct and complete metabolism of the fat soluble vitamins A, D, E and K. Correct and continuous bile flow is therefore an important aspect of excellent digestion and is one of my major goals in liver cleansing, this is why many herbs and nutrients we recommend in liver cleansing are "cholagogue" by nature, meaning they help to promote the flow of bile through the bile ducts. Gallstones, bloating, gas and attacks of pain after eating fats are signs of a sluggish gallbladder. This is the reason I like people to complete a liver and gallbladder flush after a detox.

Improved Blood Sugar Control

Your liver will control your blood sugar in multiple ways; did you know that your liver has a large storage capacity of a substance called glycogen? Glycogen is stored blood sugar, and when you body needs a burst of energy the adrenal gland releases the hormone cortisol which in turn liberates stored glycogen which then becomes converted to blood sugar which is then utilized as an energy source by the millions of cells in your body. Your liver is very clever, because it can also help convert other forms of sugar into glucose, the preferred fuel for your body's cells, such as the conversion of fructose (fruit) and galactose (dairy) into glucose. The clever thing about an effective liver cleanse is that it improves the body's ability to metabolize blood sugars, making this process much more efficient. This more effective balancing of blood sugars will in turn prevent episodes of hypoglycaemia (low-blood sugar) that commonly occur in those with congested livers. The other important point worth mentioning here is that sugar cravings are more easily controlled with more effective blood-sugar control, reducing the likelihood of those sweet cravings and weight gain that many men and women experience.

3

Improved Immune Function

Did you know that the liver has a very high concentration of white blood cells, and is a primary immune organ in its own right? Your liver possesses a very high concentration of natural killer cells and macrophages that play an important role in preventing any infection or illness due to toxins, or xenobiotic chemicals from spreading to the rest of the body.

Some experts state that as much as a quarter of all the liver cells are white blood cells, designed to allow the liver to work most effectively as a filter. By regularly completing a deep cleanse you are ensuring that your liver remains vigilant and highly efficient at performing its task optimally. By reducing your total toxic load and completing the 3-stage detox annually you are well on your way to preventing the many different chronic degenerative diseases which affect all too many people prematurely.

Improved Skin Tone

The skin is your body's biggest organ and is affected very much by the underlying toxins of a body that has been overloaded over a period of many years. Perspiration is one way your body effectively deals with toxins, and this is why sauna therapy is an important part of an internal cleansing regime. Many patients I see in their 40's and 50's complain about accelerated ageing, and I explain that an accumulation of free radical damage over the past twenty to thirty years (chemicals, alcohol, drugs, nutrient deficiencies, toxins, sunshine, stress, etc.) takes its toll on the skin resulting in wrinkles through the loss of elasticity and collagen.

A healthy and vibrant liver can help the body deal with free radicals much more efficiently, and you will notice that those who do not smoke, drink, take any drug and lead a healthy stress-free life always look many years younger (their biological age) compared to their real age (their chronological age). Did they have Botox or a face-lift? NO, their ageing was reduced because their liver was more able to clear out the damage before it was inflicted on their skin. Just take a look at a woman who worships the sun and who smokes, by the time she is 50 her skin can look quite old and wrinkly. Now look at the peaches and cream complexion of a woman who avoids the harsh sun and who has never smoked in her life, pay her a visit on her 50th birthday and sit her next to the sun goddess. You will be quite shocked to see such an incredible difference in skin tone. To prevent accelerated ageing is why many people take anti- oxidants like vitamins A, C and E, zinc, selenium, alpha lipoic acid, resveratrol, pine bark extract, etc.

Regular liver cleansing will certainly improve your liver's ability to move out those free radicals thereby allowing the body to produce collagen more efficiently which in turn will keep your skin looking healthy and vital in spite of your age. And all this can be accomplished without the need of a plastic surgeon or Botox.

- Stop taking the Colozone (or magnesium powder) but continue on with the Vitamin C powder, 1 teaspoon a day in water after you get up (before breakfast). Reduce dosage if your bowels remain too loose.

- After the bowel purge, the liver's two main detoxification pathways are supported during this stage, allowing cleansing to take place on a deeper level.

- Some patients may desire to undergo a liver and gallbladder flush after this detox (before they undertake the Stage 3 Repair), to release accumulated sludge, bile and gallstones.

- If you are aiming at weight-loss, this is the all-important stage. It is worth bearing in mind that the liver is the main fat burning organ!

Liver Tablet or capsule

Take 1 tablet or capsule of a good liver formula with meals for the first 7 days. For the next 7 days, take two liver tablets or capsules three times daily with meals. This tablet may contain various herbs and nutrients of benefit to cleansing your liver. My favorite liver cleansing nutrients include the nutrients Choline Bitartrate, L-Methionine, Inositol, Betaine, Lecithin, Niacin (vitamin B3), and the herbal medicines Taraxacum (Dandelion root), Curcumin (Tumeric), Silybum Marianum (St Mary's thistle), and Cynara (Globe artichoke)

Liver Cleansing Tips:

- Follow the liver friendly tips below

- It is important to consume plenty of water (1.5—2 liters) per day.

- Do the liver/gallbladder flush at least once per year, it is best achieved right now, after you deep cleanse of the liver and before Stage 3 – The Digestive Repair.

How Can You Encourage A Healthy Liver?

- Watch out for coffee, alcohol and bad fats

- Reduce ingested toxins such as wine, beer and spirits.

- Reduce chocolate.

- Reduce your intake of paracetamol and pharma drugs in general.

- Reduce processed, refined and junk foods.

- Increase omega 3, vitamins A, C and E.

- Get into time management and reduce stress.

What Foods Can Encourage A Healthy Liver?

- Bitter foods: rocket, endive, chicory, capers, olives

- Best herbs & vegetables: beetroot, garlic, Brussels sprouts, fennel, artichoke, carrots, broccoli, onions, fresh ginger, dried turmeric

- Glass of warm water with lemon juice before breakfast

- Dandelion root coffee

- Herbal tea, green tea – instead of regular tea & coffee

The Royal Flush – The Liver And Gallbladder Flush

After you have completed the first 2 stages of detoxification, it makes a lot of sense to give your liver and gallbladder a good cleanse. I have included a few pictures of gallstones that I have received from different patients who have attempted this flush. The Liver and Gallbladder Flush should not be attempted by pregnant women, children, very elderly and frail persons, insulin dependent diabetics, those with severe liver disease or those with an acutely inflamed gallbladder.

I have placed several hundred patients on this protocol over the years and have never once experienced any bad outcomes with people. Occasionally, some people may suffer with discomfort such as abdominal cramps, diarrhea, nausea or vomiting before the gallstones are passed. The liver and gallbladder flush should not to be attempted on a constipated person. If in doubt, discuss this procedure with your health-care professional. Here is what you do :

 Drink 2 to 3 liters of a good quality apple juice daily for 2 days before the flush is attempted. This is best done between 8.00am and 4.00 pm, for example, one glass every four hours. It is best that you consume NO FOOD for the two days prior, just eat apples (green are best) and drink the apple juice.

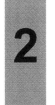 Freshly squeeze 300mls of citrus juices such as grapefruit, lemon or lime. Plain grapefruit or 100% lemon juice works best. Plain citrus juices may aggravate those with liver congestion, causing headaches and some nausea, dilute with 40% water if necessary. The mixture will be bitter, and needs to be in order to stimulate the bile flow from the gallbladder and liver.

 Grate and press a small onion and one clove of garlic, add the juice to the citrus mixture. The allium family of vegetables contains sulphur compounds known to aid in the detoxification of toxins via the biliary route.

3 At 6.00 pm, mix together the 300mls of citrus juice along with 300mls of extra-virgin olive oil. Drink/sip this mixture over the next 2 hours, have sips every 15 to 20 minutes. A warm castor-oil pack over the liver region will be found to be beneficial, or a hot-water bottle. Some prefer to sit in a warm bath. All these will help to relax the digestion and stimulate bile flow from the bile ducts.

4 Retire as normal, after the mixture is finished, lying if possible on your right side with a pillow elevating your right hip slightly. This will allow the mixture to more effectively promote expulsion of the sludge and stones from the gallbladder and liver.

5 You may desire to collect your bowel motions (they will probably be quite loose) into a suitable container and wash/strain through an old colander. You may be quite surprised to find several dozen or even over one hundred small stones remaining. Gallstones can be easily seen in the toilet bowl however, as they will probably float and be greenish in color.

Now that you have completed the flush, it is time to do the final stage, the Digestive Repair Stage. Did you manage to pass any gallstones? Many people do, here are a few pictures from a couple of different people.

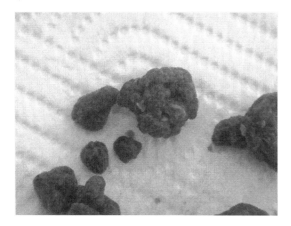
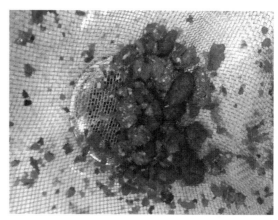

Repair – Digestive Repair (14 days)

If you want to do a bacterial, parasite and yeast cleanse, now is the time to begin the removal of adverse microbial pathogens the bad guys and start with the replacement of beneficial organisms known as the friendly bacteria in the gut. For some who have completed the Candida Crusher Program and are feeling great, they may not want to do the parasite cleanse but go straight into taking the probiotics, it is entirely up to you.

It is essential to remain on a great probiotic for some time after you have completed this stage, and I prefer you take one capsule twice daily for at least eight to twelve weeks after you have completed stage 3. This is to ensure you have fully established a small army of friendly bacteria inside your body, protecting your digestion and helping to keep any invading organisms under control.

You provide the nutrients and herbs that remove the bad guys and also the probiotics that sustain the growth of the beneficial bacteria.

Anti-Parasite And Anti-Microbial Capsule Formula

■ Take a good anti-parasite and anti-microbial formula with meals for the first 7 days, like the Candida Crusher Formula. For the next 7 days, take of 2 these three times daily with meals. Reduce with discomfort or any aggravation. See section 4 of this chapter for a more detailed description of the best dietary supplements to take.

Probiotic Capsule

■ Take 1 capsule of a top quality probiotic formula twice daily like the Candida Crusher probiotic, take one on rising (when you get up in the morning) and take one on retiring (on going to bed).

Digestive Repair Tips:

- Be sure to read the information in section 4 of this chapter 7, Understanding Special Foods, Supplements and Herbs.

- Keep up with the probiotic for at least 8 – 12 weeks on completion.

- It is important to consume plenty of water (1.5—2 liters) per day.

- If you want to do the Liver and Gallbladder Flush, it is best to complete it before you start on Stage 3 detoxification, although you can do the flush later if you so desire.

Suppress and Reduce the Yeast

Candida albicans generally affects a person's digestive tract first. It may colonize the digestive system and stay there causing all manner of digestive problems, or it may migrate out and cause problems in other parts of the body. The main treatment for candida is directed at overhauling the gastro-intestinal tract first, regardless if the condition is digestive or systemic, and the best way to achieve this is with the Candida Crusher Diet as well as the Candida Crusher Program for the best results. I used to like to use the word "kill" instead of yeast reduction when it came to candida treatment, but killing is not really necessary.

Wars never solve problems, they just create more wars, so today I rather suppress yeast and gently inhibit thereby reducing the numbers and at the same time build good bowel flora. I have found this a much more satisfactory method and just as effective long term as those programs that "kill" candida rapidly, without seriously aggravating the patient. After having examined and used many different candida programs, I believe that most programs just don't work effectively enough because they don't use the right products, recommend the right dosages, advise the correct diet or lifestyle or just don't engage the person quite long enough to really make a difference to that digestive system. Others try to kill the candida too rapidly, some kill too hard, some too soft, and some programs will treat for a week or two and others for up to two years. One of the best ways to learn something is by making mistakes and realizing that things have to be done differently, and I can tell you, I've made plenty over the years that I won't make again when it comes to eradicating a yeast infection.

"What is die-off? (Herxheimer reaction)

You will often find that candida treatment can cause in many cases, but certainly not all, the rapid death of large numbers of yeasts, during which great amounts of toxins are released from the dead candida microorganisms. These toxins can also cause allergies in many people. Some patients prematurely abandon their candida treatment under the mistaken belief that this die-off reaction and its associated allergic reactions are an indication that their candida overgrowth and treatment is worsening rather than diminishing.

On the contrary, I have found that this is sometimes used as a diagnostic tool, particularly with chronic candida. When you kill off a large population of candida all at once, all of the toxins that are currently stored in them are released into your system all at once. As there are usually significant amount of toxins stored in candida cells, these toxins when released will causes a temporary increase in yeast symptoms (and sometimes including new symptoms as new toxins are released), followed by a considerable lessening of symptoms.

The technical name for this experience is a *Herxheimer reaction* ; which is more commonly referred to as *"die-off" or "flare-up"*. This experience is similar to as when you have eaten a "forbidden" food that you have avoided when you actually have candida. In both cases, candida releases its toxins and it can be hard to differentiate whether you are killing it or feeding it.

Some people (prematurely) abandon their candida albicans therapy under the mistaken belief that this "die-off" reaction and its associated allergic reactions are an indication that their candida albicans over-proliferation is worsening rather than diminishing.

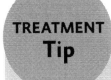

TREATMENT
Tip

In order to tell the difference between die-off symptoms, a food allergy or candida yeast symptoms in general, it is very wise to keep a food diary or journal of what you eat and what anti-fungal products you take, so when you get a change you will know which it's likely to be.

If any die-off is caused from treatment, the aggravation will usually last from few days to 2 weeks depending of what anti-fungal you use and the state of your digestive system. As you reduce almost all of the candida the die-off effect will generally subside. Even if you don't get die-off it does not mean that candida is eradicated from the body. It is possible that amount of candida killed in your system (and their associated toxins being released) is too small to produce massive die-off. Then, you should either continue the same anti-fungal for few weeks to finish it off or even better still, change to new anti-fungal product. Also, the dosing of the anti-fungal treatment and the effectiveness of these products on your system can be established by observing die-off effect.

The other thing to bear in mind is that the colony of yeast in your digestive system can be greater than the amount of yeast metabolites in your digestive system and circulation, and this can affect the severity and nature of your die-off. In my experience, the people who experience the greatest amount of die-off are the ones with a heaviest digestive load of yeast who kill the candida too fast, too soon. Another type of aggravation I see is when the body has a heavy load of metabolites in the circulation or outside of the digestive system, and the person's immune system starts to attack these chemicals. So how can you tell the difference?

Here's how

1 High digestive load of yeast, bacteria and parasites, small amount of metabolites in peripheral tissues such as the circulation and other organs adjacent to the digestive system. These people have a mild case of leaky gut and tend to experience local aggravations, such as vaginal thrush and digestive problems. Their aggravations are more inclined to be local but they can also experience fatigue. A stool test will reveal what their SIgA levels are like, (generally low), their beneficial bacteria, pathogenic bacteria and parasites as well as the amount of yeast in their digestive system.

2 Low digestive load of yeast in comparison to larger amounts metabolites in peripheral tissues such as the circulation and other organs adjacent to the digestive system. These folks may have significant leaky gut and lots of symptoms that may at first appear unrelated to a yeast infection, even neurological complaints. Again, a comprehensive stool test will reveal all. It will tell you how leaky the gut is, if there is any inflammation and how high or low their levels of good and bad bacteria are.

Some Cases Are Complex And Chronic

An intelligent interpretation of the comprehensive stool test results can give you a clue as to what is really happening inside, and take away much guesswork. You may think that I seem presumptuous with my clinical observations, but comprehensive stool testing has taught me how to treat yeast infections and avoid most all cases of aggravations or die-off with patients. It gets really tricky if the patient has inflammatory bowel disease (IBD) like ulcerative colitis or Crohn's disease, or is a celiac on top of their yeast infection. These chronic digestive conditions throw a spanner in the works and can really complicate cases, they most certainly delay recovery and it is easy for these patients to aggravate and have repeated bouts of die-off. With chronic yeast infections, especially is you are a complex chronic case, find a health-care professional who can assist you with a stool test, and work with a good laboratory and you will short-cut you treatment by less than half. Don't even think about home-treatment if you have IBD or are a celiac and have a yeast infection as well. You may get some results, but you will be glad you paid a visit to somebody who is expert in these cases and who has plenty of experience.

Symptom Aggravations Versus Allergic Aggravations

Don't be confused with a worsening of your yeast infection symptoms when taking an anti-fungal dietary supplement as opposed to the aggravation experienced when you eat or drink something that may also cause an allergic reaction instead. This is easily done and can be confusing, for this reason I want you to stay rather strictly on the Candida Crusher Diet and thus eliminate this situation from occurring. The Low-Allergy

Diet is starting to make more sense, now you can see why an elimination of any potential allergenic foods makes a whole lot more sense. Most all people with a yeast infection have some degree of leaky gut, and it is easy to have a food reaction when you are going through the Candida Crusher 4-month Program, and I don't want you thinking that this food reaction was because of yeast dying off. It may make you stop supplementation or cut the dosage, and this will delay your recovery and could give yeasts and bad bacteria the upper hand they have been waiting for!

When you follow this line of treatment and experience any aggravation, you will know whether it is caused by a food or the supplements. Keeping a food diary is therefore a good idea, and by following the Candida Symptom Tracker (chapter 3) you will soon see if your aggravation is from a food or dietary supplement.

You may experience some degree of die-off, but the effect of the anti-fungal should not be intolerable. After having read the signs and symptoms of a yeast infection in chapter 3 and you suspect that you have a severe case of a yeast infection, then you are probably experiencing die-off and the severity of the die-off will usually be in proportion to the dosage of the Candida Crusher supplements you have been taking. If die-off effect is too strong, the dose of anti-fungal treatment should be decreased, and to decrease the effect of die-off, try this flush out tip at the beginning stages of treatment:

Avoiding Aggravation Tip

Sometimes an aggravation is unavoidable, and you may experience a die-off reaction. To avoid or minimize any potentially unpleasant side effects, I recommend initially flushing out the gastro-intestinal tract before taking anti-microbial remedies.

I recommend taking a vitamin C powder that boosts your immune system and takes the dead or dying microbes immediately out of the body, greatly minimizing any discomfort. Repeat the flush for two to three days. Usually the reaction in the first three to four days to "die off" is the strongest.

An alternative approach that I favor is to start with a low-dose of the Candida Crusher Formula (anti-fungal/microbial) and increase only very slowly. In this way any die-off symptoms you experience will be much milder, but unfortunately may also remain low-key for several weeks longer. You can abate this by ensuring that you take the Candida Crusher pro-biotic twice daily if you decide to go slow. It is my favorite method and seems to work very well but with this method it is especially important to maintain your strict diet, and for prolonged periods of time especially in the early stages of treatment. I generally prefer the vitamin C flush method, but if you cannot use that for any reason, then try the go low and go slow approach.

Effective Treatments For A Herxheimer Reaction

I often find that supplemental digestive enzymes such as pancreatic amylase, bromelain, chymotrypsin, lipases, papain and trypsin can dramatically aid in the reduction of aggravations and reduce the discomfort caused by the Herxheimer reaction. Take an enzyme, probiotic and antifungal/antimicrobial.

Candida Crusher Formula Take as required, but reduce if any aggravations occur.

Candida Crusher Digestive Enzymes work well, ensure one with each meal.

Candida Crusher Probiotic. Take one three times daily.

Charcoal (20 - 30 grams per day) absorbs the toxins produced by candida albicans in the gastrointestinal tract, thereby counteracting the Herxheimer Reaction. Take if you experience headaches, severe digestive problems, or feel spaced-out, unreal or have brain fog. Your stool may appear darker when you take charcoal, so don't freak!

Congratulations!

This brings you to the end of your 3-stage Candida Crusher Detoxification Program. Since you have worked so hard to regain wellness throughout this detox, I'd like to make a few recommendations to keep you in the wellness zone, so to speak.

- Eat less sugars, breads, alcohol and refined carbohydrates.

- Stick closely with the principles you learned with the MEVY Diet.

- Eat less food not more, and always strive for quality and not quantity.

- Occasionally say "No thanks" to a meal and eat light. The best exercise is to push the plate away from your belly at night.

- Pay attention to your digestion, appetite, sleep and energy levels and make appropriate changes you have learned so far in this book to bring these areas back into balance.

- Be aware of chemicals in your life and take appropriate action to minimize any unnecessary exposure.

Repeating a detox once per year is a very smart idea and a great way of maintaining your health and wellbeing. You could get your annual check-up including blood tests after your detox; your doctor will be most impressed. Anytime during the year when you feel sluggish, you can do a mini 7-day cleanse as outlined in the Big Clean-Up.

Best Kept Secret – The Kidney Flush

The kidneys are a regulatory organ, they help to control the levels of electrolytes, and when salt is dissolved its elements sodium and chloride become important electrolytes, responsible for transferring the electrical activity within your body.
The kidney is also responsible for blood pressure regulation as well as ensuring you have a correct acid base balance (pH levels); kidneys even stimulate the production of red blood cells within your body. Each day your kidneys process a staggering 230 litres of blood (400 pints) and manage to remove an incredible 2.2 litres (4 pints) of wastes!

Without optimal kidney function, toxic wastes would simply build up in our blood stream causing infection, inflammation and we would soon develop kidney stones or they would fail altogether causing premature death. It is important to remember the kidney damage takes place slowly and gradually – and without symptoms, and if left untreated, kidney disease can become irreversible leading to kidney failure.

The kidneys are also responsible for excreting many different waste products, toxins and chemicals from your body. These toxins are many and varied and can come from a wide variety of sources, including chemicals and toxins in your food and water, pharmaceutical drugs, environmental chemicals (pesticides, etc.), alcohol residues, various forms of pollution and radiation and many other potential toxins. When the kidneys fail to function optimally, these toxins can potentially cause many different health problems like headaches, high blood pressure, nausea, itchy skin, fatigue and a host of other problems.

I have always found it amazing that a lot of emphasis is placed on liver and bowel detoxification, but nobody ever speaks of kidney detoxification of cleansing.

There are many different herbal medicines, juices and different dietary supplement formulations that will help tone and detoxify the kidneys; some of these include parsley, basil, black cherry, celery, watermelon (rich in potassium and very high in water), golden rod and corn silk.

Kidney Cleansing

- **Drink adequate water every day**, this is the most important part of your kidney cleansing regime. Without adequate water, your body is unable to expel wastes through the urinary route efficiently.

- **Wash a small bunch of parsley, add to 600 mls of water (a pint) and simmer** (with the lid on) in a non-aluminium pot for 4 minutes.

- **When cool, drink half a cup** (about 125ml) and keep the remainder in a glass container in the refrigerator. Drink 125 mls twice daily for seven to ten days.

- Better results are obtained when you **add the (carefully) cleaned roots of a parsley plant that is two years old.** This will give your kidneys a good flush.

- **Take a good quality probiotic capsule three times daily before meals** to help repopulate your urinary and digestive tract with beneficial bacteria.

- **Drink in addition during this week a glass of apple juice** (certified organic) to which you have added some kidney herbs. Ask your local herbalist to make you up some liver herbs, be sure to shake them well before use as kidney herbs are mineral rich and these minerals will sink to the bottom of the container they are dispensed into.

- **Eat more of the following kidney-friendly foods**: watermelon, celery, red bell peppers, cabbage, cauliflower, garlic, onions, apples, cranberries, blueberries, raspberries, strawberries, cherries, red grapes, egg whites, and fresh fish.

- **When kidney cleansing, reduce consumption of the following**: red meats, white flour and sugar products, rich foods, junk foods, peanuts, spinach and chocolate, all detrimental to a kidney cleansing routine and kidney congesting foods.

- Now that have read section 3 of chapter 7, let's put the detoxification concept together to form a plan. You will get a better result if you stage your detox to include the liver and gallbladder flush as well as the kidney flush. By follwing this protocol as I have outlined in the box below, you will be ensuring that your body has had the most thorough cleanse, and you should feel amazing. Why not follow this procedure annually?

Staging Your Bowel, Liver, Gallbladder And Kidney Cleanse

1 Do the 3-stage Candida Crusher Detox Program once per year. The first time is the hardest time, once you have successfully detoxed, it will be easier to repeat the process. Tell yourself that your health will improve dramatically after you have completed this entire process.

2 Do the Liver and Gallbladder Flush after Stage 2. Do the detox first, and then do your liver and gallbladder flush before you do the Digestive Repair. Repeat the flush if you have noticed many gallstones, some patients have completed the flush many times and have noticed continual improvements with each flush.

3 Do the Kidney Cleanse after the Liver and Gallbladder Flush. This is the final stage of your detoxification regime but never the less a very important (any often entirely overlooked) stage of cleansing your body. Kidneys can harbor many tiny stones and gravel that can in some cases represent perfect hiding places for parasites, yeasts and bacteria. Flush them out and keep them clean by regularly performing the kidney flush as outlined.

Heavy Metal Detoxification

An area of concern to many is the possibility of heavy metals in the body, particularly mercury, being an underlying cause of a chronic yeast infection. There is no doubt about it, there is a connection between mercury in a person's body and candida, but there is a whole lot of ridiculous information online about it as well, my advice is to be cautious about any information you act on, and if you are going to make any decisions on what I write below then do consult your holistic doctor and mercury-free dentist. Don't make any quick decisions, take your time and do your homework first.

Do A Hair Analysis First

Dr. Trowbridge ("The Yeast Syndrome") wrote that some doctors who specialize in yeast infections have reported that over 90% of chronic candida patients have mercury toxicity. I would certainly agree with this statement after having examined the test results of several hundred patients with chronic yeast infections. I have discovered not only an elevated mercury level, but also an elevation of the other sulphydryl metals arsenic, lead and cadmium.

I have also noticed in the hair test an elevation of copper and/or zinc. This occurs due to a metal binding protein called metallothionine inside your cell. This protein loves the sulphydryl-loving metals mercury (Hg), lead (Pb), arsenic (As) and cadmium (Cd) but also loves the metals zinc (Zn) and copper (Cu). Sulphydryl loving metals are metals which are attracted and bind to compounds attracted to substances containing sulphur. Knowing this helps us to understand what agents are best used to help remove these metals, like garlic. Aluminium detoxification for example is quite different from mercury detoxification, as aluminium is not sulphydryl.

As mercury levels increase, copper and zinc elevation in the hair test results may increase. The reason for this is that as the cell's sites become increasingly occupied by mercury, copper and zinc are literally kicked-out of the cell as metallothionine's binding affinity for Hg is many hundreds of times greater than it is for copper and zinc. Some practitioners who then interpret their patient's hair analysis reports with elevations of copper and zinc state that the patient has a "excess" of copper and zinc in their body, when in fact the opposite applies, they have a deficiency. The patient's hair is showing elevated levels when in fact they have low intracellular levels of these two vitals metals. Have you done your hair test yet? Ask your practitioner, and do check in the back of this book for different laboratories I recommend.

Mercury certainly was one of the leading causes with my chronic yeast infection when I was in my twenties, I had all of my mercury amalgam fillings replaced with new mercury amalgam fillings. Not long after, my yeast infection took a turn for the worst and my health plummeted. It wasn't until a year later after I completed a hair analysis that I discovered how high my hair mercury levels were. Over the next eighteen months I replaced all my thirteen mercury fillings for white composite fillings and then undertook a heavy metal detox.

If you are serious about your health and have mercury amalgam fillings you may want to consider having these fillings removed and replaced with white composite fillings, particularly if you have noticed a sharp decline in your health and an aggravation of your yeast infection after a lot of dental work.

With a hair analysis, you can either request a head hair or pubic hair test. Head hair is the preferred sample, but if your hair is dyed, permed or bleached in any way or has had any treatment in the past several months then do a pubic hair sample. Those in trades like jewellery, sheet metal workers, printers, welders, mechanics, bus drivers or people who are around metals or chemicals are best to complete a pubic hair test I feel. This is because their head hair may have a certain amount of external contamination.

My concern with heavy metals is that most all medical practitioners are not interested in toxicity with their patients, and many natural health care professionals (at least in Australia and New Zealand) simply don't have the right kind of training to know what to do with their patients who may be affected with heavy metals, pesticide toxicity or who are generally toxic in other ways. A quick two-week detox just won't cut it I'm afraid, nor will a detox out of a box ready made detox kit that some practitioners market to their clients. There is no simple solution, but by undergoing a cleanse as I have suggested above, you will be going a long way to reducing your toxic load, and by cleansing annually you will be making even greater strides forward. Living the clean lifestyle is one of the best ways forward. Seek out health-care professional with experience in heavy mental dextoxification if you need help here.

Urinary Provocation Testing

Your practitioner may want you to undertake a further test, a urinary provocation test, particularly if your hair test results have revealed high levels of mercury or other heavy metals. You will be given a "challenge" substance which maybe something called DMSA (orally) or an intravenous solution called DMPS. These provocating agents liberate heavy metals and cause them to be flushed from your body through the kidneys, a urine sample is collected after the provocation and sampled for heavy metals including mercury, arsenic, lead and cadmium, the four most common heavy metals found in a person's body. It is not the scope of the Candida Crusher to delve too deeply into this topic, but it probably will be in the second edition.

Why Is Mercury Bad?

Professor Boyd Haley from Kentucky, USA, has been studying the effects of mercury on human health for decades and is considered one of the world experts in mercury toxicity. His website www.mercuryexposure.info is packed with information and is certainly worth a read if you are interested in learning a great deal more about the connection between mercury exposure and your health in general.

Mercury has a particular nasty effect of the membranes of the cells of your body. It has the ability to disrupt the cellular membranes and negatively effect the essential fatty acids in these membranes themselves. Mercury binds to sites inside and outside your cells which should be occupied by other metals like copper and zinc, disrupting cellular function on many levels. These sites then become inactive and various cellular functions no longer occur.

3 Reasons Mercury Can Cause
And Help Maintain A Yeast Infection

1 Proteins inside your cells and their membrane walls become oxidized (damaged) which makes your cells less effective in general. The cells also begin to lose the ability to communicate with each other due to this damage. As their cellular membranes become increasingly compromised, the immune system increasingly begins to lose its effectiveness. White blood cells produce chemical messengers such as cytokines which allow cells to communicate. With damage to the cells membranes, this signalling becomes impaired which has a negative effect on the cell's ability to control bacteria, viruses and yeasts themselves. The cells become increasingly defenseless against attack not only from external sources, but also from chemicals and wastes produced by the cells and your metabolism in general. This is one of the reasons those with yeast infections can become so fatigued.

2 Secondly, mercury amalgam fillings have the ability to continually release a vapor containing methyl mercury, which is a more toxic form of mercury than the mercury contained in those fillings. You will find an interesting You Tube video showing the actual vapor coming off a mercury filling. It is believed that this methyl mercury is one source of food in your intestines for candida albicans. Why would you want to feed the yeasts in your digestive system? You have taken the sweet foods, alcohol, refined carbohydrates and the yeast containing foods from your diet and now you may well have up to a dozen or more mercury amalgam fillings which are potentially feeding the candida. I'm certainly not suggesting that you have your fillings all removed, it is a costly, painful and time-consuming process, but if you can't seem to recover like I couldn't recover, then maybe getting yourself checked out carefully is a good option. People with a chronic yeast infection of many years duration may need to consider the option of dental work. Either way, you are always best to talk it over with your holistic doctor before you make any decisions.

3 Thirdly, one of the most plausible theories is that mercury and other heavy metals such as lead, cadmium and arsenic, place a huge load on the body's immune system. They slowly but surely lodge in the nervous system and the endocrine glands including the adrenal glands, thyroid, hypothalamus, pituitary gland and many other places of the body. Candida and many different kinds of bad bacteria, parasites and viruses wil find it much easier to proliferate in a body under such a toxic load. Not to mention any other environmental toxins such as pesticides, carbamates, organochlorine residues and VOCs (volatile organic compounds). We certainly live in a toxic world, and this is why I encourage you to determine your toxic load and undergo regular detoxification. It certainly makes sense.

Frequently Asked Candida Detoxification Questions (FAQs)

What Is The Difference Between A Herxheimer (Candida Die-Off) Reaction And A Detoxification Aggravation?

Some patients I have known over the years have complained about a bad case of "die-off" (otherwise known as Herxheimer reaction) which occurs when large numbers of candida yeast organisms are killed off, releasing large amounts of antigenic compounds (your white blood cells produce antibodies towards these) as well as various toxins, usually in excess of the liver's capability of dealing with them.

During this die-off, the patient will typically experience a worsening of their symptoms. It is therefore important to support the liver before, during and after and strong yeast-killing program. For this reason, I'm not a big fan of strong candida yeast killing programs, but prefer the more gentle approach. This is also one of the reasons why I do NOT advocate the use of any anti-parasite, anti-yeast or anti-bacterial dietary supplements or herbs for the first two weeks of the Candida Crusher Program. Does this make sense? Just focus on diet initially, then bring the products in slowly, that way you won't overwhelm the liver and create a Herxheimer situation.

There is a difference between killing off the yeast and suffering from the effects of "die-off", as opposed to suffering from the aggravations of detoxification. It is important for you to remember that when you kill off a large population of candida all at once, the toxins that are currently stored in them are released into your system all at once – you will feel bad quickly. As there are usually significant amount of toxins stored in candida cells, these toxins when released will causes a temporary increase in yeast symptoms by way of overloading your liver in particular. Your symptoms that you have been experiencing will probably worsen and can do so suddenly in that case. When you suffer from the effects of a detox aggravation, it is more likely to be less "violent" or extreme in nature and tends to be a low-grade (could be high for those who are extremely toxic) sensation of feeling sluggish, headachy and unmotivated. This is a big contrast to the candida die-off reactions which some patients will experience when they push their body too fast, too soon and just too hard through the "kill" phases of the program. If anyone advocates a strong "kill program", walk away or be warned – you may experience the wrath of your liver and develop a full-blown Herxheimer reaction.

How Long Will The Detoxification Program Take?

Good question, the exact duration of the program will depend on how ill and/or toxic you are and how well you system responds. Most people require anywhere between 3 weeks right up to 6 months with an on-going maintenance program.

How Much Will Detoxification Cost Me?

Owing to dietary changes, you may well save money on your grocery bill. Supplementation varies according to the individual program, but on average it will cost between $5 and $12 per day. Considering how important this program is to your overall health, this is a very worthwhile investment. Are you worried about a few hundred dollars? In my experience, many people spend more money on their health in their last 3 months of their lives than in their whole lifetime– and by then it is generally too late.

Will The Detoxification Make Me Feel Ill?

When cleansing the body with a detoxification program, you may experience some temporary reactions in the first 2 or 3 weeks. These symptoms will be short lived (a week at the most – generally speaking), and are quite normal. Adequate water intake is essential al least 1.5 to 2 litres daily. Reactions may occur while the body attempts to physiologically balance the body chemistry and revitalize your immune system. With some people, as they enter the second stage (phase 2) of the liver detoxification program, they may feel they get worse after an initial improvement. This is quite ok! Remember in chapter 6, at the beginning when you read "How people think they get well" as opposed to "How people get well"? If you have skipped this chapter, you may want to go back and read the first few pages. The longer your toxicity or nutritional deficiencies have existed, the more prevalent this response is likely to be. Corrective reactions that may occur include: skin rash, excessive flatulence, runny nose, mild dull headaches, insomnia, increased thirst and/or urination, weakness, lethargy, loss of appetite, loose bowel motions or constipation, dizziness, nervousness, and various mild body aches and pains in your joints or muscles. If these reactions do occur, (if at all possible) ensure you have a restful couple of weeks at this time.

You can be assured that your body is making positive changes toward an improved state of health. By recognizing these as part of the corrective 'healing crisis', it will be easier to accept them as steps on the road to better health, and any lost ground will be quickly regained when the program is maintained.

What Are The 3 Primary Reasons For These Detox Reactions?

The Toxic Dump: By far the most common reason. Your body has an amazing cleansing system for eliminating toxins that accumulate in it, as long the conditions are right for it to do so! Your system can become inefficient and lazy, allowing toxins to build up and be stored, especially in body fat, rather than being eliminated. Once this natural cleansing system begins to work more efficiently, reactions can occur. These reactions result from the stored toxins being released faster than the liver, kidneys, skin and lungs can remove them from the body. These temporary reactions are a small price to pay for the long-lasting health benefits you will gain long term. Ongoing toxic burden can result in fatigue, sleeping problems, dull headaches, countless digestive complaints, feeling unwell often, weight gain, depression, easily angered and more irritable.

2 Poor Immune Response: When your body is exposed to long periods of emotional, physical and environmental stress (such as heavy metals, additives in your foods, pesticides, petrochemicals, and the many other chemical exposures) combined with an inappropriate or nutrient depleted diet, your natural defense system can become compromised and less efficient. Ongoing poor immune response can result in you being more prone to colds and flu, sore throats, poor wound healing, and frequent skin, urinary tract or respiratory infections.

3 Allergic-Type Reactions: Allergic-type reactions can be caused by a 'leaky gut', and/or a deficiency of hydrochloric acid in the stomach and/or by dysfunctional or exhausted liver, thyroid and adrenal glands. Antibiotic prescriptions can add to this burden, and are frequently prescribed for all manner of acute infections. Ongoing poor immunity can result in you being more prone to an increased incidence of allergies such as eczema, asthma, sinus and hay fever, skin rashes and shortness of breath and sensitivities to certain foods. Do any of these above problems sound familiar to you? Chances are you have some now, and this is why we recommended the detox.

I Have Detoxified Before - Why Is This 3-Stage Program Any Better?

Detoxification must be conducted in a well-defined sequence if it is to work properly. Many other programs concentrate on the liver, with no preparation for the rest of the digestive system. Others I have seen just recommend a "colon flush" without a liver cleansing stage. This can result in toxins being released from the liver, only to be reabsorbed by the "leaky gut", so that no long-term benefit is gained. Many 'detox-in-a-box' programs are available, and have a very limited and short-term effect. One I have seen involves swallowing up to 50 capsules a day! Following my carefully designed program will ensure maximum therapeutic effect for a complete and long-lasting result. My aim is also for you to become aware of *where* your toxic burden has come from, to *avoid* a future 'build-up', as well as to *educate* you in terms of adopting and maintaining a healthier diet and lifestyle long term.

Is The Detoxification Program Safe For Children?

Yes, providing the dose is modified appropriately. Children will not generally require liver detoxification, but may well benefit from the bowel repair program after gastroenteritis or antibiotic treatment. Because their systems are still relatively new to the world, they will usually respond very quickly and easily. At first, you may have to be strict regarding food choices, as children do not have the foresight to understand that "a stitch in time saves nine". Once they feel the benefits of a healthy digestion, they will be happy to continue the program.

Is This Program Safe During Pregnancy And Breast Feeding?

The answer is an emphatic NO. Most internal cleansing programs mobilize stored toxins that may affect the growing baby. For this reason, we do not recommend detoxification during pregnancy or breastfeeding. It is however a wonderful preparation for healthy conception. Ideally both prospective parents should undertake a 3-month detoxification before even thinking about conception.

Will I Lose Weight On This Detox?

This program is not about weight loss– although detoxification is an important part of a weight loss program. Depending on your initial condition, the dietary modification that I recommend and the detoxifying effects of the program may cause the shedding of some unwanted kgs. It is also a fact that larger people, (who carry more body fat) are also more toxic. Therefore, people on any weight-loss program would do well to undergo detoxification. The presence of toxins in the body causes fluid retention. As you remove any toxins (and fat), you will also release that fluid. You may notice that you pass more urine during the program.

But What If I Start To Lose Weight? I'm Already Too Thin!

When you follow the program exactly as instructed you need not be concerned. The only weight loss in these cases is usually toxic fluid accumulation, in addition to some potentially toxic fat stores. Such loss can be followed by a healthy weight gain when there is proper adherence to the program.

What If I Get Constipated When I Stop Eating My Usual Diet?

Make sure you increase your water intake to eight 200ml glasses daily. Add ground flax seeds (2 tablespoons daily) on top or your vegetables. You can also obtain LSA mix (linseed, sunflower & almond ground up into a powder) from your health-food shop. If your bowels still do not move increase your fibre intake. You could also take Colozone again for 1-2 nights, and perhaps one or two doses of Aloe Vera juice in water daily.

Can I Continue To Exercise Throughout The Program?

For optimal results, it is recommended that during this program you do mild exercise regularly, as well as get adequate sleep. Both adequate rest and light physical activity facilitate cleansing, detoxification and restoration. At the very least, allow some time each day for yourself to relax: breathe deeply, listen to some nice gentle music, relax in a bath, take a yoga class, or a walk in the park. Give your body and mind the break they need to cleanse and heal. If you are used to a strenuous exercise routine, such as daily running, gym or swimming, you can continue as per usual. However, do not do this program if you are increasing your exercise routine in preparation for a competitive event. If you have a competition planned, wait at least 10 days after the event to start this detoxification program, and listen to your body's guidance! This area may need to be discussed more with your practitioner, in order to achieve maximum results

Shouldn't My Mercury Fillings Be Removed Before I Begin The Candida Crusher Program?

No they shouldn't, first concentrate on your total body burden. You have enough to worry about with your current yeast infection, and you don't want to be doing a mercury chelation program at the same time you are making such radical diet changes and trying to eradicate the yeast overgrowth. It is just too much in my opinion, and after having worked with many patients who have tried to get rid of their of their mercury load while at the same time trying to eradicate and kill their candida I can tell you that it just isn't worth it. Do one thing at a time and do it right, you have plenty of time to work on mercury after you have reduced your candida overgrowth.

First, remove as many "obstacles to cure" as you can, see the end of section 5 for more complete information what is mean by obstacles to cure. Have you improved your diet? Have you adopted the lifestyle recommendations? Have you taken the Candida Crusher supplements? If you have done all this then you should be feeling a whole lot better. But, on the other hand, if you have done all this and to the best of your ability, there just may be the possibility that a mercury toxicity is part of the cause of your ongoing yeast infection. You may be one of those patients who are so loaded with mercury and possibly other heavy metals, that the methyl mercury just keeps on feeding the yeast in your digestive system.

In this case, go and see a mercury-free dentist and get evaluated like I did. A dentist who is familiar with mercury removal can do an electrical reading of your teeth to see how many "negatively charged" teeth you have and how they could be affecting your brain, nervous and immune system. I had one tooth with a negative 14 charge, which is apparently quite extreme. No wonder I was having such severe depression when I had everything to live for, no wonder I was having headaches almost daily. And all my medical doctor wanted to do was to send me to the psychiatrist, because he thought all the problems were in my head. They were in fact, but in my mouth and not in my emotional state. Have you done that Hair Test yet? A hair analysis is another way you will be able to determine how much mercury your body is carrying.

How Do I Detoxify From Mercury And Other Heavy Metals?

There are different ways you can do a heavy metal detox, and it is not the scope of the Candida Crusher to go into detail with heavy metal cleansing. There is a lot of nonsense written online about this topic I've noticed! I urge you to pay very little attention to most forums and blog sites when it comes to serious detox. You really should consult somebody in your area who is expert when it comes to heavy metal detox. You should certainly not see a lay practitioner (unqualified) at the very least, and preferably a practitioner with at least ten years of clinical expertise in heavy metal detoxification methods.

Some of the more popular methods of heavy metal detoxification include chelation (oral or intravenous), cilantro (coriander), chlorella preparations, zeolite, alpha-lipoic acid, glutathione, N-acetyl-cysteine, and garlic extracts. You may also have heard about EDTA, DMSA or DMPS. Mercury detox is not something ou really should do at home unsupervised, get expert help, you will be glad you did.

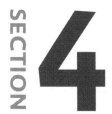

SECTION

Candida Crusher Eradication – Understanding Special Foods, Supplements and Herbs

Candida Crushing Suggestions

In this section I will describe what the best foods, supplements and herbal medicines that in my experience have the best effect on the inhibition and eradication of candida, including unwanted bacteria and parasites from the body. Some of my suggestions you will have heard and may already know, others you will have not. Towards the end of this section I'll outline the core Candida Crusher supplementation program.

The three categories you will find in this section are as follows:

1. Candida Crushing Foods,

2. Candida Crushing Dietary Supplements

3. Candida Crushing Herbal Medicines

1 Candida Crushing Foods

Get Your Yeast Infection Under Control With These Fungus-Fighting Foods

When it comes to inhibiting and even eradicating a yeast infection there are several foods you will want to know about. Most people who see me with candida ask for the best supplements or herbs to kill candida, but forget that there are several foods they can easily get from their local grocery store which have an excellent effect in getting rid of a yeast infection.

I have found over the years that some foods are better than others, and I like to call them "Candida Crushing" foods. If you incorporate these special foods into your diet on a regular basis, you will be well on your way to getting rid of your yeast infection and if you keep on eating these foods and adopt the dietary and lifestyle principles I've outlined in the Candida Crusher then you can be confident in knowing that there is little chance of a recurrence.

Make sure you also read the information in this chapter (chapter 7 - section 1) about fermented and cultured foods, and by eating the candida crushing foods I'm about to explain along with the fermented and cultured foods in your diet, you will be doing all you can in terms of your diet to ensure a complete eradication of your yeast infection.

While the candida crushing foods inhibit and kill candida, the fermented and cultured foods encourage the proliferation of friendly bacteria. Remember the saying: "Let food be your medicine and medicine be your food"?

The MEVY (Meat, Eggs, Vegetables and Yogurt) diet I recommend is wholesome and nutritious, but by including these extra special candida-busting foods into your eating regime you will be turning your diet into a powerful yeast killing tool. What I wanted to achieve with this section of Candida Crusher is to place in your hands the correct dietary information you need to treat your yeast infection at home

Key Candida Crusher Steps:

1.   Do the Big Clean-Up first.

2.   Do the MEVY Diet for 2 – 3 weeks.

3.   Do the Candida Crushing foods and incorporate Fermented & Cultured foods.

4.   Do the Hypoallergenic Diet.

5.   Do the Food Re-Introduction Diet.

6.   Take the recommended Dietary Supplements appropriate for the different stages.

Candida Crusher # 1 Garlic.

Allium sativum, commonly known as garlic, is a species in the onion genus, *Allium*. Its close relatives include the onion, shallot, leek, and chives. With a history of human use of over 7,000 years, garlic is native to central Asia, and has long been a staple in the Mediterranean region, as well as a frequent seasoning in Asia, Africa, and Europe. Garlic was well known to ancient Egyptians, and has been used for both culinary and medicinal purposes for many thousands of years.

Garlic is one food that has powerful anti-bacterial and anti-fungal properties and several scientific studies have found it to be as effective as the popular anti-fungal pharmaceutical drugs Ketoconazole and Nystatin in destroying candida albicans. Garlic in my opinion is the number 1 food that counters a yeast infection and should be consumed daily. One important difference between taking drugs like antibiotics and antifungals, and taking garlic, is that bacteria and fungi are not likely to develop a resistance to garlic. This is great news for you, and one the drug companies are not likely to tell you.

Garlic is one of my favorite and most effective anti-candida measures, and although I use this herb as part of my supplementation regime, I 'd like to explain it under the special foods section because it is really a food you will want to consume most days.

The day I can finally convince a patient to eat fresh garlic daily along with increasing their intake of onions, leeks, spring onions and chives is the day their "luck" turns for the better; it often spells the beginning of the end of their yeast infection. Garlic suppresses, inhibits and destroys most every single form of detrimental fungi, bacteria, protozoan and viruses. I have for many years had a large bowl of garlic cloves on my kitchen bench and use fresh cloves in most of my cooking along with plenty of fresh herbs such as oregano, sage, basil, thyme, and parsley. These herbs were introduced into cooking many thousands of years ago to inhibit bacteria and eliminate parasites, not actually to flavor foods like most people believe. Do you eat garlic daily? It can help your digestive, circulatory and immune system in so many different ways. Will it cure your yeast infection? It won't all by itself, but as part of my Candida Crusher Program I consider it one on the major pillars of strength.

The best way to eat fresh garlic is to have a bowl handy with many cloves, take a small clove of garlic and carefully crush it to remove the skin, then get a small knife and score the garlic down one side. This is done to allow the digestive juices in your stomach and small bowel to have access to the inside of the clove; otherwise you would pass the small clove straight through the digestive system. The outer layer of the garlic clove is high in silica; your stomach's digestive juices may find it hard to penetrate through this layer. Scratch the outer layer and your digestive system will have no problem. Whilst you can supplement with capsules of aged or odorless garlic, fresh is again the best. You can use garlic in salads, egg dishes, etc. Can't tolerate garlic? Then get the odorless capsules. If you buy fresh garlic, please make sure you *avoid* any garlic grown in China (high in heavy metals). Buy locally grown or grow it yourself. And, the best time to plant garlic is on the shortest day of the year, in winter. The best time to harvest garlic is on the longest day, in summer.

Tip

How do you get rid of the smell of garlic?

The best way to eliminate the pungent garlic smell from your breath after you have eaten is to chew on a sprig of fresh parsley soon after. Parsley neutralizes the smell of garlic. You can also try chewing on a sprig of fresh mint, and I have found that this works just as well if not better than parsley.

How Does Garlic Work Against Candida?

Russian scientists long ago discovered that when they introduced a garlic extract into a colony of dysbiotic (bad) bacteria and yeasts that the bacteria and yeasts ceased to function literally within minutes. They used fresh garlic extract in these experiments. There has been much study completed on the health aspects of garlic, and much has been even written in mainstream medical journals about the virtues of garlic. Garlic is a most effective agent against fungi and yeast as well, and should be high on your list of foods that inhibit and kill yeast in your body. Garlic was confirmed in reports back in the 1980's to be more active against human ringworm (a fungal infection) than conventional pharmaceutical drugs.

Research at the University of Indiana in 1979 revealed that the therapeutic value of garlic against candida fungal infections is great, and that an extract of garlic bulbs has the ability to inhibit many aspects of fungi. The unfortunate thing about garlic unfortunately is that not everybody is keen on consuming it, with many finding its odor and taste unpleasant. Trust me, the more you consume garlic the more you get used to it and can tolerate it.

Part of your anti-candida program, and an important part of the Candida Crusher Program is the inclusion of fresh and supplemental forms of garlic. Eat as much fresh garlic as you can, and anywhere from one to a half a dozen cloves of fresh garlic is an excellent way to get what you need. Slice it finely over cooked vegetables, crush garlic and finely chop it before adding to a fresh salad or add several cloves to a roast meal.

The Therapeutic Uses Of Garlic In Yeast Infections

It is important for you to realize that you will get the best benefit from garlic by taking it in fresh as well as supplementary form. That way you will be taking it in as both a food and a more concentrated form as a dietary supplement. There are many therapeutic uses for garlic when it comes to a yeast infection.

- **Fungal infections of the skin** (including ringworm, jock itch and athlete's foot). Ringworm and jock itch respond to treatment with garlic juice that is applied directly to the skin. You don't need a high concentration so mix with a little water and try first – it may initially feel unpleasant. Garlic juice will be required with a higher concentration (straight and undiluted) to be effective against athlete's foot. You will find that fresh garlic is as effective (or even superior) against athlete's foot as is the medicine Lamisil. Just crush a clove and apply the juice neat to the affected area once per day. You will be amazed at the result! I have "cured" countless cases this way.

- **Fungal overgrowths of the digestive system.** A study (1999 Arora) revealed that garlic was more effective against candida albicans than the antifungal drug Nystatin. Carefully peel 1 clove of garlic and then make a neat slice down the side of the clove with a small paring knife. This will allow the digestive juices to open up and digest the clove. Otherwise you may well pass the clove through undigested due to the silica present in the outer layer of the clove, which is quite resistant to digestion. Raw garlic is superior to cooked garlic, which destroys the allicin content.

- **Vaginal yeast infections.** You may want to read the other sections of the Candida Crusher that is more relevant to this common women's complaint. Naturopathic doctor Tori Hudson (USA) who specializes in women's complaints recommends using garlic tampons. Be careful not to cut the clove but thread a string carefully through the end of a peeled clove. Insert and leave for 8 hours.

- **Earaches and itchy ears.** Place a drop of onion or garlic juice into the ear. Works wonders for earache too, especially in young children prone to earaches.

Good Tip

Take Garlic Before Full Moon

Here is a more unusual but very effective health tip that works. People for generations have planted and harvested crops according to the moon cycle, and smart hunters and fishermen know that they will increase their catch significantly when they look at the moon cycle. Try to target yeast, bacterial and parasite eradication with garlic especially in the two days leading up to full moon. The best times to take garlic for two days before full moon, on full moon and a day or two after are at dawn and dusk. Take one clove on rising or at dawn, and one clove on dusk.

In addition, have some grated beetroot and carrot and also pumpkin seeds and treat especially three days leading up to and including full moon, but have this with meals and away from the garlic. Don't laugh, bacteria, fungi and parasites have shown to have an increase in activity with the waxing moon. You will get better results treating in the week leading up to the full moon as opposed to the week after full moon.

Garlic Recipe: Hummus

Chickpeas (garbanzo beans) are very versatile and highly nutritious, and hummus is one of the tastiest ways to eat chickpeas, especially when you add fresh garlic. I prefer to have the chickpeas fresh, but you can use canned chickpeas. Just soak a cup full of plump, large chickpeas overnight. The following day drain and simmer for two hours. Drain, cool and blend. Hummus is very versatile; you can use it as a dip or on pitta bread with a filling of your choice. There are many possibilities. Great with falafel too

Ingredients

- 400g canned chickpeas, drained and rinsed (If you prefer the real thing, use 1 cup of dried chickpeas)

- 2 garlic cloves

- 2 - 3 tablespoons water

- 2 tablespoons of tahini (sesame seed paste)

- 2 tablespoons of olive oil

- The juice of 1 lemon

- Black pepper

- Paprika powder, to garnish

Method

- Process the chickpeas, garlic, water, tahini, olive oil and lemon juice in a food processor until smooth.

- Add more water or lemon juice if necessary, be careful, only a little at a time.

- Season with black pepper or chili to taste.

- Transfer to a bowl and refrigerate.

- Garnish and serve with a sprinkling of sweet paprika

- Enjoy!

Candida Crusher # 2   The Allium Family

Did you know that garlic and onions both belong to the same family of plants, the allium family? If you have candida, make it a point of including plenty of onions (brown and red), leeks, spring onions (scallions), shallots, chives as well as garlic in your diet. This will significantly increase your body's ability to fight bacteria and candida. Many books on yeast infection talk about garlic and fail to mention that you really should be eating more of the allium family in general, and by eating a full complement of allium foods you will be ensuring that you really do use your food as medicine.

How Does The Allium Family Work Against Candida?

The allium family contains many different types of natural yeast-fighting compounds including organic sulfur. Sulfur has been used for centuries to rid the body of infections and to purify the blood. It is a natural liver cleanser as well.

They allium family exhibit antibacterial and antifungal activity, and a study that was conducted in 2006 in Iran that certainly validates this fact.

The study: By using an agar dilution assay, the antifungal activity of water-based extracts prepared from allium cepa (onion) and allium sativum (garlic) were evaluated against candida albicans (19 strains), other candida species (12 different strains) as well as 35 strains of various dermatophyte species (a fungi that cause skin, hair, and nail infections) and compared with the activity of a known antifungal drug, ketoconazole. The onion, garlic and ketoconazole solutions were found to be able to inhibit growth of all fungi tested in a dose-dependent manner with maximum of 100% at defined concentrations. The results indicate that onion and garlic are equally promising to ketoconazole in treatment of fungal-associated diseases from the pathogenic genera candida including dermatophytes.

Reference: Shams-Ghahforoki, M., et al. In vitro antifungal activities of Allium cepa, Allium sativum and ketoconazole against some pathogenic yeasts and dermatophytes. Fitoterapia. 2006. Department of Mycology, Faculty of Medical Sciences, Tarbiat Modarress, University, Tehran, Iran.

Candida Crusher # 3   Oregano

Oregano (origanum vulgare) is a perennial herb growing to a height of 20 inches, with purple flowers and spade-shaped, olive-green leaves. It is native to warm-temperate western and southwestern Eurasia and the Mediterranean region.

Oregano is well known in the Mediterranean world (Greece and Crete) for its ability to slow down food spoilage through its anti-bacterial, anti-fungal, anti-parasitic and anti-oxidant activity. It was used many centuries ago, and still is today, in conjunction with meat dishes to stop contamination of bacteria from spoilage, long before the discovery of refrigeration.
The related herbs thyme and marjoram are also effective when used as antimicrobials, but possess little of oregano's miraculous healing properties. Thyme is an excellent herb for coughs however, and I have recommended it in cases of whooping cough for many years, it works particularly well in curing coughs that appear to have settled into the chest for ages.

Oil of oregano is a completely natural substance derived from wild oregano species. The plant grows in remote mountainous regions free of pollution. Only the leaves of the flowering plant are used and they are picked precisely when the plant is highest in essential oil. Ideally being grown wild, top quality oregano oil is grown chemical-free and the oil is extracted via a completely natural process without the use of chemicals or solvents. The oil is the source of virtually all of the plant's active ingredients.

I have been recommending oregano oil for candida and all manner of digestive problems for over ten years, and find that it really works well with people who complain of candida yeast infections, small intestinal bowel overgrowth (SIBO) and those who complain in general of gas, indigestion and bloating. It is a good idea to complement oregano oil with a top quality probiotic. These natural products are compatible with each other and will often hasten recovery, especially when used in conjunction with the Candida Crusher Program. You will be interested to know that I am developing a unique Candida Crusher yeast eradicator, which includes wild oregano oil of the highest quality.

It is important to remember that you will NOT get the full benefit from oregano just by eating the leaves of the herb you have bought at your local garden center, or by eating a few oregano leaves on your pizza or in your salad. Unlike garlic, eating fresh oregano will not give you strong therapeutic benefits and it is best that you take an oregano product which contains a high quality wild-crafted oregano oil. Watch this space, i'm working on it!

Anti-Bacterial And Anti-Fungal Agent Extraordinaire

Oregano is a superb antibacterial and antifungal herb; it contains many different volatile oils that are highly active against the majority of pathogenic bacteria and yeasts, including staph, strep, and E.coli. Furthermore, just like garlic, fungal resistance to oregano oil is exceptionally rare, it just doesn't happen and the drug companies will never let you in on that secret. Oregano is such a potent antifungal agent that it is capable of destroying even resistant fungal forms such as the mutated fungi which result from antibiotic therapy, I have noticed this on many occasions when treating resistant cases of yeast infection. I'm a big fan of oregano oil in cases of yeast infection and believe that the best results come to those who use the powerful double-hitting combination of an allicin rich garlic extract AND a carvacrol rich oregano oil. You just can't beat nature!

Keep an eye out for my Candida Crushing formulations, one of the formulations will contain the highest quality oregano oil, and by joining our mailing list you will be the first to know of my new product releases.

How Does Oregano Oil Work Against Candida?

Oregano oil is antiviral, antibacterial and antifungal and has even got anti parasitic qualities. It has a strong antioxidant and anti-inflammatory effect and is therefore the ideal natural medicine to use by those who suffer with yeast infections.

One of the main reasons oregano is so powerful is that it contains a chemical called a phenol (primarily carvacrol) which works in extremely low dilutions, even as low as 1 part per 50,000! Carvacrol has the amazing ability to destroy Candida albicans, the Aspergillus mold, Staphylococcus, Campylobacter, Klebsiella, E.coli, Giardia, Pseudomonas, and even Proteus. Another phenol constituent, thymol, boosts the immune system. These two compounds also act as free radical scavengers (preventing oxidative stress, or damage) thus preventing further damage while encouraging the body's natural healing response.

The Therapeutic Uses of Oregano Oil in Yeast Infections

- Fighting and killing candida & yeast, fungus (skin and blood-borne)
- Improving digestion, stimulating bile flow (gas and bloating)
- Supporting & boosting immunity, allergies, hay fever, and sinusitis
- Supporting infections (cold and flu)

Internally: **(caps)** Take one capsule of oregano oil daily with meals, build up to two or three capsules daily with meals. Take for 14 days straight then STOP, repeat as required but wait one week between the two-week cycles. **(Use liquid oil or open a capsule)** Use the oil on or in the body. It is strong, so when using it internally, <u>start with small amounts</u>, like one cap daily with meals or start with two drops of the liquid oil twice daily in vegetable juice or with a meal. If in doubt or if you have a major yeast infection or you feel you are a sensitive person then please go LOW and start SLOW with liquid oregano oil, it will save an aggravation. Try taking one drop twice per day working your way to one drop four times per day then start on the caps if you can take four drops or more daily without too much drama. Mix with one teaspoon of olive oil to improve palatability and compliance. Take for a period of two weeks and then stop for one week. Then repeat the process. Don't give up in a hurry, it can take a while to get used to oregano oil but it certainly works! Don't be scared of pushing the boundaries and if you can take more temporarily – then do so.

Externally: **(use the liquid oil or open a capsule)** Oil of oregano may also be applied (sparingly - avoid use around the eyes) topically to treat itches, infections of the skin, gums, teeth, and just about any orifice in the body. Exercise care if you use it in the genital region where it is best mixed with olive oil or coconut oil before application (1 drop per teaspoon of olive oil or coconut oil/butter).

From what I believe, and in my experience, there are no side effects and oregano oil is compatible with any other natural remedy or prescription drug.

Candida Crusher # 4 Cloves

Cloves are the aromatic dried flower buds of a tree in the family Myrtaceae, Syzygium aromaticum. Cloves are native to the Maluku islands in Indonesia and have been used as a spice all over the world for many centuries. Cloves are harvested primarily in Indonesia, India, Madagascar, Zanzibar, Pakistan, and Sri Lanka. You may have heard about the effect that cloves have on toothache; the oil in particular has a numbing effect on mouth tissues such as the gums and help to soothe nerves of teeth that are affected by toothache. What you may be less familiar with is that even in the tiniest of concentrations, clove oil is a very powerful antibacterial and antifungal agent.

How Do Cloves Work Against Candida?

The main compound that is the effective antibacterial, antifungal and anti-parasitic is eugenol that comprises up to 90% of the essential oil extracted from cloves. Eugenol is the compound most responsible for the strong medicinal effects as well as for the characteristic aroma of cloves.

The good thing is that even commercially available clove oil has been analyzed by scientists and found to have a high concentration of eugenol (over 80%), and it is cheap and readily available. But you must take care when using clove oil! You will be able to read more about caution when using clove oil further ahead.

There are numerous studies from India and Asia that have revealed the yeast suppressing and yeast killing effect of cloves in both the oral cavity as well as in the digestive tract. Clove tea, made by steeping the dried buds in boiling water can help to ease nausea and indigestion. Tincture of cloves as well as oil of cloves helps to heal many types of fungal infections such as athlete's foot and ringworm.

A laboratory study in 2009 has found clove oil and its active component to be effective antifungal agents against candida and other fungal pathogens Researchers at the University of Porto, Portugal, studied the composition and antifungal activity of clove essential oil. The researchers found that both whole clove oil and eugenol showed inhibitory activity against all the fungal strains tested. They discovered that yeast cells were ruptured and even died due to the damage inflicted by cloves, but even better news was that they discovered that cloves almost entirely prevented the production of hyphae by candida albicans. (Hyphae are branching filaments that extend out from the cells of candida albicans and other fungi and can penetrate tissues in the body). It is these hyphae that are know to penetrate the walls of the small intestine and are known to contribute to an increase in intestinal permeability (leaky gut syndrome).

Clove Oil Kills Yeast That Have Become Resistant To Anti-Fungal Drugs

The conclusion from the Portuguese research was that cloves and eugenol in particular have demonstrated a considerable antifungal activity against many fungal strains, including candida albicans (including fluconazole resistant yeast strains) and that clove deserves much further investigation into its use into the clinical applications for a wide variety of yeast infections. It is impressive that clove oil is effective against fungal strains that have become resistant to fluconazole (Diflucan), one of the most common and well known of the antifungal drugs your doctor will use. Make sure that a product you take to inhibit and kill candida contains a compound of clove, and you will be pleased to know that I'm working on a Candida Crusher product as I speak which contains a high quality organic clove oil compound with a 90%+ eugenol content. One of the biggest benefits of clove is that it is cost effective and when appropriately used is virtually side effect free when compared to the commonly used azole drugs.

Reference: Pinto E Vale-Silva L Cavaleiro C Salgueiro L (2009) Antifungal activity of the clove essential oil from Syzygium aromaticum (Eugenia caryophyllus) on Candida, Aspergillus and dermatophyte species

Spices like cloves have long been known to possess medicinal value, in particular, antimicrobial and antifungal activity. An Indian study was completed in 1999 that compared the sensitivity of some human pathogenic bacteria and yeasts to various spice extracts and commonly employed antibacterial and antifungal drugs. Of the different spices tested, garlic and cloves were found to possess the main antimicrobial and antifungal activity. The bactericidal effect of garlic extract was apparent within 1 hour of incubation and 93% killing of staphylococcus and salmonella was achieved within 3 hours. Yeasts were totally killed in 1 hour by garlic extract but it took 5 hours with clove. The interesting thing is that in this study some bacteria showing resistance to certain antibiotics were highly sensitive to extracts of both garlic and clove. When Nystatin was trialed against garlic, it was discovered that garlic as well as cloves have a greater anti-candida activity than Nystatin. This study has once again showed that commonly used household spices might have a greater potential to be used as antimicrobial agents than is commonly thought.

Reference: Arora, D. S., et al. Antimicrobial activity of spices. Int J Antimicrob Agents. 12(3):257-262, 1999.Department of Microbiology, Guru Nanak Dev University, Amritsar, India

The Therapeutic Uses Of Clove Oil In Yeast Infections

o   Fighting and killing candida & yeast, fungus (skin, digestive system and blood-borne)

o   Improving digestion (nausea, restores appetite, reduces gas)

o   Supporting & boosting immunity, antiviral, antifungal, antibacterial, anti-parasitic.

o   Reduces inflammation (rheumatoid arthritis and osteoarthritis)

o   Pain-relieving (toothache, has an anesthetic effect)

Internally: (caps) Take one capsule (of a compound dietary supplement formulation containing dried clove bud amongst other herbs, spices, vitamins, etc.) daily with meals, build up to two or three daily with meals.

CAUTION: Take clove in a dietary supplement that contains a very small percentage. I do NOT recommend the use of straight clove oil orally (unless you use it on a cotton bud or tip applied to your gum or tooth when you have a toothache) because liquid clove oil is a known hepatotoxin (toxic to the liver) and it is an inhibitor of blood clotting. Make sure you take clove either in the form of a candida dietary supplement (which contains several other ingredients and clove is NOT the primary ingredient, it is a minute amount) or in the form of a clove tea which you can at times get from your health-food shop.

Any product containing clove will be strong, so just like when starting out with garlic or oregano, start with small amounts!

Externally: (use the liquid essential oil or make clove tea)

CAUTION: Oil of clove can easily cause skin irritation and should never be used in concentrations any higher than 1% when applied directly to the skin. Like oregano oil, it is best mixed with olive oil or coconut oil before application (1 drop per tablespoon of olive oil or coconut oil/butter). Some people can take more (anywhere from 2 to 10 drops per tablespoon), and some can take less, like any essential oil, it is all about trial and error. You need to especially careful with clove oil around the face/eyes and genitals. I once had a tiny amount very close to my eye and it was a most terrible experience I wouldn't wish on anyone, so be warned! Apply the tiniest amount sparingly on your wrist and see if there is any reaction and if there is, take extra care.

Athlete's foot and toenail fungus application

I recommend that you try this oil blended with oregano oil if you have a particularly difficult case of toenail fungus or athlete's foot. Mix five drops of clove oil with five drops of oregano oil along with a tablespoon of olive oil. Apply to the affected areas very sparingly twice daily. Reduce the clove oil if too strong and add a few drops of lavender oil if you want to mask the clove oil smell.

Jock itch clove tea

I saw a patient some years ago who successfully got rid of his jock itch by using a concentrated tea made from clove buds. He washed his groin each evening with this strong tea made from 1 teaspoon of clove buds that had been steeped in boiling water (about 250 ml) for 20 minutes. It only took two weeks to make a change, and along with a diet very similar to the MEVY diet he eradicated jock itch within two months.

Essential oil fungal foot massage

Clove oil is an essential oil that blends very well with other essential oils. It's strong penetrating and spicy odor blends well with lavender, Spanish rosemary, nutmeg, thyme, cinnamon and basil. Each of these oils will only add to the antiseptic quality of clove oil and I recommend you start by blending with just one oil initially to find out which combination you like the best. My favorite oil to blend with clove oil is good quality lavender oil, a 50/50 mix is excellent and a fantastic fungal foot massage can be had by rubbing a combination of these two oils into the feet vigorously each evening. It is important to always remember with clove oil that less is better. The smell is too overpowering if you have too much oil in the blend and you will soon be put off this fantastic essential oil. By the way, always rotate the pairs of shoes you wear and place a few drops in the tow and heel area of your shoes once per week if you have athlete's foot or toenail fungus and go bear foot when you can.

Caution With Clove Oil

As I have mentioned previously, be careful with clove oil, as it is very strong, it can cause skin irritations in some and should NEVER be consumed in the straight liquid oil form. Always get the opinion of your health-care professional regarding the use of clove oil during pregnancy or breastfeeding. Occasionally I've noticed that a few patients may have an allergic reaction to cloves, although this is very rare, so it is always best to start with a small dose.

Candida Crusher # 5 Coconut

The coconut palm, *Cocos nucifera*, is a member of the family Arecaceae (palm family). This amazing "tree of life" as it is called is found throughout the tropic and subtropics and is well known for its incredible versatility as can be seen in the many domestic, commercial, and industrial uses of its different parts such as the husk, oil, water and copra.
Coconuts are an important part of the daily diet of many people around the world.

Like garlic, you will inhibit the reproduction and even kill-off candida particularly well if you include some coconut oil and coconut cream in your diet each day. Coconut contains fatty acids that inhibit candida, and contains many beneficial properties that help prevent bacterial and viral infections. It is also a fabulous antifungal and it tastes great! It supports immune system function, supplies important nutrients necessary for good health and improves digestion and the absorption of nutrients from proteins and carbohydrates.

The saturated fat in coconut oil is easily digested and absorbed, unlike the unnatural man-made hydrogenated fats or oils that act just like plastic in the body. Coconut oil places very little strain on the digestive system and provides a quick source of energy necessary to promote healing.

The big difference is that coconut oil, cream and butter are absorbed into bloodstream directly from the intestines through the lymph system, whereas other fats require pancreatic enzymes and bile to break them into smaller units and then they transported to the liver, where they are processed before entering the bloodstream. That is why these excellent saturated fats put very little strain on the digestive system, even for people who have had difficulty digesting fats, have gall bladder problems or if they do not have a gall bladder. I have found women who have had their gallbladders removed can easily tolerate coconut oil without the reflux or nausea experienced with other oils or fats. When buying coconut oil look for one that is cold or expeller-pressed, unrefined, unbleached, un-deodorized and non-hydrogenated. Coconut oil is highly resistant to spoilage and has a long shelf life (2 years at room temperature), so it is not kept refrigerated. It is kept in the cupboard or on the kitchen counter. Many people freak out when I tell them to consume more coconut oil and cream, when in fact coconuts have been consumed for thousands of years by many cultures that lived long and healthy and productive lives. We have been led to believe that all saturated fats are bad for our health, which is far from the truth.

Like other saturated fats coconut oil goes solid when cooled below room temperature. Coconut oil has a high burning point and is the perfect oil for cooking. It can be used alone, or mixed with butter, a little lard or other good fats for cooking and frying. Coconut oil can be taken by the spoonful with meals to aid digestion or melted on cooked foods. The most common healing reactions are stomach upsets and diarrhea because coconut oil is antifungal so it kills off candida and also helps clean out toxins. Stomach upsets are caused by candida being killed off, and diarrhea is a way for the body to get rid of toxins. Other healing reactions may include increased mucus in the intestines, throat, nose, sinuses, lungs, etc.

How Does Coconut Work Against Candida?

Coconut oil and milk contain three principle fats (medium chained fatty acids, otherwise known as MCT's): caprylic acid, capric acid and lauric acid. These three fatty acids have been shown to be anti fungal in action and are the prime reason why you should seriously consider coconut oil (due to its higher content of the fatty acids) in particular in your anti-candida regime.

All of the MCTs found in coconut oil have the potential to kill yeast, viruses and bacteria, the most potent being lauric acid and caprylic acid. Capric and caprylic acid in particular have shown to exhibit the strongest anti-microbial and anti-fungal activities against candida species, and they do so by weakening and disrupting the yeast cell's membrane. Once the membrane (the outer edge of the yeast cell) becomes weakened, the cytoplasm (the inside of the cell) becomes exposed to your immune system that can then attack it more effectively. A good book to read on the topic of coconut and health is Naturopath Bruce Fife's book entitled *The Coconut Oil Miracle (New York: Penguin, 2004).*

My two favorite anti-candida foods are fresh garlic and extra virgin coconut oil, and it makes a lot of sense for you to incorporate both of them into your diet each and every day. Regular supplementation with specialized anti-candida dietary supplements which contain allicin (garlic) as we as capric and caprylic acid (coconut) along with the daily consumption of foods containing these natural candida crushers makes a whole lot more sense. I'll soon be launching my Candida Crusher range of specialized products that contain the very best quality of MCT's along with high-grade allicin, oregano's carvacrol and several other notable candida crushers based on my research.

Health Benefits Of Coconut Oil

Most of the health benefits of coconut oil can be attributed to its high content of medium-chained saturated fatty acids (MCT'S) such as capric acid, caprylic acid and lauric acid. Unlike most other dietary oils, coconut oil (if it is not hydrogenated) does not contain trans-fatty acids due to its low content of unsaturated fatty acids.

"Bad" For The Heart?

Research from years ago found coconut oil to be "toxic" or not good for health due to the research being based on hydrogenated products, and there are still people today who believe that coconut oil is "bad for the heart". There are no polyunsaturated fatty acids in coconut oil, and it therefore does not contribute to heart disease. In fact, virgin coconut oil has been shown to reduce total cholesterol, triglycerides, phospholipids, LDL, and VLDL (the bad) cholesterol levels and increased HDL (the good) cholesterol in serum and tissues.

It is important to remember that only extra-virgin and unadulterated coconut oil should be used if you want to achieve the best effects for your health, whether it be for your heart health, weight-loss or to cure your yeast infection.

100 grams of coconut oil contains:

- Capric acid 6,000 mg

- Caprylic acid 7,500 mg

- Lauric acid 44,600 mg

Health Benefits Of Coconut Milk And Coconut Cream

Like coconut oil, the health benefits associated with coconut milk and cream are attributable to their content of caprylic acid, capric acid and lauric acid, but in this case there are much less of these active therapeutic acids present in coconut milk and the cream on a gram for gram basis. Coconut oil is therefore a much more potent anti-candida product and the logical choice when it comes to inhibiting and killing your yeast infection. Coconut milk is nevertheless still worth having, and a great way to take in coconut milk and cream is to use it when making curries or smoothies. It is delicious when blended with ice cubes and berries (use a Vitamix) and served on a hot summer's day.

100 grams of coconut milk contains:

- Capric acid   1,187 mg

- Caprylic acid   1,494 mg

- Lauric acid   9,463 mg

Avoid The Coconut Detox If You Have A Yeast Infection

Are you desperate to get rid of your yeast infection, desperate enough to want to attempt the Coconut Detox? This is NOT the way to go if you have a yeast infection and want to beat it. With this diet you consume 2 tablespoons of Extra Virgin Coconut Oil (EVCO) every two hours, and take up to 12 or 14 tablespoons of EVCO daily. Nothing else. One website stated that the author had a severe case of candida and did the Coconut Detox and experienced "the most horrible healing crisis to date, I experienced vomiting, diarrhea, racing heart, shivering, severe bouts of pain, massive insomnia and severe anxiety" and went on further to say "I imagine a heroin withdrawal to be like this". Well folks, this is NOT how to get rid of candida from your body and certainly not a method I endorse, it is almost as crazy as the Lemon Detox Diet. Crazy and extreme diets will only give you crazy and extreme results, and by following the Candida Crusher Diet I can assure you that you will certainly NOT experience the extreme reactions that the gentleman did as mentioned above! Interestingly, he mentioned that even after the severe reaction he is still not well and is seeking another method to get rid of his yeast infection. The best way as I have mentioned several times so far throughout the Candida Crusher is to stick with a clearly defined plan and stick with it long enough to see it through. You should experience minimal (if any) aggravations and notice a slow but steady improvement initially and a full and complete recovery in time.

Coconut Oil And Your Weight

Some patients I see who have a yeast infection are also interested in losing some weight. Is that you? Are you interested in dropping a few pounds and dress sizes? If you are, then I'd like you to sit up and pay attention to learning this "secret" about coconut oil. There are many studies that have discovered that coconut oil (not the cream or milk) helps you to lose weight due to the concentration of MCTs.

Not all saturated fats are "bad", and even though 1 tablespoon of coconut oil contains 120 calories and 14 grams of fat it can actually aid in weight loss believe it or not!

Those on the Candida Crusher Diet will find that coconut oil is an excellent way to boost up their calorie intake and whether you are slim or carry a little too much weight, coconut oil will help to maintain your metabolism and maintain your regular and natural weight more easily. You should lose weight naturally on the Candida Crusher Diet (if you are overweight) but if not, see your health-care professional; your thyroid or adrenal glands may need attention. For those who are underweight, they will find that coconut oil will help them maintain their weight more easily.

Cooking With Coconut Oil

Cooking with coconut oil is an excellent way to consume more of this incredible oil. Use it as a substitute over other types of fats and oils you may use in cooking. This oil is especially stable at high temperatures and will not readily break down into those unhealthy trans fatty acids. You will find that the best coconut cooking oils are the extra virgin and organic coconut oils, see your health food shop.

The Therapeutic Uses Of Coconut In Yeast Infections

Do you like coconut oil? You may want to develop a taste for it if you have candida, because coconut oil contains 7500mg of caprylic acid per 100 grams and is an excellent adjunct in your anti-candida diet approach, along with caprylic acid supplementation. To minimize healing reactions or die-off start taking coconut oil at a low dose (1/2 to 1 teaspoon 3 times a day) and gradually increase the amount every 4-5 days, or more depending upon your die-off symptoms, until you reach the maximum therapeutic dose of 5-6 tablespoons per day. It is also important to take coconut oil in divided doses during the day and not all at once. Try it in a drink or smoothie, with a fruit meal or dessert or just on its own, the way I like it.

My recommended therapeutic dose for candida sufferers or anyone who is unhealthy is 3-6 tablespoons per day, in divided doses, preferably with meals that contain protein. Remember, since coconut oil (like fresh garlic and oregano oil) is a potent antifungal, anti-parasitic, antibacterial and antiviral, etc; it may create die-off or healing reactions in people who are very unhealthy and toxic, but it may be particularly pronounced in severe candida sufferers, so go easy when you first start to take this food into your diet, particularly if your system has never had coconut oil in it previously. Start slowly and gradually build up over a week or two. You will soon become a coconut convert like I have years ago. The taste and smell are amazing and before you know it you may go nuts for coconuts!

- **Fungal infections of the skin** (including ringworm, jock itch and athlete's foot). When it comes to local treatment and coconut oil (your skin, feet, hands, scalp, nails, etc.) you don't need to slowly step up treatment, just when you take it internally. Coconut oil absorbs well into your skin and is therefore an excellent treatment for all manner of local fungal infections. It is important to remember that coconuts are often used in the beauty industry in moisturizers and body butters as well as suntan lotions because coconut oil is easily absorbed into the skin. Use the straight coconut oil and rub well into the affected areas of the groin, scalp, hands, feet, nails, etc. In addition, you can also use coconut oil to which you have added a few drops of oregano oil, which is particularly effective for stubborn or hard to cure cases affecting your hands, feet as well toe or fingernails. Apply twice daily (sparingly) and NEVER give up until fully cured! (See Cassandra's Case Study # 21 below)

- **Fungal overgrowths of the digestive system.** Coconut oil (go easy initially) and coconut milk are perfect for intestinal yeast overgrowth, consume some of the milk (1/2 – 1 cup) daily and begin with a few teaspoons and gradually build up the coconut oil. Remember, the oil is up to 6 times as strong as the milk so go easily accordingly. You may notice that your bowel motions may change when you first start with coconut, this is normal and should give you no reason to be concerned.

- **Vaginal yeast infections.** You may want to read the other sections of the Candida Crusher that is more relevant to this common women's complaint. You can use a tampon that you have soaked in warm extra virgin coconut oil and leave for 6 – 8 hours. For stubborn yeast infections, you can also try using coconut oil in which you have infused some freshly crushed garlic.

Case Study #21
Cassandra, 46 years

Cassandra is a dairy farmer who came to our clinic with athlete's foot and toenail fungus approximately two years ago. This was by far the worst case of athlete's foot I have ever seen in my professional career as a naturopathic doctor, in fact, here heels were split, cracked and bleeding in places. It looked as if her heels were coming away from her feet. Her doctor had prescribed her a fungal cream called Lamisil that was not effective in her case; he then referred her to a medical specialist who was talking about an operation, at this point she decided to seek my help. I told her that I couldn't promise anything but would try my absolute best and would only work with her if she followed all of my instructions to the letter. I make it a point now to work with people who really want to get well and get tired of those who half-heartedly will "give it a go" and see what happens. In most cases I've found that the more severe the case and the more desperate the patient is, the better the compliance understandably becomes. Desperate cases call for desperate measures, and Cassandra's case was the worst I've seen, it looked like leprosy of the feet.

These are the "impossible" fungal foot cases that a practitioner may see once in a lifetime and will most probably refer onto a doctor or podiatrist. I immediately recognized this to be a seriously bad and neglected case of fungal infection and it was not hard to see why this had occurred. Cassandra has been a dairy farmer for over twenty years and spends many hours a day in damp and moist environments; her feet were almost constantly in large rubber boots. Here we can see a poor case of ventilation and the perfect breeding ground for a yeast infection – dark, warm and moist environment.

Cassandra admitted that she wears socks 24/7 because her feet always feel cold, and so do her hands. She even sleeps with her socks on each night. I noticed that her neck was swollen and that the outer edge of her eyebrow was non existent and then it became apparent that she had been suffering from hypothyroidism for some time, and we have successfully treated this issue as well since then.

We worked with the Candida Crusher Diet right away and removed the copious amounts of bread and wine this lady was consuming; I included raw garlic into her diet as well as a small amount of coconut oil each day that we built up over time.

My first recommendations were to work on her hypothyroidism which in her case turned out to be a lack of iodine, and once we supplemented her with adequate iodine her hands and feet soon warmed up. I asked her to never wear socks in bed and to go barefoot when possible, even for a walk outside. This was excruciatingly painful at first so we had to compromise and she wore leather sandals initially. Her feet were to be thoroughly rubbed three times daily with extra virgin coconut oil in which she had added 5 drops of oregano oil per tablespoon of coconut oil. Results can slowly but surely over the months. I got her to throw her original boots away which smelled like rotten cheese and also asked if she could get three brand new pairs of rubber boots and rotate them daily, and to add a few drops of tea tree oil into the toe and heel of the boots each week. The boots were to be exposed to sunlight whenever possible. I asked her to wear her boots initially only for an hour a day, no more. This was when she used a hose and strong cleaning agents in the cow shed, the rest of the time she was to wear sandals.

After about two months I noticed that the heels looked so much better but her toenails were not getting any better. That is when we went to applying one drop of pure oregano oil on each toe in the evening and one drop of tea tree oil on each toe in the morning. After about six weeks for this regime we saw an amazing improvement, we then stopped treating the nails and then just recommended she rub her feet and toe nails with the coconut oil to which she had added some oregano oil. After about five months of treatment we stopped because we didn't need to continue on, Cassandra had fully recovered. As you can see, it can take a long time to recover from a serious case of athlete's foot and toenail fungus but it IS possible. I doubt that your case will be as severe as Cassandra's case, and it may only require you to work diligently for one, two or three months to effect a cure. Remember, you need to work on your diet, your lifestyle and do the local treatment – daily, for as long as it takes.

It has been two years now, I have seen Cassandra on several occasions since and I'm amazed to see that her feet are a nice healthy pink color. Her doctor has still not spoken to me and probably never will and I'm OK with that too, I just hope her doctor has learned that natural medicine can work.

More Candida Crushers

Cruciferous Vegetables:

Bok choy, broccoli, Brussels sprouts, cabbage, cauliflower, collard greens, kale, radish, rutabaga, turnip, and watercress.

This family of leafy vegetables rank highly when it comes to improving the health of your digestive system, and I recommend that you consume them regularly. Dr. William Crook wrote about the importance of cruciferous vegetables many years ago due to their high fiber and phyto-nutrient content. These vegetables are rich in nutrients such as indole-3-carbinol and are loaded with fiber, and it is this fiber that is all-important to have in your large intestine to allow your body to re-populate the large amounts of friendly bacteria you need to crowd out the bad bacteria and yeast. This group of vegetables also acts as a pre- biotic solution to your diet, and prebiotics are a food that feed the pro-biotics.

Good Tip

Don't Consume Cruciferous Vegetables Raw

I recommend that you avoid eating the cruciferous vegetable family raw, but cook them lightly like steaming. Cooking cruciferous vegetables reduces the goitrogenic substances by almost three-quarters, and this is important. Eating raw broccoli for example may help to block the production of thyroid hormones in your body and may contribute to hypothyroidism. Incidentally, the fermentation of cruciferous vegetables (like cabbage as in sauerkraut for example) does not reduce goitrogens, but because fermented are typically eaten in such small quantities and not daily, consumption of them is OK as long as your diet is rich in iodine which allows for the production of the all important thyroid hormones T4 and T3. Be sure to include some kelp or other forms of seaweed in your diet if you do eat cruciferous vegetables, this is a clever idea and will take care if you do happen to inadvertently eat any raw cruciferous vegetables.

Olive oil

Olive oil has shown to be effective against yeast infections, and in particular has the ability to prevent the transformation on candida to its mycelial form. Olive oil is rich in a substance called oleic acid, which has an effect on candida not unlike the B-vitamin called biotin. Take between four to six teaspoons per day, and there are several ways you can supplement your diet with olive oil. For example you can mix it with lemon juice and fresh garlic to make up a salad dressing. You can also cook more with it and even pour some (or spray it) on your steamed vegetables.

Almonds

Almonds are an alkaline nut and good to eat if you have a yeast infection. They are rich in many minerals and high in protein and you will find that by eating almonds (just like the cruciferous vegetables) you will be also supplying your intestines with a prebiotic food that will aid in re-establishing beneficial bacteria in your digestive tract.

Omega 3 Containing Foods

Those with a yeast infection may well have an increased level of inflammation in their digestive system, and it is not is uncommon either for those with candida to have food allergies or leaky gut syndrome. These are manifestations of an up-regulated immune system which could do with calming down, and omega 3 is one important nutrient we can add to our diet to quell such inflammation. What are some of the best foods to include into our diet if we want more omega 3?

- Fatty fish (flounder, albacore tuna, sardines, trout, herring, salmon, etc.)

- Walnuts and walnut oil

- Venison (deer meat)

- Flaxseeds or flaxseed meal (linseed)

It is important to reduce the amount of red meat you consume in favor of fatty fish, because consuming red meat is associated with increased inflammation and increasing fish protein (especially fish high in omega 3) in your diet is associated with a decrease in inflammation.

 2 # Candida Crushing Dietary Supplements

There are various dietary supplements and herbal medicines I recommend depending on the case at hand, but in saying that, there are certain supplements in particular which I tend to recommend routinely to most patients with a yeast infection because the protocol I have come up with over the years has simply proven to work for the vast majority. Before we launch into the different products I'd like to explain a few different points regarding supplements which I think are important to raise, points like take care when buying products, especially online purchases, why to avoid budget products and more. Let's cover these areas first and then come back and outline some protocols and products.

I often get frequently asked questions, and I will answer them all for you in this section a little later on. You may find some of my suggestions differ from what you may have been told by your health-food storeowner, your health-care professional or from what you have read in candida books or read online. The replies I have given to these questions are based on my experience in treating candida for many years including several thousands of patients.

> *The best doctors give the least medicines.*
> Benjamin Franklin

Be Careful With Self-Medicating, And Stick With The Game Plan

When people who have a yeast infection become unwell, most will begin to look for a solution, some look for a natural solution while others will seek a drug solution. Some will attempt to self-medicate, others will seek out assistance from a natural health-care therapist and yet others will follow the advice of their medical doctor. The problem in self-medicating is that it is hard to know the best things to take in your particular situation, what dosage to take and how long to take it. Seeing a natural therapist (especially someone with experience in yeast infections) is likely to give you a better result because he or she will have seen many patients just like you and will have gained experience in knowing what works and what doesn't, but you have my commiserations if you decide on seeing a conventional medical doctor, unless of course he or she is conversant with natural medicine. Don't despair, that is why I wrote Candida Crusher, I figured that you wanted to treat yourself and did rather not have to visit a practitioner or wanted to partner up with somebody with an open mind. You can visit your practitioner and use this book at the same time too, however, especially if you tell your practitioner what you are doing and what my recommendations are in terms of diet, lifestyle and the appropriate products.

There are too many reasons why people with yeast infections relapse and drop out of treatment. Perhaps the person may initially get a result (feeling initially worse, but the inevitably better after a week or two, which is common), but will often experience bouts of improvement along with periods of aggravation and then become disillusioned as he or she feels worse and ends up on the doorstep of yet another practitioner. Many patients we see today go online looking for answers and some websites may offer reasonably sound advice whilst others offer advice ranging from the sublime (high quality and sound advice) to the totally ridiculous (completely laughable and in some cases dangerous), advice such as "vodka is fine to drink when you have a yeast infection, just avoid beer and wine" or "eating fruit is fine during the entire yeast program, it is a natural part of life".

Yes, and so is mercury and uranium but we don't want to consume them daily either. Many online products I have seen are either therapeutically worthless or just too expensive to maintain for too long, and even if they are effective, as soon as you stop taking them all yeast infection related problems recur. Let's get one thing straight right now; the whole idea of taking a dietary supplement or an herbal medicine in your quest to conquer candida is to get well and then to stop taking the product, it's as simple as that. The important thing is to stay with one clearly defined plan that incorporates a well-balanced lifestyle along with a sound diet and a few high quality supplements. And then to stay with this game plan long enough to get the desired results. The object is not to be flashy and brilliant in the short run and then drop out when the going get's tough, (and believe me if you are a chronic yeast sufferer it will get tough at some stage) but to stick with the principles I have outlined in Candida Crusher. You certainly can win this yeast infection game, but you will need to learn the rules and apply them carefully along the way. Break the rules and pay the price so be warned.

What you will most definitely discover is that recovery is achieved much more rapidly to those who look further afield than just dietary supplements. I want to stress that you will do well to follow the advice of eating well in terms of taking out the foods candida thrives on and including those foods and drinks that candida hates, this concept along with your carefully selected supplements will get you what you are after, and this is why I'm pleased you decided to get the Candida Crusher because my plan is based on the all-important holistic treatment concept. It is all about balance between foods, lifestyle and supplements, and it was this balance which was previously tipped in favor of candida, that's why you initially developed this yeast infection. Let's restore the harmony once and for all by adopting a balanced approach.

Caution with Online Purchases

Much online advice for a yeast infection today is centered on a particular product, and if you just take this product then "all your candida problems will be solved rapidly". Sorry folks, if it only were that easy, I suppose if you buy a lottery ticket then all of your dreams will come true as well. Just like in wealth, miracles (cures) occasionally happen spontaneously but in 99% of cases this is just wishful thinking and you actually have to work smart and hard it you want to make it in this life. If the sales page sounds totally over the top stating an "instant 12 hour yeast infection cure" and you actually buy this nonsense then you deserve to quickly part with your money. I once read somewhere that "It is morally wrong to allow suckers to keep their money".

Without wanting to appear condescending, most candida yeast infection websites and e-books have been written by self positioned experts who have actually never seen a patient themselves and tend to be either very product or very diet focused, most never talk about making the appropriate lifestyle changes or a combination of all three. OK, they may have had a yeast infection themselves which they cured with a special diet and supplements, but have they treated several thousand cases of yeast infection from mild toenail fungus right through to those with a potentially life-threatening systemic yeast infection? Have they worked through several hundred cases of women with a vaginal yeast infection and found out what protocols work and what are a complete waste of time? Have they also discovered that the most "perfect" candida protocol and product is totally useless unless the patient engages fully in the treatment? In my humble opinion, it's not until you have seen countless cases, understood human nature of why and how people get sick and have used just about every product you can get your hands on that you get a true feel for what a yeast infection really is, how it can affect somebody on so many different levels, and the best way to conquer the beast called yeast.

A particular word of caution is to be careful with online dietary supplement sales; it pays to deal with a reliable and reputable business established for many years.

Ask yourself these questions before you enter your details and click the green button in the shopping cart:

- Does the website have plenty of quality articles to read with excellent information?

- Are the articles or pages just centered on products and their specifications?

- Does the 75/25 rule apply? (75% information on the site is about diet and lifestyle changes, 25% is about products)

- Has the person who wrote this website treated or worked supplying specialized products to several thousands of yeast infection patients and inspires you with confidence?

- Is the article original or just rehashed from somebody else's website? (A common occurrence called plagiarism)

- Is the company easy to contact and great to deal with?

- Is the person selling the product an actual therapist (or employs experienced therapists) or are they just another online reseller?

- Do they have a most knowledgeable helpline and super-fast delivery?

- Can you talk with somebody if this product does not live up to its expectations? etc.

Lifestyle And Diet - 80% Of Cure.
Supplements - 20% Of Cure

Sometimes the best advice I have given somebody is "a good talking to" for not having the self-discipline to stop his or her crappy diet or ridiculously unnatural lifestyle. In most cases, it's the simple changes that will have the most profound effects on a person's health and wellbeing long-term. Small lifestyle and diet changes along with a few carefully chosen good quality products will generally do the trick.

Although I don't like using the "cure" word in my clinic, what I'm about to explain with this word is just to illustrate a point. The many books I have studied over the years on natural health have made me aware that lifestyle and diet modification account for about seventy five percent of the cure, and that dietary supplements or herbal medicines account for roughly twenty-five percent of the cure. That is why in the Candida Crusher you will find that I have apportioned around 80 percent of this book to lifestyle changes such as self-discipline, stress, sleep improvement, rest, relaxation, exercise, environmental considerations such as mold and toxin awareness, detoxification, why humor and positive thinking help the healing process as well as plenty of detailed information about your best approaches to eating and drinking if you want to fully recover and stay well.

About 20 percent is devoted to teaching you about the special foods, dietary supplements and herbal medicines that have the most profound effect in healing your body from a yeast and bacterial infection.

I position myself not as the guru of candida by any means, but as a naturopathic doctor with a high level of specialized knowledge relating to yeast infection treatments for the reason that I have treated several thousand patients with yeast related issues for over twenty years, I've developed highly specialized anti bacterial and anti fungal products for companies in the field of nutritional medicine and associated with many expert practitioners who know this area very well. I've written and researched about yeast infection ever since I graduated and do believe that this is one area I feel entirely confident in when it comes to natural medicine treatments. There is not much I haven't seen when it comes to difficult candida presentations so I do consider myself with having a reasonable amount of knowledge in this area.

Some Yeast Infected Patients Take Over Two Dozen Products

Some patients I have seen complain of many years of bloating, bowel and skin problems, perhaps recurrent ear, nose or throat infections and having taken repeated anti-biotics. For some women it could be an endless cycle of thrush and vaginal irritation, for others it may be anxiety, sugar cravings and bad PMS. For others it may be no interest in sex, joint pain, depression, toenail fungus or cracked heels, an increasing allergy to many foods and plenty more.

It all begins with one product recommended by a website, magazine, health-food shop, friend or a practitioner, and after a few years the products just keep on coming. You are thinking: "I'll try this one for my digestion" or "This one will make me sleep better". And so the list goes on. You soon find that you can't keep them on the kitchen bench top; they are starting to take too much room so you put them in a box or container. Have you ever worked out the daily cost to you? Have you noticed yet that all these pills aren't making that much difference when it comes to getting rid of your yeast infection permanently?

I believe that the more products a person takes, the more product focused they will eventually become and the more likely that they become "symptom prescribers"; i.e.:

- This one is for my digestion
- This one is for my bones
- This one is for my joints

- This one is for my pain

- This one is for my eyes

- This one is for my libido

- This one is for my hot flushes

- This one is to stop me getting a cold

- This one is for my urinary tract infection

- This one is my Magnesium supplement

- This one is my antioxidant

- This one is for my skin

- This one is for my constipation

- This one is to help me lose weight

- This one is for my sleep

- This one is for my fluid retention

- My daughter told me to take this one because I keep forgetting to take all these pills!

Does this sound a bit over the top to you? Well not to me, you see, I've seen many patients who have told me exactly what you read above, "This one is for my…" It is certainly not uncommon to see somebody take more than ten different products in one day.

Here is a list I received from a yeast infection patient recently, it is true and has not been altered in any way, and I just retyped the medications and dosages from a document she emailed to me:

Pharmaceutical drugs	Dose
Nystatin 500,000	3 tabs TID
Bi-Est Cream 2.5mg/0.1ml	0.1ml QAM; 0.2ml QHS
Testosterone Cream 1.0mg/0.1ml	2mg Mon/Wed/Fri AM
Progesterone Cream 20% ¼ tsp. (1gram)	1/8 tsp. QHS 3 weeks out of
4 E2 0.05mg E3 2mg/GM vaginal cream	0.5 gram QHS
Armor Thyroid	60mg QAM

Dietary Supplements	Dose
A.D.P Oil of Oregano	50mg BID
Candaclear (4 different supplements)	1 QD of each
Ortho Biotic Probiotics	2 caps QAM
Digestzyme V	2 caps with each meal
Betaine HCL 1.3gr	3 caps with each meal
Pepsin 260mg	3 caps with each meal
B Complex # 5	1 cap QD
Berberine Complex	2 caps BID
Boron	3 mg QD
Super Bio Buffered C	1500mg QD
Cal Mag Citrate Powder	1 scoop QD
Super Bio-Cucurmin	400mg QAM
Vitamin D3 Liquid	5000 i.u. QD
DHEA	25 mg QAM
Gamma E-Tocopherol	359mg QD
EPA-DHA liquid	5600mg QD
Glucosamine Sulphate	750mg BID
Grape seed Extract	100mg QD
Iodide Oligo Element	2/3 dropper QAM
Super K with K2 Complex	2100 mcg QD
L-Glutamine Powder	3.8 gr scoop 2 scoops QAM
Super R-Lipoic Acid	300mg QD
Magnesium Citrate	140mg/cap 4 caps QD
OsteoGuard + Ipriflavone	2 tabs bid
Pregnenolone	100mg QAM
Super Selenium Complex	200mcg QD
Opti Zinc	30mg QD
Super Zeaxanthin	1 cap QD
Avipaxin	2 caps BID
DL-Phenalanine	1000mg/2 caps 2 caps BID
Travacor	2 caps BID

Well, I just counted thirty-seven different dietary supplements and drugs. Imagine having to take all that in one day, not to mention the cost of it all. But the interesting thing here is when I asked her how she felt on this regime her reply was: "terrible". Why is it that people keep on taking supplements and even adding more yet keep on feeling unwell?

Most chronic candida patients I see have well and truly had enough of feeling sick and have been from one end of the country to the next, from doctor to specialist and then to several naturopaths, faith healers, color therapists or herbalists and more in order to finally get rid of their multiple health problems. Many of these patients I have seen over the years bring along with them several bags or boxes of dietary supplements from many different sources, from health care professionals, health-food shops as well as online purchases. I could write a rather large paper on the many hundreds of different products I have seen yeast infection patients trial over the years to assist in their recovery.

I've always looked for the most efficient and cost-effective way for my clients to recover, and can tell you that it doesn't have to involve several dozen products simultaneously. Why waste you money on all these products from many different sources, when the best solution is to aim for a few select products of very high quality which are targeted to eliminate your candida yeast problems sooner rather than later?

Case History # 22
Sally, 38 yrs

In February 2012 I had a Skype consultation with a lady by the name of Sally from Sydney, Australia (not her real name, but certainly a real female patient living in the Australia) Sally contacted me through yeastinfection.org after feeling unwell for several years. She is a busy real estate agent who along with her partner runs a very busy company. Her hours are crazy, and it is not unusual for Sally to work 10-hour days, seven days a week. She has been suffering from vaginal thrush since her early twenties and gave up on her medical doctor a number of years ago after taking antibiotics and using vaginal applicators for over ten years. Sally has visited many nutritionists, naturopathic and chiropractic doctors for many years as well, and each visit included the addition of several dietary supplements that she continuously takes and re-orders. Sally was taking close to 30 different dietary supplement products when she first contacted me, and was still taking antibiotics as well, her regime including doctor visits was costing her over a thousand dollars a month and yet the crazy thing is that she was feeling no better for it all!

This is like buying an increasing number of lottery tickets in the belief that the more you buy the bigger your chances will be of winning the game.

The first thing I recommended was the Candida Crusher Diet, including the MEVY Diet, the low-allergy diet and then we worked with the re-introduction phase. I took Sally off ALL her supplements and just worked with diet and lifestyle changes with her for the first three months, and guess what? She improved out of sight! We slowly started to work with an anti-candida formula and a good probiotic and increased them as she improved. The only supplements I had Sally take were a good multivitamin, and omega 3, a digestive enzyme, and an anti-candida product. The results have been amazing, we caught up on Skype recently, in November this year (2012), and she is delighted with her progress. And best of all, the amount of money she is saving will mean a luxury holiday to New Zealand, and then she will be able to see me in person as well as enjoy a fantastic trip down to the South Island for some well deserved rest and recreation with her husband.

Budget Products Return Poor Results, Costing You Money and Time

I have experimented and trialed hundreds of different dietary supplements and herbal medicines with candida patients and found from experience that many companies make fantastic claims about the effectiveness of their candida kill products and beneficial bacterial strains, but unfortunately many have failed to deliver on that promise of delivering the real and long lasting results I was aiming to achieve with my patients. I feel certain now that I have found the right protocol, easy to follow, not too expensive or involving dozens of dietary and herbal medicine supplements either.

You may think that you can beat candida without nutritional or herbal help – there is no doubt, you can, but you may want to reconsider, it will take considerably longer this way and many patients literally struggle for years trying to eliminate candida from their system by diet alone or by using budget supermarket dietary supplements. Believe me, I have verified this with hundreds of patients, particularly the more money-conscious ones, but have invariably found that most end up taking a quite a lot products this way including the cheap ones to begin with, and then end up purchasing the better quality ones in the end due to the sheer frustration because of a lack of anticipated results. The problem lies here - inferior products made from poor raw materials simply don't give the same kind of results, meaning you end up spending more on the products in the long run that you originally expected and this ends up costing you a lot more money. Do it once, do it right is the motto I now believe in with yeast infections.

If you want to follow the line of not taking any products whatsoever because you are certain diet can treat all diseases, (let food be your medicine, and medicine be your food) then you will need to be super disciplined with your diet and lifestyle habits for a minimum of 6 months to a year or longer, much longer that if you were to take the right supplements and adopt the correct protocol from the beginning. And if you want to take no supplements at all, then I would recommend a slightly different dietary approach from the one I recommend in this book. You would need to consume considerably more of the foods that not only help to inhibit and kill a yeast infection, but also to eat plenty of fermented or cultured foods.

Can you now imagine how quick you could restore optimal health if you decided to adopt this strict dietary approach, made the appropriate lifestyle changes AND decided to take the right dietary supplements? I've seen some women with a chronic vaginal yeast infection recover fully after as little as eight weeks by taking this kind of approach. No bull, you get out of your treatment protocol whatever you are willing to put into it. The same goes for tackling anything in your life that is worthwhile. Get the good stuff to start with and get those results you are looking for sooner rather than later, then get on and enjoy the rest of your life.

Holistic Treatment Is The Permanent Solution To A Yeast Infection

Taking quality candida specific products will not only ensure that you get back on track fast, but that you stay on track. It will also keep you in better health if you take a regular candida specific product until your diet and lifestyle habits have become fully engrained into your life. The "secret" is to keep the candida yeast infection at bay by developing and adopting the right lifestyle and dietary habits conducive of an excellent digestive system.

As I have previously mentioned, not only should your candida overgrowth disappear and never return, your health will improve to the point of being outstanding, like it hasn't been for as long as you can remember. I have experienced this with many patients, and one of the most rewarding aspects of being a naturopath is watching patients go from a serious health dilapidation and literally cast on the scrap heap by doctors - "I'm sorry, but there is nothing more we can do for you" or "You will have to stay on those drugs for the rest of your life". The truth is, you can improve and gain incredible health with the right treatment. "Wow, I would have never thought that after all these years I could ever feel this great again". One case of a lady in her late 40's comes to mind to illustrate this point perfectly:

Case History # 23
Tracey, 48 years

Tracey came to my clinic many years ago seeking help for vaginal thrush that had plagued her since she was 18 years of age, almost all her adult life. The first thing I noticed how depressed and anxious this patient was, she clearly didn't look happy and I wasn't sure if she was ready to take my advice, after all, she had been to so many doctors and other health-care professionals, I was just another person she came to for advice. However, the difference in this case was that I had seen a younger sister of Tracey about 6 months before she came to see me. Patricia from California had come over to stay with Tracey for a while and had come to see me with a recurrent urinary tract infection that had been causing her concern. We soon had this cleared up and it gave Tracey the confidence to come in and ask for my help.

Tracey's yeast infection was chronic and had caused her so much concern that she had not had a relationship for over ten years, something I found incredible. The first several consultations were difficult as Tracey cried and displayed much grief and anger over a complaint which was wrecking the quality of her life and at one stage she had even become suicidal because nobody could help her find any real solutions. Antidepressants were offered along with a sleeping pill each night. What a mess!

Like many chronic cases, Tracey started on the oral contraceptive pill in her late teens and stayed on this drug for over a decade. She drank copious amounts of alcohol, smoked cigarettes and worked rotating shifts as a nurse from the age of 20 up until she was 38 years old. Her lifestyle was frequently stressful, as she liked to work in the emergency ward of the hospital because she "enjoyed the buzz'. Meanwhile, her health deteriorated as her adrenal glands became increasingly fatigued and her immunity suffered due to this hectic and stressful life. Her boyfriend at the time was a doctor who would routinely give her antibiotics, and over the years in the hospital she must have taken over one hundred rounds of various types of antibiotics.

Where was I to begin with this case? The most challenging thing I found was to try and break through to this patient and give her the confidence that her body could and would right itself if the correct conditions were met. But it would take time, lots of time to repair the damage. This damage was on many levels including emotionally and well as physically. You see, when you have slowly developed a seriously chronic case of a yeast infection like Tracey over the years, it will first affect you on the physical plane (fatigue, vaginal thrush, recurrent infection, etc.) and slowly but surely as the health improvements are not forthcoming after seeking expert help it will begin to affect you on the emotional plane (grief, anger, anxiety, etc.). This explains why many chronic cases I have seen come to me with a plethora of drugs and dietary supplements.

I worked with Tracey for over 18 months and what I noticed was that with each visit from about nine months into the Candida Crusher treatment her mental and emotional disposition changed for the better, it made me quite emotional myself to see a woman (looking old before her time) go literally from a wilting flower to a woman in full bloom. Her smile became radiant, you could even see the change in her posture, and her new wardrobe was a reflection of how she was now starting to feel inside – full of hope for a beautiful new life. I love cases like this and they reconfirm what I've really started to take note of in the last ten years of my work, that it is critical to see this deep inner change if you are to expect a full and complete recovery in chronic cases.

The dietary supplements I had Tracey taking were a top quality multivitamin twice daily with meals, an Omega 3 fish oil twice daily with meals, a digestive enzyme with each meal, two different candida crushing supplements and a high quality probiotic. The products she took most often and regularly (and for the longest period of time) was the probiotic.

Helping patients improve their lives has kept me going for over twenty years in the clinic and it is one of the biggest reasons I get up each morning and love the work I do, I just couldn't imagine doing anything else in my life. Treating many cases has also made me aware of just how insidious yeast infections really are, and how they can so seriously affect the many different aspects of a person's health and wellbeing. Tracey's case was an eye-opener in that sense, and I'm sure that some of you out there may be able to relate to her story.

There is no true healing unless there is a change in outlook, peace of mind and an inner happiness.
Dr. Edward Bach 1936 (The Bach Flower Remedies)

Candida Crusher Products – Online Soon

If you are considering purchasing from a company which you suspect may not deliver the quality of product or service you are looking for then do click off, consider my Candida Crusher products, soon online for you to purchase. I first wanted to get my book into your hands so that you could make the appropriate lifestyle and dietary changes as well as get a good understanding on the best foods to rid your body of candida. It is my desire to create the most effective and yet highest quality yeast infection products possible and have these available online in 2013, so do keep an eye out for the Candida Crusher product releases and be sure to join my mailing list and you will be the first to know. The Candida Crusher product website will have fantastic support and an excellent back-end system so you won't be disappointed.

The Right Supplements And Herbal Medicines To Take

It is very important at the onset of discussing a highly effective candida treatment program to stress not only the importance of the quality of your lifestyle and diet, but also the quality of the dietary supplements and herbal medicines you take to eradicate a yeast infection promptly and effectively from your system in the most efficient possible way without any residual side effects.

Ultimately it is up to you what dietary supplements you can afford, but also how urgently and effectively you want to finally get rid of the health problems that have been plaguing you for many years. If you can identify with many of the typical signs and symptoms of a candida yeast infection and strongly believe that you have this problem, then the most effective program, including diet, lifestyle and the right products will ensure you achieve you aim of great health sooner rather than later.

Are Dietary Supplements Really That Necessary?

I have often have candida patients ask me if nutritional supplementation is really necessary to inhibit, control and successfully eradicate candida. Many people don't really understand that dietary supplements are needed to protect and nourish their cells against damage during the cleansing phase and correct any underlying deficiencies during the strict diet phase and in addition to assist in the re-colonization of their digestive system, and then further to maintain a prolonged state of wellness. Why you ask can't we obtain all we need from a balanced diet, why can't we just eat better or "100% organic" foods and get well? We all know that good foods contain the necessary calories and essential nutrients our bodies need to maintain optimal function. Good foods contain the building blocks which support a healthy body, but when our bodies are in a state of digestive chaos and gut dysfunction such as with a yeast infection it becomes critical that we supply all the main elements and minor elements to get us back on track and to help us stay that way. Yes, you can just work with diet but it will certainly take longer and the ride will be rougher along the way.

But Don't Dietary Supplements Just Create Expensive Urine?

William Kaufman, MD, a medical doctor with a PhD in nutritional biochemistry as well, wrote: "Those who believe that you can get all the nourishment including vitamins and minerals you need to sustain optimal health throughout life from food alone can be very smug. They have the equivalent of an orthodox religious belief that 'food is everything.' They don't have to concern themselves with the fact that the nutritional value of foods their patient eats may be greatly inferior to the listed nutritional values given in food tables. The two-liner 'we get all the vitamins we need in our diets' and 'taking supplements only gives you an expensive urine' completely overlooks the significant benefits vitamin supplements can produce in our bodies long before being excreted in our urine.'

To me, the term expensive urine is a rather bizarre argument because a one-hundred dollar restaurant meal including a fancy desert and a nice bottle of wine is in reality what leads to expensive urine, but no one seems to complain about this! There are numerous studies that have shown that high quality nutritional supplements do increase people's blood levels of those nutrients leading to a greater state of health and wellbeing.

The main problem that many of us face is that we just don't eat a balanced diet rich in all the micronutrients our bodies require to build and then maintain great health, and once we have a digestive system overloaded with yeasts and bad bacteria, specific natural products incorporated into our diets are vital to help restore the balance – from products which help thoroughly clean the inside of the digestive system through to potent anti-oxidants which help protect cells inside our bodies during the transition from poor health to good health, essential fatty acids to boost aspects of immunity and specialized nutrients which help heal and re-populate the intestinal tract are all an important part of a good anti-candida program.

The 10 Proven Nutrients and Herbs to Fight Yeast Infections

Here is a list of what I believe to be simply the best nutrients and herbal medicines to take when it comes to beating a yeast infection. I will explain them all for you and tell you why they are a necessary part of my Candida Crusher Program. You will find them in my Candida Crusher formulations available online soon.

There are many other herbs and nutrients that are effective in yeast infections of course, and I could write many volumes on the many remedies available, but here follows ten of the best.

Do keep an eye out for my product releases and be sure to join my regular Candida Crusher newsletter, that way you will learn all about what and how to supplement in addition to what dosages are best in your situation.

Also, watch out for the many You Tube videos out soon which will help you significantly, I'll be answering the many questions I get and explain many concepts you may have read about in the Candida Crusher book.

1. Garlic Extract
2. Oregano
3. Caprylic Acid
4. Undecylenic acid
5. Grapefruit Seed Extract
6. Colloidal Silver
7. Pau d'arco
8. Clove
9. Golden Seal
10. Biotin

Candida Crusher # 1 & 2

Caprylic Acid and Undecylenic Acid
My Two Secret Weapons To Fight Candida

Many organic fatty acids and medium chained triglycerides (MCTs) are fungicidal and have been used literally for centuries as antifungal and antimicrobial agents. It was centuries ago discovered that soaps made up from fats were great cleansers, but only 50 years ago that they had other properties about them apart from cleansing; they were also antimicrobial and antifungal. Caprylic acid is an MCT that comes from the coconut and undecylenic acid is a monounsaturated fatty acid that comes from the vacuum distillation of the castor bean. Let's take a look at both and then I'll explain why I like using them, especially when combined with GSE (grapefruit seed extract) and other antifungals.

After treating many candida patients over the past twenty years or more, one tends to experiment and try different products out. You use and recommend what works and tend to move on from those products that give poor or average results. Caprylic acid and undecylenic acid have now become some of my favorite and key anti-candida products, because they effectively inhibit and kill the growth specifically of candida yeast infections in the small and intestine and are very well tolerated – without creating very strong reactions in patients. I like to use what works and stop using products that give consistently very average results, this combo works, but even more so when carefully combined with several other key antifungals as you will see.

Beware Of Die-Off With Many
Yeast Infection Supplements

Die-off is also known as a Herxheimer reaction. You will often find that successful candida treatment can cause in many cases, but certainly not all cases, the rapid death of large numbers of yeast organisms, during which time great amounts of toxins are released from the dead candida microorganisms. These toxins cause problems in their own right, but are often attacked by an over zealous immune system, and can also cause allergies in many people. In my clinical experience, I have found that caprylic acid and undecylenic acid do not cause this die-off that so many talk about, and this is something I have witnessed with many patients in my clinic taking all manner of candida products. Of course not everybody who takes these acids will avoid a reaction, but in my experience it is much less common.

Caprylic acid and Dr. William Crook

Caprylic Acid is designed to nutritionally support the needs of those who want to maintain optimal balance in their friendly flora; it has anti-fungal properties and is widely recognized as one of the key candida supplements. Dr. William Crook, author of the famous book on internal ecology, "The Yeast Connection", first made caprylic acid popular. Dr. Crook found caprylic acid to be the most effective anti-candida supplement in the 1980's, and today it is still just as effective, I believe that there is little need to take the latest "scientific discovery", chances are you are most probably paying more than you should for a product without the impressive 50 year track record of caprylic acid. My Candida Crusher product contains high-grade caprylic acid.

Undecylenic Acid Or Caprylic Acid?

We once used to recommended just caprylic acid as a stand-alone candida treatment, and then just undecylenic acid as a stand-alone treatment, but have since discovered that a combination of undecylenic acid and caprylic acid to be a much more effective product combination in most all candida cases. My naturopathic clinic has tried well over one hundred candida kill products and I've consistently found undecylenic acid and caprylic acids when used on their own or combined to be considerably less effective than when grapefruit seed extract was used in addition. So now I tend to recommend the combination of all three: undecylenic acid, caprylic acid AND grapefruit seed extract. A killer triple combination, and one I've recommended many times over because it just works.

I think I've discovered why this is such a potent combo, it's because the combination of different fatty acids together with the potent anti microbial and anti fungal action of GSE have a powerful broad-spectrum effect on the many (19) different species of candida as well as the literally hundreds of other strains of yeast and bacteria which populate the gastrointestinal tract of many patients with chronic yeast infections. Do you really need the latest whiz-bang enzymatic product? I don't think so; you just need to figure out the right combination of nutrients that have proven themselves over the past 50 years in therapy.

Caprylic acid inhibits the growth of detrimental yeasts such as candida albicans within the intestines. It exerts this effect via its incorporation into the cell membranes of yeasts, the cell membranes then rupture that effectively kills the yeast cell. Caprylic acid is an 8 carbon-chained MCT (medium chained triglycerides), and MCTs have an excellent stability of oxidation, and most top quality dietary supplements containing this acid have a two-year shelf life. Capric acid is similar to caprylic acid, but is a 10-carbon chained MCT, and the best candida formulations will contain both of these fatty acids. Besides being great antifungals, caprylic and capric acids are also beneficial in treating bacterial infections. Due to their relatively short chain length they have little difficulty in penetrating fatty cell wall membranes, hence their effectiveness in combating certain bacteria, such as Staphylococcus aureus and various species of Streptococcus.

Always Looking Out For The Latest And Greatest?

Some practitioners tell me that garlic, caprylic acid, grapefruit seed extract and even Lactobacillus acidophilus are all old hat and that it's time to "upgrade" the candida product lines I use in my clinic. Such opinions generally stem from dietary supplement wholesalers who convince their customers (the health-care professionals) that the most effective products are the latest ones they release every year. I don't like entertaining sales reps that don't teach me something of actual use to my patients, but rather just try to sell me the "latest and greatest" product out, yawn.

The practitioners I know who continually look for "the latest thing out" still use good old Zinc, Vitamin C and B Vitamins. They still recommend Echinacea and Golden Seal as well. But aren't these herbs and vitamins a little "old hat" too? We still recommend them because we know they work, just like they did fifty years ago. Besides, their patients don't really change much either; they still like beer, chocolate and take antibiotics – just like they did fifty years ago. Their habits, diets and lifestyles are much the same; the causative factors for yeast infections haven't really changed much either. And in my opinion, the most effective candida treatment protocol is still the one that uses what has proven to work in the past, along with an excellent understanding of human nature and the actual causative effects of candida.

So why do we continually need to look for the "latest and greatest thing" when it comes to yeast infection supplements? Maybe as practitioners it's because we are more focused on trying to make a buck out of products instead of actually spending time with our patients and instructing them on the right ways to live, no profits there, the medical profession worked that one out many years ago. As cynical as it may sound, there is little profit in getting people well, but plenty of profit in managing their sickness with drugs or dietary supplements.

Dietary supplement companies are focused on their bottom line, profits, not on patient outcomes, and their customers (practitioners) needs to always bear this point in mind. There is nothing wrong with taking a dietary supplement to recover from a yeast infection, but there comes a time when you won't need these products anymore because they have served their purpose. And let me tell you, the latest and greatest won't necessarily get you there any faster. Expect to pay more too.

> *The doctor of the future will give no medication, but will interest his patients in the care of the human frame, diet and in the cause and prevention of disease.*
> **Thomas Edison**

Many folks with major yeast infections just like me back in the 80's and 90's recovered from candida without the help of all these "amazing" candida formulations that seem to come out each year. I'm interested in herbs and dietary supplements with a solid track record, products that have proven themselves over many decades of use, used by many tens of thousands of yeast infection sufferers, and that's why I still recommend supplements like caprylic acid and GSE, just like Vitamin C and Golden seal. Now, let's take a closer look at two great candida inhibitors, caprylic and undecylenic acid.

Caprylic Acid Is Tasteless But Undecylenic Acid Is Certainly Not

Unlike undecylenic acid, a monounsaturated fatty acid, a big plus is that MCTs are known for not having any taste, scent or color whatsoever and also aid in weight loss. MCTs are derived from coconut oil, and naturally occur in breast milk, goat's milk and butterfat. Capsules or gel caps containing undecylenic acid should preferably not be opened, as the average person will certainly not appreciate the taste and odor! Besides, the oil can be quite irritating to the mucous membranes.

Undecylenic Acid Can Be Tricky To Use With Candida

Undecylenic acid is an 11-carbon mono-unsaturated fatty acid that comes from the castor bean. It has proven to be a most effective antifungal agent and is the active ingredient in many over-the-counter antifungal preparations.

Just because something is difficult to use doesn't mean it should be avoided, sometimes you just have to learn a work-around, and I've discovered by studying and trial and error that there is an excellent work around with undecylenic acid.

Even though the antifungal activity of undecylenic acid has shown to be more potent than caprylic acid, the problem is that this mono-unsaturated fatty acid is much more sensitive to pH imbalances commonly found in those with candida. Many people with candida have shown to have alkaline pH issues with their small intestine in particular, directly due to the yeast infection and dysbiosis. Many practitioners who recommend different formulations of this fatty acid, whether it is the oil found in gel caps or in a powder (in case of its salts), are not even aware that there are potentially serious delivery issues with undecylenic acid, it is more difficult to use most effectively than caprylic acid with candida. That is, I find it easier to get a good result with caprylic acid than with undecylenic acid but prefer the combined action of both. All you need to do is to add a good quality digestive enzyme along with it or include a little betaine HCL with the supplement itself. Let me explain.

Unlike caprylic acid, studies have shown that undecylenic acid works best in a predominantly acid environment. To ensure that undecylenic acid works best in the small bowel, I have included a small amount of time-release betaine hydrochloride in my Candida Crusher formulation. This ensures that the undecylenic acid will work exactly where you want it to, in the duodenum and ileum, the two parts of the small bowel mostly effected by candida, thus avoiding the release of excessive bicarbonate (an alkaline solution) produced by the pancreas which would potentially render this fatty acid useless.

Many people with candida have multiple issues with their digestive system, including their stomach, pancreas, small and large intestine. As the yeast infection subsides, the digestion slowly but surely improves in health.

Fatty acids work better if you take between one teaspoon up to one dessertspoon of extra-virgin olive oil daily as well.

Is Your Candida Product Sustained-Released And Balanced?

A big downside of nearly all candida products I have trialed is that they are not "sustained release" like my product, The Candida Crusher. A major benefit of The Candida Crusher is that it delivers the highest concentration of the purest form of caprylic and capric acid in a controlled and sustained released form to both the central and lower intestinal tract out of any comparable product currently available.

The Candida Crusher contains (in addition to many other nutrients and herbal medicines) a specially buffered sustained release compound in a very well tolerated form which can be reliably used time and again, even for long periods of time, without inhibiting the growth of normal gut bacteria necessary for optimal health. This is an important feature, because many candida product brands I have trialed over the years were simply too strong and actually added to the problem by inhibiting the reproduction of the friendly bacteria, and others were just too weak to be effective enough to inhibit the reproduction of the several candida strains some folks have when they present to my clinic with a major yeast infection.

I've learned from many other products that the best product acts on several levels on both the 19 different strains of candida and other yeast species as well as the many different types of bad bacteria and parasites that populate the human digestive system in those with a yeast infection.

Experience has shown me, after analyzing hundreds of stool tests:

- The best natural medicines to use when it comes to a yeast infections
- What proportions of each to use in my formulations.
- To use standardized forms or herbal medicines to ensure actual potency.
- To use the highest–grade vitamins & minerals.
- To ensure slow-release of the formula, ensuring a 2–3 hour delivery.

As you are aware, I specialize in candida treatment and have found caprylic acid to be extremely well tolerated by even the most yeast-sensitive patients and very effective for the inhibition and control of the several strains of candida in both the small and large intestine, but it is important to understand that it is best used in addition to several other key nutrients in order to get a broad-spectrum effect. That way you will not have to rotate several anti-fungal formulations but just stick with the one top quality and proven formula.

You save money and complete the job of permanently eradicating your yeast infection in much less time.

A Study Released In PubMed:

"The susceptibility of candida albicans to several fatty acids was tested with a short inactivation time, and ultra-thin sections were studied by transmission electron microscopy (TEM) after treatment with caprylic and capric acid. The results show that caprylic and capric acids cause the fastest and most effective killing of all three strains of C. albicans tested, leaving the cytoplasm dis-organized and shrunken because of a disrupted or disintegrated plasma membrane".

Ref:http://www.ncbi.nlm.nih.gov/pubmed/11600381

The Candida Crusher contains a blend of both caprylic and capric acids and is one of the best candida crushing products on the market.

Candida Crusher # 5 Grapefruit Seed Extract

The Most Powerful Natural Antibiotic Available

Grapefruit seed extract (GSE) is made by converting grapefruit seeds and their pulp into a highly acidic liquid. After processing, filtering and distillation a yellow, viscous and quite bitter liquid is left to which a sweet vegetable glycerin is added to improve the taste. GSE can be obtained in both liquid and dry form, and you will find it in The Candida Crusher product.

Dr. Jakob Harich in Florida, USA, discovered grapefruit seed extract in 1972. He found that the extract from grapefruit seeds not only inactivated viruses, but also yeasts, other fungi and parasites.

Its commercial use initially began in the agricultural industry after scientists found out it could stop the growth of mold on foodstuff. Hospitals began to use it as an antiseptic and to clean surgical equipment and it has even been used in swimming pools as an alternative to chlorine to kill harmful microbes. GSE has been extensively researched, but mainly on farm animals and widely used since the 1980's in both Europe and the United States. The renowned American Research Institute has found GSE to be effective in the treatment of over 800 different bacteria and viruses and over 100 yeast and fungi species, in addition to inhibiting and killing many different species of parasites.

I have been using GSE increasingly more in my practice over the past ten years, and consider it to be in my "top three" when it comes to candida. But why would I rate it so highly? Simple, it works, and it works consistently and reliably time and again. But there is a further reason and that is I've noticed that most all of the stool testing I have completed over the years have revealed that candida is very susceptible to the effects of GSE, as well as caprylic acid. These three two appear to consistently rank the highest in the sensitivity panels of the CDSA x 3 tests (Comprehensive Digestive Stool Analysis x three stool samples).

GSE Is A .45 Caliber Yeast Killer

Let me give you an example of candida killing power. I have a patient who hunts deer in the South Island of New Zealand who once told me of a particular rifle that he favors, and the more he has gone deer hunting using various other high powered rifles, the more he favors this particular rifle. He has been hunting deer for over 30 years and has a collection of over two-dozen different hunting rifles, but there is one particular gun that he likes overall. When I asked him why, his reply was simple: "It's the most consistently reliable gun I've ever owned, it is accurate in a wide range of conditions and outperforms most of the other rifles. It is half the price of my best rifle yet I've had more kills and trophies with it than any other gun". This is how I feel about GSE and candida, it outperforms most all other anti-candida products and it has a consistent and reliable mode of action with a wide variety of pathogens like yeasts, bacteria and parasites, even when compared with those expensive cutting-edge candida supplements that seem to come out every year. I've tried them all but keep coming back to GSE as part or my Candida Crusher Formula when it comes to killing yeast. Why settle for a water pistol when you can get a .45 caliber? Be sure that your candida formula contains GSE, the Dirty Harry of yeast killers.

How Does GSE Work?

Recently, Scientist Dr. Sung-Hwan from Korea discovered by electron microscope that GSE works by altering the cell membranes of bacteria and yeasts, and the loss of the cell membrane can actually be seen under high magnification, in addition, he also discovered that GSE inhibits the pathogenic cells enzyme activities. How exactly it work on viruses remains to be seen, since viruses are incredibly tiny cells which are coated in a protein that is virtually impossible to penetrate. We do know that GSE does work on a virus, as there have been some good successes in using GSE with hepatitis for example.

Although we know little about its mode of action, we do know a lot more about how GSE is effective in so many different conditions. Does it matter? We started using Aspirin as a medicine in 1899, but only since the 1960's have we really understood how this anti-inflammatory works.

Once we really understand how this incredible natural antibiotic called GSE works, it will far surpass Aspirin, antibiotics, and the many other current expensive and patented wonder drugs that are quickly becoming useless against bacteria, creating superbugs like MRSA.

The Many Uses Of GSE

GSE can be used in the treatment of many different conditions, and it can be used even more successfully when used in conjunction with other candida products such as caprylic acid, capric acid and undecylenic acid.

The most effective uses of GSE, apart from candida and intestinal complaints, are as follows:

- Colds and influenza

- Ear, nose and throat complaints

- Urinary tract infections

- Nail and skin fungal problems (see chapter 4)

- Acne

- Vaginal thrush (see chapter 5)

- Chronic fatigue syndrome

- Decreased immunity

- Parasites. Take this stuff when you travel to Asia or Central America, don't leave home without your liquid GSE; it could save you from much misery.

No Friendly Fire with GSE

It is amazing how many soldiers in battle end up dying by way of friendly fire; accidentally by their own troops. This collateral damage occasionally does occur unfortunately, and it is sometimes difficult to avoid. No such problem with GSE, this is one powerful yeast killer that will not cause any collateral damage. A comparison with more than 30 commonly used antibiotics and anti fungal candida supplements gave similar results GSE, however, the difference being that GSE is not detrimental to the immune system and unlike antibiotics, GSE does NOT destroy any beneficial flora.

Caution, GSE Contains Naringenin

If you decide to take GSE as a candida supplement on its own, more so if you want to take GSE in very high and sustained dosages, it pays to be cautious if you are taking certain prescribed medications, if you recognize any of the drugs below that you may be on, then check with your doctor first before you go out and buy liquid GSE drops. Although the Candida Crusher formulation which you will be able to purchase soon does contain GSE, the level is sufficiently low enough not to interact with your medication, this caution applies primarily to eating grapefruits, drinking grapefruit juice or taking GSE in high dosages for weeks on end. I consider a high dose to be 15 – 20 drops up to four times daily in water or juice.

The same goes with drinking grapefruit juice or eating grapefruit regularly, which is not a good idea if you take certain drugs as listed below. What you do on a short-term and irregular basis will not generally pose a problem, it is when you do something sustained and prolonged that it could be an issue.

Grapefruit and grapefruit seed extract contains a flavonoid called naringenin. Naringenin is a natural compound found in fruits such as grapefruit, oranges and tomatoes especially, which has antioxidant and anti-inflammatory effects. Only grapefruit contains the highest levels of naringenin, this is not so with oranges or tomatoes, so don't worry about them.

It is important to keep in mind that naringenin can interact with a number of pharmaceutical drugs, altering and influencing their blood levels.

Naringenin has been shown to have an inhibitory effect on a certain liver enzyme (human cytochrome P450 isoform CYP1A2) which can change the way some drugs work in your body by making them much more toxic than they normally would be, even resulting in creating carcinogens (cancer causing) of otherwise relatively harmless substances. We call this "upregulation". In France and some other countries, immunosuppressive or antiviral drugs are administered along with the advice to drink small amounts of grapefruit juice regularly to allow the drugs to remain longer and at more sustained dosages in the body.

Drugs Affected By Grapefruit Include:

- Statins used for cholesterol control

- Calcium channel blockers used to treat high blood pressure

- Non-sedating antihistamines such as Hismanal (astemizole)

- Anti-anxiety drugs like Valium (diazepam), Xanax (alprazolam), Halcion (triazolam), and others

- Immunosuppressive drugs used to prevent rejection of transplanted tissues organs

- Antiviral agents used to treat HIV/AIDS

Is GSE Safe To Use?

Don't freak, I don't want to needlessly alarm you and frighten you away from using GSE. Just like anything high-powered, in the wrong hands it can be a hazard but when used skillfully it can be one of your best friends. Is this stuff safe to use? Absolutely, it has been estimated that you would have to take 4,000 times the normal adult oral dose to risk a 50% chance of poisoning. But there are a few precautions you should take nevertheless. I am more concerned with adults taking Acetaminophen (Paracetamol) that kills over 450 people each year in the USA, according to the FDA.

- Do not use for sustained periods of time at high dose. I consider a high dose of the liquid to be 15 drops, 4 times daily. There is nothing wrong with this dose for a week, but you are best to keep the dose down to 15 drops per day if you want to treat ongoing with liquid GSE. If you are using a dry compound then the general dosage suggestion are from 200 up to 700 mg per day. I've found dry to work as well as the liquid and with less concern for the bitter taste as well, besides, it can then be blended with several other compounds to create a powerful antimicrobial compound.

- Do not use undiluted on the eyes, nose, mouth, ears or other sensitive areas. Careful with the skin or mucous membranes, GSE may cause irritation.

- Keep it away from the eyes!

- Keep it away from children; you don't want them to swallow this stuff undiluted.

- Do not use in pregnancy.

- Be sure to dilute it in water or a dilute juice before using, if you use the liquid.

Candida Crusher # Colloidal Silver

Colloidal silver is yet another potent antifungal and antibacterial product you can use. Again, I find it best to use colloidal silver as part of a formula and not in isolation. Before penicillin was discovered in 1934, silver was one of the main things used to fight infectious disease. It is interesting how antibiotics have been showing increasing resistance, but colloidal silver shows no such thing!

I've been recommending colloidal silver in my clinic for over twenty years for all manner of infections, cuts, coughs and colds, all eye problems, ear, nose and throat and more recently for yeast infections.

How Does Colloidal Silver Work?

There are several ways how colloidal silver works in yeast infections, but here are the most common ways:

1. Colloidal silver has a strong antibiotic and sterilizing-like activity against many species of bacteria and viruses. As soon as it comes into contact with any anaerobic bacteria it starts to kill them. Silver has been known to purify and cleanse for over one hundred years.

2. Colloidal silver is an antifungal agent in its own right, and has proven to be more effective than even Fluconazole when it comes to yeast infections.

3. Colloidal silver has a supporting effecting on wound healing and can heal many different types of inflammations and wounds, both internal as well as external.

A Potent Antifungal

A Korean study published in the Journal of Microbiology and Biotechnology demonstrated that colloidal silver is an excellent antifungal in its own right and showed potent activity against clinical isolates of various fungal strains. Research revealed that silver nanoparticles (colloidal silver) were very effective against Candida species (yeast infections, vaginal thrush) as well as Trichophyton species (athlete's foot, jock itch and ring worm, hair, scalp and nail fungus).

It is interesting to note that colloidal silver in this study was shown to be equally effective against fungal strains as Amphotericin B, a very potent antifungal pharmaceutical drug. Even more interesting is that it was found to be superior to Diflucan, a widely used drug otherwise known as Fluconazole, widely prescribed to women with vaginal thrush.

Careful Of Die-Off

I'm not a fan of recommending colloidal silver on its own in the treatment of chronic or severe yeast infections, for the simple reason that most people who do use it, simply use too much at the beginning and experience strong aggravations as their yeast infection dies off. For this reason, if you are going to use colloidal silver internally, the dosage should be small at first, only once per day. After three days step it up to twice daily, and at the end of the week try three times daily.

I use and recommend a silver supplement with a minimum potency of 40 ppm and with a micron size of no more than .001.

Is Colloidal Silver Safe to Use?

Yes, there is a lot of nonsense written about the toxicity of colloidal silver, but tap water is probably more toxic, especially if you live in a big city and drink plenty of it. You may want to check out the silversafety.org website and work out exactly your own daily, weekly or annual limit of how much is OK to use.

Dr. Jeffrey Blumer, M.D., Ph.D., Director of the Center for Drug Research (the world's largest clinical research center for drugs) and former director of the Greater Cleveland Poison Control Center, has this to say about colloidal silver:

"Common substances like table salt and aspirin are harmless with normal use, but excessive intake can become toxic and even life-threatening. With normal responsible usage, silver supplements are entirely harmless to humans."

Candida Crusher # 5 Biotin

I first started to recommend the vitamin called biotin with yeast infection about three years ago after I read some interesting studies into its use, and especially after reading about biotin written by an experienced doctor who had been recommending it for years for candida. Biotin is an essential coenzyme that assists in the making of fatty acids and in the burning of carbohydrates and fats for body heat and energy. Additionally, it also aids in the utilization of different amino acids, folic acid and vitamins B5 and B12. It is a potent stimulator of healthy cells of your body.

Good Tip

Avoid Raw Eggs

Avoid raw eggs if you don't want a deficiency of biotin. Egg white contains a protein called avidin, and this protein binds extremely tightly to biotin and prevents it being utilized by the body. Cooking egg destroys the ability of avidin to bind to biotin, so cooked eggs are fine but raw eggs are not.

Dr. Orion Truss Recommended Biotin

Not many people know that candida organisms are dimorphic, meaning they exist in two different forms. Candida can change its round yeast-like form into a puncturing mycelial form. What are mycelia? They are tangled masses of fine branching threads that make up the invasive fungal form of candida, and it is this form that can penetrate into the cell looking for food.

Dr. Orion Truss (The Missing Diagnosis, 1983) stated that candida in its normal rounded state is sugar fermenting, actively reproducing and non-invasive. Dr. Truss mentioned that good dietary sources of biotin include egg yolks, brown rice, liver and kidney and soybeans (which were not genetically modified in the 80's) along with dietary supplements of biotin may well help to prevent candida from converting into its invasive fungal form.

Dr. Truss recognized even 30 years ago that people were deficient in biotin as it was lacking in the typical SAD diet back then as it is today (Standard American Diet). Today it is worse than in the 1980's, with yet even more people eating higher amounts of refined diets lacking in biotin, include white flour products, French fries, soda drinks, deep fried foods, candy, pastries and other similar depleted or fake foods. These foods not only allow candida to thrive, they are deficient in biotin and have the potential to allow candida to more easily morph into its more invasive form.

Biotin and the Inhibition Of The Mycelial Form Of Candida

Dr. Luc De Shepper was one of the first physicians to write about the connection between biotin and candida in the 1980's, his book opened my eyes to the amazing effects of biotin with yeast infection: "Candida, The Symptoms, The Causes, The Cure", it is worth a read by anyone serious about yeast infections. But as early as 1974, researcher Dr. Yamaguchi noted that when candida albicans was cultured on a biotin-poor dish, it quickly changed into its invasive mycelial form.

Biotin And The Development Of Candida Albicans*

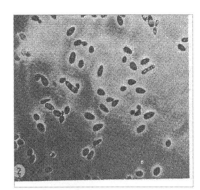

Candida albicans (400x magnification) grown in a medium containing biotin at a concentration of 10ng/ml. The round form of candida can be clearly seen in this image.

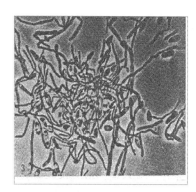

Candida albicans (400x magnification) when grown in a much lower medium of biotin. (0.1ng/ml). The mycelial form of candida can be clearly seen in this image.

*Yamaguchi H. Sabouraudia. 1974 Nov;12(3):320-8.
Mycelial development and chemical alteration of Candida albicans from biotin insufficiency.

How Does Biotin Work With Yeast Infections?

There are a few reasons why it makes good sense for you to have biotin in your yeast infection treatment protocol, and here are three good reasons:

Biotin has the ability to halt candida from turning into a hyphal or mycelial form, which is a lot harder to get rid of than the yeast itself, and potentially more serious in your body. According to medical doctor, acupuncturist and homeopath Dr. Luc De Shepper, biotin taken in the amount of at least 3 milligram will cut the transformation cycle from the yeast to the fungus form. In order avoid the spreading of the mycelial form of candida into the bloodstream (and thus giving the opportunity for the yeast cells to invade almost all of the organs, including the brain), the interruption of the vicious cycle is a must and a priority and biotin will halt this progression. There are certain people who may have a biotinidase deficiency who may have an increased risk of a yeast infection. Biotinidase is an enzyme that helps to recycle biotin in your body.

Beneficial bacteria in your digestive system help to produce B vitamins, including biotin. A primary source of biotin is the healthy bacteria in the intestinal tract. Because these are often compromised by a candida albicans overgrowth, candida sufferers are particularly prone to a biotin deficiency. People with yeast infections often have altered bowel flora and have a harder time making their own B vitamins, and this is one of the big reasons they get so tired. Carbohydrates need B vitamins to be metabolized efficiently, and those with chronic yeast infections eat too many carbs and always seem to be B vitamin deficient, especially biotin. And if little to no biotin is pro**duced then you need to rely solely on dietary sources and that can be hit and miss.**

The Low Carbohydrate-Biotin Self-Test

This test can be performed in conjunction with other tests I have recommended for achieving optimal results if you want to know if you have a yeast infection or not.

This candida test was recommended to me by natural medicine expert Dr. James Wilson from Arizona, Doctor Wilson is the world's authority in adrenal fatigue.

Strictly avoid carbohydrates and take 3000 micrograms of biotin (3 milligrams) per day for 3 days and see if any of your yeast infection symptoms improve. If symptoms improve, especially dramatically, you are probably suffering from a mycelial candida overgrowth in your intestines and/or circulation. Make sure your candida supplement contains sufficient biotin in divided doses and take with foods.

I have included biotin naturally in The Candida Crusher Formula that will be available in 2013.

3 Candida Crushing Herbal Medicines

I could write an entire book just about the virtue of herbs and yeast infections, but I won't! There are so many different herbal medicines that have a positive effect on inhibiting and destroying a yeast infection, but I do believe that the most beneficial herbal medicines discovered in my research are the ones I have highlighted below in bold. Herbal medicines are best purchased through your herbalist. Herbal medicine is literally the mother of all medicines and has been in use for thousands of years. Be sure to visit an herbalist with experience, and preferably one who is registered with a professional herbal association and experienced with yeast infections.

I have already discussed garlic and oregano oil above in the special foods section, and will cover Pau D'arco, Golden Seal and Tea Tree Oil below.

Best Herbs For Gastrointestinal Yeast infection

Andrographis, Aniseed, Barberry, Black Walnut, Cinnamon, Echinacea root, **Garlic**, **Golden Seal**, Grape Seed, Green Tea, **Oregano**, **Pau D'arco**, St Mary's Thistle, **Tea Tree** (use the essential oil externally)

Herbs For A Vaginal Yeast Infection

When it comes to vaginal yeast infections, be sure to read chapters 4 and 5. There are many ways you can use herbal medicines when it comes to vaginal thrush, but the most common ways are to make a strong decoction (simmering and using the solution) or infusions (making a tea) of these herbs to ease itching and burning; use either internally as a douche or apply externally with pads or tampons that have been soaked in the solution. It is always best to treat internally (The Candida Crusher Program) as well as externally with any yeast infection.

Andrographis, Aniseed, Chaste Tree, Echinacea Root, **Garlic** (topically), **Oregano** (topically), **Pau D'arco** (topically), **Tea Tree Oil** (use the essential oil externally), Thyme (use the essential oil externally)

Candida Crusher Herb # 1 Pau D'arco

This herb is also known as LaPacho or Taheebo. Pau D'arco (Tabebuia avellanedae) tea is an herbal tea prepared from the inner bark of a rainforest tree from South American. The tree is not killed during harvesting process, and only the inner bark is used. This herb that has a long folk use in the treatment of infections is an excellent adjunct in candida infections. While I wouldn't recommend it as primary therapy, it is brilliant to use in conjunction with the Candida Crusher Program.

The native Indians of Brazil traditionally used the inner bark for a wide range of health problems including boils, ulcerative colitis, bedwetting, fevers, sore throats, snakebites, various wounds, and several types of cancers including cancer of the tongue, prostate, esophagus, lung, bowel, and head cancers. LaPacho was also traditionally used for ulcers, constipation and many types of digestive problems, poor circulation and arthritis.

How Does Pau D'arco Work?

Several compounds from Pau d'arco have demonstrated strong anti-candida effects. Lapacho, the other name for this remarkable rainforest tree, has often singled out of all the herbal medicines as one of the premier treatments for candida or yeast infections and after many years of laboratory research by the mid 1970's, the list of nutrients in Pau d'arco that inhibit Candida albicans and other fungi had grown to several dozen. An interesting application has been reported in which toe and fingernail fungi infections are hugely relieved and disappear by soaking them in lapacho tea off and on for a couple of weeks.

Adulteration And Misunderstanding With This Herb Is Common

I have found that the big problem with Pau D'arco is that it is one of the very few herbs that is also effective in cancer, and whenever an herb is popular in cancer and in very high demand you can bet your bottom dollar that there are a lot of unscrupulous operators out there who offer inferior and totally fake or entirely useless substitutes. This is especially so with the quality rainforest herbs like Pau D'arco. Some websites I have looked at are obviously fradulent in their offerings, so buyer beware!

And secondly, due to a lack of quality control and confusion about what are the best portions of this tree to be used (many of the chemical analysis have been performed on the tree's heartwood, while the inner bark was always used in South American folklore), it is most likely that consumers and herbalists are being supplied with the wrong and generally ineffective product.

You will need to take particular care that your Pau D'arco is the "real McCoy", and if it is you will certainly notice the benefits when used as a tea or vaginally as a douche. Herbal medicines DO work, but when you use fakes you will be disappointed I guarantee it. Now you can understand why there is so much skepticism with the mainstream scientists when it come to herbal medicines and effective treatment.

How To Use Pau D'arco With Candida

The most effective ratio is 3 level tablespoons of Pau d'arco tea with four cups (1 litre) of purified or filtered water. (You can also use 1 tablespoon tea with 1 1/3 cup of water). Add the tea to a saucepan (glass or stainless steel) of cold water. After water starts to boil, reduce heat and simmer very low (with the lid on) for at least 20 minutes. Then add a little more water to bring liquid level back to start level. You can make it a bit stronger or weaker if you are uncomfortable with the taste. Do not use aluminium or tin pots or storage containers! Strain the tea through a piece of linen cloth, tea strainer or coffee press device. Serve luke warm or cooler. Store the tea in a glass container.

The incredible thing with this herb is that the tea does not deteriorate in time because the herb is totally immune to mould and fungus. You will find Pau D'arco a most effective tea for your digestive and immune system in general. Many studies now show that it is potentially a useful cancer treatment as well.

For those with a yeast infection, drink at least one cup daily; better still have one cup twice daily between meals.

How To Use Pau D'arco For Vaginal Thrush

The precise dosage I recommend is based on a lapachol content of between 2 – 4 percent. Boil 15-20 grams of the inner bark in 500 milliliters (or 1 pint) of pure water (Don't use tap water) for 10 to 15 minutes. Bring to the rolling boil then cover and very gently simmer. Do not use an aluminimium saucepan, use stainless steel. A tampon that has been soaked in this tepid solution is perfect to most effectively treat any vaginal infection. Insert the tampon and change every 24 hours until resolution. This treatment works, especially if you get the real Pau D'arco and not a fake product. I've repeated this same information for your convenience in chapter 5, Crushing Chronic Vaginal Yeast Infections.

Candida Crusher Herb # 1 Golden Seal

My personal favorite herbal medicine when it comes to any acute infections in my clinic is Golden seal. The plants that share similar indications when it comes to effective yeast infection treatment are Golden seal (Hydrastis canadensis), Barberry (Berberis vulgaris), Oregon grape (Berberis aquifolium), and Goldthread (Coptis chinensis). But what do these plants all have in common? They all contain a high content of berberine that is antibacterial, antiparasitic and antifungal that is an effective immune enhancer. Golden seal or barberry are best used as part of a candida formula, and not relied upon as a single agent.

How Does Berberine Work?

Golden seal and barberry in particular contain high levels berberine that has positively stimulating effect on the immune system. This effect is strongest no doubt is in mucous membrane tissues found in the vagina, mouth, and especially the digestive system. Berberine has been shown to possess excellent antimicrobial activity against a wide variety of microorganisms some of which are found in the vagina, like candida albicans, e coli, staph aureus and many others. Different types of preparations of Golden seal and barberry especially have been used both orally in teas, capsules and in liquid herbal extracts, and intra-vaginally in douches and as suppositories.

I don't think of berberine containing herbs as candida specifics, but more adjuncts, meaning they are perfect to add to a candida cleansing and inhibiting dietary supplement because they:

1. Enhance the activity of stronger antifungals like caprylic and undecylenic acid.

2. Work in the background by killing bad bacteria and parasites, allowing stronger antifungals to do they job more easily.

3. Unlike most antifungals, they support the mucous membranes and have an immune enhancing and cleansing effect on the mucosa of the throat, vagina and digestive system.

4. Act as liver tonics and help the body secrete bile, good to use when detoxing.

Intestinal Parasites

Berberine has demonstrated growth inhibition of Giardia, Entamoeba histolytica, Trichomonas vaginalis, and Leishmania donovani as well as several other well-known parasites and many different types of detrimental bacteria. Studies of berberine have shown in particular that it markedly decreases the parasitic load and can rapidly improve somebody's immune system profile. Test tube studies have revealed that berberine inhibits the multiplication and inhibits the maturation of parasites. It is a most effective anti-parasitic herbal medicine and in my opinion is a must when treating any chronic yeast infection.

Rifles and shotguns

Because of its ability to affect both yeast but especially parasites and bacteria, Golden seal and/or Barberry are a logical choice in cases where multiple infectious agents in any yeast infection are involved. And when a person has a chronic yeast infection, they won't just have a candida overgrowth, they most probably will have a case of dysbiosis and have an imbalance of many potentially "bad" bacteria, fungi and parasites at the same time, and this is where berberine is effective, just like GSE. Instead of one shotgun we now have two shotguns when we go hunting for candida. I tend to see garlic, tea tree oil and oregano oil as rifles (strong and specific high powered anti-fungal action) and GSE and berberine as shotguns (a more widespread action on bacteria, yeasts and parasites). What a blast, no pun intended ;-)

Precautions with Berberine

Don't take a berberine extract by itself for more than two weeks, it is OK to have berberine as part of a formula in a lower dose for more than two weeks but you wouldn't want to take for example straight liquid Golden seal or Barberry for any longer than two weeks. The reason being is that they are quite potent and may irritate the mucous membranes. Also, don't take when pregnant.

Candida Crusher Herb # 3   Tea Tree Oil

The indigenous people of north-eastern New South Wales (Australia) had known about the healing and disinfecting properties of tea tree oil for thousands of years, long before the development of any pharmaceutical drugs. They applied poultices of crushed tea tree leaves to cuts and wounds and inhaled the volatile oil from the crushed leaves to alleviate congestion and respiratory tract infections. The scientific discovery of the plant's virtues came in 1923 when the leading state government chemist, Arthur Penfold, tested the oil of the tea tree and determined its antiseptic action was about 12 times stronger than the widely used carbolic acid. Extensive clinical trials with medical and dental colleagues in London and Sydney led to glowing reports in the distinguished scientific journals of the day.

The Near-Perfect Antiseptic

Indeed, the 1930's and 1940's saw tea tree oil widely acclaimed as a "near perfect antiseptic", so much so that during World War II Australian soldiers were issued with tea tree oil in their first aid kits. The troops also sang the praises of tea tree oil's insect repellent and anti-fungal properties. At home, it was put to an amazing spectrum of uses from shampoo, toothpaste and smelly feet to boils, acne and head lice.

Sadly, this remedy from nature was forgotten for almost 30 years as cheap, synthetic antibiotics flooded the world's medicine markets and became a way of life. The tea tree industry collapsed by the 1960's and the oil became a rare commodity. But, in 1976, Eric White became the latter-day pioneer of the Australian tea tree industry. Convinced of its applications in modern society, Eric chose the alternately flood-washed and drought-baked Bungawalbyn Swamp, near Coraki in northern NSW, for his first crops. After four years of painstaking research and lobbying, a crown lease was granted. It arrived on a Thursday in 1976, and this was the day "Thursday Plantation" brand of Tea Tree Oil was born. It is still one of the best; the original is generally always the best.

I would recommend that you always keep a bottle in your medicine cabinet; you will be amazed at how many uses you will find. This is my top antifungal when it comes to topical (skin or nail) applications and I believe it to be the best when it comes to vaginal thrush as well.

How Can I Use Tea Tree Oil in Yeast Infections?

One of the best things I have found with this remarkable oil is that it has many and varied applications with candida patients. It is so effective with topical (skin) applications, on the toenail with discolored toenails or tinea, as a vaginal cleanse/douche for vaginitis (thrush) and those whitish skin patches that candida patients sometimes get.

Toe Nail Fungus

Place one drop on each affected toe after your bath, make sure some oil gets under the nail. Apply each day. Stay with it, it can take a few weeks but watch the difference it makes!

Ringworm

Apply the oil neat to the affected areas three times daily.

Jock Itch

Read the section about male yeast infections in chapter 4 entitled QUICK START, The Candida Crusher Guide.

Vaginal Pessary and Douche

Tea tree oil is one of the best things you can use when you have a vaginal yeast infection, its just one of those medicines that works consistently time and again. A Tea Tree Oil douche has ben used and recommended by alternative medicine doctors for over 50 years now for vaginal yeast infections, literally since the discovery of the remarkable natural anti fungal.

Use from eight to ten drops of the pure Australian Tea Tree Oil in 500 milliliters (or 1 pint) of tepid purified or distilled water. Douching in between pessary applications seems to be the best solution in ridding your vagina from the discomfort including the burning and incessant itching of a candida vaginal yeast infection. You will find this information on the tea Tree Oil pessary and douche combo repeated in chapter 5, which contains more information about vaginal yeast infections, if this is your problem then be sure to read this chapter.

You may be able to purchase a Tea Tree Oil pessary from a good health-food shop or maybe a natural drug store in your region or online (pharmacy or chemist). Incidentally, the Tea Tree Oil pessary can be used for either vaginal thrush or in the anal passage for a stubborn case of hemorrhoids as well. If you can't get hold of the pessaries, you can make your own using a 2% solution of Tea Tree oil in a cocoa butter base, which will most effectively kill the yeast infection without disturbing the body's natural flora.

Are There Any Other Uses For Australian Tea Tree Oil?

I have recommended and used Tea Tree oil for over thirty years, and know first hand about how powerful this natural healing product really is. Australian Tea Tree Oil (Melaleuca alternifolia) has been proven to be more effective that the New Zealand Tea Tree Oil. Here are a few recollections of my use and recommendation of Tea Tree Oil over the years:

- I can remember when I was twenty years old (1980) and had a motorcycle accident that resulted in a severely gravel-rashed back and shoulders. Tea Tree oil was applied and all was well within four days, I used up a whole 50ml bottle on an old towel and it allowed me to avoid a doctor's visit. The healing power of this oil in **truly amazing, no scarring, no pain and quick healing.**

- I took a bottle of Tea Tree Oil with me on my journeys around Australia in the mid 1980's and found it to be **wonderful for insect bites and to ward off mosquitoes in general.** Excellent for cuts, grazes and a good general travel medicine. This is one medicine I tell my patients **never to travel without.** Get the 25ml bottle of Tea Tree Oil; it is the first thing you place in your natural medicine first aid travel kit. You will find that you will be treating fellow travellers as they get **sore feet or blisters**, etc.

- I like to use Tea Tree Oil Toothpaste, it is most pleasant and has a **very good effect on your gums** and will help to keep them in top shape.

- I brought several large bottles of Tea Tree Oil with me to India in 1994, as I knew I was going to do voluntary work for several months in Mother Theresa's slum clinic in Calcutta. This is where I saw first hand just how powerful this **amazing natural healer** was first hand, **severely infected** patients were responding remarkably well in a hospital setting with natural medicines.

- I have always used Tea Tree Oil with my family and particularly with my four children - ranging from everything to **cuts, skin rashes, acne, lacerations** and even when my eight year old was attacked by a rather savage cat and had four major **puncture wounds** to his lower arm. We soaked a cloth in Tea Tree Oil and applied it. No doctor, No tetanus shot and No long waiting in the emergency department of the hospital.

- I have even used Tea Tree Oil with our three cats, **saves those expensive veterinary bills.** Our cat was attacked and bitten around the head, which resulted in several wounds of which a few went septic. I injected Tea Tree Oil into the wounds and let them drain. Within one week it was healed, **no infection, no puss** and I saved a few hundred dollars - more than I have probably spent on this remarkable potion over the years.

- I have even recommended it with patients presenting with tongue cancer **and have seen fantastic results here as well.**

Why Use Tea Tree Oil Products for Toe Nail Fungus and Athlete's Foot?

When put to an independent test supervised by The University of Western Australia, the Department of Microbiology concluded that Tea Tree Anti-Fungal gel performed equal to or, for the most part, better than other products tested. Products evaluated were Daktarin, DaktaGOLD, Canesten, Canesten Once Daily Bifonazole, Lamisil and Bio-Juven Foot Care Anto-Fungal Gel. The results as seen below, clearly show that Tea Tree Anti-Fungal Gel was the most effective product against *Candida albicans* and second only to Lamisil against *Trichophyton rubrum (tinea)*.

Are There Any Precautions With Tea Tree Oil?

Like any strong essential plant oil, there are precautions.

- Avoid contact with the eyes.

- Avoid internal use, use topically (externally) only.

- Do not place Tea Tree Oil in any plastic container as it may dissolve the container!

- Keep out of reach of (very young) children.

General Supplementation Recommendations

In section 1 of this chapter 7, the diet and nutrition section, you will have read about the supplementation recommendations. As I have mentioned earlier, while nutritional supplementation is not absolutely necessary, it does play a crucial role in fully recovering from a yeast infection. They will not only speed-up your recovery, but in many cases they will be found necessary for a complete and deep-seated recovery from the dysbiosis (bowel overgrowth of yeasts, poor bacteria, and parasites), leaky gut, fatigue and brain fog, food allergies and many other chronic health problems associated with a chronic yeast infection.

The Candida Crusher supplements I have chosen and personally developed have been specifically selected based on my extensive experiences in working with many patients with chronic yeast infections for their cleansing, healing and deeply restorative effects. I will explain the significance of these formulations because it is important for you to understand why these supplements have been included as part of your Candida Crusher Program, and the necessity of taking them regularly. But let's start first with some general dietary supplementation recommendations first.

The Go Low and Go Slow Method

Experience has taught me that in most cases of candidiasis it is best to start with low dosages of all supplements, especially in severe cases, and to take it easy the first week or two in particular. If at any time you feel uncomfortable or experience any die-off, be sure not to increase the dose but to stay on this level (or just under this threshold) for a few days until you stabilize. Many with a mild yeast infection may be OK on the recommended dosages though, but I would still err on the side of caution.

If you increase the dosages at any stage and find the adjustments too uncomfortable, simply decrease the dosage again and stay at this reduced dose for three days before trying to increase it again. This rule applies to all supplementation. There is no "right" or "wrong" dosage and the correct dosage for you depends entirely on what adjustments or healing your body is going through at the time, and it also depends on your own personal level of tolerance you have towards any discomfort. Some people with a yeast infection can put up with a lot, others with a very minimal level. You will need to decide what is right for you, because there are no rules here.

Some Will Treble The Dosage In The Belief They Will Be Quickly Cured

Some folks have rather strange ideas about supplementation dosages, because they think that they will "quickly cure" their candida by taking double, treble or quadruple the recommended dosage, sorry folks, it doesn't quite work like this! I once worked in a health-food shop as a naturopathic student, it was some the best early learning in my career before I started to actively see clients in my practice, and I highly recommend any person starting out in our industry who is serious to do the same. You will also learn that there are folks who take either way too much product or way too little, besides those who take the right amount. A man came into our shop distraught once, after telling me that an ambulance had just taken his wife to hospital after a serious epileptic fit which she had never previously experienced of this severity. He said that she had been purchased bottles of Vitamin E capsules (500 iu) for her mild epilepsy and was taking 30 capsules a day to "improve brain circulation". Yes, that's right, thirty capsules of Vitamin E 500 IU a day. I saw a man once take twenty or more B Complex tablets daily for weeks "to give himself a boost" and then come into the shop complaining about chronic palpitations and insomnia which he had never previously experienced. I've more recently had a lady complaining in my clinic about her three year old child with rotten teeth, she was completely perplexed and couldn't understand why, her child was not having any sweets, juice nor any soda drinks. But she was sprinkling dry ascorbic acid powder on his various foods several times daily "to boost his immune system".

Take It Easy On Yourself

As naturopathic practitioners we see patients every day in our clinic and sometimes take it for granted that they will take the correct dosages of the products we recommend. I have learned over the years that there is no "right" nor "wrong" dosage in many cases, it is finding the right dosage for you without causing any unwanted effects like requiring hospitalization, insomnia and palpitations or rotten teeth. Potentially anytime you take a dietary supplement or pharmaceutical drug you will be causing changes to occur inside your body. The more you take (the larger the dose) and the more often you take it (frequency of dose) the higher the likelihood of an adverse or unwanted effect. For this reason, I recommend you go slow to begin with and gradually step the dosage up. Does this make any sense to you? Can you remember when you last got all enthusiastic about exercise? Maybe you went to the gym or joined a class. Were you not told to gradually "break in" over a few weeks, to take it easy at first and then gradually increase the pace? It is important to remember that your body does not like very quick change, whether it is taking a supplement, drug or begin an exercise program.

The Sensitive Person And The Ultra Sensitive Person

A few good tips I'd like to share with you regarding dosages is that it is important to look at your sensitivity levels and body size when you are considering what dosage to take. There is no point for example for a practitioner to recommend an 80-pound woman take the same dosage as a 220-pound woman. In addition, I am always on the lookout for the sensitive and the "ultra" sensitive patient. But how can I tell the difference? I just listen to what the person tells me and ask questions; after all, they know their body and its reactions the best. A sensitive person will tell you that he or she reacts to different foods and drinks and needs to be careful as things may react. Sensitive people are careful people, more cautious than the average person.

An ultra sensitive person will be quite different in that she will explain "violent" reactions and be very suspicious or careful about any supplement indeed, she may even be paranoid or highly anxious when you recommend various dietary supplements. She will have experienced significant aggravations in the past with even the smallest dose of any dietary supplement or drug. She will have been like this for most of her life and be a real challenge in the clinic. There is little you can do with the ultra sensitive patient in terms of dosage recommendations, it is best to give her a few tablets or capsules to take home in order for her to work out her sensitivity to these substances, otherwise they will return the product within three days. I figure that about ten percent of the population is sensitive, and about two percent of this group is ultra sensitive. Its what keeps us on our toes as practitioners, and the longer you see people like I have the more you will be familiar with sensitive and ultra sensitive people.

Do I Take My Dietary Supplements With Or Away From Meals Or Snacks?

We always get asked this question. The answer to this is quite simple, because vitamins and minerals are naturally found in foods, in most all cases you should take them with meals or snacks. Digestive enzymes are best taken at the beginning of a meal, but if you take several then take some at the beginning, during, and at the end of the meal. Omega 3 supplements, vitamin D and any fat-soluble vitamins are best taken with a bit of oil or a fatty meal for enhanced absorption. Multivitamins are best taken in the middle of a meal.

Probiotics are best taken on rising, retiring and before lunch. A lot of this is also trial and error; some can only take supplements away from meals, others only with. In the long run, it does not really matter, because if you are taking a supplement for several months you will absorb what is in it if you eat well, chew foods well and rest up.

Are You Aggravating Even On The Lowest Possible Dose?

It can happen, and if you find that even at the lowest possible dosages on supplementation program I have outlined below. If you are having any problems even with the lowest dosages, some of these measures may be helpful:

1. **Activated Charcoal.** A good option if you have an upset stomach or are suffering from gas or bloating during the Big Clean-Up, it helps to absorbs toxins from the digestive tract. When using activated charcoal, it is best to take it between meals and a few hours before or after taking any medications or supplements, as it is so effective in absorbing things that it may interfere with the action of these. Take with water only. Good to take if you go travelling or to a party and feel that you have an upset digestion after food when you are on the Candida Crusher Program. Don't freak if your stools turn a black color, as this is normal with charcoal supplementation.

2. **St Mary's Thistle.** A great herb to use in conjunction with any detoxification program. Good if you experience any nausea when you are on the Candida Crusher Program. Helps the liver with clearing toxins, assists in bile production and clearing. Good for skin problems when on the C.C. Program.

    Epsom Salts. This is also known as Magnesium sulphate, it is perfect for the Bowel Purge when you start The Big Clean-Up, just before you commence the C.C. Program. Can also be used very effectively for constipation, and can also be used to clear the digestive system gently anytime you feel you are aggravating, just use a small dose.

3. **Filtered or Pure Water.** Quite bad aggravations? Just drink water, avoid all other beverages including herbal tea and just drink good quality water. This is a good option if you have been experiencing a major aggravation and want a quick resolution. Keep your diet basic and simple and rest up plenty; your aggravation will soon pass.

3. **Aloe Vera Liquid.** Aloe Vera is an excellent aid when it comes to aggravations. It helps to soothe the lining of the stomach and intestines and supports natural digestion. Aloe can help maintain healthy intestinal bacteria throughout the C.C. Program, and supports the immune system and is excellent in both constipation and diarrhea. It ticks all the boxes when it comes to supporting the digestive system during any yeast infection treatment aggravation. It is one of my favourite natural medicines with detox in particular.

I don't recommend that you do all of these 5 options, and this is just a rather small list of some of your best natural aids to support your digestive system if you aggravate.

The Candida Crusher Supplementation Recommendations

These are the five supplements I recommend you to take during the program. You should find that if you include the Candida Crushing foods previously outlined in the chapter, along with these supplements, that you really should not need to take any additional products for the duration of your yeast infection treatment.

The Candida Crusher products will be released in 2013, you will know of their release by joining our mailing list or by visiting yeastinfection.org or candidacrusher.com

1. The Candida Crusher Formula

2. The Candida Crusher Multi Vitamin

3. The Candida Crusher Digestive enzyme

4. The Candida Crusher Probiotic

5. The Candida Crusher Omega 3

The 4-R Program Outlining Supplementation

1 **Remove** offending foods, crush candida and correct nutritional deficiencies: Follow the 3-Stage Candida Crusher Diet as outlined in section 1 of chapter 7. Consider antimicrobial, antifungal, and antiparasitic treatment in the case of opportunistic/ pathogenic bacterial, yeast, and/or parasite overgrowth (the Candida Crusher Formula). Take the Candida Crusher Multi to correct any deficiencies.

2 **Replace** what is needed for normal digestion and absorption: Take the Candida Crusher Digestive Enzyme to significantly improve digestion and absorption.

3 **Reinoculate** with favorable microbes: Take the Candida Crusher Probiotic to enhance the growth of the favorable bacteria, supplement with prebiotics such as the correct fibers in your diet.

4 **Repair** digestive system cells: Repair the leaky gut and the immune system. Reduce the inflammatory response by taking the Candida Crusher Omega 3 and the Candida Crusher Probiotic.

How Long Should You Take The Supplements?

There are many factors that account for how long you will need to take the supplements for. I don't like to put time frames on anything really. There always seems to be some unforeseen circumstance like moving house, a job change, marriage, a sudden acute illness, etc.; that can come out of nowhere, have you noticed? Such events or happenings in our lives place additional stresses on us and can cause setbacks with our treatment. It is the unpredictability of life with these unforeseen circumstances that may mean that we need to take additional nutritional support for longer than we initially think.

Basically, you take the products for as long as you need them, some will need them for two months only, others will require them for six months or longer. As a general rule, I would say that four to six months is about the right time to take the Candida Crusher formulations, in varying dosages depending on your situation. Some people will want to stay on a maintenance dose of most of the products on/off for some time until they have a permanent resolution from their yeast infection, and with severe or chronic cases this can take twelve to eighteen months.

When can I stop taking them? You stop taking any dietary supplement when you no longer derive any or limited benefit from it. It is simply wrong for any company to suggest that you need to stay on supplements continually. Stop them periodically and see how you feel, then recommence. If you notice an improvement on recommencement, you may want to stay of this particular product a little longer.

1 The Candida Crusher Formula

The Candida Crusher Formula is the cornerstone and key product in the Candida Crusher Program, a product that helps to reduce the reproduction and assists in ridding the body of yeasts, bacteria and parasites. This is an excellent formulation that works time and again, consistently, and when used as directed without causing any unnecessary aggravations.

The time to start taking this product is not the very first day you begin the Candida Crusher Program, I'd recommend you do the Big Clean-Up first. (see section 1)

The Candida Crusher Formula dosage will be one a day (with supper/dinner) for three days, then take one with lunch and one with supper for three days. On the third day, take one three times daily, i.e. one with each meal. The duration of treatment varies widely, some people may want to use it for a month whereas others may still wish to take it after one year, but the average duration of treatment with this product is three to six months.

Some people believe that a formula such as this cannot be taken with a probiotic, this is not the case. Pharmaceutical antibiotics kill beneficial bacteria as well as bad bacteria, whilst allowing yeasts to thrive. The natural antifungal and antibacterial agents like garlic, oregano, caprylic and undecylenic acid don't, but it still is best to take this Formula with meals and the probiotic between meals or away from foods. I prefer that patients take the probiotic on rising (before breakfast) and on retiring (before bedtime) for that reason, the Candida Crusher Formula is a powerful product and you may get some degree of friendly bacteria inhibition if you use it at the same time as the probiotic, so just take them apart to be on the safe side.

You may want to join my mailing list or keep an eye on You Tube to find out when it will be released. The formula contains all the nutrients and herbs I have described in this section.

2 The Candida Crusher Multivitamin and Mineral

The Candida Crusher Multi Vitamin & Mineral is a synergistic and comprehensive combination of vitamins, minerals, trace elements, herbal medicines including specialized nutrients which have been carefully formulated and specifically designed to offer the most comprehensive nutritional support in those affected by bacterial overgrowth, parasites and in particular a yeast infection.

It is important if you have a yeast infection that you get the right nutrients to maintain good health and for the optimal functioning of the body's structure and its various systems, including gastrointestinal and immune system.

The Candida Crusher Multi Vitamin & Mineral was specifically designed with the yeast infection patient in mind, it contains the correct and balanced proportion of vitamins, minerals, trace elements along with other more specialized nutrients without the danger of long term side-effects or a harmful build-up of nutrients. Particular consideration has been given to the absorbability as well as the synergistic action of each ingredient, because those with yeast infections often have compromised digestive, gastrointestinal and immune systems.

Certain ingredients such as antioxidants are in higher amounts due to the critical role they play in protecting your body from the toxins produced by candida, other ingredients have been increased to ensure constant energy production, because those with candida have a tendency to become fatigued more easily.

The Candida Crusher Multi Vitamin & Mineral offers intensive support for the optimal functioning of a body affected by yeast, bacteria and parasites, in addition to vitamins and minerals, it contains additional specialized nutrients and herbal medicines targeted to support, protect and defend the body under stress of a yeast infection.

Healthy people generally have healthy levels of beneficial bacteria providing a symbiotic relationship in their digestive system, ensuring that they get additional nutritional benefits from this healthy balance. Those with a yeast infection tend to have a more disturbed balance and lack these benefits and often have lower intestinal numbers of the friendly bacteria. Therefore The Candida Crusher Multi Vitamin and Mineral even contains additional probiotics to ensure that a more harmonious balance is maintained, I really don't believe that you can take too many probiotics when you have candida.

3 The Candida Crusher Digestive Enzyme

One of the very first places candida takes a foothold is in the digestive system where it creates an environment that allows it to thrive. But this comes at a cost to the you the host as it compromises various digestive processes, preventing it from fully absorbing vitamins and minerals, increasing acidity in the intestines, allowing other bad bugs like disease causing bacteria and parasites to thrive and reducing enzymatic activity. By allowing these processes to take place, candida to become established in the digestive tract, weakening the person's overall health due to potentially creating mal-absorption of many of the nutrients critical for the countless chemical processes to occur in your body. The pH of the digestive system becomes slightly altered, allowing an unfavorable environment for of other pathogens while the digestive enzyme levels become compromised creating several problems for the body.

Digestive enzymes are essential when you have a yeast infection, they allow foods to break down into useable nutrients, and especially where there is a candida overgrowth that potentially affects digestive enzymes in the stomach and small intestine. The best digestive enzyme dietary supplements contain enzymes that support the digestion of protein, carbohydrates and fats.

Supplemental pancreatic enzymes (amylase and pancreatin in particular) and supplemental protein-targeting enzymes (known as proteolytic) will reduce the discomfort caused by any Herxheimer (die-off) reactions. Some of the most beneficial digestive enzyme products contain betaine hydrochloric acid and pepsin.

It normally takes anywhere from two to six months to seriously improve the health of the digestive system, and as I have previously mentioned, even longer in severe cases, I have know some patients with chronic yeast infections who required treatment with digestive enzymes for a two full years. These are frequently the patients who have long been given up and "discarded" by many other health-care professionals as being "impossible" cases. They seem to react to everything in their environment and have a diet limited to a half a dozen foods. They have little or no energy, mood disorders, and generally an extremely poor quality of life. They have had every test known to man performed on them, all to no avail, and they are sometimes seen as "mental cases", when in fact they are in serious need of full digestive rejuvenation.
Yes, I have seen such impossible cases improve considerably, and sometimes all these seemingly impossible folks need is an ongoing digestive enzyme, probiotic and multi vitamin. Make sure if your digestion does not improve to try the Stomach Tolerance Method outlined soon.

Why Should You Take an Enzyme Formula?

There are several different reasons why you would want to take an enzyme formula when you have a yeast infection, but the three main reasons are:

1. Digestive Reasons: to assist in the breakdown and absorption of foods.

2. Candida Crushing: to assist in the breakdown of candida itself.

3. Inflammation: to assist in healing the gut

After using digestive enzymes with yeast infection patients many years ago, I started to work out that they are best taken if you are serious about recovering from a yeast infection. The Candida Crusher Digestive Enzyme has been designed to work synergistically with the other four Candida Crusher products. You take this product just before a meal, and if you need several (after having completed the "stomach tolerance method", see below) just spread them out at the beginning, during and at the end of the meal. There is no advantage taking these enzymes between meals, take the probiotic rather away from or in between meals.

Enzymes For More Than Just Digestive Reasons

I have discovered that many patients with yeast infections seem to feel that much better when they take a good enzymatic formula. Their digestive system becomes damaged and inflamed by a yeast infection overgrowth and supplemental enzymes can assist with the healing process and facilitate gut healing which increases recovery time. That's why it is especially important that you take the digestive enzymes not only when you begin the Candida Crusher Diet, but throughout the whole C.C. Program and beyond, as these dietary changes may be quite foreign to your body and the habits you learn through the whole process may take some time before they become fully engrained into your daily life.

There may be slight pH changes in your digestive system and shifts in the bacterial population, and initially there will be the regular garbage that needs shifting out of your bowel, it's a bit like sweeping a floor that has not been cleaned thoroughly for many years. Many people will notice that they pass out bowel plaques, some mucous and either an increasing amount of bowel motions or larger stools, especially those who were on processed or diets high in refined or junk foods to begin with. Do enzymes assist in the cleansing process? I know they do because of the feedback I've received from the many patients who have undergone The Big Clean-Up before starting the MEVY Diet.

As far as inflammation is concerned, your digestive system is quite a dynamic place with many areas that can become potentially damaged by the inflammatory responses of a leaky gut, food allergies, parasites, and bacterial in addition to yeast overgrowth. Enzymes will help counter this inflammation, assist in breaking down any garbage and even help to counter the yeast overgrowth.

How Long Do I Need To Take The Digestive Enzymes?

This will vary from person to person. I've found that it can take about 4-6 months on average to heal the gut, especially if the diet is adhered to and probiotics are taken as well. But in some severe yeast infection cases I've worked with it has taken as long as 12–18 months for the healing to take place. I do urge you to take them and give them a good try; it may cut your recovery time by as much as half. Everybody seems to think that a good probiotic formula and a candida kill product are all you need when you have a yeast infection, but I believe that this is not the case, and trial and error with many patients especially the past few years has shown me this.

Some people find they need enzymes with every meal, some with every meal as well as any snack foods they consume whereas others will find that they only require them occasionally with meals, especially meals containing meats. It's all about trial and error, and only experimentation will reveal your individual requirements so you may want to experiment to see which method gives you best results.

For the average yeast infection patient I recommend that they take one dose of the Candida Crusher Digestive Enzyme twice daily for the first three to four weeks to assist digestion as well as to assist in the elimination of yeast toxins, particularly once they start the MEVY Diet. This is primarily because they will be changing their diet and increasing the amount of protein (meat, eggs, chicken, fish, etc.) as well as vegetable matter they will be eating. Generally this means that they supplement with the digestive enzymes with lunch and dinner.

Increase or decrease the dosage to suit your own needs, and your bowel motions and level of digestive comfort will generally be a good guide as how much digestive enzyme to take. Unless you eat a high protein breakfast, it is best to take a digestive enzyme with your lunch and evening meal, but for those with known food allergies try one with breakfast, lunch and one with dinner. I have found that digestive enzymes are particularly effective for those with food allergies and food intolerances.

You may like to try the "stomach tolerance method" to determine how many digestive enzymes you need, especially if you have any signs or symptoms of hypo-chlorhydria (an underactive stomach). I have found this common in those with chronic candida, especially in those over the age of fifty.

Signs and Symptoms of Low Stomach Acid

- Stomach aching/pain/ discomfort or bloating after meals

- Feel unwell/fatigued right after meals

- Food or water 'sits in stomach'

- High protein or fat foods cause nausea/stomach upset

- Undigested food in stool

- Reflux and/or heartburn

- Poor appetite or feel overly full easily

- Poor fingernail health/splitting easily/white flecks

- Multiple food sensitivities

- Trouble digesting red meat

- Constipation

- Low iron levels

- Frequent low-grade nausea

- Nausea/reflux after supplements (e.g. fish oil)

- Burping after meals

- Thin, weak or fragile hair

Good Tip

The Stomach Tolerance Method

The best way to determine how much digestive enzyme supplementation you require is to do the Stomach Tolerance Method. Capsules are taken in increasing doses with meals until symptoms of excess acid are evident, at which time you would cut back on how many capsules or tablets taken. This is what a typical digestive enzyme "tummy tolerance" program would look like:

Meal 1 – Take 1 cap or tab at the beginning of your meal.

Meal 2 - Take 2 caps or tabs at the beginning of your meal.

Meal 3 - Take 3 caps or tabs at the beginning of your meal.

Meal 4 - Take 4 caps or tabs, two at the beginning of your meal and two in the middle of your meal, and so on, up to 8 capsules per meal.

NOTES: When taking several caps or tabs they will help you more if you take them throughout the meal (beginning, middle and end). For individuals that are daring and want more rapid results, you could increase the dose by two tabs or caps each meal instead of one. If any irritation occurs (heartburn, stomachache, heaviness, nausea), you can take baking soda in water to neutralize the excess acidity (1/2 teaspoon of baking soda in 250mls of warm water), but sip it only long enough to alleviate the symptoms. At your next meal you would take 1-2 caps or tabs less than the number that caused symptoms. Sometimes small meals (or those with little protein) do not require as many caps or tabs as required for a larger meal. Remember that symptoms of high stomach acid are exactly the same as low stomach acid, i.e. heartburn, stomachaches, a sense of heaviness behind the sternum and low-grade nausea.

Precautions

Avoid The Candida Crusher Digestive Enzyme if you have a peptic ulcer or take an anti-inflammatory drug like aspirin, Inodicin, Motrin, or Butazolidin.

4   The Candida Crusher Probiotic

What Are Probiotics?

A probiotic is a microorganism introduced into the body for its beneficial qualities. There are many different types and strains of beneficial bacteria, and the Candida Crusher Probiotic contains some of the best strains that have proven to excel in repopulating the digestive system and discouraging the pathogenic bacteria from returning. Unlike many probiotics on the market, the Candida Crusher Probiotic is stable at room temperature with a shelf life of two years.

Normally the intestinal wall is densely covered with over 500 hundred different species of microbes grouped essentially in three types:

The Beneficial Bacteria. The good guys, you may have heard of beneficial bacteria such as Lactobacillus acidophilus or Bifidobacterium bifidus, these are but two of the many different bacteria which are beneficial and essential to our good health.

The Commensals. These bacteria form a symbiotic relationship in which the entire bacterial population of the digestive system is benefitted, but the other bacteria are neither benefited nor harmed. Commensals can go good or bad depending on the level of beneficial or pathogenic bacteria. I call these guys the "politicians" of the gut; they can swing weight either way depending on the majority.

The Pathogenic Bacteria. These are the nasty guys; they can harm other bacteria but are kept in balance by the beneficial bacteria. When we take beneficial bacteria (probiotics) continually during candida treatment, the bad bacteria will find it more difficult to get a foothold on the intestinal wall and the commensals tend to swing more towards behaving themselves rather than misbehaving, and with a good anti-fungal supplement such as the Candida Crusher Formula along with the Candida Crusher Probiotic, the pathogenic bacterial population will decline and a harmonious balance will be maintained once again in the intestinal tract.

Therefore we must first make some free space in the digestive system by not only taking the Candida Crusher Formula which will inhibit and control the yeast infection, but also include in our diet specialized anti-fungal foods like which you can read about at the beginning of this section. With more space and a less hostile environment, the beneficial probiotic bacteria can more easily occupy the vacated spaces at the intestinal wall, and crowd out the yeasts and bad bacteria.

Why Should You Take A Probiotic When You Have A Yeast Infection?

Try not to consider the probiotic supplement as a supplement, but rather as a beneficial food instead. That way you won't think to yourself "Well, I'll just take these pills for a few weeks, and when I feel better I'll stop taking them". Is that how you feel about beneficial foods like yogurt, garlic and coconut too? We tend to view dietary supplements as just that, something to supplement our diet with for a short period of time and then to discontinue them. But probiotics are different in that they are beneficial bacteria that have spectacular effects on our health and their fragile populations are easily compromised due to the very way we eat and live. You will find that by taking them for a long period of time that your will miraculously appear to keep on improving in many different ways, and that's because they are involved in so many different processes affecting your health.

It is therefore important to take a high quality probiotic supplement like the Candida Crusher Probiotic in addition to regularly consuming live yogurt and other fermented and cultured foods (see section 1) as part of the Candida Crusher Diet, that way you are guaranteed to continually re-populate your digestive system with these friendly bacteria. This "Body Ecology" concept as promoted by leading health experts such as Sally Fallon (Nourishing Traditions, New Trends Publishing Inc., 1999) and Donna Gates (The Body Ecology Diet, Body Ecology Publishing; 1996) becomes a very important consideration when you have a yeast infection. If you are serious about a permanent resolution of your yeast infection, and I assume that's why you purchased this book, then you will most certainly want to develop a life-long habit of encouraging the continual reproduction as well as growth of many species of the beneficial bacteria. Can you recall in section 1 that we spoke of the "bad bugs are calling your name"? this implies that the yeasts within you are hungry and want you to consume food for them in the form of refined carbohydrates and simple sugars. These sugar cravings (often after a meal) are not unlike owning a cat the cries out to you each time you come into your kitchen, you love your cat, so you give in and feed the cat, don't you now?

When Do You Take Probiotics?

Some experts say to always take probiotics away from foods while others I have spoken to say to always take probiotics with meals. So what do you do? Well, the most important thing to do is to, just take the pro-biotics. But because you are not taking the probiotic in isolation to other products, but you are taking the probiotic with a product (the Candida Crusher Formula) that strongly inhibits and actively eradicates bad bacteria and yeasts, it does pay to separate them.

Some people believe that beneficial bacteria are degraded and destroyed in the stomach, and that nothing survives the stomach bypass because the "acid kills all the beneficial bacteria". A long time ago, people used to eat foods rich in lactic acid and loaded in beneficial bacteria and did not ever have to rely on taking pro-biotics. My grandmother used to make large quantities of sauerkraut in summer that would be consumed all winter long. Do you think she paid any attention to when the sauerkraut was to be eaten? It was eaten as a side-serve along with foods like sausage, mash and gravy; sometimes it was eaten alone, sometimes with meat.

Take your pro-biotics with food, or away, in my opinion it makes little difference especially if you take them long-term and on an on-going basis. Like any dietary supplements, the hard part is just to remember to take them regularly every day and if you take a supplement long enough, you will get in into the system.

And for this reason I'm not that happy with the refrigerated kind of probiotics, and much prefer a "non-refrigeration" and dairy-free product. Are you going to remember to go to the refrigerator twice or three times a day to take your probiotic? Can you take the refrigerator with you on your journey?

The dosage is one capsule twice daily with meals. Take on an ongoing basis with candida. How long? I recommend with serious cases for at least 6 and sometimes for as long as 12 months continually, seven days a week.

Good advice is to introduce the Candida Crusher Probiotic and the Candida Crusher Formula about ten to fourteen days after you commence the MEVY Diet, no point taking these products during The Big Clean-Up; you are trying to purge and clean the bowel out and will only be wasting your money and efforts. Give yourself a week or two on the diet and then commence with these two supplements.

Stay On The Probiotic, Especially With Carb Re-Introduction

By taking the Candida Crusher Formula with meals and the Candida Crusher Probiotic on rising and retiring over a prolonged period of time, you can over time regenerate a healthy intestinal flora, especially if you understand the concept of a healthy balance in your life of work and play, exercise, relaxation, healthy foods, etc. However, if you don't follow up your yeast elimination with the Candida Crusher Probiotic, then as you are on the road to recovery and you slowly begin to ingest increasing amounts of carbohydrates (especially the refined ones, the sugars), the yeast overgrowth may quickly multiply and fill the empty spaces again. This often occurs when a patient I see starts to notice significant improvements and then starts to eat bread again, drinks wine and slowly slides back into the dietary behavioral patterns they originally had which caused the problems. All of a sudden they feel terrible and experience a reoccurrence.

However, with more serious and chronic yeast infections, it may take much longer to eliminate the spores and fungal roots growing through the intestinal wall. Therefore we need to be particularly careful vigilant and continue avoiding or minimizing drugs, alcohol, sweet foods and many different kinds of chemicals, and use a suitable diet as I have outlined in section 1 of this chapter. Sometimes it can take as long as a year or more of being hyper-vigilant if you have been seriously unwell, but there comes a time when you will most certainly is able to return to your old self again, all in good time.

Don't Be Quick To Stop Taking The Pro-Biotics

Some books I have read on yeast infection treatments say not to give the pro-biotics *until after* the treatment phase. I do believe this is a mistake. If you have not re-established beneficial bacteria, and candida still prevails in your intestinal tract, then candida may potentially re-grow after each dose of anti-fungal medicine, and it may take longer to control it. You may be eating commercial chicken again (containing commercial antibiotics) or be taking a pharmaceutical drug contributing to bad bacteria again at this stage.

As candida is naturally present in small amounts in a person's digestive tract, it is not desirable to eliminate all of it from the intestines, nor is it really possible – it will simply grow back to the state it was before you developed the overgrowth. The key point is that the dominant species will remain dominant unless we do something that kills the over population of the bad bacteria and the candida fungus. And with an imbalanced bowel flora, the dominant species can either be the friendly bacteria or the unfriendly ones.

Don't be quick to stop taking the pro-biotics, these should be the last nutritional supplements you continue to take, and continue with them until you feel really well, and when all symptoms abate then take them for at least a month or two longer. I have always found it beneficial and highly advisable to recommend pro-biotics regularly during the prolonged anti-candida therapy, and especially *for some time after* completing the therapy. These are the patients who stay better for longer.

Are You A Sensitive Yeast Infection Patient?

For the sensitive patients, i.e.; those who react quite strongly to any anti-microbial treatment, for once a day you may like to try to take the Candida Crusher Probiotic 30 to 60 minutes *after* the Candida Crusher Formula and *definitely before* consuming any carbohydrate foods or drinks. Alternatively, frequently consume lactic acid fermented foods like yoghurt and/or sauerkraut, miso soup, tempeh, quark, etc. After finishing the anti-microbial therapy continue to take the pro-biotics for one to two months before breakfast (on rising) and after dinner (on retiring). The last four to eight weeks of pro-biotic treatment just take a dose before bedtime.

Even after what you and most probably your health-care professional deem as successful therapy, candida spores and dormant microbes may remain in your body and re-emerge when we you chronically stressed, just like the herpes virus. As your immune system gets stronger, you will eventually get over the candida. Therefore, repeat the pro-biotic treatment whenever candida or gut infection-related symptoms re-appear. Remember – don't be in a hurry to stop the pro-biotics, most patients do in my experience and this is one of the key ways to fail with treating a case of chronic candida successfully. The "rebuild" phase is in many ways more important than the actual "kill" phase along with the dietary changes that most practitioners seem to focus on. It can take many, many months to rebuild and often just one to several weeks to kill candida. Please be a *patient* patient!

I have found that the "extremely sensitive" patients with multiple allergies and multiple food intolerances generally should proceed very slowly indeed, good advice for them is remain on the Hypo-Allergenic (stage 2) Diet, use anti-inflammatory remedies, such as slippery elm powder before meals and ginger with meals, and introduce probiotics, lactic acid fermented food and anti-microbial products only *very gradually* over a four week period. They may not even be able in some cases be able to tolerate the Candida Crusher Formula for a month when they start therapy, but eventually will. Either way, all dosages of supplements need to be very carefully and slowly increased over time.

 5 The Candida Crusher Omega 3 What is an Omega 3 Supplement?

Omega-3 fatty acids are considered essential fatty acids, they are necessary for human health because your body can' t make them, you have to get them through your diet. There are many different types of Omega 3 fatty acids, but the two predominant ones are eicosapentaenoic acid (EPA) and docosahexaenoic acid (DHA). Also known as polyun-saturated fatty acids (PUFAs), omega-3 fatty acids play a critical role in normal growth and development as well as brain function. They are also important in reducing the risk of heart disease, cancer, arthritis, diabetes, and many other chronic and degenerative diseases.

Omega 3 fatty acids are concentrated in the brain and nervous system and have proven to be important for cognitive (brain memory and performance) and behavioural as well as mood function. Symptoms of omega-3 fatty acid deficiency include fatigue, poor memory, dry skin, heart problems, mood swings or depression, poor circulation, reduced immune function and an increased risk of an imbalanced inflammatory response in the body.

We Get Too Much Omega 6 In Our Diet, And Not Enough Omega 3

The correct ratio of fatty acids is important to have in our diet. For example, omega 3 helps to reduce inflammation whereas most omega 6 fatty acids tend to promote inflammation. A typical diet in most Western nations can contain 20 or even 30 times more Omega 6 fatty acids than mega 3 fatty acids, which most nutritional experts consider to be much to high in favour of Omega 6. The ideal ratio is 1:1, and many years ago before fats and oils were highly processed as they are today, people consumed a healthier balance of these two fatty acids..

What Are The Best Dietary Sources Of Omega 3?

I recommend that you take the Candida Crusher Omega 3 as well as supplement your diet with dietary sources of omega 3. While you can get omega 3 from your diet, you won't generally consume enough of the omega 3 rich foods to get the inflammatory response you are looking for with this wonderful supplement.

There are many sources of obtaining Omega 3 through your diet, but fish, plant and nut oils are considered to be the primary sources. The omega 3 fatty acids eicosapentaenoic acid (EPA) and docosahexaenoic acid (DHA) are found in cold-water fish such as herring, sardines, tuna, halibut, mackerel and salmon. The other important fatty acid is called alpha linolenic acid (ALA), it is found in flax seeds, canola (rapeseed) oil, walnuts and walnut oil, purslane, pumpkin seeds and pumpkin seed oil, soybeans and soybean oil as well as perilla seed.

Fish, plant, and nut oils are the primary dietary source of omega-3 fatty acids. Eicosapentaenoic acid (EPA) and docosahexaenoic acid (DHA) are found in cold-water fish such as salmon, mackerel, halibut, sardines, tuna, and herring. ALA is found in flaxseeds, flaxseed oil, canola (rapeseed) oil, soybeans, soybean oil, pumpkin seeds and pumpkin seed oil, purslane, perilla seed oil, walnuts, and walnut oil. Most of the health benefits from omega 3 are conferred by DHA and EPA, but ALA can be converted in the body to EPA and DHA although many people have problems with this conversion pathway that is dependent on many nutrients

Why Would You Need Omega 3 With A Yeast Infection?

I believe that omega 3 supplementation with a yeast infection is one of the best-kept secrets, and not commonly promoted as being necessary. All the focus appears to be on antifungals and probiotics, but you rarely hear about the necessity of taking omega 3 supplements when you have a yeast infection.

Omega 3 can help your digestive system in different ways when you have a yeast infection; there are four main reasons why I believe omega 3 is essential with candida:

1. To protect cell membranes from damage due to yeast toxins.

2. To reduce inflammation in the digestive system due to yeast.

3. To boost immune function in general.

4. To directly inhibit and kill candida albicans.

Cell Membrane Protection

Omega 3 helps protect your cell membranes from many different types of toxins, and as yeast cells die they produce various toxins that can irritate and inflame the cells lining your small intestine in particular. These are the kinds of reactions that can cause subtle aggravations, and omega 3 is known to counter reactions such as these.

Reducing Inflammatory Responses

In addition, omega 3 oils have substantial anti-inflammatory properties, and one of the most important reasons to supplement with omega 3 during the Candida Crusher Diet is to reduce the impact of any potential inflammatory reactions that may occur in your digestive system and anywhere else in your body, especially if you have a chronic or serious yeast infection which may have become systemic.

Having an imbalance in your digestive tract of the beneficial and pathogenic microbes and yeasts may spell an inflammatory response, and a CDSA (functional stool test) may well reveal an elevation in an inflammatory marker such as lysozyme or calprotectin. To understand more about CDSA or stool testing for yeast, please go to chapter 3.

An elevation of lysozyme or calprotectin (biomarkers of inflammation, labs may use one or the other marker) is an indication of intestinal inflammation, and it may be an indication of inflammatory bowel disease (ulcerative colitis or Crohn's disease), but may be found in celiac patients as well. I have found these biomarkers elevated in those with a yeast infection as well, especially with serious cases. It is important to rule out inflammatory bowel disease or gluten issues, so keep an eye out for the yeast panel and see how many out of the three stool samples contain yeast. (You did ask for a CDSA x 3, didn't you?) You will generally find an elevation of yeasts in two or three samples out of three tested, and in addition the key signs and symptoms of a yeast infection.

Immune Support

Omega 3 EFAs have such a positive effect on several aspects of your immune function, and supporting your immune system makes good sense if you are trying to beat your yeast infection and fully recover. One of the best ways to counter digestive inflammation is to ensure you have a regular intake of omega 3.

Yeast Killing Potential

A study* involving oral health in Kentucky, USA in 2010 revealed that omega 3 EFAs could have a positive therapeutic effect for improving oral health via their antifungal and antibacterial activities, besides their anti-inflammatory effects.

The omega 3 fatty acids EPA, DHA) and ALA, were analyzed for anti fungal and anti bacterial activity against oral pathogens. The experimental data indicated that omega 3 and their ester derivatives exhibited strong anti fungal and antibacterial activity against various oral pathogens, including Streptococcus mutans, Candida albicans, Aggregatibacter actinomycetemcomitans, Fusobacterium nucleatum, and Porphyromonas gingivalis.

I have read other similar studies and believe that omega 3, just like other fatty acids such as caprylic acid, undecylenic acid and even olive oil, all have the capability to inhibit and kill candida. Are you consuming these regularly? The more you do and the wider range of healthy fats you consume the more you will be increasing your chances of permanently eradicating your yeast infection.

- Huang, C. B., et al. A novel bioactivity of omega-3 polyunsaturated fatty acids and their ester derivatives. Mol Oral Microbiol. 25(1):75-80, 2010. Center for Oral Health Research, College of Dentistry, University of Kentucky, Lexington, KY, USA.

Dosage

Take one capsule of the Candida Crusher Omega 3 twice daily with meals. You can take this product from the beginning and continue on until well after you have recovered from your yeast infection. The omega 3, probiotic and the multi are three dietary supplements you will want to continue on for as long as you can, they are cornerstones and form a foundation for a great level of continual health and wellbeing. Why stop taking a supplement that keeps you feeling great and reduces your chances of chronic ill health?

SECTION 5

Candida Crusher Lifestyle – Understanding the Healthy Lifestyle

> *Your lifestyle - how you live, eat, think and express emotions will determine your health. To prevent disease, you may have to change how you live.*
> *Brian Carter*

Your lifestyle should be your main concern as far as yeast infection recovery is concerned, and that is why I have left some of what I consider to be some of the best information until last.

As far back as 1983, Dr. William Crook (*The Yeast Connection*) pointed out that the influence of lifestyle was paramount in both the creation and the ultimate recovery from a yeast infection.

Dr. Crook's writings of almost 30 years ago mentioned that unless those with yeast infections changed their lifestyle to reduce the causative factors, complete healing was seldom accomplished. I have certainly discovered this to be the case in my practice and have noticed that those patients who are the most committed to recognizing the causes of their yeast infection and make the appropriate diet and lifestyle changes long-term are the ones who get the best results.

But how long does it take you ask, how long do I have to keep eating the diet, how long do I have to change my ways until I get well? When can I get back to the foods I love to eat like ice cream, refined foods, alcohol, candy, etc.? If you are starting to think like this you are probably not going to really recover and you probably don't have what it takes to fully recover either, to be perfectly honest. I don't want you to think that you need to be looking at delayed gratification with your new diet and your new lifestyle, these are going to have to be modified and stay modified until you are 100 percent and then some more. Once these new elements become so engrained into your being they will most probably stay like this and become part of the "new you". You will be able to adopt some of your former ways again, but wait until you have fully recovered, that way you will be able to discover the true nature of cause and effect more easily, i.e.; if you start to eat Twinkies, chocolate, or drink beer every day again and get itchy, feel bloated and have gas, then that is cause and effect, simple as that!

Lifestyle elements are frequently both the primary cause as well as the maintaining causes of a yeast infection that stand squarely in the way of healing. When you come to recognize and understand these particular factors in your own lifestyle, then you will have finally discovered that the power is really in your own hands to fully recover, by making the necessary changes long-term.

Then why you are asking is the lifestyle section the last section in this chapter?

I wanted you to get a really good grasp of the other concepts such as eating the right foods and avoiding the wrong ones, understanding about how stress affects your immune system, learning how to clean up your body through detoxification and learning about the best special foods and supplements which help to eradicate your yeast infection.

If you have read sections 1 – 4 of this chapter carefully, then you will have noticed that these sections contain many elements of lifestyle modification already.

Take your time and read this section all the way through because if you can fully grasp the message contained and implement the suggestions herein, I promise you that happiness and a much greater state of health will be awaiting you.

The Pareto 80/20 Concept

Healing yourself from a yeast infection requires a combination of things we have spoken about at length throughout the five sections of this chapter, but most importantly, it requires some kind of balance. The eighty/twenty balance is a concept that can help you put these factors into perspective.

An Italian economist named Pareto created a mathematical formula in 1906 to describe the distribution of unequal wealth in his country at the time. Pareto noticed that twenty percent of the population owned eighty percent of the country's wealth.

This 80/20 principle can be applied to help you manage your yeast infection, and your life in general more effectively.

The 80 Percent

Spend eighty percent of your time concerning yourself about your lifestyle habits, including ways you can balance your work and home life and work to live (not the other way around), how you can include plenty of healthy activity and exercise into your daily life, what you do to relax every day and interact in a positive way with those around you. Family or friends may know you better than you know yourself and they on occasion give you feedback if you appear tense, stressed, anxious or get angry or impatient at times. It is more important for me as a practitioner to have you address these issues than it is to worry about what kind of fruit or grain is better for your digestive system. By spending a proportionately bigger chunk of your time working on *you* rather than on *your yeast infection*, you will have understood the immense healing power that can come from within rather than from outside your body. You body's innate ability to heal, leading to a recovery from your yeast infection may quite surprise you.

Look at ways of healthy eating we have spoken at length about in section 1, such habits include eating away from computers and TV screens, slowing down when you eat, chewing foods, etc. Do you ever leave the table feeling eighty percent full, and twenty percent empty? Or do you eat until you are almost full, and then go back for more? You should never have to go back for second helpings; it means that you are probably overfilling your stomach. By leaving the table while you are still capable of eating more, your stomach will be much more capable of processing any foods in it, and also allowing the enzymes and hydrochloric acid to deal more efficiently with the yeast infection. I wrote about the analogy of the cement mixer and the stomach in section 1, this is an important concept for you to grasp, because a cement mixer works best when it is only filled to three-quarters of its capacity just like your stomach.

As you can see, the 80/20 concepts just keep on coming up. Now is the time to drop the word "diet" from your vocabulary, it can have negative connotations and for some it means eating a certain way for a while, and then slowly sliding back into their regular eating pattern. I use the word Candida Crusher "Diet" to show you the healthy eating principles which are not only important overcome a yeast infection, but to remain in great health for many years to come. Once you customize and adopt many of these eating habits into your own life, you won't think of your newly adopted habits and food choices as a diet but rather as an eating style that makes you feel consistently great.

The 20 Percent

Spend about twenty percent of your time being more focused on your health complaints, and look at the potential issues that are building up your health, as well as issues involved right now which may be breaking down your health, maintaining your yeast infection. Are they diet related, lifestyle related, stress related, etc. Remain objective, and focus your attention from a positive and not a negative perspective, concerning yourself about the best possible ways of tackling your particular yeast infection. You may need to ask for some professional help, and don't be afraid to do so.

Unfortunately, some people with chronic yeast infections can pursue stressed-out lifestyles, thinking about how candida is affecting them, lamenting to anybody who wants to hear how bad they feel and maintain a strong focus on yeast eradication by way of a super-strict regimented diet and dozens of supplements, rather than lifestyle enhancement. And I can perfectly understand why, it's because they have not really found much long-term relief with many of the treatments they have tried, and have most probably not been taken too seriously by their doctor.

Others may become entirely absorbed in taking supplements or drugs with the aim of conquering the yeast infection almost like some sort of inner battle has to be waged. There may not as much concern with leading a balanced and relaxed lifestyle than taking products or special foods, and may pay lip service when it comes to healthy eating, including a token piece of lettuce and tomato next to their fries and glass of wine, thinking that a bunch of pills might get things right. Unfortunately, this too is not a wellness-centered approach, it is very hit and miss and will give temporary results at best. This scenario is more common than you think; I see it all the time in the clinic.

Here is a picture taken of the dietary supplements a person with a chronic yeast infection has been taking. There are more than 60 different kinds of dietary supplements, herbal and homeopathic medicines taken for years on a rotational basis. This is an extreme example of being disease focused and not wellness centered, and it is not unusual for a person who has had a yeast infection for several years to have a cupboard full of such products. And yet they still have their yeast infection, albeit with a lighter wallet.

A balanced approach to diet and lifestyle and supplementation is critical, it can get boring when you eat a perfect diet one hundred percent of the time, and some folks may begin to see you as a pain in the butt. I gave up preaching to family and friends years ago, and the only people who get my health sermons today are the ones who pay for my services, or when I give presentations to the public or at colleges.

Here Is A Brief Summary Of How 80/20 Rules Can Apply To You

- Devote eighty percent of your efforts towards your lifestyle and dietary habits when it comes to recovering from a yeast infection. Spend 20 percent of your efforts concerning yourself with the actual diet itself and treatment of inhibiting and eradicating the yeast infection by way of specialized foods, dietary supplements, essential oils and herbal medicines. Follow the Candida Crusher Diet principles and taking your dietary supplements.

- Devote eighty percent of your diet to the vegetables that grow above the ground primarily, the leafy greens and colored vegetables. Twenty percent of your diet could be a combination of animal proteins like white meats, eggs, the grains (quinoa, amaranth, millet, brown rice) nuts, and seeds as well as starchy vegetables.

- Devote eighty percent of your diet towards alkaline foods, and twenty percent towards acid based foods.

- Leave the table when you are eighty percent full, leave twenty percent of your stomach empty in order for efficient digestion to occur.

Staying In Control

> *Never let circumstances control you. You change your circumstances.*
> *Jackie Chan*

When it comes to lifestyle, your recovery is contingent not only on the foods you feed your stomach, but also on the thoughts you feed your mind and even the very beliefs you base your life on.

The important thing about the Candida Crusher Program outlined in this book is that the protocol gives you complete control over your recovery process because it has a strong focus on your attitudes and belief systems and the fact the you will need to accept full responsibility for your yeast infection. You can modify this program, customize and design it and continually adjust it as you improve to suit your personal preferences and lifestyle situation, because you are in control.

When it comes to treatment, it is best if you can work in with your health-care professional, but for many patients this may not be a reality due to many factors such as cost, travel or other specific issues.

No doubt, many of you who read this book will become your own physician, nevertheless don't be afraid to ask for help but do remain in control of your recovery at all times, and accept responsibility, you are an adult after all!

Accept Full Responsibility For Your Health

> *There are two types of pain you will go through in life, the pain of discipline and the pain of regret. Discipline weighs ounces while regret weighs tons.*
>
> *Jim Rohn*

As part of your healing process, it is important to see for yourself how you are contributing to your own yeast infection problems and how you can take charge of your own life to create the kind of health you really want. Unfortunately, some folks I've seen with yeast infections don't appear to have a strong sense of personal accountability for their own health.

But this evidence is quite obvious when it comes to health in general and not just yeast infections, because there are many high-risk behaviors such as smoking, drinking alcohol daily, eating take-out too frequently, surviving on nutritionally depleted, refined or highly processed foods and living a sedentary lifestyle which are all potentially predisposing factors in a number of chronic diseases such as diabetes, heart disease, stroke, and cancer.

I'm always optimistic nevertheless that I can encourage patients to overcome many of these high-risk behaviors and move into wellness behavioral patterns if they choose to do so.

I'm going to let you in on a secret, *are you paying attention?*

Learn to act upon the conviction that *your* health is primarily within *your* own hands, not the doctor's, your mother-in-law's, your partners; it's in *your* hands. That's what self-responsibility is all about, and so is a full and complete recovery from a yeast infection.

But why you ask is everybody around me telling me that somebody they knew just got diagnosed with cancer or heart disease? Isn't that just a consequence of getting older? Not really, there are just too many people today developing seriously chronic and avoidable diseases prematurely, self-responsibility clearly hasn't caught on in any big way and it is because many people just keep on living without any thought of the future when it comes to their health. One of the biggest factors accounting for insufficient self-responsibility in our society today is a clear lack of effective health education.

You may not have been taught a lot of the dietary and lifestyle concepts you will read about in Candida Crusher, and I encourage you to investigate your current diet and lifestyle and ask yourself why you are not getting the permanent results you desire. Maybe it's time for a change, and while I can't persuade you unless you are committed and ready to make those necessary changes, you will almost certainly discover that the amazing benefits of asserting your sovereignty and autonomy will be more than sufficient to reward your efforts.

You can have amazing health if you want to!

The 6 Principles Of Self-Responsibility

" I find your lack of faith quite disturbing. "
Darth Vader

Why should you take on the responsibility of your own health? It is too easy to get caught up in the trap of non-responsibility like some folks with a yeast infection have. Some patients I have seen believe that they are controlled by their circumstances or by their partner's choices, and not by their own choices. When you create these loopholes and booby-traps for yourself it is too easy to create destructive health patterns like avoiding exercise, eating convenience foods on the hop, drinking too much alcohol, all the while knowing that "things could be a whole lot better", but you have made the decision to defer your healthy habits until the kids move out, until you have a better job, until your finances improve, until you have left your partner who takes you for granted, or any one of a million other reasons such as "I'll wait until the 1st of January next year, that's when I'll go on a detox".

Here are 6 principles that can help you shape some more self-responsibility if you only let them:

1 **Be motivated by a desire to be happy.** You can pursue a high level of health for the sake of wanting to feel great about your life. Focus on the positive in your life and never the negative, and always know that people are as happy as they make up their minds to be. I like people to always imagine that their future will be the best time of their life. When your mind is encouraged to think positive on a daily basis, "miracles" just seem to happen. You may like to read "The Secret", a self-help book written in 2006 by Rhonda Byrne.

2 **Take control of your life.** Some of my favorite quotes are from Jim Rohn, and this is one of my personal favorites: "If you don't design your own life plan, chances are you'll fall into someone else's plan. And guess what they have planned for you? …. *Not much.*" While your family, friends, boss and co-workers may have an influence in your life, you will ultimately make your own choices and need to accept full responsibility for what good or poor health patterns occur in your own life. When you finally decide to come to terms with this level of reality, only then will you be free from the need to find lame excuses, scapegoats, or victim mentalities. At that point you will most certainly discover that the relationship between diet, lifestyle and yeast infection are inextricably linked.

3 **There is only one you.** This is very important to understand. Even though similar factors apply when it comes to people developing a yeast infection, your individual path to recovery and wellness in your situation will be different from anybody else. Try to picture yourself as being extraordinary in every way, your immune system, brain, body-build, likes and dislikes, occupation, lifestyle and diet, in fact everything is different from anybody else. This is why you will need to shape and form the Candida Crusher program to suit your own unique and individual needs. As in disease development processes, similar principles apply to most people like diet, lifestyle, stress management, exercise, etc., but you will have to tweak things to suit your own unique needs.

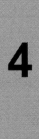

Do you have a sense of purpose? Do you have an aim in your life? If you do, having an aim and clear set of goals in your life can give you the rewards of feeling centered and content as your life progresses. For example, one of my goals was to complete the Candida Crusher and to get it into your hands, and I have achieved a great sense of satisfaction by having achieved this. What is one of your goals? I'm sure that a permanent solution to your yeast infection is on your mind, that's why you bought this book. Dr. Hans Selye (*Stress Without Distress*) discovered and documented in the 1930's that stress made people sick, always believed that a goal or definite purpose in a person's life was one of the most important and fundamental principles to positive health and wellbeing. Write down your goals and think about your purpose, your immune system will certainly benefit and so will your recovery from candida.

Don't make decisions when stressed. Postpone making any decisions until you feel better. Some patients make big or important decisions during an aggravation of their candida treatment or when they are undergoing a detox for example. These are the wrong times because you can be emotionally charged and your feelings and thoughts may be clouded with negativity or a sense of pessimism.

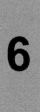

Start Today! Don't postpone the inevitable, start right NOW by making simple healthy changes and don't tell anybody about it either. How many people have you heard tell you: "I've just started a diet, I'm going to the gym now and eating healthy". Next week they have a wine glass in their hand and don't mention anything about the exercise. Just do it don't talk about it, actions speak louder than words. You will have a lot more self-respect and people will respect you more too. It's the little things you do everyday that count. Start today by moving your body more, and doing something that brings you joy and pleasure every single day. The biggest journey starts with the smallest steps – today.

Why 21st Century Living Encourages Yeast Infections

It is not hard to see why living today encourages a yeast infection. Many of us tend to live stressed and hurried lives, we eat the wrong kinds of foods and too many of them, we eat too quick, we even eat in front of TV or computer. An interesting survey recently mentioned that 1 in 8 people today globally are on Facebook and 1 in 5 people in America eat one meal of the day, either breakfast, lunch or dinner, while checking their Facebook page. This is like sending a text message while you are driving, you can your brain be engaged with eating and digesting a meal when the mind is concentrating on something else! Soda drinks and alcohol as well as copious amounts of coffee and tea are drunk every day by millions.

Many people still live in damp or poor ventilated housing or what we known in New Zealand to be "leaky buildings". Others routinely take an antibiotic or the oral contraceptive pill, antacids, statins or anti-inflammatory drugs.

There are so many reasons why we live in an age today which is just as conducive for the development and maintenance of a yeast infection as it was in the 1980's, and I suspect in the year 2050 that folks will be just as susceptible to a yeast infection. It has been estimated that over 60 million Americans alone have yeast infections.

But there are many ways we can avoid getting into this mess in the first place, and the first and foremost thing that we can do is to look carefully at what we are eating and drinking everyday, it's as simple as that.

After having read section 1, the Candida Crusher Diet, you will have gained a good understanding on avoiding certain yeast-loving foods, section 4 explains about yeast inhibiting and yeast killing foods. You will have read about raw foods, a pH balanced diet as well as importance of including those fermented and cultured foods in your diet. By implementing these dietary strategies I've outlined you are doing everything you can in a diet sense, but this is not enough!

It is especially important that you grasp the final section of this chapter, section 5, Understanding The Healthy Lifestyle. Health-care professionals are generally great at telling their patients what to eat and what to avoid as well as the correct supplements or products to take that will help to eradicate a yeast infection, but this is not enough to prevent it from coming back.

Remember what I mentioned earlier on, the 80/20 rule? Recovery will mean that you need to be focused and eighty percent of your efforts need to go into positive diet and lifestyle changes, there is little point in eating a nutritious and healthy balanced diet if you eat it in front of your widescreen every night, or you have lunch while checking how many friends "like" your comment or recent photos on Facebook.

I've learned years ago to keep away from screens when it comes to eating. I also learned to slow down and relax more and to accept that jobs I accomplish are OK at 75% and don't need to be 100% perfect! I'd like to explain about how stress can negatively impact on your immune system and the importance of relaxation when it comes to yeast infection recovery, this piece of information may be your tipping point when it comes to not only recovering from candida, but from many other health complaints that may have plagued you all your life.

Are You Fussy?

This is not meant to be derogatory at all, but some patients I've seen over the years are just too plain fussy or way too anal about even the smallest of details.

Some people with candida fuss too much about their diet, or place too much emphasis on eating this or that kind of grain or certified spray-free produce - until they eat out at a café, a wedding or somebody else's place. Others with a yeast infection are hyper critical about mobile phone use, adorning their bodies with strange gadgets designed to clear negative vibrations from their living environment - until they step outside and are bombarded by microwaves from all directions.

Some folks are always looking for the holy grail of yeast infection killing products, and discover that every six months the latest and greatest product has just been released and they just have to have it because it will solve all their problems – but then realize that it made absolutely no difference. Many eventually end up with a cupboard full of expired stuff.

Yet others shun all plastics and are totally absorbed by reading every label to exclude every possible chemical from their life - until they step outside and breathe in the air or communicate wirelessly. I have a friend who is a staunch anti-fluoride campaigner but drinks beer, uses a mobile phone and has a poor diet, but nevertheless passionately believes that fluoride is carcinogenic substance that should be banned.

Can you see how lop-sided many of us have become? Having a chronic yeast infection can make us rather anxious about our health and the things that can affect it, and this then becomes a self-fulfilling prophecy.

Isn't it is time to focus on the real issues and the bigger picture here, your lifestyle and diet and the causes of your yeast infection, and not to become too anal or entirely focused about just one aspect of this until it consumes you?

There is no point spending a big part of your day fussing about trivial details, worrying or even developing anxiety about one aspect of your diet or lifestyle that you feel is important and may hinder your recovery, it will only hold you back.

Let's take look at stress and your digestive system.

Stress And Your Digestive System – The 6 Main Factors

The six main factors today affecting stress and your digestive system:

Time Urgency – convenience and fast foods rule today, they have become acceptable to many simply because we "do not have the time anymore". And when we do eat, we eat hurried and just eat to get it over and done with. We don't chew foods properly and many times don't even look at our foods, up to one third of us look at a screen when we eat.

Eating Under Stress Or Tension – Many families eat under stress or when tense, and many eat whilst at their desk or at work. Today, many families are single parent and there are not enough good family times when everybody sits around the table enjoying a meal and each other's company.

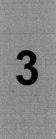

Not Eating Breakfast – You would be surprised how many women skip breakfast! My guess is, as many as one in two or three working women with kids just don't make enough time to have a decent breakfast. By the time morning tea comes around they are hungry, and by 6.00pm they are starving and eat too much, affecting their digestive systems at night. People who skip breakfast are more prone to a higher carbohydrate intake later in the day for an energy boost, especially coffee and chocolate. They will also find themselves having more mood issues.

4 Eating Too Late – placing stress on our ability for our digestive system to adequately break down and absorb our meals. We eat at a time when our body is preparing to rest for the evening.

5 Too Many Stimulants – Many people rely on tea, coffee and caffeinated drinks today whilst others rely on alcoholic beverages. These stimulants and depressants can wreak havoc with our nervous and digestive systems. We end up getting caught in a no-win situation of fatigue and energy.

6 Multi-Tasking – A bit similar to time urgency, this term was unheard of when I grew up in the sixties, today it is seen as the norm if you can complete several jobs at once. With the global economies in financial crisis at present, companies are downsizing and placing more strain and workload on their existing employees. The result is that fewer remaining staff are expected to increase their work output and yet get the same pay rate. The end result is that people have less time for food or relaxation breaks, and many work over their lunchtime, arriving home later and more stressed. Teachers are a prime example here; just ask one about their never-ending workload!

What You Can Do

- It is important in stress not just to treat the physical manifestations of stress, but to also to allow help through proper stress management or counseling. Good lifestyle recommendations for those with stress or burnout include regular relaxation exercises, yoga, tai chi, meditation, massage swimming and walking. I will expand a lot more on the important areas of why relaxation later on.

- Nutritionally it is best to follow section 1 of this chapter.

- Slow down when you eat, belly-breathe and if possible eat in a relaxed environment. It can make the world of difference.

- Although there are many specific and effective herbs, minerals and supplements such as amino acids available for stress, whenever I treat a patient presenting with stress, fatigue, burn-out, and poor immunity associated with stress, I recommend adrenal fatigue treatment, look at section 2 in this chapter where I discuss stress, immunity and the candida connection. In most instances, pharmaceutical medicines are not required.

- Complete Holmes Rahe Stress Test further ahead in this section, this test will give you an insight into how much stress is affecting your body.

- Follow the 80/20 concepts.

Many people with digestive problems who have a yeast infection have one or several underlying stress related problems. In order to truly heal, it is necessary to tackle not just the surface manifestations of the stress, i.e. the physical symptoms by taking an "acid blocker" drug or a sleeping pill from your doctor, but to understand and treat the actual causes of the stresses, whether they be of psychological, emotional, nutritional or toxic origin underpinning your physical complaints.

How Stress Affects Your Immune System – The Walking Wounded

Did you read Section 2 of this chapter entitled Stress and Immunity? It will give you a good overview of how your immune system copes under stress.

I've found that the kind of chronic candida patients who come to us for help appear to be continually in a state of sickness or unwellness, often with a poor immune system, are those folks who have a tendency to suffer from long-term and low-grade continual stress. I call them the walking wounded, they are not necessarily "sick", but they never seem to have abundant energy, they hardly ever seem to smile or fully embrace life.

They don't appear to enjoy life much and see it as some sort of drudgery they have to go through, and many such folk are not really happy with the quality of their lives or rather what has become of it. The thing with a yeast infection is that it can affect so many systems of the body and create dysfunction across the board that it truly is a systemic problem for many, is it any wonder a person with a yeast infection feels so terrible, and so do the people around him or her? Many of the really sick candida patients, like I used to be, can even be considered "social lepers", they go nowhere, can't eat out, have minimal friends and can feel like an outcast. They become stressed, and it is this chronic state of stress that will ensure they don't recover anytime soon.

Among adults, job and financial worries are often among the leading contributors to stress, but increased crime, violence, peer pressure leading to substance abuse (alcohol and drugs like ecstasy, cannabis and methamphetamine), social isolation, loneliness, and family problems can also create stress-related problems. Stress is not only creating problems with adults, but is increasingly causing health problems among children, teenagers and especially the elderly.

When I grew up in the 60's, stress didn't seem to be the buzzword that it is today. Sure people did drugs, but nothing like the drugs of today; alcohol was a problem - now alcohol related problems like domestic violence and automobile accidents are quite chronic and regular daily events. Sure there was violence, but nothing like today, now we accept violence on most all of our TV programs and computer games and even children's cartoons are just about all violence. Bad language is now kosher on TV.

Remember the 1950's when children could walk to school and high-school massacres were unheard of? In the 21st Century, it seems that we have become an increasingly violent, hurried, stressed, time poor, worried, politically correct and sick society. Baby boomers today are more prone to stress related illness like diabetes, heart disease and cancer than their forebears, the silent generation, were.
It is your immune system that is particularly affected by chronic low-grade stress, and it is the walking wounded as patients we see in the clinic on a daily basis.

We see patients with all manner of disease due to a compromised immune system like recurrent cough and colds, skin infections, recurrent allergies, autoimmune diseases and many different types of cancers.

As I mentioned earlier that we see a certain group of patients who always "always sick" or who are chronically fatigued from the hurry and worry of modern life. Their conventional doctor may label them as being depressed or anxious and prescribe a drug, after all, the test results appear to be fine, it must be in the patient's head.

When no test results can account for the way a patient with a compromised immune system feels, these are the folks in particular who need to make the necessary lifestyle changes as well as look at their adrenal health before they take any form of prescribed (drug-based) medications.

A compromised immune system can mean that you could become a sitting duck for a bacterial or a yeast infection, because your resistance will be lowered and your susceptibility will be increased. All you need now is a prescription for an antibiotic drug to tip the balance and precipitate a yeast infection, especially if you drink alcohol or have a sugar rich diet to cope with your stressful life. It is the convergence of several factors which most always account for a yeast infection, but it generally stems from an immune system which was compromised in the first place which will not only ensure the beginning but the continuation of candida, and sometimes indefinitely.

Most people today associate stress with worry, but stress has a much broader definition to your body. I have always noted that patients don't generally see themselves as living under much stress, or even feeling stressed. Dr. Wilson, the adrenal fatigue expert, once said to me "anybody with a pulse and breathing will suffer with stress in their lives". I recall telling him that I didn't feel particularly stressed and his reply was this: "But Eric, you have just told me that you have a wife and four teenagers, you certainly will have lots of stress in your life!"

Any kind of change, whether it is emotional, environmental, illness, hormonal or just pushing yourself too hard, can be stressful to your body. Even positive events, such as getting a promotion at work, winning a large sum of money or just taking a vacation can be stressful and can gradually weaken your health before you realize what is happening. If you have recently experienced a change in your sleep patterns, feel fatigued, anxious or a lack of enjoyment for life, or have multiple aches and pains, it is highly likely that you are overstressed.

Unhappy Lives Create Inner Stress And Eventually Illness

Research by Dr. Hans Selye, the first scientist who discovered that stress actually made people sick found something quite amazing – that animals, which were simply restrained, died quicker from stress than animals that were physically injured.

How does this relate to humans? Women for example who are living in a situation of constraint, such as a new born baby or perhaps in an unhappy relationship tend to feel constrained, that there is no light at the end of the tunnel. The same goes for the teacher trying to teach a class of unruly students, or the air traffic controller with too many decisions to make under high pressure.

When my elderly mother was placed in a nursing home at 78 years after a stroke it proved to be more than a handful for my brothers and created a huge amount of stress and tension in our family.

After a life of independence she was not able to relinquish control and felt very stressed until her passing, almost like an animal in Dr. Selye's experiments that was restrained to a chair. I have no doubt that the stress of her "imprisonment" as she called it only hastened her demise, because her high blood pressure, which she never previously had and brought on by stress, ensured that a second and fatal stroke occurred during a period of time when she felt the most reliant on the nursing home staff.

Research has found that psychological stress in human beings can take a hefty toll on the immune system by reducing the concentration of cytokines, highly specialized proteins that help to ward off infections. Cytokines are proteins that are produced by certain white blood cells of the immune system in order to regulate the body's response to disease and infection.

It was recently discovered that people under chronic low-grade stress had above normal levels of interleukin-6 (IL-6) that promotes inflammation and has been linked with heart disease, diabetes, osteoporosis, rheumatoid arthritis, severe infections and certain cancers. It appears that stress increases levels of IL-6 that in turn accelerates a variety of age-related diseases.

Stress can weaken a person's immune response leaving them much more susceptible to infection, including a yeast infection, and can lead to unhealthy lifestyle habits which only serves to increase the severity and duration of the yeast infection. For instance, stress often leads people to overeat, lose sleep, and neglect exercise, drink alcohol and coffee and become dependent of drugs all of which can create health problems in their own right.

Stress Increases Your Chances Of An Infection – Any Infection

In one study, skin wounds on the arms of women who had higher levels of the stress hormone cortisol had lower levels of key compounds released by the body to mediate healing. Stress may make it easier for germs to infect skin wounds as researchers have proved. Investigators created skin wounds in mice that were exposed to stressful living conditions. The researchers then applied Streptococcus bacteria to the wounds, and compared the healing rates of the stressed mice with those of mice with skin wounds that were also exposed to the bacteria but did not undergo the same levels of stress.

Mice that had been stressed out prior to wounding and infection showed a 30% delay in wound healing at 3 and 5 days compared with the mice that were not stressed, the report indicates. In addition, the investigators found that after 5 days, the stressed mice had 100,000 times more opportunistic bacteria in their wounds than the non-stressed mice. Seven days after the bacteria exposure, about 85% of the wounds in the stressed mice were infected, versus about 27% of the wounds in the non-stressed mice. In this study, stress increased the rate of wound infection by threefold. Stress disrupts the body's equilibrium, in turn significantly impairing its ability to control and eradicate bacterial infection during wound healing. Chronic stress, which has been called our number one health problem, is not something to take lightly, it can have profound effects on your immune system and your overall health.

Stress-Related Health Problem – The # 1 Reason People See Doctors

Estimates have placed stress-related problems as the cause of 75 percent to 90 percent of all primary care physician visits. Psycho-neuro-immunology is a whole new field that studies the effects of psychological stress on the immune system. Scientists in this area have demonstrated alterations in the normal function of immune cells in animals during times of stress. For example, excessive physical stress changes your immune cell profile. Increased upper respiratory tract infections occur in athletes who over-train, and a decreased cell-mediated immunity has been demonstrated in such athletes. Without a properly functioning immune system, your body is vulnerable to invasion by opportunistic germs such as candida, viruses and bacteria.

It is not practical to advise you to avoid stress because, let's face it; we all have stress in our lives from one degree to another. What is practical, however, is to emphasize to you the importance of recognizing stress in yourself and others and more importantly in dealing with stress before it takes a toll on your health. There now exists ample scientific evidence to suggest that stress impairs the immune system, which allows underlying infections to cause damage.

Relaxation And Meditation Calm The Mind And Fight Stress

Relaxation techniques can also be useful when stress becomes overwhelming. Yoga is a discipline I call meditation in motion, it can lead to mental clarity, greater self-understanding, and a feeling of well being, along with improved physical fitness. Many people experience benefits not only because of the physical stretching and muscle strengthening but also because of the meditative state that is encouraged. Have you ever considered Yoga or Tai Chi? They are both wonderful and will add a whole new dimension to your life.

Meditation is another technique that will allow you to calm your mind and fight stress. Meditating can help you to focus your thoughts on relaxing images or principles.

It can also help you to examine your daily life and determine what activities are contributing to your stress.

The bottom line is that stress shuts down either the recruitment or the function of those immune cells needed to fight infection. Awareness of adrenal fatigue along with the correct treatment can significantly help by supporting the hormonal control of the body under-pinning stress. This highly effective protocol along with the correct dietary and lifestyle changes as outlined in Dr. Wilson's ground breaking book entitled "Adrenal Fatigue: The 21st Century Stress Syndrome" can offer you the greatest chance of overcoming stress before it takes control and ruins your health.

Is it any wonder that most Western countries are now experiencing soaring rates of cancer, the ultimate immune disease? It is important for you to recognize that stress can be a good thing; we call this eustress as opposed to distress that leads ultimately to disease and death. For example if you are going for a job interview, a driving test, or are going to give a speech at a wedding, this type of positive short term acute stress will actually boost your adrenaline level and gives your body a natural push to get things done, your mind has a bit more clarity and you feel more alert. The key is to be aware of your stress level and get things under control if stress starts to take over.

The Holmes-Rahe Stress Test

In 1967, two American doctors formed a do-it-yourself stress test after studying the effects of stressful events and illness on several thousand patients in a hospital setting. They examined the stress of a person by measuring what they called Life Changing Units (LCU), and these included events occurring in a person's life ranging from going on a vacation (a LCU rating of 13) through to the death of a spouse (a LCU rating of 100). I have included this stress test here so you can complete it right now, and by adding up your score you will be able to predict the likelihood of a stress related illness in your own life.

Have you noticed something when you look at the events, especially the top five most stressful events? They all have to do with a person who is close to you. As I stated earlier, it is the *emotional stresses* that have the most lasting and profound effect on our health and wellbeing.

1. Death of Spouse

2. Divorce

3. Marital Separation

4. Jail Term

5. Death of a Close Family Member

Try to complete the test below, your total score will show you how your risk will be of a stress-related illness or accident within a two-year period.

- Total LCU less than 150:   35% increased risk

- Total LCU between 150 - 300:   51% increased risk

- Total LCU greater than 300:   80% increased risk

What events have happened to you in the past 12 months, and what is your score? The higher the score the more likely you are heading for stress related health problems.

The Holmes-Rahe Stress Test

Life Event		Life Value	Your Score
Death of Spouse	_	100	
Divorce	_	73	
Marital Separation	_	65	
Jail term	_	63	
Death of close family member	_	63	
Personal injury/illness	_	53	
Marriage	_	50	
Fired from work	_	47	
Marital reconciliation	_	45	
Retirement	_	45	
Change in family member's health	_	44	
Pregnancy	_	40	
Sex difficulties	_	39	
Addition to family	_	39	
Business readjustment	_	39	
Change in financial status	_	38	
Death of a close friend	_	37	
Change in number of marital arguments	_	35	
Mortgage/Loan greater than $10,000	_	31	
Foreclosure of mortgage/loan	_	30	
Change in work responsibilities	_	29	
Son/daughter leaving home	_	29	
Trouble with the in-laws	_	29	
Outstanding achievement	_	28	
Spouse begins work	_	26	
Start or finish school	_	26	
Change in living conditions	_	25	

Revision of personal habits	_ 24	
Trouble with boss	_ 23	
Change in work hours, conditions	_ 20	
Change in residence	_ 20	
Change in school	_ 20	
Change in recreational habits	_ 19	
Change in religious activities	_ 19	
Change in social activities	_ 18	
Mortgage/Loan less than $10,000	_ 18	
Change in sleeping habits	_ 16	
Change in number of family gatherings	_ 15	
Change in eating habits	_ 15	
Vacation	_ 13	
Celebrated Christmas	_ 12	
Minor violation of law	_ 11	
Your Total Score:		

If your score is 200 points or more and you have not been feeling well, it might be wise to have a check-up. If your score is 200 or more and you're feeling good, you are probably handling the changes rather well.

Reference: Dr.Thomas Holmes,

Dr. Richard Rahe. Journal of Psychosomatic Research. 1967, vol. II p. 214.

Recognizing Stress in Yourself

I believe that the real key is to recognizing stress and how it affects your body, and this differs from person to person. Here are some typical stress warning signals; can you recognize any of them?

- Feeling unable to slow-down and relax

- Explosive anger in response to minor irritation

- Anxiety or tension lasting more than a few days

- Feeling that things frequently go wrong in your life

- Can't focus your complete attention

- Regular or continual sleeping problems

- Aching neck and shoulders

- Lower back pain

- Regular indigestion or heartburn

- Heart palpitations or awareness of your heart beating

- Increased consumption of alcohol

- Overeating, especially of sweet foods

- Frequent low-grade infections

- Shortness of breath

- Constipation or diarrhea

- Loss of appetite or low-grade nausea

Can you recognize more than four of the above 16 different stress warning signals? If you can confidently say "YES" to at least four of the above then you are certainly suffering from acute stress *right now*. Changing well-established habits is never easy. Because stress is accumulative, reducing any strains on your body is beneficial, and you will find it considerably easier and more effective to work on the smaller stress-related issues in your life right now than wait until they eventually develop into a full-blown health crisis like a heart attack.

Sorry, but hiding the symptoms of stress will not get rid of the strain on your body. Early treatment of stress-related health problems is most effective, especially if you want to prevent premature illness. Feelings of irritation or anger, tension in your neck or shoulders, sweaty palms or heart palpitations, tossing and turning at night and so forth are all early warning signs that your body is keeping itself unnaturally "revved up", and it is your sympathetic nervous system which is at work here.

It is clever for you to understand that if you focus your attention to stimulating your parasympathetic nervous system that you will be able to bring peace and harmony back once more, and restore the balance.

Stress is increasingly becoming recognized as a major contributor to heart disease, cancer and strokes, and these three are some of the most common causes of death and disability in my country and no doubt in your country as well. They may be traced, in part, to how we mismanage the stressors in our lives. Let's take a look at how stress can aggravate certain yeast infection symptoms.

Recognizing Stress-Related Yeast Infection Symptom Aggravations

The typical stress warning symptoms above apply, but what you may well notice is an exacerbation of some of the key problems you have been experiencing. Two of the most common aggravation areas with candida and stress are the *digestive system* and the *skin*. I have found that the gut often becomes affected with stress, because as you will soon read, your sympathetic nervous system reduces the blood supply to the digestive system in favor of routing the blood to the larger skeletal muscles of the body in case you need to escape from a stressful event. The movement of stool in the large intestine is slowed down (inhibition of peristalsis), Your digestive secretions (pancreas, stomach and small intestine) are reduced likewise, because you don't need an optimally functioning digestive system when you were running away from a dinosaur a long time ago. Today we are not so fortunate, we can run but we never really seem to recover from one stress to another.

Digestive System Aggravations

The digestive system is a key area for those with candida, and under stress yeast infection sufferers may notice a significant amount more gas, cramps, bloating, constipation or diarrhea.

So, if you regularly get an exacerbation of your symptoms, ask yourself what kind of stress were you facing the day of the week before, this may well explain a few things! I'd like you to observe the cause (e.g. your mother-in law, son, daughter, partner or your boss) and the effect (e.g. your sudden indigestion, gas, constipation, nausea, etc.)

Remember, the major and even minor emotional events or conflicts we have with people often can bring on aggravations. By understanding the relationship between any potential stressful events in your life and their physical outcome, you will be in a much better position to avert such potential problems by a two-fold nature.

- You will learn the art of cause and effect, and will be more able to understand that any stressful event could be potentially underpinning some of the key digestive complaints you experience when you have a yeast infection. Knowledge is power.

- By applying the knowledge you are about to learn below with regard to the autonomic nervous system, that stressful events effect your sympathetic nervous system, and that by increasing the activity of your parasympathetic nervous system you will be able to reduce all yeast infection related symptoms caused by stress and bring your body back to a state of harmony.

Skin Aggravations

Likewise, your skin may be affected, because stress causes your blood vessels to constrict (goose bumps) and increases the activity of the sweat glands. I've seen many patients with a yeast infection that affected their skin with key areas including the armpits, groin, ears, hands, feet as well as the finger and toenails. Warm and moist perspiration will certainly encourage a yeast infection only more as it will give candida exactly what it wants, a warm and moist and damp atmosphere to thrive in.

Excessive sweating in not a pleasant thing to occur in those with a bad case of jock itch or yeast related rash affecting the armpits. By recognizing the stressful events in your life and any subsequent aggravations to these keys areas of your body you will be able to learn about any potential cause and effect. By increasing your parasympathetic nervous system's dominance you can calm the skin down by reducing the body's ability to perspire as well as increase the blood supply to your skin, and this especially important if you want your body to heal your skin more rapidly. Blood is an effective carrier and will help to remove wastes from the areas that need healing, it helps to boost the oxygen and nutrient supply as well which it carries to each and every cell.

So now you understand why stress can be a bad thing if you have a yeast infection both in the sense of the unnecessary aggravations you will probably be experiencing as well as the delayed healing that takes place when a person is under the effects of stress. Once you understand the candida-stress connection and master the ability to balance your autonomic nervous system, you will experience considerably less symptom aggravation and speed your healing response.

Case Study # 24
Emma, 69 years

Emma came to see me with a bad yeast infection of the skin under her arms, around her groin and under her breasts. She has had problems in these areas for several years that were manageable, according to her, but more recently it had become unbearable. The patches were huge and the discomfort, especially in summer, was significant.

Her doctor had referred her to a Dermatologist who prescribed at first an antifungal cream, after discovering that it was a significant skin yeast infection, but then later a combination of a steroidal cream and antifungal cream, all to no avail. That is when her daughter referred her to me.

I found Emma initially to be tense, defensive and only interested in a "natural side-effect free cream" that was going to cure her yeast infection. I immediately realized by her body language that this problem was a lot more than just a skin-deep issue! I was particularly interested to hear that she was having some issues with her son in law who she never took a liking to, and mentioned that her daughter should have married somebody with "more brains" than a truck driver, after all, her other daughter was married to a lawyer, and they had bought their own home in a "nice" area.

Her daughter who was renting, recently had her first child, and Emma was paying a lot of attention to her new grand daughter and also having to interact with her son in law, and it was at this time that her skin flared up significantly.

Attention to a strict diet had made a big change, but not enough to improve her yeast infection to a satisfactory level. It was about a month after we had Emma as well as her daughter and husband in my room and had a frank and open conversation (including tears and suppressed anger) that the improvements came. We treated Emma with several dietary supplements as well.

Emma has made peace with her son in law at last, and the most impressive thing for me is that after one month her yeast infection now was the best it has ever been. It never ceases to amaze me how powerful the effects of stress can be on a person's immune system.

Emma's cortisol levels were significantly elevated after we had initially completed a salivary cortisol test, and it was because of these test results along with an explanation of the cause and effect of stress, adrenal gland health and a suppressed immune system, that we could help Emma to bring about a positive change to her situation. This case has been one of the most spectacular cases I've seen yet in terms of recovery and I am delighted to say that today Emma has not only changed on the inside, but on the outside as well.

Can you remember Dr. Edward Bach's saying? "No true healing can take place unless there has been a change in the patient's outlook".

Anxiety

Laugh and the world laughs with you, cry and you cry alone.
Ella Wheeler Wilcox

The clue here is adrenaline, a powerful hormone produced by your sympathetic nervous system. The question is why should the body produce excess adrenaline out of the blue, causing us to have "unexplainable" anxiety attacks, and heart palpitations and many other symptoms? As mentioned earlier, When we are faced with a dinosaur or a tiger, or when we encounter any kind of trauma, grief, rejection of a loved one and so forth, the body floods the circulatory system with adrenaline, the most powerful hormone of strenuous action and fear or fight. This hormone helps us to deal with the 'danger', but this danger can be real or imaginary. Those with chronic candida are caught up in a real Catch-22 situation, they have several chronic symptoms which may be causing them plenty of ongoing anxiety and stress, like finding it difficult eating out with friends, fatigue, brain fog, recurrent vaginal thrush or any one of several other problems. These health concerns become a stress in their own right and in turn stimulate the sympathetic nervous system to continually produce low levels of adrenalin and cortisol. Eventually the body's many cells become resistant to the continual production of these powerful hormones and even higher levels become produced. Depletion occurs and adrenal fatigue sets in, yet another health problem to add to the pile.

In the initial stages of a chronic yeast infection, I find that many patients present with higher levels of anxiety (higher levels of adrenalin and cortisol) than those who have had a chronic yeast infection for many years, these patients tend to show the classic signs of adrenal fatigue, and now you know why. Their endocrine glands (the adrenal glands and thyroid especially) have become increasingly exhausted from years of worry and anxiety about their unresolved health problems. In time the patient becomes increasingly despondent and exhausted and will wonder if she is ever going to get well. I've learned that when a person's hope for a healthy future is fading, when she feels that "no one is listening" and that every day brings little joy but fear of the yeast infection symptoms she may experience, that the patient's attitude becomes more disease-focused and not wellness-centered.

Is it any wonder that chronically affected yeast patients stay unwell? Now that you understand a little more about stress, attitude, and recovery, ask yourself this question: "How have I been thinking about my recovery, am I positive and truly believe that one day I will beat this thing entirely and feel fantastic once again?" Or, are you just barely getting through each day, focusing on the negative rather than the positive aspects of your health and life?

By now you may understand why I have written a great deal about stress, anxiety and yeast infection in the Candida Crusher. A person's emotional state is generally most always affected when they have had a yeast infection for several years, and most all books I have studied on this topic have very little to say about stress and a person's emotional state when it comes to candida. I think it is because most of the focus is on diet and killing a yeast infection. Your mind and emotions rule your nervous system that in turn rules your immune system.

An intelligent person is more interested in treating the cause of their yeast infection rather than the effect, and in many instances a person's emotional state can in fact be one of the primary maintaining causes of their yeast infection, believe it or not. Sometimes I see the "light go on" in a patient's eyes when they begin to understand this information in my room, it can be their tipping point. Here are a few solutions when it comes to anxiety and tension.

6 Tips On Dealing With Anxiety And Tension

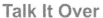 *Anxiety's like a rocking chair. It gives you something to do, but it doesn't get you very far.* "

Jodi Picoult

1 Talk It Over

Why do you think many people with a yeast infection come to see health-care practitioners? My guess is to talk about their physical as well as emotional yeast-related problems. This is because every patient will naturally want to talk about the physical symptoms they present with (like thrush, itching, burning, bloating, gas, etc.), and will generally launch into how they feel and issues they face with family, friends and employers, etc. because of their health condition. Many confide about what is really bugging them, and by talking it out it helps to relieve the strain and tension. Communication allows a person to see their worries and concerns in a different light. You may notice yourself that by talking about your worries and problems with somebody you trust you will often begin to see a clear path. Bottling things up only creates destructive "self-talk" with problems going round and round in your head. Poor communication like this can lead to all kinds of problems, and it forms the basis for most personal and business relationship failures as well. You will become a lot less tense, stressed and anxious by discussing issues affecting you, so talk it over with someone you trust.

2 Escape For A Little While

Have you ever lost yourself in a good movie or book? Escaping mentally is a great way to alleviate mental pressure and stress. If you have a really important meeting or engagement coming up, escaping for ten to twenty minutes before the event can work miracles in terms of you being more focused and centered on the mental task at hand. A brief trip like a walk in the park or along the beach is wonderfully refreshing and only takes minutes and can take your mind off that chronic itch, at least you'll be away from a website telling you how terrible you must feel! Why escape with a glass of wine or rely on recreational drugs and physically punish yourself and only aggravate your symptoms thereafter? Making yourself stand and suffer after you opened that bottle because you couldn't switch your mind off without booze? Why do you think half the world is stoned on some form of prescribed or recreational drug? People want to free their minds, and by allowing your mind to escape with a book, a musical instrument, prayer, a walk or whatever technique you have developed you will have your own pressure release valve from the stress and strain of day-to-day living.

3 Work Off Your Anger

Have you ever felt so angry that you hit an object like a cupboard door, or thrown an object on the ground whilst swearing and cursing under your breath? Well, you are not alone. If you find yourself using anger as a general pattern of behavior, it is important to remember that anger will always leave

3

you feeling sorry and foolish in the end. A chronic yeast infection can create a lot of physical, emotional and mental problems for a person, including anger and anxiety. If you feel like screaming or lashing out at somebody, try to hold off for just a few minutes, and like most strong emotions it will soon pass. The thing to do for example is some physical exercise like gardening, a long walk or a game of tennis. Working the anger out of the system this way, along with talking it over will leave you much less tense and more prepared to handle your conflicts and problems more intelligently. Stress has a way of working in on the psyche making some people literally snap, this is how many acts of violence such as murder are committed. If you regularly "defuse" your anger, you will find that you can act calmly and rationally even under the toughest conditions and tension can't build under these conditions.

Are You A Perfectionist?

4

Is your way the highway? Then give in occasionally. Have you noticed that sometimes it is just easier to agree with somebody, even though you know they are wrong and you are right? When you do, it will make you realize that winning doesn't really matter, but keeping the relationship does. Do stand your ground on what you believe is right, but do so calmly and make allowances for the fact that you could be completely wrong. The result will be a huge relief from tension along with the satisfaction of achievement and maturity. Are you going to still act like a child and "always have to be right"? You will lose a lot of friends if you never give in. Who cares in the end if you really were right or wrong, one of my favorite sayings: "People may forget what you said, but they will never forget how you made them feel". If you truly care about your own stress levels, be aware that when you engage in conversation with somebody else that their stress levels will very much influence yours. If you stay calm and the conversation remains calm, you both leave calm and stress free with a lot less tension. Does everything you do have to be 100% perfect or you can't relax? Some people like me are just born perfectionists, and they can be hard on themselves or others if perfection is not regularly attained. These patients are the ones I see who often go onto develop thyroid and adrenal fatigue issues, because of the extreme demands they place on their physical bodies because their minds just can't seem to switch off.

Case History # 25
Mandy, 36 years

Let's look at Mandy who is a dynamic young mum with two small children. Mandy has boundless energy, is perfectly proportioned and whizzes about like a pocket edition of Wonder Woman, and was the driving force behind two successful businesses before she reached the age of 30. Mandy works out at the gym most mornings, breeds purebred dogs, drives a convertible sports car and belongs to a few women's groups. When I first saw her as a patient, she had just become the assistant editor of a most influential New Zealand magazine. Mandy's love life has been a disaster with several failed relationships.

Mandy is an extroverted perfectionist with excess energy, what I call a full throttle person with the foot flat to the floor for up to 12 hours a day. What Mandy hadn't worked out yet was that her super high achievement lifestyle never seemed to bring her that "state of bliss" or knight in shining armor she was so desperately looking for. She is always making new friends and literally wearing out her old ones. I had spoken with Mandy about the importance of the pursuit of moderation, and instead of her undertaking 20 things in one day, to say no to ten of them and allowing more "Mandy time". This lady's thyroid gland was hyperactive, and is it any wonder?

Mandy also liked to drink white wine and she came to me with a rampant yeast infection which had been driving her crazy for over five years. I spent a considerable amount of time with her showing her different ways to relax and the difference it made in time absolutely amazed me! It took less than six months for her yeast infection to go completely, and along with that I noticed a more calm and serene Mandy who finally realized that her major priorities were not her career, but her relationships with those she cared the most about.

I saw Mandy about two months ago and was pleased to hear that she had finally got married and maintained her daily relaxation sessions and cessation of alcohol. But the biggest change was not just a disappearance of her yeast infection; it was in a complete turn-around in her Grave's disease (hyperthyroid) and perfectionism, as she has become to accept the fact that near enough is good enough.

Do One Thing At A Time

5

When I grew up as a baby boomer in the 60's I never heard of a word called "multi-tasking", we certainly had no mobile phones or computers. We seem obsessed these days with being able to do two or more things at once, and keep lists of all the tasks we want to complete. Many people are so busy with their own lives but manage to keep on saying "yes, I can do that" and later think "why the hell did I say yes, when I've got so much to do?" so before you promise to do something for somebody else, first think the important tasks you have set for yourself for today and if you won't be putting yourself under a lot of stress by taking on that extra work.

To people under tension, an ordinary workload looks so huge that it's almost painful to tackle it. Whenever you feel overwhelmed, try to tackle the most important task first then you will find that rest flows easily. Say for example you have ten things to do, just write them all down and mark them in priority with 1 being critically important, 2 moderately and 3 can wait a few days to a week. You have just clarified your priorities and set your mind at ease. And doesn't it feel good when you can cross that list off?

Do one thing at a time and do it well, then move on. By learning when to say no and completing tasks you set yourself you have more time to relax, more "you" time without that feeling that you have to be continually doing something. Are you obsessed with checking emails continually? Learn to slow down and be less accessible by way of phone or email, it is important to remember that you need time to work and time to relax. Try not to blur the whole thing; it can get a bit messy that way and you and your family will suffer. Work hard and then relax even harder, that's my motto these days.

Go Easy With Criticism

How hard and critical are you with yourself and others? I have found that tense people are often critical people. They can tend to be hard on themselves and others. Do you expect a lot from others and then get disappointed when they don't deliver? It could be your partner, or a child who you are trying to squeeze into your preconceived plans or maybe even try to control or take over to suit yourself. Some tense people I have observed can even be considered to be control freaks at times. Instead of being critical of tense people, search out and point out their good points and help them develop their weaknesses without exposing them. Nobody likes to be criticized, do you?

6

I often ask a patient if they have a family member or friend who they are at conflict with regularly, or who they don't often agree with. Do they dread going to a social family event like a wedding or a family Christmas party because aunt Mary or uncle Frank will be there? If you deal with somebody regularly who you do not get on with like perhaps the "out-laws", become aware how your may body tense up, how the muscles in your face may tighten up, or do your shoulders become tight when you are around this person? Emotional stress and tension is often felt subconsciously with thoughts and feelings about events or people creating mind-body patterns such as jaw clenching or teeth grinding later that night in bed, perhaps insomnia and muscular tension throughout the body the next day. In addition, emotional stress also causes adrenalin to be released causing muscles to fire up and be tense resulting in pain, more anxiety, your heartbeat quickens and blood sugar levels may increase which can make you feel "hyper". By being nice to others, they in turn will be more pleasant towards you and will feel more relaxed because less conflict will occur, and the result means less tension. Adrenalin then will not be released and you don't get the physical responses either. There is plenty of research showing that tense and anxious people are more prone to all forms of chronic illnesses, because the hormonal systems underpinning our system are geared towards restoring our bodies after any kind of stress. These hormonal systems affect every part of our being, so it stands to reason that when this stress defense mechanism itself breaks down that we become ill and may eventually even die as a result of continued stress and conflict.

Stop Worrying About Your Health!

Have you had your gluten-free, low caffeine, biodynamic, spray-free and non-irradiated breakfast yet? Had you eight hours of sleep, 5 + serves of vegetables, exercised for an hour and cut right back on saturated fat?

Have you noticed that there are countless websites, books, health-columns in e-zines and magazines and endless talk shows that have become the "health-police"? They dictate what you should and should not be eating and how you will stay in optimal health. A friend of mine recently gave up on a subscription o a well-known international magazine, because he was sick and tired of reading about how high his risk of cancer was from various foods and normal daily habits. He said, "If I haven't got cancer now, they'll make sure I get it by keeping it under my nose every month."

When I grew up, my mother used the word "hypochondriac" a lot because a friend of our family was always worried and perpetually complaining about his health to anybody who would listen. He would visit his doctor almost weekly with yet another symptom like palpitations, bad breath, gurgling sounds in his abdomen, itchy back, and so the list went on. Some patients I have seen are just like this, they worry and fuss over their health continually and just don't seem to get on with their lives. Ironically, but I've noticed that some people I see with the most amazingly healthy diets appear to be the ones in the worst state of health. Those who do everything "just right" can't seem to get their health just right.

Many folks live in the belief that they must continually strive to attain perfect health, but "perfect health" is a myth and most of us are living far healthier lives than we realize. Once you develop a yeast infection you certainly become more focused on your health, but failing to live by the health rules set by the "health police" can be a major source of stress, anxiety and guilt, especially for women I've found. The goal is to live for as long as you can with the best quality of life, but some women I meet are absolutely scared to death about their diet and lifestyle, they simply must exercise every day and eat a perfect diet, because there always seems to be a some woman who looks so much sexier and skinnier than she does.

A lot of women have lost sight of what it means to be healthy I think, the point is to use common sense and if you feel good then all is well, in spite of what you eat and how much you exercise, regardless of what those websites or magazines may tell you. Recovery from a yeast infection is straightforward and you should notice improvements all along the way, cut yourself plenty of slack along the way. Remember, your life is a journey and not a destination!

Don't become overwhelmed by that ocean of health information out there written by all those armchair experts, just enjoy your life for what it is, your recovery will be that much quicker if you can just *stop worrying about your health*. And if you worry less there is less chance you will verbalize these anxious thoughts you hold, and that has to be a good thing.

> *Common people ascribe all ills that they feel to others;*
> *people of little wisdom ascribe to themselves; people of much wisdom, to no one.*
> *Epictetus*

Stress and Your Autonomic Nervous System.

What you are about to read is something I will often try to explain to patients who pay me a visit, it is an explanation of the autonomic nervous system (ANS) and how it can bring you a lot of joy or a lot of grief in your life. When you understand this system reasonably well, you will be in a good position to be able to more effectively balance your ANS and bring about harmony to your nervous system that in turn can have a tremendously positive effect on your immune system.

The stronger your immune system, the better your body will be able to resist a yeast (or any) infection and the quicker it will be able to recover from illness.

I consider this information to be priceless and one of those gold nuggets you will find in the Candida Crusher. For those in particular who have had a chronic yeast infection for many years, a healthy, well-balanced ANS which in turn can build and powerful immune system will be worth more than the most powerful dietary supplement or herbal medicine you could ever wish to buy.

The best awareness you can have is self-awareness of how stress can push your buttons and what you can do about it. Your autonomic nervous system is the system that automatically regulates your body in times of stress, and then helps to de-regulate your body and chill it out after any stressful event. The sympathetic nervous system is the accelerator of stress, it primes your body in preparation for any upcoming stressful event, no matter how small (like hurting your toe) or how big (like jumping out of a plane) and your parasympathetic nervous system is the brake and will help to normalize your body after any stressful event. Now let's look at this fantastic system a little more closely. Your autonomic nervous system is a part of your nervous system that regulates key involuntary functions of the body, including the activity of the heart muscle; the smooth muscles, including the muscles of the intestinal tract; and the glands. The autonomic nervous system has two separate divisions: the sympathetic nervous system, which accelerates the heart rate, constricts blood vessels, and raises blood pressure, and the parasympathetic nervous system, which slows the heart rate, increases intestinal and gland activity, and relaxes sphincter muscles.

Of all of your body's systems, your nervous system is most probably the most fragile. Its delicate balance is easily affected by emotional, physical and chemical factors or more commonly by a combination of these stresses. As a result of an imbalance, you can readily suffer from a wide variety of health problems, and because your entire body is controlled by your nervous system, chronic stress has been linked with just about every single illness known to man.

Emotional Stress Affects Your Nervous System The Most

What I have noticed after having treated many patients with stress-related illness is that powerful emotional events occurring in that person's life are frequently linked with the actual cause of their poor health.

When I carefully look at the patient's time line, and ask the question: "When can you last remember feeling truly well?" the person can generally recall one or several stressful events which took place before they became unwell. If you have been unwell for several years, ask yourself what happened in your life *before* you became sick. An event may have occurred up one year prior, but typically it will have been in the months leading up to you becoming unwell.

With a yeast infection, the onset was often precipitated after taking an antibiotic for some type of infection due to poor immunity. The person's immune system may have been struggling for some time and I've typically seen a patient developing a yeast infection after a few rounds of antibiotics. What I've also seen is a cluster of stressful events occurring in a patient's life which started to cause adrenal fatigue, and then their immune system became increasingly compromised leading to leaky gut syndrome, small intestinal bacterial overgrowth and a rampant yeast infection. See section 2 – Understanding Stress and Immunity for more comprehensive information on adrenal fatigue).

Stress Is A Nervous System Reaction

Your autonomic nervous system (ANS) is the part of your nervous system that maintains harmony and a sense of inner equilibrium inside your body. Whatever you feel, your ANS will be feeling, and in fact, anything you feel "automatically" your ANS will be responsible for. For example, your appetite, your mood, your ability to think clearly and even your sexual urges are all controlled by your ANS. If you feel excitement, dread, fear, anger, hunger and sleep all have their home in the ANS. But as you are about to see, the ANS can bring us to heaven as well as make us feel like we are in hell!

It is important to understand that your ANS is divided into two distinctly separate nervous systems, one which stimulates the nerve fibers, the sympathetic nervous system or SNS, and the other which sedates nerve fibers, the parasympathetic nervous system or PNS. It may be easier for you to remember that the SNS is the accelerator and the PNS is the brake.
It is the ANS that gets our body ready to rally for any likely emergency it may face, and this will occur whether the emergency is real or imaginary. It makes no difference really, for your brain cannot tell the difference between a real or imaginary stress. The well-know "fight-or-fight" response as discovered by the famous endocrinologist Dr. Hans Selye, is the main system that is stimulated by any potentially stressful event in the body, the sympathetic nervous system.

When your body is in a healthy state of balance, there is a smooth transition between the sympathetic and parasympathetic nervous systems not unlike a considerate and courteous driver who gently accelerates and then gently brakes. It is a pleasure travelling in a vehicle driven by a person who understands the gentle balance between powering a motor car up when required, but has learned equally when to power it down smoothly. The example I like to explain of a healthy balance is the reaction between a cat and a dog; it illustrates both parts of the ANS and how in the natural world they can work in perfect harmony.

When a cat comes into contact with a dog, its sympathetic nervous system will go on red alert, the cat's body is fully and automatically mobilized in a fraction of a second. Its eyes open up and the pupils dilate, its fur stands on end and all her muscles straighten and tighten up, it hisses violently and prepares for attack with claws and fangs bared. The cat's heart rate will have gone up considerably and it is prepared to do battle, all in less than a quarter of a second! If the dog is smart, he will remember the last painful encounter he had and move away. In a flash, the cat's parasympathetic nervous system will kick in and it will lie down and stretch out and begin licking its fur.

This is a wonderful display of a healthy balance between the sympathetic and parasympathetic nervous systems, but in reality it is not what happens to humans! Cats don't drive cars, pay hefty mortgages or have to worry about taxes.

You see, in a healthy and balanced body these two branches of the ANS maintain perfect harmony. The SNS allows us to act and effectively deal with any kind of stress in our lives, its responses sharpen the mind, quicken the pulse, tense our musculature and move blood to the areas we need in order to escape the threat (constrict the blood vessels). But after this danger has passed, the PNS will take over and calm our mind, relax the blood vessels (dilate), decrease the heartbeat, move blood back to our digestive organs, stimulate our immune system and clear away any metabolic wastes like residues of adrenalin and lactic acid.

This is how it should happen, but in reality it doesn't really occur this way in humans. Tension and action should be followed by relaxation and inaction, a yin and yang balance. In today's world many of us have to stay on guard and rarely find downtime or "me" time. If the imbalance becomes chronic it can often lead to a whole variety of stress-related symptoms. And for those with a yeast infection it can spell one aggravation after another.

Many people with a chronic yeast infection I have seen don't seem to realize that great health requires great balance, harmony and equilibrium between the body and the mind.

Muscular Tension Is Common With Stress

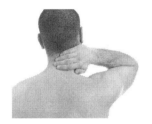

Do you suffer with a sore lower back, tight neck and shoulders or have tension headaches regularly? What I've noticed is that many people I've seen with yeast infections of several years duration also complain of sore and tight muscles, and these muscles can differ from person to person. There happens to be six hundred and twenty different skeletal muscles, but there are also a lot of smooth muscles found throughout your body, for example in your digestive system. There are many blood vessels in addition which have smooth muscles, and many of these can potentially go into a state of contraction with sympathetic stress overload, resulting in cramps, spasms and the many and varied other symptoms produced by circulatory insufficiencies.

If your parasympathetic nervous system is unable to maintain a steady balance to counter the effects of the sympathetic nervous system, toxins and stress by-products can build-up as they become trapped in muscles, and your muscles can become even more tense, contracted and painful.

But if your parasympathetic nervous system could be activated and maintain a regular state of balance, a whole new world will open up to you.

It's time to explore the wonderful world of the parasympathetic nervous system, the PNS. While a sympathetic nervous system can make us feel like we are in the fires of hell at times, the parasympathetic nervous system has the ability to make us feel like we are in heaven.

The PNS brings us to that contented place of peace and harmony and allows us a much greater sense of well-being, it expands what was contracted, it calms what was tense, it clicks things back into place and pulls things back into line that were overstretched.

The PNS is even responsible for great nights sleep and will have you waking feeling thoroughly refreshed. This nervous system calms and relaxes the mind, it is conducive to creative and imaginative thinking, allays anxiety and banishes depression. It slows the heartbeat and steadies the pulse; it improves your immune system's capabilities and improves your digestion by encouraging the production of digestive enzymes and the movement of foods and wastes through the gut. It relaxes all the muscles, blood vessels and internal organs so that the movement of nutrients and wastes are encouraged.

Boosting Your Parasympathetic Nervous System

The important point to understand is that we do need the sympathetic response, but more than anything, we need to maintain a balance between the nervous system that activates (SNS) and de-activates (PNS) our responses. As a culture, in the Western world we have literally trained ourselves to override the ANS in favor of a more convenient and faster and electronic computer-based lifestyle.

Even for the sake of physical fitness, many people today are encouraged to engage in exercises that are challenging and physically demanding, and these are often high-intensity exercises can be exhausting and quite stressful on the sympathetic nervous system.

I have found on many occasions when I ask a patient what she does to relax, she may well reply with "But Eric, I exercise every day" It is interesting how most folks don't see exercise as being a stressful activity on the body, and in my opinion it needs to be balanced out with regular and daily less stressful activities. Even though regular exercise and keeping in top form will allow you to have much more control over your autonomic nervous system, it is important to understand that a healthy balance between exercise and relaxation will keep your ANS in a much better form than if you just do the one and forego the other.

Even though most of us do not enjoy the more extreme effects of sympathetic dominance such as sweaty palms, muscular tension, headaches, palpitations, anxiety and sleepless nights, unfortunately many of us are unwilling to sacrifice our lifestyles of staying up late at night, eating poorly and working 24/7 which all contribute to the dominance of our sympathetic nervous system. Others enjoy the buzz of base, bungee or parachute jumping, various motor sports, white water rafting or jet boating, jet-skiing or any one of a dozen or more such extreme sports. All of these activities significantly boost the sympathetic nervous system.

There are many different kinds of therapies and exercise that are aimed at boosting your PNS. So how can you increase your parasympathetic responses and what are some of the best ways for you to gain this balance back into your life? I'm glad you asked, and now I'll explain some of the best ways to boost your parasympathetic nervous system. Unlike conventional medicine which relies on anti-anxiolytic drugs to calm a person down, natural medicine can be highly effective at strengthening the parasympathetic nervous system, and there are many different techniques and treatments that can be of assistance like meditation, self-hypnosis, various breathing and relaxation techniques, yoga, tai chi, and Chi gong, reflexology and various massage techniques all of which can make you feel relaxed and calm and in control of all of your bodily functions.

Buteyko Breathing

I am a convert and a big fan of the Buteyko breathing method and regularly refer patients to a Buteyko specialist. Were you aware that many people in fact over-breathe (hyperventilate), and all too many believe that deep breathing is one of the best ways of stimulating the PNS when in fact it stimulates the SNS, the stress response!

Professor Konstantin Buteyko was born into the small farming community of Ivanitsa (about 150km from Kiev) in 1923. In 1946, he enrolled into the First Medical Institute in Moscow to train as a medical doctor. In 1953 Dr. Buteyko was given a practical assignment that involved monitoring patients' breathing, and spent many hundreds of hours recording their breathing. It was during this time that Professor Buteyko discovered that incorrect and deep breathing caused a wide range of health problems. There after, most of his professional medical life was devoted to researching, studying respiration and refining his breathing method that has helped thousands of people throughout the world to overcome their asthma and other breathing conditions.

Breathing is one activity that has a most profound effect on your parasympathetic nervous system, and most people will be quick to tell you that deep breathing is the correct way to induce relaxation, and that to practice deep breathing on a daily basis is most advantageous during times of stress and anxiety. Currently, a very popular e-book on yeast infection states that "Correct breathing is deep breathing", when in fact deep breathing is *not* the right way to breathe; Buteyko in fact states (after studying respiration and its effects on human health for 50 years) that "the essence of my method is in decreasing the depth of breathing". Professor Konstantin Buteyko, a Russian physician, developed a slower breathing method that has been named the Buteyko breathing method; it has been used since the 1940s to alleviate many different health conditions. Buteyko found that hyperventilation is the primary cause of many medical conditions and thus his program is based on *slowing down breathing rates* to within normal parameters. The Buteyko program includes guidelines for correct diaphragmatic breathing and learning to breathe in and out through the nose only.

> " *The essence of my method is in decreasing the depth of breathing.* "
> Professor K. Buteyko

The reason that slow breathing is so effective is that during times of stress, heart rate and respiration rapidly increase as the sympathetic nervous system takes over.

Correct breathing (which helps to balance the correct oxygen/carbon dioxide level) helps convince the body there is no immediate danger and allows the parasympathetic nervous system to regain control.

The Buteyko breathing method is a strategy to retrain dysfunctional breathing based on the theory that many diseases result from an abnormal breathing pattern. To be more specific, conditions such as asthma, high blood pressure, sleep apnea, panic disorders, high blood pressure, etc. are believed to be the body's responses (a defense mechanism) to hyperventilation or in simple terms; over-breathing. The Buteyko theory is based on the understanding that over-breathing disturbs the balance of oxygen and carbon dioxide in our lungs, according to Professor Buteyko, more than 200 different chronic diseases are essentially just one, which he called "the deep-breathing disease". By simply decreasing the depth of breathing, thus allowing carbon dioxide in the lungs to reach the desired level of 6.5, breathing normalizes and symptoms can disappear. Though most people may think of it as a poison, carbon dioxide may, in fact, be the "breath of life".

If you want to really learn how to breathe properly and overcome excessive yawning, coughing, sneezing, sniffing, sighing or any one of a host of breathing related problems then I can highly recommend that you get in touch with your local certified Buteyko practitioner. This technique requires only a small amount of practice each day and will soon become second nature.

Here are some of the benefits of the Buteyko method of breathing:

- Deal with stress and anxiety quickly and effectively

- Enjoy more energy and a happier state of mind

- Control the feeling of panic attacks

- Safely reduce or eliminate medication in time

- Sleep soundly through the night

- Have a clear nose - experience the joy of being able to smell again

- Eliminate snoring for a better night's sleep for you and your partner

- Monitor your condition without gadgets or machinery

- Return to activities or places you love, but have avoided because of your health

- Enjoy physical activity without fear of asthma attacks or other breathing problems

- Improve your athletic performance, stamina and recovery time

- Have freedom from symptoms related to chronic conditions

- Reduce snoring, sniffing, wheezing, shortness of breath

- Gain knowledge about your medication and its side effects

- Eliminate sore throats and hoarseness

- Reduce the incidence of headaches, earaches and stomach aches

- Enhance exercise and sports performance, have more stamina

- Greatly reduce your absentee rate at work or school

Nasal Breathing, Not Mouth Breathing

The Buteyko method emphasizes the importance of nasal breathing, which protects the airways by humidifying, warming, and cleaning the air entering the lungs. Many people breathe through their mouth however, do you? By keeping the nose clear and encouraging nasal breathing during the day, nighttime symptoms can also improve. Nasal breathing only during any physical exercise is another key element of the Buteyko method, and you will find that your performance will improve if you adhere to this.

Reduced Breathing Exercises

The main focus of the Buteyko method involves controlling your breath, and to consciously reduce your breathing rate and volume that is in contrast to deep breathing exercises recommended by most. Once you have spent time practicing and retraining yourself it will become instinctive and you won't look back. The Buteyko method uses a measurement called the CP or controlled pause that means the amount of time you can hold your breath comfortably after you exhale, until you need to breath again. The MP or maximum pause is the same, but with specially taught exercises that distract your brain, you learn to push out your controlled pause. Success comes as you are able to comfortably hold your breath in the out position for a minute or longer, and this will signify that you are breathing for one person. The less you can comfortably hold your breath for, the more you are over-breathing and the more people you are breathing for.

Abdominal Breathing

This is the most natural form of breathing but not familiar to most. If you have ever watched a baby or an animal breathe you will notice that their way of breathing is slow and that their belly rather than their chest expands. Supplying air to the lower part of your lungs is what belly breathing is all about and it is almost impossible for you to be tense and stressed and belly-breathe at the same time.

Lie down or get seated in a comfortable position that supports your entire body and place your hands (palms down) on your abdomen just below your belly button. Close your eyes and slowly inhale (remember, nose only, keep your mouth closed at all times). Imagine you have a balloon inside your lower abdomen you are trying to blow up where you have placed your hands and as you breathe in you are slowly inflating the balloon; and as you exhale; you are deflating it. Concentrate on your belly and not your chest as you inhale. I imagine that I'm at the beach and that when I breathe in that a wave is coming into shore and when I breathe out that it is going back out again. I can even hear the sound the ocean makes and have found that this relaxes me within two minutes. This exercise is best practiced daily for about five to ten minutes and before you know it, you will soon belly breathe when you are not even aware of it. Abdominal breathing is in my mind of the most powerful ways to induce the parasympathetic response and should be practice daily. The best time to do this exercise is between two to four in the afternoon, this is the time when your adrenal glands are in the low part of their 24 hour cycle and you will naturally feel a little tired and relaxed. Now try to incorporate this breathing technique as part of your TPM (twenty Peaceful Minutes) sessions I'm just about to outline.

TPM Sessions

Meditation? That word has always had strange connotations and sounds more like some weird kind of cult activity to me; I prefer the term TPM or Twenty Peaceful Minutes. I read a book written by Jack Canfield, Mark Victor Hansen and Les Hewitt some years ago called The Power of Focus that described this relaxation tip, and the TPM term kind of stuck. This type of relaxation tip is something I've been recommending in my clinic for over twenty years and I get great feedback from those who have taken this technique on board.

Ok, so this is where I am asking for a commitment, I would like you to start regular relaxation sessions for yourself at least three times weekly for about twenty minutes at a time. Now tell me honestly, is sixty minutes a week too much? Some folk may spend three times more time than this much just watching sitcoms, "liking" somebody's stuff on Facebook, talking on the phone or wasting time by not planning what they are doing next. How would you like to have a sense of inner calm and reduced tension and irritability like you haven't experienced for years? It is so simple, just find a carpeted floor (not a bed, you are not going to sleep, you are just having a rest) and lie down on your back. Take your shoes off and loosen your waistband. Make sure you won't get disturbed - no kids, people, computers or especially telephones of any description around you, etc. I want you to just relax and take a nice slow deep breath in, being sure to breathe in as I have mentioned above – abdominal breathing, don't breathe in a shallow pattern into your chest. It's all a bit weird and foreign at first, I know, I can assure you that very soon you will get the hang of it, and that these mini siestas will rejuvenate your energy, allowing you to stay relaxed and focused well into the evening instead of collapsing on the sofa never to stir again until bedtime. This extra burst of energy will allow you to spend time with your family.

The ultimate time to have your TPM sessions are between 2 – 4.00pm, this is because cortisol (a main stress hormone) is then at its lowest point of production during the day and you will naturally feel a sense of "three thirty-itis". With these sessions, your heart rate will drop, your digestion will relax, your immune profile will increase and you will soon start to experience a sense of inner calm and serenity. With a sense of inner calm comes a release of tension – you will actually become aware of the muscles that tighten up when you are more relaxed. Twenty minutes is about the right time, and when you do these sessions you may want to take advantage of visualization, just visualize that your yeast infection is entirely gone. All those pesky signs and symptoms are no more and you see yourself as health and radiant. The most successful people in this world are those who believe in themselves and never gave up believing. Have the courage and belief that your yeast infection is only temporary and the your are getting better every day in every way.

> " Ordinary people believe only in the possible. Extraordinary people visualize not what is possible or probable, but rather what is seemingly "impossible. And by visualizing the impossible, they begin to see it as absolutely possible. "
> Cherie Carter-Scott

I believe that it is as important to schedule these relaxation TPM sessions, as it is to schedule your regular business meetings. The most progressive organizations realize that people pushing themselves until they drop does not achieve a highly productive workforce. You don't need to lower your performance standards; you just need to recognize that being at home with the kids or being at work and expecting a high level of productivity requires a high amount of energy which in turn requires your body to recover as well. Look at the big picture, how much time do you take off each week? And how many weeks a year do you schedule for fun? Are you happy with your life?

"I must be available 24/7" is the passionate excuse today for having a smart phone. Do you really have to monitor those "urgent" calls, most of which aren't urgent at all? By slotting in regular TMP sessions you can dramatically help to reduce the amount of self-induced stress and tension in your life and you will soon realize that being available at all times can be a big trap as well as a continual source of stress. Check your emails twice daily, not hourly!

How on earth did our grandparents survive I sometimes think without mobile phone technology or Facebook I'll never know, but I think they coped fine and always appeared to have the time to talk, unlike most of us today who are just too plain busy all the time. By making sure you take regular "time out" from your busy life, and by engaging in regular TPM sessions, you will start to begin to replenish your mental and emotional energy levels and actively diffuse tension in your life.

The Quiet Pond

I like this parasympathetic nervous system boosting tip, and it is one I got after I read Dr. Wilson's book on adrenal fatigue. Have you ever sat by a quiet pond and just gazed into the water? You look at the ducks, feel the sun and wind and listen to the noises of nature as you let you cares and worries slip away off your shoulders. It is amazing just how refreshing a walk in the local park can be, and just to sit beside the pond and forget about the world.

Once you've been to the pond (or beach, mountains, etc.) a few times, take it all in and let your senses bathe in the splendor that nature has provided us with, those wonderful sounds and smells and feeling of the elements like the sun and wind, it becomes easier to go to your imaginary quiet pond in the comfort of your own home, or even at a busy airport, during a train ride or any other place you may feel a little tense, stressed or nervous. Just sit down, close you eyes, and smell those smells, and feel those elements and instantly transport your mind back to that place of serenity. Remember, your mind doesn't know the difference between a real or imaginary place. Everybody has the capability of carrying his or her own quiet pond around within, and once you have used this technique several times you will find it easy to do. I fly frequently and have found this technique to be wonderful after the seatbelt signs go off and we are in the air, I close my eyes, feel and see the beach, I can hear the crashing waves and seagulls and even feel the squelching sound that sand makes as you walk on it. I can smell suntan lotion and the salty air, what a wonderful yet imaginary experience. My quiet TPM pond is something I always do on the flights, and once I arrive at my destination I feel relaxed, focused and fresh.

You can find your quiet pond every day, just move away from your computer, stay seated and drop your shoulders, close your eyes and take a few slow breaths in through you nose and into that belly. Imagine that pond or mountain, beach, forest or your special place and feel the sun on your face, and the sound of birds and smells of nature. Bring your senses into play as you fully relax your body, the long-term memory for the sense of smell is one of the strongest, so be sure to smell with your imagination. By doing this exercise at a particular time of day, just like breakfast, your body will soon know when it is time to do your regular relaxation session, and don't be surprised if your mind starts giving you a few subconscious signals. Find your quiet pond every day and refresh yourself, regardless of where you are and what is going on around you.

Chewing Food Properly and Slowly

Did you know that the act of slowing down when you eat foods and chewing your foods slowly and carefully has a stimulating effect on your parasympathetic nervous system? I'll bet you didn't. Did you also know that up to one third of people eat their main meal in front of the wide screen? Tell me how you can concentrate on your meal and digest it properly if you are watching some show about a serial killer? This is absurd as thinking you are capable of texting while driving your automobile at sixty miles an hour.

A 2012 study* revealed that a randomized trial of 120 patients who had had abdominal surgery had a reduced level of inflammation in their digestive system from chewing gum before and after surgery, when compared to those who did not chew any gum. It was noted that their autonomic nervous system (the parasympathetic nervous system) had become greatly activated leading to a decrease in pro-inflammatory mediators and an improved immune profile in their digestive system. This "down-regulation" of the immune system's inflammatory cascade (via stimulation of the vagus nerve) enhanced postoperative recovery by reducing the chances of any infection, pain and inflammation. And all of this was achieved simply by the act of chewing!

* Tim M P Berghmans, Karel W E Hulsewé, Wim A Buurman, Misha D P Luyer Faculty of Medicine, Maastricht University, Maastricht ER 6229, The Netherlands. June 2012; 13:93. DOI:10.1186/1745-6215-13-93. Source: Pubmed.

Do you slow down when you eat your meals, or do you gulp your food down in twenty to thirty seconds flat? Try this trick, record how long it takes you to eat your meal, and then to double the time it normally takes you. That will allow you to chew your food more slowly and thoroughly and will help to stimulate your vagus nerve to give your PNS a boost. When your parasympathetic nervous system becomes increasingly activated, it will ensure a good production of saliva, increased motility of food and stool through the digestive system and relaxed sphincter muscles that will enable easier swallowing, digestion and defecation. The bottom line is that your digestive system will work better if you slow down and chew your foods more thoroughly. Your bowel will work better too, and I've heard many patients over the years tell me how amazed they were with just this one single tip. All common sense and basic 101 digestive physiology stuff, but who teaches the basic stuff in the 21st Century when we think we are smarter than nature?

Laughter Is The Best Medicine!

What is there to laugh about when you have a yeast infection you might say when there is plenty to laugh about! The best outcomes come to those who remain positive and optimistic and who begin to enjoy life once again.

You could laugh about the fact that you have just invested in the Candida Crusher program and have started to implement the strategies outlined in the five sections in this chapter. This will put you miles ahead of those who just commonly tend to focus on anti candida foods and anti candida pills, because if you follow my program your recovery is almost assured, and that should bring a smile to your face.

Have you noticed that when you smile it triggers a smile in those around you? When you laugh others will in turn laugh. Happiness and laughter when shared will cement your relationships with family and friends and is a powerful trigger for strengthening your immune system. A great sense of humor will help to pull you through some of your darkest days of your yeast infection, and if you can't laugh about your own situation, just hang out with a friend who laughs and smiles a lot, because she will be like a breath of fresh air or the sun on your shoulders when all is dark around you.

> *Through humor, you can soften some of the worst blows that life delivers.*
> *And once you find laughter, no matter how painful*
> *your situation might be, you can survive it.*
> *- Bill Cosby*

My wife and I have a friend called Theresa, a single mom on her own with six kids who would happen to be one of the happiest ladies I know. I've never seen Theresa without a smile on her face and even when she speaks on the phone you can feel that radiant smile and hear her laughing. Not that Theresa has a lot to laugh about, at times she hasn't even got enough money to pay the power bill she still manages a smile. This is in contrast to another lady I used to know who along with her husband have long retired after selling their manufacturing business for millions when they were only in their early fifties. Judy never seemed to smile and perpetually complained about the cost of living and how has kids never seemed to visit. They have overseas holidays twice annually, the very best home and cars and are in good health. Yet never a smile, a nice word to say about anybody and certainly no joy in Judy and Neil's life. I don't cultivate friendships with people anymore that are no fun to be with, life is just to short to associate with folks who walk around with a face like a slapped backside.

Have you noticed that money does not make you happy? It can make you life easier, but happiness is a state of mind, and like all states on mind it can be cultivated.

Anatomy Of An Illness As Perceived By The Patient

> *If people only knew the healing power of laughter and joy, many of our*
> *finest doctors would be out of a business. Joy is one of nature's greatest medicines.*
> *Joy is always healthy. A pleasant state of mind tends to bring*
> *abnormal conditions back to normal.*
> *Catherine Ponder*

One book I'd like ALL of my patients to read is called "Anatomy of an Illness" by the author Norman Cousins. This best-selling groundbreaking classic book was written by a person with a life-threatening illness and how he overcame his health-challenges through having a sense of humor.

Go to Amazon and buy it, it will change the way you view laughter and having a sense of humor and your recovery from ANY illness, including a chronic yeast infection.

Anatomy of an Illness was the first book by a patient that spoke about taking charge of our own health. It started the revolution in patients working with their doctors and using humour to boost their bodies' capacity for healing. When Norman Cousins was diagnosed with a crippling and irreversible disease, he forged an unusual collaboration with his doctor, and together they were able to beat the odds. The doctor's genius was in helping his patient to use his own powers: laughter, courage, and tenacity. The patient's talent was in mobilizing his body's own natural resources, proving what an effective healing tool the mind can be. This remarkable story of the triumph of the human spirit is truly inspirational reading, I recommend you get a copy.

Laughter Is Medicine For Both Mind And Body

Laughter and having fun have an amazingly powerful effect on so many aspects of your health and wellbeing, if the effects of this "medicine" could be made into a drug it would make a company like Pfizer billions in annual revenue. Unlike pharmaceutical drugs, laughter is not toxic or addictive to the body in any way, shape or form. But best of all, laughter is free, fun, easy to use and has no known side effects, maybe apart from sore ribs or falling off a chair from laughing too much.

> " *A good sense of humor prevents hardening of the attitudes -* "
> *Anonymous*

Laughter can be the perfect antidote when you have a yeast infection; it works faster than a drug and can instantly transform your mind away from those annoying and aggravating symptoms. With this renewed power to stimulate and heal your immune system and consequently renew your body, having a sense of humor can be a tremendous resource for those with candida. Laughter lightens your burden, allows you to more easily connect with others and keeps you more centered, alert and focused on your real problems like avoiding the real causes which maintain your yeast infection, allowing you to make those powerful and corrective changes to your attitude, your diet and your lifestyle.

When you smile and laugh a lot more like Theresa, you will find that people will naturally be attracted to you. Theresa has many friends who help her out at a moments notice, when her garden needed attention and it was overgrown (her landlord threatened to evict her), about twenty volunteers turned up and after one day her rented property looked absolutely amazing! When you frown and complain a lot, people tend to avoid you, regardless of your material wealth. Judy has only one real friend, a lady with plenty of money also. She has to find her happiness through travel, fancy clothes and all the material things in life that rarely bring inner happiness.

5 Reasons Why Laughter Is Good For Your Health

1

Laughter Dispels Stress. Research has shown that those who laugh regularly have less chance of developing a stress related health challenge like heart disease or cancer. Dr. Ian Gawler is well known as an Australian pioneer in Mind-Body Medicine and therapeutic meditation. He is a long-term cancer survivor and an articulate advocate for a healthy and balanced lifestyle. The author of 6 bestselling books, Ian has spent the last 30 years developing a wide range of self-help techniques that integrate lifestyle practices, such as a healthy diet, regular exercise, positive thinking and affirmations along with meditation combined with contemporary Western medical cancer treatments. Dr. Gawler noticed years ago after having put tens of thousands of cancer patients through his cancer retreat that most all patients had one or more significant emotional stresses in their lives from twelve to eighteen months before their cancer diagnosis.

2

Laughter Relaxes The Body. A good laugh dispels tension and stress and can leave you feeling relaxed for up to on hour after. Having an orgasm with sex as well as laughter both tend to have similar effects on the body, they both help the body released stored up tension and can induce a deep state of relaxation thereafter. One of my patients is a certified laughter therapist, how awesome is that? Her facial expressions can make me laugh that much my sides hurt!

3

Laughter Boosts Immunity. Laughter boosts the parasympathetic nervous system that in turn down regulates and balances the production of the stress hormones adrenalin and cortisol. A well-balanced adrenal gland system in turn can assist in boosting the production and activity of lymphocytes, specialized white blood cells that produce infection-fighting antibodies.

4

Laughter Triggers Endorphin Release. Researchers at Loma Linda University in Southern California found that laughter stimulates the production of beta-endorphins, the body's natural painkillers, as well as human growth hormone, which help improve a person's immune system profile and assist in the regulation of a person's metabolism. Endorphins make you feel great and temporarily help to reduce the pain and sensations you may be experiencing with your yeast infection.

5

Laughter Protects Your Cardiovascular System. Research spanning many years has shown that those with a sense of humor tend to have a lot less problem with their heart and circulatory system as they grow older. A reduction in inflammation occurs with laughter that improves a person's immune profile, and this reduction in inflammatory mediators is thought to help dramatically reduce one's risk of a heart attack or stroke.

Laugh And Stay Emotionally Healthy

I grew up in a household with a father who had a good sense of humor, but my grandfather was outrageous when it came to having a laugh and my dad and granddad would always play tricks on each other. It's the funny things in life, as well as the tragic events, that you never quite seem to forget. Have you ever done anything crazy in your life that made others laugh out loud?

Emotional happiness leads to a state of physical happiness and is the basis for mind over matter. It has been said that people are as happy as they make up their minds to be, so, have you made up your mind to be like Theresa or to be like Judy? It's your life and you only get one of them.

Having a positive sense of humor will make recovery from your yeast infection that much easier because you remain more optimistic and will be able to see a clear path to recovery, humor will help you through those tough days when you feel terrible. It will help you when you feel disappointed and annoyed because of unmet expectations because your recovery may be delayed or protracted due to unforeseen circumstances that invariably arise. I have noticed that those who laugh a lot develop the courage and strength to go on, and on, and on.

Those who laugh will find it difficult to feel anxious, tense or angry. Humor has an incredible way of shifting your perspective and allows you to engage with others in a much less threatening way, have you noticed? Your relationships with others, including your health-care practitioner, partner, family and friends will improve because your positive and humorous attitude helps to foster a stronger emotional connection. It is almost impossible to disagree with somebody when you are in a positive and happy mood too, by the way.

12 Opportunities For You To Laugh

1. Become a person who plays practical jokes occasionally on others, but know when to goof around and when not to! Again, it's all about balance and knowing when the time is right. Have you ever dropped a plastic ice cube (complete with a fly in it) into somebody's glass, given a friend a sandwich which contains a rubber fried egg in it, or had itching powder put in your T-shirt? Ever tried wearing a pair of those Groucho Marx glasses and popped a cigar into your mouth when you went to a party? I like going into those gag shops were you can still buy all this kind of stuff.

2. Go to watch a live comedian, these people just make me laugh every time, I have my favorites and can sometimes laugh so much it hurts! Do you live in a big city? Then go to your local comedy club.

3. Host a fancy dress party and give a prize for the most outrageous costume!

4. When you talk with somebody, make sure you ask what they did today that made him or her smile or laugh.

5. Host a games night with a bunch of friends, invite only those people that make you laugh. An evening like this will do you more good that a month of antibiotics.

6. Read funny books or buy some books with gags and jokes and read them out to others.

7. Invite a few friends to your place and have a food fight. Make up a heap of spaghetti and have cream pies for dessert, you'll laugh that much your sides will split open. I'd suggest you eat outside. My 14 year-old son had a fantastic time shoving a cream pie in my face during his birthday party. Talk about some father-son bonding time! You may think of these suggestions as weird or downright crazy, but they sure do make you laugh!

8. Spend time with young children, they haven't forgotten how to laugh and have lots of fun like their all-too-serious parents often have.

9. Play with your cat or dog, especially with a young pet, just like young kids, they still know how to have a good time and not take life too seriously!

10. Read the funny pages of your newspaper or magazine.

11. Do something crazy like you did when you were a pre-teen! I'm known to do strange things at home and never take life too seriously.

12. And lastly, get involved in fun activities like bowling, skating or skiing, go-kart racing, water skiing, karaoke, mini golf or clay pigeon shooting if you are that way inclined. Whatever turns you on is fine, as long as you are having fun with a bunch of other folks and nobody gets hurt.

Conclusion

It is important to understand that understand that humor and laughter are powerful parasympathetic nervous system stimulators. I tell patients that is important to focus on the positive in life and not the negative, because negative beliefs and thoughts are a barrier not only to forming meaningful relationships with those around you, but to recovery from a yeast infection as well.

Are things really that bad that you can't at least smile once a day? Is your yeast infection that serious that it has become the entire and negative focus of your life? Is your yeast-related health problem completely irreparable and incurable? Are you that ill that you need to concern and upset people around you regularly with bad news flashes? I'll bet you answer a big NO to all these questions. Then why worry?

Here are a few ways to kick-start your laughter therapy, try practice smiling at least once each day, it is easy and you will find that by smiling you will break down barriers and others will smile too. Just take a look at your life and count your blessings, there are plenty of things in your life to be grateful for when you really think about it! Be happy that you will soon recover from your yeast infection and think about others who have medical conditions that are terminal; a yeast infection is certainly not a terminal condition. Spend time with people who make you feel good and who have a sense of humor and avoid negative or toxic people in your life. It may mean that you will have to leave one or two people behind, then so be it. Just like chemicals and toxins in your body, toxic people are best avoided and purged from your life when necessary. Don't take yourself or life so seriously, life is just too short when you think about it, it is important to have fun and enjoy your life while you can. How boring and mundane your life would be without humor!

Vacations And Unstructured Time

Vacations are an important time for you to take each year as they give you the ability to have plenty of unstructured time. During your vacation, leisure replaces your work as a priority and you become filled with the enthusiasm to explore, travel and learn new things. So indulge in laziness and enjoy spending times with those you care about the most, spend time with the ones you love, you will be hooked once you feel like this and then will realize the importance of the vacation and unstructured times.

These lazy and self-indulgent days pay big dividends to your health and well being, and once you are back at work you will find yourself more refreshed and focused on the task at hand. I always like to clear my desk and tidy my office up so that when I'm back on deck I can start with a clean slate.

How much time do you take off each week? How many weeks a year do you schedule for fun family time? If you do plan to take a day off, then make sure it is a full twenty-four hours. No emails, no calls, NO business of any kind, just fun and relaxation time. Many business folk are confused about time-out, they think it means no office but mobile phone. Many at-home mothers are also confused, and think that time-out means no washing, cooking or cleaning when in reality it would be great for them to get away for a whole two-days (48 hours) with their girlfriend and to leave the kids with somebody else, like their caring partner, friend or relation.

Schedule your vacation time on your calendar at the beginning of each year and decide when you want to take major breaks and reserve this time, make sure you set your goals because I've found if YOU don't structure your time, somebody else will structure it for you! The important thing here is to develop the habit of regularly creating some total relaxation time, so that when you return from your break you will feel well rested and completely refreshed. This also has the other major benefit of boosting your immune system by way of re-charging your adrenals glands, and this can only be positive for those with a yeast infection.

The other point I didn't mention is that you will sleep plenty when on vacation, as relaxation leads automatically to a very important element in your healing process – a deep and relaxing sleep, and that's the next topic.

Sleep And Insomnia

Laugh and the world laughs with you, snore and you sleep alone.
Anthony Burgess

Up to 30% of the population have a problem sleeping. Do you rely on sleeping pills? In most cases, drugs are not necessary to help you sleep. You have many other options. You may find some of the material on this page helpful if you either can't get to sleep or frequently wake up during the night.

Isn't it funny how many of us want to "take" things to improve our sleep, when what we really need to be looking at is improving the simple things first like going to bed when we are actually physically or mentally tired, avoiding stimulants like caffeine and depressants like alcohol if we have regular sleeping issues, and also trying to exercise regularly. Poor sleeping patterns affect so many people I see with yeast infections, is your poor sleep affecting you?

Most people with a chronic yeast infection at some stage during their lives will suffer from insomnia particularly during the rough times, but when this pattern happens for weeks, months or years on end, it needs sorting out. Working and thinking too much, worried about treatments, stress and sleeplessness feed on each other. When you suffer from stress and fatigue, anxiety or depression, you will have more difficulty in getting a good night's sleep.

By following the self help tips mentioned; you will be surprised how much the quality of your sleep and your life can improve.

The Less Sleep, The Less You Will Cope With A Yeast Infection

The more tired you become, the less you are capable of coping with stress and the more stressful life seems and more you have a problem going to sleep. Many patients we see in the clinic are victims of the wear and tear of modern 21st century lifestyles, and appear to be caught in this "no-win, no-rest cycle, yet they are probably blissfully unaware that simply doing too much and stress is actually sabotaging their efforts to get a good night's sleep.

Research in the 1970's revealed that stress decreases the time spent in the deepest and most restorative sleep stages and disrupts dream or "rapid-eye-movement" (REM) sleep.

In one study, chronic insomniacs reported that during the time their sleep problems began, they also experienced a greater number of stressful life events than in previous years. These problems include marital problems, financial worries, health problems and the death of a close person or losing their job.

Many patients I have seen have cited causes such as "I have not had a regular sleeping pattern since having my children" or "since my separation or divorce", "since my husband died", etc. These sleeping patterns can be changed, you do not have to be plagued with insomnia all your life and having to stay reliant on sleeping aids. It is so true that you don't really appreciate good health until you have a lack of it, what bliss it is to sleep deeply and soundly night after night!

Researchers have associated lack of sleep with a range of damaging physical and psychological conditions. Not getting enough sleep can increase your risk of diabetes, heart problems, depression, substance abuse and anxiety. It can also make you fat, reduce your sex drive, impair your immune system and make it harder for you to pay attention or remember any new information. You need plenty of sleep; especially good quality and deep sleep on a very regular basis, if not you will soon get sick and delay your recovery from a yeast infection. Could you imagine if you had a poor sleep pattern for years, and how this could affect your immune system and consequently delay your recovery from candida?

There are no hard or fast rules really in terms of exactly how much sleep you need, and it is unfair to say that you need 8 hours each and every night no exception. Thomas Edison who invented the light bulb amongst other things, slept apparently only a few hours a night yet was one of the most prolific inventors ever, no doubt he would have had an afternoon nap. Albert Einstein, on the other hand, said that he needed eleven hours a night and was at his most creative when he slept from eleven to twelve hours. Have you worked out your individual needs?

You may want to experiment and particularly once you get into the habit of the TPM sessions like I have, you may find that you can get away with going to sleep later yet awake most refreshed an 6.30 am because your mind and body were rested the afternoon before.

Ask Yourself These 7 Sleep Questions:

1. Do you fall asleep within 15 minutes of going to bed, or does it take you ages to go to sleep?

2. Do you always need an alarm clock to wake up to?

3. Do you naturally wake within 15 minutes each day at the same time?

4. If you lie down for a nap in the middle of the day, are you in a good sleep within 10 minutes?

5. How are your sleep patterns on the weekends as compared to during the working week?

6. When you go on holidays, do you sleep a lot for 2-3 days in the first week?

7. How does my partner's snoring affect my sleep?

Answers:

1 A healthy person takes about 10 – 20 minutes before they are really asleep. You don't generally get into a healthy deep-sleep pattern by sleeping "as soon as you head hits the pillow". This is because your mind will first go from the beta brain wave (busy thinking & conscious thought patterns) into the alpha brain wave pattern (relaxed, dreamy, "floating", half-asleep/half-awake pattern) Later on in the night you slide into the very refreshing theta brain wave state, and then into the theta brainwave pattern, called the "rapid eye movement" or REM state. This is the important phase as far as feeling great when you awake is concerned. The delta state is even deeper, and a healthy person is in this state for up to 60 minutes. Those who say: "a bomb can go off and I don't wake" are generally in the deeper states such as the delta, because arousal is much more difficult in this state than it is in the alpha. Healthy sleep consists of a combination and repetitive phase of the four above mentioned brain wave states. Interrupting a cycle can have negative consequences. Remember sometimes just as you dose off that you remember something important? This is because the alpha state allows your mind to be more creative and think "peripherally" about minor trivial problem-solving issues, and you are less focused on the main problems in your life.

2 A good indication that you are getting enough sleep is the ability for you to wake most mornings without an alarm clock. This generally means you are getting enough sleep. In my experience, most people simply don't get enough rest, they tell me they sleep fine, but do they really get the quality of sleep they need? If during the week the alarm wakes you and you turn over, you need more sleep! Using your alarm clock is a good measure for this.

3 Waking up close to the same time each morning, and not waking early (from midnight to 5.00am) and then having a disturbed sleep pattern thereon, tells me that your hormone patterns are well balanced. If you have a problem with your morning or afternoon energy levels then you may well have a sleeping problem. People with sleeping problems have energy problems, and people who are always fatigued have sleeping issues, have you noticed? This is a typical presentation in my clinic and I don't generally treat insomnia, I prefer to treat for a lack of energy that tends to improve a person's sleeping pattern profoundly.

4 This is similar to question 1, if you fall asleep rapidly when you lie down in the day you need more sleep. But only when the tiredness is not in relation to meals, i.e.; well away from meals, because if you get tired after eating a meal containing carbs like bread or pasta, it could mean you are a bit low in blood sugar and you may naturally feel a bit tired, Try sleeping for 8 hours a night for 1 week, and if wake up feeling refreshed then try these afternoon naps and you will find that it takes generally much longer to easily sleep in the afternoon after a 5 minute lie down.

5 If you don't get quite enough sleep, your brain will want a catch-up in the weekend generally. If these "catch-ups" continually occur, you may find it harder to function on a Monday morning, because you are starting to shift you waking and sleeping patterns and are pushing them ahead by an hour or two. It is important to get to bed by 9.30pm - 10.00pm at the latest for most people. Get to bed when you feel naturally

5 tired, don't have a nap at 8 or 9.00pm and then stay up until 12.00pm – 1.00am. This is very common today, as we try to squeeze every last drop out of our day due to our increasing workloads. And we prop these habits up with coffee and tea to keep us "topped up" with energy. Are you starting to "droop" at 9 – 9.30? Then go to bed.

6 If you find that you need more sleep whilst you are on holidays, you are over-working yourself, end of story. If you are away from the stressors and go "phew" when you are away, it would be best to create a sanctuary at your home, a place where you can escape and relax away from phones, kids, computers, and stop always saying yes to people. How much "you" time do you set aside each day or week? Sleeping more on holidays and weekends indicates an underlying problem with sleep debt, your sleep back account is going into the red fast and you will soon be bankrupt (burn-out) unless you service this debt. I recommend to patients that they slow down one week before going on holidays, what is the point of sleeping for two days when you take a week off?

7 If your husband and you are fine in your relationship but he snores and it drives you crazy, it could be really be affecting the quality of your sleep cycles. Your brain needs to be in a combination and repetitive pattern of different brain-wave patterns to allow sleep to be refreshing and fully restorative. If his snoring has bumped you out of a deep sleep state, it could have severely interrupted your sleep cycles. Remember, deep sleep improves your daytime serotonin (the feel good hormone) cycles, which allows you to wake up feeling positive, happy and motivated. Try separate beds for a week or two to see how the quality of your sleep improves. If there is a marked change for the better, consider him getting his snoring sorted, there is help available and by speaking with your doctor you will be able to get a referral for appropriate help. I recommend Buteyko breathing for chronic snorers, and also weight loss that can help chronic snoring tremendously.

Poor sleep in turn makes coping with a stressful lifestyle more challenging. In time, trying to get by despite sleeplessness can lead to depression, anxiety and other psychological problems.

Developing Regular Habits Will Improve Your Sleep

Try to get into the habit of regular sleep to keep your biological clock in sync. By going to bed around the same time, and getting up at the same time you will soon see that your body starts to fall into the pattern of regularity. Travel can really throw you out, and here again; keep to regular times with eating and sleeping. Learn to understand how important a good night's sleep is to your health, it is one of the most important foundations apart from good nutrition and good emotional health. Learning to develop regular healthy habits in general will pay big rewards in the years ahead as you age, but in the short term if will mean you will recover much faster from a yeast infection than those with poor or sloppy habits.

> " *Those who think they have no time for health today will sooner or later have to find time for illness tomorrow.* "
> *Edward Stanley*

14 Ways To Beat Insomnia

1 Exercise will help by allowing your body to deal with tension and stress more effectively, allowing your body and mind a chance to unwind. It could be something as simple as a twenty-minute walk, swim or bike ride at least three times weekly. What's the big deal? And you tell me that you "haven't got the time"? There is an old saying that "those who don't make the time for good health now, will find plenty of time for ill health in time" is a classic. If you get stressed and tensed at work, the ideal time to exercise is later in the day like late afternoon. Exercise when it suits your lifestyle – either early morning or late afternoon. Exercise is a classic example of investing your time in an activity that is guaranteed to give you rewards later on. A one-hour exercise session makes your other 23 hours so much more effective and the spin off is that you will sleep much more deeply and soundly. Like Nike tell you, Just Do It!

2 Never go to bed Completely worn out or very hungry this is a big mistake that some make, going to bed too tired will mean that you are not going to get a good night's sleep. Eating a big meal too late will interfere with your sleep as well. Your digestive system may well play up too, giving you plenty of gas, flatus and tummy rumblings. Another tip is not to go to bed on an empty tummy; you may well wake up due to low blood sugar levels, especially if you suffer from adrenal fatigue. Sometimes eating a small snack, even a little piece of cheese can do the trick.

3 Watch the caffeine. No coffee at least 6 – 8 hours before bedtime if you have sleeping problems and like coffee. Coffee, tea or chocolate may stimulate you for several hours after, causing a disturbed or a restless sleep. Be aware that caffeine containing foods or drinks may in addition clash with certain prescription drugs causing sleep issues, so check in with your doctor here. Are your teens up at all hours? I'll bet they have developed a taste for those caffeinated soft drinks.

They were unheard of when I was a teen, I was told I had to be 15 before I could have a cup of coffee, and now we let kids as young as 7 or 8 have cans with as much caffeine as two cups of coffee! Time for adults to wake up to the reality of energy drinks with their kids. And you wonder why they are bouncing off the walls at times, funny that!

4 Sleep on a good bed. This is a BIG one. You are less likely to get a good night's sleep on a worn out old bed, or one that is too hard or soft or too small. I know from experience, I replaced my bed recently and what a huge difference it has made. Do you wake up regularly with a sore neck or back; is your bed sagging or creaking? Time to replace it, and remember how much time you are sleeping, so why do you put up with a crappy bed? Apparently, American folk on average replace their bed every ten to twelve years, but New Zealanders wait up to twenty years! If you go to bed tonight and say to yourself" Eric is right, I hate my bed" then I don't think it is a silly idea to invest in a nice new bed. You will wonder why on earth you didn't get a good bed few years ago. It could mean the difference between a great night's sleep and a feeling like you woke up after sleeping all night in a tent. Forget the one-week in the Bahamas this winter, buy the bed instead. Ooh, by the way, don't forget to replace that pillow every year.

5 Are you a sleeping pill taker? A 30% increase in the number of sleeping pills being taken by New Zealanders has one of our opposing political parties calling on the government to look at prescribing habits of doctors in my country. In 2005 more than half a million prescriptions for sleeping pills were dispensed, up by a third on 1999 figures. We should be concerned that more people are feeling enough stress to the point where they feel they need sleeping medications, and we need to be vigilant we are not setting the scene for drug dependency issues down the track. Get your stress sorted sooner rather than later, because stress leads to sleeping issues, which in turn stimulates stress, a real Catch Twenty Two situation. See your naturopath or herbalist for non-drug options to help you sleep at night; I use herbal medicines like passiflora, avena sativa, valerian, and various others depending on the person's requirements.

6 Smokers don't sleep as deep as non-smokers. Research has shown that those who smoke heavy take longer to fall asleep, awaken more often and spend less time in the REM (deep) sleep phase. Because nicotine withdrawal can last two to three hours after their last puff, smokers may actually wake in the middle of the night craving a cigarette. Ask a reformed smoker, and most will tell you how much their sleep has improved since they kicked the habit.

7 Drink in moderation. Many people think that a drink will help them get to sleep and stay asleep, but drinkers don't sleep as well as those who drink in moderation or not at all. According to many different studies, even moderate drinking can suppress REM sleep, the deep sleep we need in order to wake up refreshed. Ever noticed that the nights you drink moderately heavy you wake up feeling "groggy"? Too much booze with dinner can make it hard to fall asleep, and too much later at night can harder to stay asleep. You end up sleeping in fragments and often wake in the early hours in the morning. If I have two glasses of red wine I generally never seem to sleep well and wake up at 1.00am and sleep lightly the rest of the evening, almost guaranteed. Dope smokers will certainly find that their sleep improves, the hormone melatonin increases substantially in regular cannabis smokers. But yes, there is a downside – the next day dope smokers will find that they are more tired in afternoon as a consequence and will also crave more sweet foods, the "munchies", which will create fatigue, lethargy and low blood sugar levels.

8 Go for quality of sleep, not quantity. I tell my patients that it is the quality that really counts, and six good solid hours is better than eight or even ten hours of light or disturbed sleeping patterns. Don't feel that you need eight solid hours every night anymore than you need to drink "eight glasses of water every day". If five hours does the trick several times a week, you may well find that a nap here or there for twenty minutes may be all you need. Quality counts, so experiment what is right for you.

9 Become a napper. Some people, like my wife, actually feel worse for naps. Not me, I have a chill-out session at least three times weekly for twenty minutes in my office on a carpeted floor. My TPM sessions, or "twenty peaceful minutes", you have heard me mention this before and find that it really does the trick for me. Try it yourself; these sessions involve lying down on the floor anywhere between the 2.00pm – 4.00 pm. This time slot is probably the best, due to the naturally lower level of cortisol your body produces at this time. I tell my

9 receptionist to hold all calls for this time and relax, do some relaxed abdominal breathing and can feel my mind slipping away. By the time I get up, I feel very refreshed and relaxed. It's what I call my "defrag of the mind". It is not that I lack the sleep; I need these sessions to help me re-focus and get my mind from the busy beta into the relaxed alpha state. Try it, you may find that irritability levels drop off and you become more humane around people if you are a bit anxious, easily stressed or simply try to squeeze too much into your busy life. I make it a habit of going to bed between 10 – 10.30pm every night. I wake at 6.30 every morning feeling refreshed.

10 **Time outs.** Here is a simple way to break out of the stress-sleeplessness cycle. Take regular "time-out" sessions during the day. It could be something as simple as closing your eyes. Several times a day close your eyes, take a few deep and relaxed breaths and meditate on a relaxing scene. It can work wonders. Try the Quiet Pond exercise mentioned previously.

11 **Don't worry & be more organized.** Some folks lie in bed thinking of what they should have done during the day, their mind racing and thinking about tasks they have to perform the following day. Try to deal with work related distractions *before* you hit the sack. Make a list of tasks before you go to bed may help. Write out anxieties or worries and possible solutions, this will save your mind having to do this whilst you are supposed to be resting. Tell yourself that you will sort it the next day. I tell my patients this: "when you lie down, don't think about any problem that requires a solution", it is easier said than done, but with a little practice it is easily achievable. Try not to go to bed until you resolve disagreements you care about. It is true; we all have disagreements or arguments with our partners or loved ones from time to time. The trick is in resolving the matter *before* bed so your mind can rest. Do you go to bed after an argument and lie there churning things over in your mind? Relax before you go to bed to get yourself in the right frame of mind, and if you do have indifference it is important to resolve the issue as much as possible in order to have a "clear head".

12 **Is melatonin the answer for insomnia?** Melatonin is a hormone produced in the brain that facilitates sleep, it is available freely on the Internet and I have found that many insomniacs have tried melatonin at some stage. Melatonin is very safe; I have fond no evidence of adverse effects even in those who use it for extended periods of time. When you are asleep, melatonin, which is made from the feel good hormone called serotonin, is released from the pineal gland in the brain. When you are awake, serotonin aids in many different functions including muscular contractions. Restless and fidgeting at night are often the result of a confused sleep-wake cycle and can point to a serotonin (too much) or melatonin (not enough) imbalance. Although Melatonin supplements appear to help with better sleep, it is not necessarily better quality or longer sleep. A recent study demonstrated that the differences between 0.01 and 10mg dosages were not significant. In comparison, the average adult human produces 1mg of melatonin in a 24hr period whereas most tablets available on-line come in 2, 3mg or more. Melatonin is still a controversial subject, and my advice before you take melatonin is to try other things first such as the suggestions above, especially magnesium.

Try 400 mgs of magnesium citrate before bedtime. Magnesium is one powerful mineral when it comes to relaxing the body and mind, and has helped many people I know sleep better. This is the first dietary supplement you should try if you struggle with sleep and may hold the answer to your insomnia if you need a little extra help. Always try magnesium before you try a sleeping pill. Try 400mg of magnesium citrate about half an hour before bed instead of the popular sleeping pill Immovane® (Zopiclone). Magnesium works well, especially if you drop the tea, coffee and chocolate and alcohol from lunchtime onwards.

A cup of chamomile tea can be very relaxing, it contains a natural sedative and is perfect for many people who suffer from mild anxiety, restlessness and insomnia. Have a cup about one hour before bed, and when combined with magnesium works very well indeed.

Some Final Comments On Sleeping

Work on getting to bed on time, and do look at implementing in particular some of the parasympathetic nervous system techniques I've outlined previously.

Once you start doing this as well as adopting some of the sleeping tips I've recommended, you will most certainly improve the quality and quantity of your sleep and be amazed at how your rapidly your yeast infection will improve, I guarantee it.

Isn't it funny how we always want to "take in" things to improve our sleep, when what we really need is to "take out" things to improve our sleep. By first improving the simple things like going to bed when we are actually physically or mentally tired, learning the art of relaxation (remember that PNS?), by avoiding caffeine and alcohol and also trying to exercise regularly, we are well on the way to a perfect nights sleep. Have a sleep on it.

Are you Exercising Yet?

" *A vigorous five-mile walk will do more good for an unhappy but otherwise healthy adult than all the medicine and psychology in the world.* "
Paul Dudley White

Many people over 50 are simply not active enough, and to prevent heart and circulatory disease and many other diseases of modern civilization, exercise is one of the most important factors. The good news, though, is that even modest amounts of physical activity are good for your health. There is no doubt, the more active you are, the more you'll benefit!

While I have no doubt that regular exercise is important, many people don't place enough value on the fitness that comes from everyday tasks like lifting and chasing children, lugging groceries around, spending time in the garden and even in cleaning your house. There are so many benefits of being physically active, it will open up a whole new life to you and will be worth it! You'll feel great because your metabolic rate increases resulting in an increased ability to maintain your normal, health weight. You will most certainly feel and be healthier; you will reduce your chance of getting diabetes, will have lower your blood pressure and even sleep better.

The Three Main Types Of Physical Activity

1. Aerobic or heart and lung fitness.

2. Muscle-strengthening or resistance training.

3. Flexibility exercises or stretching.

You can do physical activity with light, moderate, or vigorous intensity, and the level of intensity depends on how hard you have to work to do the activity. The ultimate is to engage in the different forms of exercise to get the maximum benefit.

How Long Do I Have To Exercise For?

For major health benefits, adults should do at least 30 minutes of moderate-intensity aerobic activity daily or about an hour of vigorous-intensity aerobic activity each week. Naturally, the best option is to do a combination of both. The more you exercise, the easier it becomes and the more you will enjoy it.

You don't have to do the activity all at once! You can break it up into shorter periods of at least 10 minutes each. Running, swimming, walking, bicycling, dancing, and doing other examples of aerobic activity.

If you have a heart problem or chronic disease, such as heart disease, diabetes, or high blood pressure, talk with your doctor about what types of physical activity are safe for you, you may need a check-up and get your blood pressure and heart rate established before you embark on any exercise program, especially if you are in your 50's.

Always talk with your doctor about safe physical activities if you have symptoms such as chest pain or dizziness before you consider any exercise regime.

Ideas For Activity Include:

1. Swimming, snorkelling.

2. Walking the dog.

3. Vacuuming, washing windows - vigorous housework.

4. Climbing stairs instead of escalator at airports, shops, etc.

5. Getting off the bus one stop earlier than you have to and walking the rest of the way

6. Golf, croquet, lawn bowls, etc.

7. Gardening - mowing, pruning, going to the dump, etc.

8. Join a gym/exercise group

Exercise Tips For Those Who Have A Yeast Infection

You may recall that we spoke about fermentation and yeast infections that affect the digestive system. I have found that those who exercise quite vigorously every day may be doing themselves a disservice and even possibly be aggravating their yeast infection because of how much stress they place on their metabolism and digestive system. This is not something I have read anywhere else; it is a personal observation I have made in my clinic after working with many athletes and patients who exercise a lot that have yeast infections.

Exercise heats up the body, and it is important for you to not only understand that vaginal yeast infections and skin yeast infections are aggravated or exacerbated by exercise due to the increased moisture caused by perspiration, I believe that any yeast infection can be aggravated by any exercise that is too vigorous or excessive.

1. Those with a vaginal yeast infection need to take extra care and shower immediately after any exercise and wear cotton undergarments.

2. Cool the body down gradually after you exercise by having a tepid then cool shower. This will prevent you body from maintaining a slightly higher than normal peripheral temperature which can aggravate a yeast infection, an increase in digestive problems and disturbed sleep.

3. Avoid having a sauna if you have a chronic yeast infection, it will heat your body core up too much, I've found that saunas frequently aggravate those with chronic yeast infections and some just feel worse and may even experience headaches, dizziness and many different types of skin and digestive flare-ups.

4. Those with athlete's foot need to dry their feet carefully in particular after showering and wear sandals preferably until the feet are completely dry. Buy a few pairs of top quality running shoes and be sure to rotate them, place a few drops of tea tree oil in the toe and heel area once per week, this will help to completely eradicate athlete's foot and toe nail fungus in time. Be patient! Apply a little tea tree oil to the nails and feet after drying them.

5. Guys with jock itch should also shower immediately after any exercise, dry themselves carefully and thoroughly and wear 100% cotton undergarments only.

6. Don't use antiperspirants! You don't want to block the flow of perspiration, and if you want to mask any body odor then use an organic product like Aubrey Organics or the brand called Jason.

7. Be especially of not falling into the trap of carbohydrate replenishing drinks if your cycle or run. Many people drink energy drinks, soda drinks or those fancy sports drinks that contain a high amount of refined carbohydrates. And I'm sorry, but you won't "burn it off" because you are exercising!

8. Keep yourself well hydrated. It is important to drink plenty of water before, during and after exercise. Water improves most all aspects of your digestive system and allows the body to fight a yeast infection all by itself generally.

Yoga

> " *The mind is everything. What you think, you become.* "
> *Buddha*

The word Yoga comes from Sanskrit that means, "to join" or "to yoke". Before I explain about yoga, let's get one thing clear; yoga is not a religion or a belief system, it is an ancient art form is based on harmonizing and developing the body, mind and spirit.

There are many different types of yoga, and I recommend that you contact a yoga teacher to find out which type best suits your needs. Some kinds of yoga are more meditative, others have been designed to help you more with flexibility and strength, and yet others have been designed to detoxify and cleanse the body. Some people who practice yoga are involved in one or even several kinds of yoga for this reason.

Pranayama for example, is a higher branch of Hatha Yoga and the main purpose of this form of yoga is to help with breath control. Using specialized techniques, those who practice pranayama have learned to strengthen and develop their parasympathetic nervous system to a very high degree, which in turn has an amazing effect at reducing your stress levels.

I've noticed with many patients I have known over the years that when they practice yoga for a length of time they develop a sense of inner peace, tranquility and wellbeing. Yoga can make you feel more in harmony with your environment and over time aids in self-development and self-realization.

When yoga is regularly performed, it helps to make your body stronger and more flexible and it certainly has been linked with improving your circulatory, respiratory, immune, digestive, nervous and hormonal systems. Like Tai Chi, yoga brings about a sense of emotional stability and clarity of the mind.

Physically I am very much in favor of yoga, it is a particularly good activity for those who want to remain active as they grow older because by regularly tuning up your body in this way you will become a lot less prone to injuries such as falls, strains and various other accidents as you age. I have an eighty-two year old patient who is remarkably flexible and young for her age after having practiced yoga for over twenty years, she came to yoga when she turned sixty! She said that yoga helped her with balance in her life after her husband had passed away and she needed to put her mind and body into something. Emotionally, yoga serves a purpose as well, those who practice yoga several times each week just feel happier and more relaxed; less easily wound-up, less given to worry and are much more optimistically inclined.

Use It Or Lose It

Maybe you are a baby-boomer like me and pushing fifty or more years, it is important to remember that old age and associated illnesses that come with it are big business today. Not everybody is sufficiently encouraged to look after him or herself, because quite frankly, folks are worth more money to the sickness industry when they are unwell. While it is true that people are living longer, the quality of life for many of our elderly citizens is far from acceptable.

It is rare today to find a person who is seventy or eighty and who is not on some form of pharmaceutical medication, and the bulk of older people are taking up to a half a dozen drugs or more. Use it or lose it, yoga has the ability to give you a quality of life that many only dream of as they age. So what are you waiting for!

Tai Chi

Tai Chi is different from Yoga, in that it originated in China, whereas Yoga originally came from India. Tai Chi is a Chinese system of slow meditative physical exercises designed for relaxing the body as well as balance and health in general. I like to call Tai Chi "meditation in motion", as it is like a moving form of yoga and meditation combined together, and would like to stress that Tai Chi is certainly not an "old person exercise" as some may think!

Tai Chi consists of a number of various *forms* (also called sets) that consist of a particular sequence of movements. These slow deliberate movements originally came from the movements of animals and birds, and later from martial arts. The movements are always performed slowly and gracefully with transitions between them.

Just like Yoga, there are different forms of Tai Chi, and most will want to do the meditative exercises for the mind and body. Others may be more interested in the combat aspects of some Tai Chi styles that are considered a martial art in their own right, just like Tae Kwon Do or Kung Fu.

Tai Chi is a traditional conditioning exercise in the Chinese community, and recently it has become much more popular in the Western societies.

The exercise intensity is low to moderate, depending on the training style, posture and duration.

Participants can choose to perform a complete set of Tai Chi movements or selected movements according to their needs, and it is even perfect for anybody with a heart or circulatory problem.

Research substantiates that Tai Chi enhances aerobic capacity, muscular strength, blood vessel function and psychological wellbeing. In addition, Tai Chi reduces some cardiovascular risk factors, such as high blood pressure and high cholesterol. Recent studies have even discovered that Tai Chi is safe and effective even for patients with heart disease, coronary bypass surgery and heart failure. I believe that this is one of the best exercises for those with burnout or who suffer from stress, as many of the movements are gentle and do not require much effort.

Chinese medicine and philosophy embrace the concept that "chi" is the vital force that animates and drives the body, and one of the main aims of Tai Chi is to enhance the health and vitality of a person by encouraging the circulation of chi.

The secondary aim of Tai Chi is to foster a tranquil and calm mind due to the slow and graceful yet precise execution of the movements. When a person learns to complete the sets and then master the movements, they learn important lessons in balance, alignment, and rhythm of their body's movements along with very finely tuned motor control of their individual muscles.

I've noticed that patients who practice Tai Chi daily have superior control over their posture including standing, walking and moving in general then folks who do not practice this ancient form of exercise. After practicing Tai Chi for a few years, you will almost certainly discover that there will be major benefits in terms of correcting your posture, alignment and many movements patterns which if faulty can often lead to tension or injury.

Tai Chi is a discipline I recommend in particular for those who have adrenal or thyroid issues, as it is calming, very relaxing and seems to have a nervous system rejuvenating power about it. I once recommended a patient many years ago with graves disease (hyperthyroidism) to begin Tai Chi, and the difference it made after several months amazed me!

I can highly recommend Tai Chi and have found it to be most beneficial for many different types of conditions, including people with chronic yeast infections. It is ideal to practice Tai Chi once or twice per day for fifteen-minute sessions.

Mold In Your Environment And Candida

An investigation in 2005 revealed that New Zealand's growing leaky building problem was causing a large increase in dangerous mold in damp homes. Asbestos awareness started off very slowly yet nobody really took the adverse health related links seriously until many non-smokers associated with this industry started to develop serious lung problems like cancer and mesothelioma. The US government and asbestos industry have both been criticized for not acting quickly enough to inform the public of dangers, and to reduce public exposure. In the late 1970s, leaked court documents proved that asbestos industry officials knew plenty of asbestos dangers since the 1930s and yet concealed them from the public.

Leaky Buildings Cause Mold

Do we really know enough about potential the dangers of mold and how many people are still living in leaky and moldy environments? The mold problem is caused by dampness that allows certain toxic varieties of mold to grow in buildings, and many countries have homes that are exposed to molds and damp conditions for many months of the year. Modern building companies utilizing the latest building materials like to make buildings watertight, and this often comes at the expense of poor ventilation and air flow as homes today are extensively insulated against the cold and wet. Many plastics and styrene have been used in housing construction which can potentially breed mold, and this coupled with defective construction, as many homes since the 1970's were built with sloppy compliance codes, can make mold lead to serious health problems. The building code has been since upgraded significantly since 2005, but we are still left with the legacy of many leaky and defective buildings that are potentially a health trap. There are many fungi which have been recognized as being quite harmful to human health including stachybotrys, which is becoming much more common. Molds feed on moisture and organic materials like carpet, wood and wallpaper and can even eat into plaster and brickwork that then have to be replaced. The popular warehouse conversions in many major cities are particularly susceptible to stachybotrys because these are quite old buildings that have never before been heated or thoroughly treated to remove any molds prior to the new construction. Such older buildings have often been hastily converted to flats or units with partitions put in, and limited ventilation and airflow creates the ideal breeding conditions for the trapped mold. In addition, the sudden heating tends to draw moisture out of the building's structure and into the inner environment.

How Does Mold Affect Your Health And Your Yeast Infection?

Many of us are exposed to mold spores every day, usually by touching or breathing them in. Because molds naturally exist outdoors as well as indoors, living in a totally mold-free environment is near impossible. You even eat foods containing plenty of the stuff like cheeses, breads, leftover foods and mushrooms that are moldy foods themselves.

As molds grow, they release microscopic spores that can then travel through the air where they can be easily inhaled. People who inhale large numbers of spores may get quite sick indeed, especially those who are more susceptible like the immune-compromised or those who are immune-suppressed from drug treatment (e.g. Prednisolone) or on recurring antibiotics for complaints like acne, those with yeast infection, those with allergies and the elderly especially.

Such infections can also affect the skin, eyes, lungs or other organs. These are considered "opportunistic" infections that usually do not affect strong and healthy people. Once again, it's all about your susceptibility and your level of resistance.

You May Have A Yeast Infection And Not A Mold Allergy

I have found that some health-care professionals get confused and diagnose patients with major mold sensitivity and allergy issues rather than the patient having candida albicans, which is itself a fungus. This is where careful case taking will uncover the real underlying cause. The signs and symptoms of mold based health problems are particularly aggravated by living in such damp environments, and in addition I've noticed over the years how several patients have told me how much better they felt when on holidays or when they lived at a friend's place (like house-sitting) even for just a few days. Not a co-incidence I believe, they just shifted to living where there was a lot less mold spore floating around and they felt better. Their immune system was not challenged and consequently their symptoms eased right off, yet their diet and lifestyle remained virtually unchanged. They were still eating bread and drinking wine but felt fine. In this case it will probably be an allergy or sensitivity to mold rather than a yeast infection, note the patient was still on the same diet yet the symptoms eased right off.

But does the person crave sugars, chocolate, alcohol and sweets in general and suffer badly in moldy, damp or smoke filled environment? Then this person needs to be checked carefully for a yeast infection, a very real possibility, but in my experience many of those who have a mold sensitivity or allergy may have a rampant yeast infection. Confused yet? With experience you soon get to understand the difference, believe me.

The hidden threat of health concerns surrounding mold are an important reason to prevent mold growth and to clean up molds, especially in our indoor environments. Have you noticed those anti-mold advertisements on the TV at night? You can bet that if it is on the flat screen it will be a big problem because they wouldn't waste their marketing dollars otherwise. These advertisements seem to target your bathroom and kitchen and make you feel that only this area is affected by mold, try looking very closely in your bedroom, you may be quite surprised! Bathrooms and kitchens are the two major areas that are potentially affected by mold. Did you know that mold could often be found growing in the kitchen? It's because there's lots of moisture in the kitchen like water running from your tap or steam from your kettle or the stove.

Mold Is Very Common In Your Kitchen

Your kitchen is a hot spot for mold; here are a few of the key areas affected and what to do about them.

The Fridge

Food that's left in the fridge for a long time frequently ends up with mold on it, did you know? When you have a yeast infection, eating ANY foods either covered in mold or containing mold is a bad idea if you are seriously trying to recover. Areas you will want to check out frequently are the bottom of the fridge, because foods near the bottom are often out of sight and forgotten about and naturally this is where any mold will thrive. The second reason mold is especially common at the bottom of the fridge is that it is not as cold here and water often ends gravitating here as well.

Did you read section one of this chapter? In this section I've mentioned that it is best to avoid all left-over foods and to throw out that collection of jars from your refrigerator when you commence treatment for your yeast infection in earnest because they are perfect little mold factories and if you have a yeast infection the last thing you want to do is to unknowingly breed and consume more fungus.

Make sure you regularly (every week) clean out your refrigerator to get rid of any mold residues, and good advice for you is to replace any fridge over five years old with a brand new one if you have a severe yeast infection. It's like moving to another home and you might be quite surprised at the difference this can make. Carefully check for any traces of any old foods left in your fridge like rotting fruit and vegetables. And did I mention the drip tray; it can often end up with mold spores as well, keep an eye on it and clean it regularly.

Mold on Dishes

If you have a yeast infection I'd prefer you use the dishwasher and not to wash your plates, cups and cutlery by hand. Mold can more easily grow this way than when using a dishwasher, which tends to typically wash at a higher temperature than you can manually and rinses better too. Don't leave plates and bowls piling up and do wash every single day, rinse dishes as soon as they are used and stack them at once in your dishwasher. All common sense isn't it?

Mold in the Garbage Bin and Compost Bin

Your garbage and compost bins are probably the most frequently overlooked areas that can potentially contain amazing amounts of mold in your kitchen.

All those food scraps and wet waste can begin grow molds in less than two days, so make sure you empty your rubbish bin every single day. If you are a severe yeast infection patient I'd recommend that you take the compostable material outside every day, throw out the compost bin from the kitchen! It is a hotbed for mold and unless you wash it out every single day (who does?) it can potentially give you a nice big dose of mold spores every time you open it.

The Cutting Board

Do you have a wooden cutting board or wooden chopping block you cut fruits, vegetables and meat on? I place my cutting boards in the dishwasher. You can scrub your cutting boards well with boiling water and give them a very good scrub. Placing them in the full sun will also help to kill mold spores. Consider non-wooden cutting boards, there is less chance of any mold contamination because you can clean and rinse these surfaces more thoroughly than you can with wood.

And while you are there in the kitchen, take the bread bin away until you recover from your yeast infection, you really shouldn't be eating any breads made with yeast until you get well

Molds Contains Spores That Circulate In The Air

According to Dr. Leo Galland, an American health expert, molds contain *bio-aerosols* that consist of microscopic living fungi and/or bacteria that can circulate freely in the air. Legionnaire's disease is one such well-known example and this disease has killed many susceptible folk over the years. An adverse reaction to mold depends largely on how much a person is exposed to, the age of the person and the person's sensitivities or allergies. The same amount of mold may cause health effects in one person, but not in another. Some mold experts like Dr. Galland believe that mold may be responsible for many hidden health problems not necessarily linked to the sick building syndrome. A study in Scotland where mold and mildew are abundant, just like New Zealand, found that those who lived in housing that was judged to be damp or showed visible signs of mildew, (particularly in the sleeping quarters) had far greater rates of sickness than those who lived in drier environments. These differences were independent of smoking, occupation or income. It is a known fact that damp homes breed both mold and dust mites more easily and indoor levels of molds can reach concentrations that are tens of thousands greater than those outside.

Symptoms Of Mold Exposure

Exposure to mold can cause a variety of symptoms, and as you will see below, a lot of these signs and symptoms also belong to those with a yeast infection. Sensitive people who have touched or inhaled mold or mold spores may have allergic reactions such as:

- Blocked nose
- Cold or flu like symptoms
- Coughing
- Difficulty breathing, shortness of breath
- Hay fever like symptoms
- Hair loss
- Itchy nose
- Itchy eyes
- Itchy ears
- Irritated or itchy skin
- Irritated or itchy throat
- Nasal congestion
- Red, bloodshot eyes

- Runny nose

- Sore throat

- Sinus congestion

- Sinus headaches

- Skin rash, hives

- Sneezing

- Watery eyes

- Wheezing

Molds can even trigger asthma attacks in people who are allergic, causing wheezing, chest tightness and shortness of breath. And when is mold at its peak? In the wet of winter, when it is rainy and damp, the same time people come down with respiratory infections, funny that. Have you gone to your bedroom yet and checked the corners and looked at the ceiling, the window sills? Do you see any silvery or dark patches in the corner of the ceiling? Check the carpets too, especially near windows.

What Mold Tests Are Available And What Do I Do?

I personally wouldn't waste any of my money on testing for mold allergies. Blood or skin testing called the RAST test can be done to show if you are allergic to a substance. The RAST test detects levels of antibodies to particular allergens and the results are highly variable indeed. Ok, so you are allergic to molds and dust mites. Big deal, what do you do now, sell your house and go live in Arizona? If you have symptoms year-round, and not just in winter or when your house is at its dampest, my first recommendation is to try to rid yourself of your yeast infection and improve your immune health in general. As I routinely say in the Candida Crusher, if you increase your resistance, your susceptibility drops. With a powerful immune system and an awareness of mold coupled with a reduction of mold in your indoor environment (if you have a problem), you should be able to significantly improve your resistance to those floating spores. If your house is particularly bad, then move out. By the way, have you checked your house out for any traces of mold and cleaned up that mold on your bathroom ceiling, in your bedroom or kitchen yet?

What to do When All Else Fails

Why Many Fail to Get Permanent Results

For most people with a yeast infection, effective treatment is simply a matter of following the Candida Crusher Program, eating the right foods, adopting the right lifestyle and taking the Candida Crushing dietary supplements. Many will finish their treatment and achieve the desired result and go on their merry way.

Unfortunately not all endings are happy, and all too many will find a returning of their old symptoms, and this is mainly the case because they have gone back to their old ways of eating and living. If you keep on doing what you have always done, there is that inherent danger of "getting what you always got" back. Common sense, isn't it? But not to many people I have seen with chronic and recurring yeast infections it seems. Some will come in for treatment only when they have uncomfortable symptoms, and as soon as these subside they slowly go back to their own ways. Others will learn and maintain healthy dietary and lifestyle changes for many years and rarely get a repeat of their annoying symptoms. It all depends on a person's ability to discipline themselves I guess.

> *Mastering others reveals strength. Mastering yourself reveals true power.*
> — Lao Tzu

Some people with yeast infections will need longer periods of treatment and some will need stronger treatments. It is hard to accurately predict and monitor the type and amount of supplements an individual will be able to tolerate. Some will have treatment aggravations and yet others may even have very strong aggravations, making treatment uncomfortable and even agonizing for the very sensitive patient. One of the smartest things you can do is to simply stay on track, work through a few difficult spots during the early phase of treatment and to especially stay on track as you notice the improvements, the more you improve, the more likely the temptation will be to stray and go off track. This is the danger zone, and I have explained this in greater detail in the introduction to chapter 7. Be sure to read "How People Actually Get Well".

What To Do If You Aggravate

I have found that most practitioners do not tell their patients that when bacteria and yeasts are killed off they may release cell wall fractions and various chemicals into the bloodstream and digestive tract. In some cases, this can weaken the immune system considerably and make the person feel very washed-out and "wasted" and is a prime reason for the side-effects of candida treatment some experience. If you follow the Candida Crusher carefully, your chances of aggravating violently will be very slim indeed, especially if you follow all of my suggestion in chapter 7 carefully.

A good way to side-step those annoying aggravations, particularly if you *know* you are a sensitive person, is to start with the minutest amount of supplements, and to *very slowly* build up the dosages until the slightest side-effects are noticeable. You may notice a slight discomfort as the yeast cells begin to die this way, and will potentially avoid any serious die-off which can leave you feeling terrible for a week or more, being barely able to function. Always remember, an increase in uncomfortable symptoms upon commencement of treatment is not a bad sign, it is a positive sign and means progress! You will find the gradually the symptoms decrease and that the treatment can be stepped up.

A further way for you to avoid aggravations is not to begin a new hobby or sport when you undergo treatment. It is not wise to go bungee jumping, skydiving, scuba diving, long-distance running or engage in a triathlon, etc. Your body is under a considerable stress when you undergo the Candida Crusher Program, your immune system will be challenged and this extra stress can only serve to lower your resistance even further an increase the chance of an aggravation. Wait until you have fully recovered before you attempt a strenuous form of any activity.

Withdrawal Symptoms

Sometimes your aggravation symptoms are not as a direct result of yeast dying or of the treatment itself, but come because of a withdrawal you are experiencing from coffee, tea, alcohol, chocolate, dairy products, sugar, wheat, corn, or even yeast itself. The withdrawal aggravation is most commonly due to caffeine, so be sure to slowly step this down during your Big Clean-Up, or better still, before you have a cleanse and well before you start on the MEVY Diet.

The withdrawal can also be due to taking an allergy prone food out of your diet, which occurs in the second stage of the Candida Crusher Diet. So it you think about it, with a bit of thought you will be able to know what it was, the caffeine or the allergy food. Did the aggravation come about not long after you stopped that coffee or chocolate, or did it occur after you went onto the low-allergy diet?

Your Greatest Weapon - Yourself

I can confidently tell you, after having suffered with a chronic yeast infection myself, and having treated many people, that the greatest weapons at your disposal are your diet, your lifestyle, the supplements but first and foremost they are patience, self-discipline, determination and the ability to stick with my program until you get the desired results. You may even become incredibly frustrated at different times, and maybe a little difficult to live with as you experience periodic setbacks, but I'd like to remind you that setbacks are commonly experienced by the vast majority of yeast infection sufferers.

There is NO such thing as a "12 Hour Cure" when it comes to a yeast infection, especially a chronic one, so please be aware that you will have to work at it but know that in the end you will have reached your ultimate goal, a complete resolution of all your yeast infection symptoms.

Potential Treatment Aggravations And What To Do

Here are some handy hints and tips on what to do if you experience any of the following aggravations that may occur during the Candida Crusher Program, especially if you have had a chronic yeast infection for many years.

Bloating and Gas. If you have gone through the Candida Crusher Book, you will have read plenty of information about dysbiosis, leaky gut, food allergies, and the many other digestive issues affecting those with yeast infections. Bloating and gas are especially common, because you have an overgrowth of yeasts inside your digestive tract and these yeasts like to eat sugars and produce gas as a result. Some people have a complete disappearance of these complaints that they may have experienced on/off for years, whereas others will begin to get them when they commence treatment.

The potential food allergies many have and leaky gut syndrome will only add to the digestive discomfort, so be aware that your level of bloating and gas may go up and down during the treatment. Make sure you do the Big Clean Up before you start on the Candida Crusher Program, it can potentially help you a lot by flushing out a lot of the bad bugs and yeasts from your system before you even begin.

Garlic is one of your best friends when it comes to bloating and gas, and so is the Candida Crusher Formula. And make sure you take it and the probiotics religiously, you should notice a significant reduction with bloating and gas if you do. Stick with my diet recommendations and be sure to look at your stress levels, as stress can affect your digestive system quite a lot. You will be able to read about the diet and stress in the appropriate sections in this chapter.

Indigestion. This is very much like the bloating and gas, and both of these digestive complaints can be as a consequence of indigestion. Be sure to take the Digestive Enzymes before or during each meal, eat smaller portion sizes and be sure to chew your foods well. Have you checked the combinations of food you are eating? Eat steamed vegetables and white (chicken and fish) proteins for a few days; this should get your digestion back on track. Keep an eye on your stress levels; stress has this way of affecting the stomach of many anxious people in particular.

Weight loss. People don't normally gain weight on the Candida Crusher Program; in fact I've found that they are much more inclined to lose it. I like people to keep on eating grains and legumes, as these will ensure that not too much weight is lost. Eat smaller meals more frequently, and be sure to eat plenty of protein as well. Have plenty of rest periods and don't do too much, anyone who expends lots of calories and cuts their diet back will be significantly more prone to losing weight. Those who worry excessively or who can't relax will find it harder to gain as well, be sure to read the lifestyle hints and tips.

Constipation. This bowel complaint may occur at any time during your treatment, and one of the main reasons it may occur is because you are changing your diet and the bowel flora become altered as a consequence.

If you come into the Candida Crusher Program with a history of constipation, I'd like you to start to eat sensibly from now on and not to revert back to what you were eating previously, and especially take a look at your lifestyle habits, because poor habits here are often at the root cause of chronic constipation.

Eat smaller, more frequent meals and avoid overeating at one sitting. Take time to eat, breathe slowly and chew food thoroughly. Are you still eating your dinner on your lap in front of the evening news? Try eating at the dinner table.

Reduce and stop your caffeine intake, caffeine is implicated in constipation and diarrhea.

Foods that lubricate the intestines. Eat foods like beet, okra (gumbo), kiwi fruit, seaweed, spinach, sesame seed, sesame oil, walnut, pine nut, almond, alfalfa sprouts, carrot and cauliflower.

Foods that promote bowel motions. Eat foods that help move stool through the intestines-cabbage, papaya, peas, sesame seeds, coconut, asparagus, and kiwi fruit.

Herbs & foods that soothe the intestines. Eat foods like marshmallow root, flax seeds, fenugreek seeds, psyllium seeds, licorice root, and slippery elm bar

Beneficial bacteria enhancing foods. Eat foods like miso, sauerkraut, yoghurt, Kim chi, kefir and quark

Decrease intake of saturated (animal) fats. Eat foods with an increased level of essential fatty acids (cold-water fish, nuts, and seeds). Take the Omega 3 fatty acid supplement twice daily.

Eat more fresh fruits, vegetables and whole grains. Did you know that a 2010 survey found that 17% of British people never eat fresh fruits or vegetables? Follow the MEVY Diet, and make sure you eat plenty of greens, they help the bowel function and you will discover that your bowels will improve significantly within weeks.

Drink more water. Do you really drink water frequently throughout the day? Warm lemon water taken before meals stimulates digestion. Try the juice of ½ a lemon in water in the morning before breakfast. REMEMBER to drink plenty of liquids. You need more fluid particularly when you have more fiber for fiber to work effectively.

Flax meal. Have 1 heaping tsp. in 8 oz. of apple juice, provides fiber and soothes the digestive tract. Follow with an additional 8 oz. of water. Linseed/Sunflower/Almond mix is excellent too. Slippery elm bark powder is good, but can be a bit pricey.

Colonic hydrotherapy. I have solved very tricky cases of constipation with recommending a course of colonics plus other complementary and alternative methods of healing. Consider visiting a professional colon therapist if you have a history of bowel problems.

Liver and bowel detox. Have you read section 3 in chapter 7? This chapter will give you all the information you need with regard to cleansing and detox. If you have been constipated for some time, get that bowel working first then consider the Liver & Gallbladder Flush.

Diarrhea. Diarrhea does occur with candida, and when it does I generally suspect parasites and bad bacterial levels, especially if there is any sensation of pain or discomfort around the belly button or to one side lower down the abdomen. Try to keep away from raw beets; they may make the diarrhea worse. Make sure you eat the raw garlic (during a meal) every day and take the Candida crusher Formula three to four times daily. Yogurt may help a lot here, and also the fermented and cultured foods, so be sure to read all this information in section 1 of chapter 7. Be sure to take the probiotics three times daily. Slippery elm bark is good and so is ground linseed.

Nausea. Although nausea does occur, I rarely witness this with patients who undergo the Candida Crusher Program. Sometimes parasites can cause nausea, particularly when they are killed during treatment. Grapefruit seed extract (GSE) can cause nausea in a very few, but GSE is just too effective to leave out of the Candida Crusher Formula, so just reduce the dose if you experience any discomfort. Sometimes taking a (yeast free) B Complex vitamin can help with nausea, especially B6. Ginger tea can help significantly, so can chewing on a thin slice of fresh ginger. Be sure to take the Digestive Enzymes a few times during the day before meals, they will help a lot and so with the Probiotics. Some folks become more sensitive to smells during treatment, or have become very sensitive to odors or fumes due to their candida overgrowth; a good idea here is to burn some essential oil like lavender. Keep your meals to small portion sizes, another good tip.

Blood Sugar Problems and Sugar Cravings. Whenever you make diet changes or are prone to stress you could develop hypoglycaemia, or low blood sugar. Signs and symptoms of low blood sugar are irritability, weakness, tiredness, headaches, sweet cravings, and shakiness if meals are delayed. Make sure you eat small meals more frequently, eat plenty of protein and avoid a carbohydrate rich diet especially. Blood sugar issues generally resolve themselves after you have worked out the right and wrong foods to eat. After you have been on the Candida Crusher Program for a month or two you will have worked out what foods suit you best, and what you should avoid.
For stubborn low blood sugar or excessive sweet cravings, take 500 mcg of Chromium picolinate before meals. For seriously heavy-duty sweet cravings, take some of the herb called Gymnema, read more about this in section 1.

Mucus. I've had some patients complain of increasing phlegm and mucus during treatment, once again, this will be cause by the change of diet and flora of the digestive system. I suspect it also has something to do with a slight change in the body's pH and digestive enzymatic levels. Be sure to get rid of the mucus-forming foods out of your diet (especially dairy products), and take a more alkaline approach to your eating, see section 1 of chapter 7 for the list of the acid and alkaline forming foods. The Digestive Enzyme formula will help considerable here, and so will lemon juice and garlic. I've found that those with phlegm tend to improve when they supplement with pancreatic enzymes in particular.

Fatigue And A Low Mood. You may not experience much fatigue or mood changes, but for the majority of patients I have seen this will not be the case. Do expect to feel tired during the different stages of treatment and be sure to allow extra rest and sleep, your body and especially your immune system will appreciate it and you will recover that much sooner. This is certainly not a good time to go to Peru for a two-week hike to see

Machu Picchu, as one of my patients did a few years ago. But it is a good time to go to a health resort and be pampered.

You may not be particularly pleasant to be around during the first two to three weeks of the MEVY Diet, bearing that in mind it may not be the best time to go to a wedding! You may be able to plan some events in your life, and if you can plan to undergo the first month of treatment away from any important upcoming social or work-related events, it will be a good decision you have made. Therefore, try to schedule the initial part of your Candida Crusher Program away from weddings, vacations or important social gatherings. Explain to the person closest to you that you are going to commence the Candida Crusher Program and that you may experience fatigue, low moods or an increase in some of your symptoms.

Good advice I can give to the chronic female yeast infection patient is to be extra kind to yourself, consider that you have a chronic health problem and to pretend you are several months pregnant. You wouldn't do anything too strenuous if you were pregnant would you? You would avoid alcohol, late nights and doing too much in general, you would be more inclined to rest up with a magazine. The "candida pregnancy" doesn't have to last 9 months though, but the kinder you are to yourself the quicker you are likely to recover fully. Give yourself permission to ease off a little and take it easy, especially on those days when you feel just drained or washed-out. For guys I usually tell them to rest up, and treat themselves as if they are recovering from an operation or a major sporting event.

Anger, Depression and Crying. Feeling lousy and even feeling angry are common emotional responses for some who are chronically unwell with a yeast infection. They are normal bodily responses to healing; so be aware that your tolerance levels may be lower than they normally are and your fuse may be a little short, especially if you have teenagers or a similar reason to get irritated. Don't feel ashamed of having a cry, it is a good emotional release as you will almost certainly be feeling more sensitive than usual, especially during the early stages of yeast infection treatment. Talking to a trusted friend about how you feel is a good idea too. Make sure you have plenty of rest and do speak with your doctor or a counsellor if you feel sad frequently.

A chronic yeast infection can make you feel really lousy at the best of times, I can recall how low I felt when I was chronically unwell, and felt quite depressed when those around me thought I was just imagining I was unwell and was just "seeking attention". St John's Wort may be a good choice for those who get the blues, but do talk to your health-care professional before you take things for emotional expressions like anger and depression. B Vitamins, Calcium/Magnesium and Vitamin C are helpful as well.

Headaches. A headache is a warning sign that something is not quite right inside your body. Is it because you stopped coffee or are going through the detox phase? The patients who get the fiercest headaches are the ones who went cold turkey on 5 cups of coffee a day. I see them regularly, and boy, what a nasty headache you can get from a caffeine withdrawal!

Are you eating enough food and drinking enough water? Blood sugar problems occur easily, your brain especially needs that glucose (blood sugar) to keep it mentally focused and a lack of food, skipping meals or eating at weird times can all help to stimulate one of those nice dull background headaches.

Are you resting enough or doing too much? Those who don't relax and stress out (especially those who worry) tend to get sore and tight muscles of face, neck and upper back. It has been estimated that over three-quarters of all headaches are caused by tense muscles, and a tension headache is also one of the most common reasons why a person would take a pain killer. Do you stress out and are you working on reducing your stress load? Maybe you have been exposed to toxic fumes or a toxic (mold) environment? Often times, those who begin the Candida Crusher Program may well experience a headache in the first few weeks, and it will be probably due to a release of toxins that were stored away in the body. These kinds of headaches tend to spontaneously disappear within two or three days.

Try a Vitamin B Complex, but also a Magnesium product, a mineral that can help to relax those tight and sore muscles.

Insomnia. I have covered this common problem in great detail in the section, just go back and take a look. You will find "13 Ways To Beat Insomnia" quite useful.

Skin Aggravations. Some people get bad breath when they detox, some get tired and develop brain fog, some get a sore throat of a cold, others develop sore joints, and then there are those who get skin aggravations. If toxins are not eliminated properly through the digestive tract or kidneys, the skin may become a dumping ground for toxins and you could find that your skin may develop pimples or an acne-like condition, itchiness, redness or various kinds of swellings. Occasionally a person undergoing the Candida Crusher program may get a stye on their eyelid or a boil somewhere on their torso. These are all signs of toxins leaving the body and should be encouraged, so don't get upset and think that you have some new skin disease; it's just the body eliminating rubbish. I have found that some people get a skin rash when they eliminate the potentially allergy foods from their diet, especially those who used to have eczema in the past. Try Vitamin C powder, 1 to 2 teaspoons per day. Aim for 3,000 milligrams a day in water in divided doses before meals. One of the best herbal medicines is Burdock (Arctium lappa), a good blood purifier when you have a skin condition. Golden seal is a good choice too; small amounts for two weeks should do the trick. Take the Probiotics twice daily before meals. Calendula cream is worth applying to these skin areas, and get some Tea Tree Oil soap for the bath. If the skin flares up considerably during treatment, then reduce the dosage of any supplements you are taking and increase your intake of water, vegetables and get plenty of rest.

Colds, Coughs And Sore Throats. Those fighting a yeast infection may be more susceptible to poor immunity, and is it any wonder? When your body is fighting a yeast infection, when it probably has food allergies and a leaky gut, you will be more prone to coming down with a cold or cough. How can your immune system work under a load of yeast and bad bacteria? And then some take antibiotics as a consequence, is it any wonder their immune system becomes increasingly weaker?

Make sure you get ample rest and avoid getting excessively cold, exposed to drafts or being in moldy or damp places. Be sure to have a fresh clove of garlic daily, take the Probiotics, the Omega 3 and have additional Vitamin C if your immune system is especially vulnerable. I recommend herbal medicines for a sore throat, and my favorite herbs here are Echinacea root, Golden seal, Myrrh and Poke root.

Trouble-Shooting - What To Do If You STILL Need Help

OK, so you have followed the Candida Crusher Program faithfully, but you are still not satisfied with your recovery. It is as is something is holding you back from getting those permanent results you have been looking for. You have been following my recommendations for three or four months and you are having difficulties recovering from your yeast infection, where to now?

Try going through the following checklist using this list as a guide:

1. Re-examine your diet. Have you faithfully applied the diet principles I have outlined in section1? Have you started to feel better and then included some of the foods that you eliminated earlier on, such as caffeine, alcohol, sugary or processed foods, or have you slipped back into your old ways of eating? Be honest with yourself.

2. Have you checked yourself out carefully for any potential food-allergies? You may need to do an IgE/IgG Elisa blood test to determine your allergy status. Have you eliminated all the foods you are allergic to, are addicted to or are sensitive to?

3. Have you incorporated the major lifestyle changes I have outlined in chapter seven? If not, make these changes right now.

4. Do you have adrenal fatigue? You may wish to read Dr. Wilson's book on Adrenal Fatigue, it may well be one of your biggest obstacles, and a major reason why you are failing to recover. Strong and healthy adrenal glands can beat a yeast infection when all else fails, so be sure to read the section in chapter seven on adrenal fatigue.

5. You may like to re-examine your lifestyle, especially consider the balance of the demands on your mind and body that you are making. Have you completed the Holmes Stress Test? Are you taking enough time out from the hectic demands of your work or family life?

6. Re-examine your exercise program. Are you moving your body at least three times a week or are you chained to your computer?

7. How is your sleep? Do you have insomnia or difficulties getting to sleep or frequent early waking? You will never have a good immune system if you have a continual sleeping problem. Read the section on insomnia in this section.

8. Have you discontinued taking any unnecessary medications from the doctor? Can you stop the oral contraceptive pill, antibiotics or hormonal treatments? These can stop your progression and set your progress right back.

9. How is your environment? Have you cleaned up that moldy ceiling or bathroom? Are you still using chemicals or exposed to fumes, poisons or any chemicals in your occupation? You may want to seriously think about finding another job. A green keeper saw me with a yeast infection and finally beat his chronic jock itch once he got rid of his job and the chemicals that went along with it.

10. Are you taking the right dietary supplements and taking them regularly? The Candida Crusher supplements have been specifically designed to complement the Candida Crusher program and will be available in 2013.

11. If you have followed all these points then let's move onto the Obstacles To Cure.

Why Do Only Some People Get Well And Stay Well?

When I wrote The Candida Crusher, it struck me that it always appears to be that the patients who get well and *stay well* are those who adopt and maintain the more holistic ways of health-care, are here are some of the major principles they adopt:

- **They do their homework.** These are the people who tend to and read & study various resources like health magazines and The Candida Crusher to gain a better understanding of their health problems and in particular the actual root causes of their yeast infection. They attend health lectures and have friendships with people who are also into healthy lifestyles. They avoid pharmaceutical drugs for all their trivial ills and have become informed about the most effective ways of using natural medicines instead of drugs. If your friends all drink, smoke and are overweight, then there's a good chance you may too.

- **They assess and change their attitude if need be.** As they become more enlightened, they become more positive and hopeful of their health and wellbeing and realize that health truly is in their hands. Instead of feeling that they are a victim of their own circumstances, they begin to actively participate in their own recovery from a yeast infection. They work out a plan of action with their practitioner and are committed and work hard to keep on track. They have learned that the glass is half full and not half empty.

- **They are committed to getting and staying well.** I have always found that those who gain the best results from lifestyle and dietary programs are the ones who are the most committed and will do whatever it takes to stay on track in terms of their health. They pursue a healthy lifestyle and avoid anything not conducive to optimal health. They have learned to live with choices, not habits.

- **They understand the importance of optimal nutrition.** Those who get well quickly from a yeast infection are those who take their diet most seriously. They plan their shopping trips and meals and make the right choices when dining out. They have learned that food is medicine, and medicine is food. They avoid the obstacles like alcohol and sweet foods until they have fully recovered.

- **They begin an exercise program.** As soon as they regain their energy levels they start to do light exercise – regularly. Those committed eat well and exercise daily, even if this means going for a half an hour walk in the morning or evening. It is important to find the kind of activity you like and to do it regularly, whether it be walking, cycling or swimming.

They understand the relevance lifestyle and adopt health habits. Getting well and maintaining optimal health and wellbeing means looking at (and be willing to change) all aspects of your lifestyle in addition to eating healthy, exercising regularly and taking relaxation seriously. Those who understand and learn the significance of stress management, relaxation techniques, the importance of balancing work and play in addition to exercise and diet will achieve the best outcomes. These are the patients I always look out for; they are a joy to work with.

Do You Have Any Obstacles To Cure?

> *Strength is not born from strength. Strength can be born only from weakness. So be glad of your weaknesses now, they are the beginnings of your strength.*
> Dr. Claire Weekes

An obstacle to cure is any body burden that continues to drain your health and is most likely an undiscovered burden. Such burdens can be like a bomb left over from a war from many years ago, they can remain buried deep and could be uncovered any day and literally blow up right in your face.

Hidden Focal Infections

Prior to the penicillin discovery in the 1940's, German research began to study chronic health problems that appeared to have obscure causes. What they found was interesting; they found that even a small problem in one part of the body could cause a disorder in a more distant part and apparently unconnected area.

Chronically inflamed areas, like a rumbling appendix, recurrent tonsillitis, and dental conditions like cracked, dead or diseased teeth all were good examples of likely culprits. However, with the discovery of the "wonder-drugs" (antibiotics) to combat infection, concern for where the infection was coming from suddenly became a lot less important than just "which particular germ" the infection was caused by. All that a doctor needed to do was to identity the specific germ and then work out which particular antibiotic was needed. Antibiotics became the rage in the 1960's, they were freely available and all the focus was on killing germs rather than balancing the good and bad bacteria. This

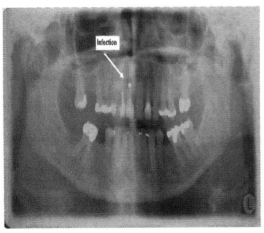

is in essence how we got away from treating the cause to just concentrating on treating the symptom.

Dental research for example has shown that inflammation of the jawbone can act as a seeding ground for a host of health problems including lethargy, poor concentration, irritability, poor sleep patterns, lower back pain, allergies and migraine. Focal infections in the head can have the strongest affect on the body, because of their proximity to the brain and the central nervous system. Root canal therapy can in some cases result long term in a "focal" infection, i.e.; an infection in some part of the body that lies undiscovered much like that World War 2 bomb. Do you see the hidden focal infection in this patient's X-ray? This is a patient with rheumatoid arthritis along with a severe yeast infection which both fully resolved after her hidden infection was dealt with.

Typical unresolved focal infections include:

- Chronically inflamed tonsils

- Chronic sinus infection

- Osteitis in the jawbone

- Root canal, dead or cracked teeth

- Abscess or cyst in the jaw

- Parasitic infection of the ileo-caecal valve (digestive system)

Be sure that your blood tests (especially the immune and inflammation blood markers) don't show anything unresolved. If you find any hidden sources of inflammation especially, be sure to get to the bottom of it, especially if you just can't seem to get that yeast infection resolved in spite of your best efforts. The following list is a list of blood tests that may help you in determine if you have a sub-acute or chronic sub-clinical infection. This is particularly so if you notice a trend and the results are consistently repeated over a prolonged period of time. Ask you doctor to run these tests, ask a knowledgeable doctor to interpret them for you, and be sure to get copies for your own records. I like people to plot their own results on a Microsoft Excel Spreadsheet, that way they have an instant overview and will be able to establish when they change something about their treatment, if the blood results change as a result too. This way you can see what works and what doesn't and you won't be wasting your time and money on ineffective treatments. Doesn't this make sense?

- Increased or decreased white blood cell counts

- Mildly increased sedimentation rate (ESR)

- Increased total serum globulin

- Increased lymphocytes

- Increased LDH isoenzyme # 1

- Elevated C reactive protein (CRP)

Furthermore, you may want to find a doctor who specializes in Live Blood Cell Analysis, this may well uncover a hidden source of inflammation.

Intestinal Dysbiosis

As you will be aware of by now, there are several hundreds of species of bacteria that live in harmony inside your digestive tract. If you really can't seem to get a handle on your digestive problems when you have a yeast infection then I urge you to get a CDSA x 3 test completed by a reputable lab.

There are several different kinds of urine, bowel, breath and blood tests that can detect dysbiosis, but in my opinion the CDSA (do three stool samples on three concurrent days) is the gold standard. This test will not only determine which microorganisms are at the heart of the problem, it will give you a sensitivity panel outlining which natural and pharmaceutical agents are best suited to eliminate them.
Find a doctor in your area who has experience with this functional test. One of the best labs in America in Doctor's Data in Chicago.

Food Allergies Or Food Sensitivities

A very common hidden and underlying burden is being sensitive or allergic to a particular food. It may take some time before your leaky gut is resolved. The tragedy is that these issues are easily treated once recognized. Be sure to read all about food allergies and food sensitivities in section 1 of this chapter. You may want to consider doing the food allergy blood test, and the best lab in my opinion is US Biotek in Seattle, USA.

Lack of Sleep

I'm amazed how many people do everything right, except find enough time to rest and sleep when they are on the Candida Crusher Program. Lack of sleep can be a particularly effective body burden because it can be a common sign of both a high or too low cortisol level in the body. Chronic lack of sleep is now regarded as a health hazard and has been associated with many different types of health conditions. Decreased immunity and an increased susceptibility to infections are much more common in those who don't sleep enough. Lack of sufficient sleep slows the healing response and prolongs the recovery phase of a yeast infection. The bottom line is that you need at least eight hours of sleep each night, and you may need even more in the first month of commencing the Candida Crusher Program.

Moldy or Toxic Environments

Have you noticed that when you moved house that your problems got better or they got worse? In New Zealand we have a particular problem with "Leaky Building Syndrome", many houses were constructed during a boom period and it has been discovered that thousands of houses in Auckland alone leak a considerable amount of water and are literally breeding grounds for molds. If your house or place of employ has a problem such as "Sick Building" Syndrome, then you may find that the best decision you could make is to leave these premises. Try moving house or changing jobs if you have a strong belief or suspicion that this may be the case, it could hold the key to your complete and permanent recovery. Be sure to read the section on mold in this chapter.

Lack of Clean Water and Fresh Air

Pretty basic stuff, but I have found that many people who just don't seem to recover don't appear to get the basics really right. Do you live or work in an environment with poor airflow or poor air exchange? Are you drinking enough pure and fresh drinking water every day, preferably filtered, which doesn't contain fluoride or chlorine, and the many other chemicals commonly found in tap water? The basic tenets of good health are high quality fresh foods, pure water and air and plenty of rest and sleep. Your body has an amazing capacity to heal if we give it the right conditions to do so.

Staying Well - Repeat A Short Candida Crusher Treatment Annually

Last but certainly not least, I recommend that everyone, not only those who used to have a yeast infection and who have recovered, repeat at least a short anti-microbial program once a year. I complete a detox each year, and have done so for over twenty-five years. It is my way of cleansing the system and keeping the bad bugs in control. Please view section 3 of this chapter for further information on detoxification and cleansing.

Many chronic diseases, including autoimmune diseases, heart disease and cancers are associated with pathogenic microbes and dysbiosis and we can prevent much disease by periodically eliminating the overpopulation of bad bugs from our body thereby restoring the delicate balance of beneficial and not so beneficial microbes in our digestive systems.

Postscript

Is candida a fictitious illness that will soon be ignored by everyone because it was disease created by a bunch of hypochondriacs? Is this a problem that is "all in your head" because test results are negative?

Candida yeast infections are possibly one of the least understood and most widespread causes of illness today, just like they were fifty years ago. Precisely because yeast infections are ubiquitous, they are generally overlooked and not even considered in many cases to be a causative factor. A wider awareness of yeast infections as a diagnosis would lead to a marked reduction to a significant amount of human suffering.

Candida Crusher was designed as a manual to help those with a yeast infection, and also for practitioners who like to help their patients with yeast infections. This book was also written to raise awareness that yeast infections are not mere trivial or imaginary problems that will not go away if we simply just ignore them.

Yeast infections do exist, whether experts believe it or not. I have absolutely no doubt about it, and based on my own experiences along with the most extensive clinical and research studies by others such as doctors William Crook M.D., Orian Truss M.D., and Sidney Baker M.D., along with countless researchers at PhD level, too many to mention in this book.

Since much of the original research dating back to the 1980's, there have been over 100,000 research papers published on the effects of candida species and their adverse effects human health. Today, only the ignorant wish to believe that yeasts play no role in illness and that only bacteria and viruses are implicated.

There will be no doubt those who read Candida Crusher and pass off my information as "unscientific" and "anecdotal", because much of my information is based on patient's case histories and my own extensive clinical experience.

In defense I would like to quote what a professor of medicine has to say:

> *Clinical experience is the gold standard on which patient care should be based.*
> Gene H. Stollerman, M.D., Professor of Medicine, Boston University School of Medicine.

I trust that you enjoyed reading the Candida Crusher and have learned a few tricks or tips that may have even become a tipping point in your life and help you on your way to health and wellness.

Just A Few Points Before We Conclude:

- Survey - Do you complete the online candida yeast infection survey at YeastInfection.Org?

- Candida Supplements - Check CanXida.com for candida supplements.

- YouTube - Be sure to check our YouTube channel https://www.youtube.com/@canxida.

- Newsletter - Are you on our newsletter mailing list? That way you will be the first to know what we've got planned? Then visit CanXida.com and sign up for our newsletter.

CHAPTER 8 FAQs & Appendixes

Frequently Asked Questions

Here are some of the most frequently asked FAQs; these are the questions I get asked time and again about yeast infection treatment. After reading the Candida Crusher, you may well have a few questions and you will probably find the answer here. You will find most of these FAQs on yeastinfection.org, and many more FAQs will appear on www.yeastinfection.org and www.candidacrusher.com in time.

Commonly Asked Yeast Infection Questions

What Are Yeast Infections?

Candida albicans is a type of yeast like fungus that inhabits the intestines of over 90% of people as well as the genital tract and mouth of the host. It is important to realize that candida albicans is normally occurring in your body, it's when an imbalance occurs and too much yeast grows that a problem develops. In women the condition migrates readily from the large intestine to the vagina.

Candida is microscopic yeast in a sub-group of fungi or molds. And molds are truly everywhere; these bugs live in and on the soil, on all plants, in the air and in fact thrive on all living creatures' great and small. You may be familiar to fungi as the green "fur" which you occasionally see on a piece of moldy cheese, bread or fruit. Molds and yeasts spread and reproduce by releasing many millions of microscopic spores into the atmosphere, they literally float on air and eventually settle on a surface and if the conditions are favourable enough, the spore will grow into another mould plant. Yeasts favor dark, moist and warm environments and there are many potential places in your body that can support the growth and proliferation of yeast.

Who Gets Yeast Infections?

Anyone from birth to old age and from any race or culture can develop and suffer from a yeast infection. People vary greatly in their ability to develop and maintain a yeast infection in their bodies. A high stress lifestyle, a life crisis or a continuing difficult situation can cause a yeast infection in even the healthiest person because these factors will lower a person's resistance and increase their susceptibility. However there are certain factors that increase susceptibility to yeast infections.

These include a diet high in take-out foods; alcohol consumption; too little sleep and rest; taking an antibiotic or the oral contraceptive pill; a diet high in refined sugars and simple carbohydrates like pasta and bread; a mother with a yeast infection during gestation and birth. Unfortunately many of these factors are common in modern life.

What Are The Common Symptoms Of A Yeast Infection?

A candida yeast infection overgrowth can potentially cause so many symptoms, the most common in my experience are:

- Fatigue and tiredness and general weakness or malaise.
- Bloating, flatulence (gas)
- Food allergies
- Itching skin such as scalp, ear, groin, armpit or vagina
- Carbohydrate craving, desire for sweet foods like candy, ice cream, alcohol, etc.
- Vaginitis (vaginal thrush) accompanied often by a vaginal discharge.
- Anxiety and depression
- Impaired memory, poor concentration
- A foggy brain with feelings of unreality of feeling spaced out.

What Are The Less Common Symptoms Of A Yeast Infection?

Additionally, numerous other symptoms may less commonly be exhibited. Of these, those I see most frequently in the clinic include:

- Cystitis/urethritis (urinary tract infection – painful, burning or "stinging" sensations when trying to urinate).
- Menstrual irregularities, loss of libido.
- Stiff, creaking and painful joints, muscle pain.
- Indigestion or heartburn.
- Diarrhea or constipation.
- Inhalant allergies and multiple chemical sensitivities.
- Mucus or catarrh, hay fever, sinusitis or a persistent cough.
- Heart arrhythmias, missing a heartbeat, fast heartbeat.
- Discoloured nails, acne and other skin eruptions, especially when itching.
- Earaches, headaches, and dizziness.

Is Yeast Infection Common?

Yes, yeast infection is a very common disorder, estimated to affect many millions of people worldwide at some point in their lives.

Where In My Body Would I Expect To Have A Yeast Infection?

You would expect yeast infection particularly in the darker, warmer and more moist regions of your body which could include the ears, mouth, nose and throat, the sinus region (AFS or allergic fungal sinusitis), the digestive system (anywhere from the mouth through to the anus), the blood, the vagina, the armpits, the groin region as well as around the toe or finger nails. As you can see, a yeast infection can affect literally any part of your body.

Can People Recover From A Yeast Infection?

Although a yeast infection may only last a short while, especially if it was caused by one transient stressful event such as one round of antibiotic, it can debilitating and last for many years – even a lifetime – without proper treatment. However, with proper treatment, most people can fully recover from a yeast infection. The Candida Crusher was written to help you overcome your yeast infection permanently, and if you follow the program you can be assured of a full and complete recovery.

Is Age Or Being Male Or Female A Factor In A Yeast Infection?

People can suffer from a yeast infection at any age, right through from newborn babies to the very elderly. Males and females are equally affected although we tend to see more women coming into the clinic seeking help.

How Often Do Bouts Of Yeast Infection Occur?

The frequency of a yeast infection occurrence varies with each person. Some people have only one episode of a yeast infection during their lifetime, some have several, and others experience chronic candida yeast infections from which they never recover. Whether a yeast infection is infrequent, or chronic, proper support will make all the difference.

Can A Yeast Infection Become Chronic?

Yes, in some people the digestive and immune systems do not return to normal levels of function without help, either because their diet and lifestyle remained poor, their stress levels were too great or too prolonged, or because their general health is poor. However, when a yeast infection becomes chronic, it is almost always because of the ignorance of factors that can be changed through the correct modification in lifestyle and diet such as the Candida Crusher Program.

How Do I Prevent A Yeast Infection From Returning And Stay Healthy?

The guidelines for keeping healthy and preventing the recurrences of a yeast infection are very similar to the overall principles of good health. A moderate lifestyle with good quality food, regular exercise and adequate rest, combined with a healthy mental attitude to the stresses of life goes a long way towards keeping your body strong and resilient. However, because modern life can be so stressful and diets can be so compromised, certain nutritional supplements specially designed to counter a yeast infection and help restore the digestive microbial balance and maintain a healthy digestive system.

What Can I Do To Prevent A Yeast Infection?

Read chapter 7, "The Candida Crusher Program" in the book Candida Crusher and faithfully follow the instructions. During your yeast infection, use the specialized dietary supplements recommended in the book for optimal support. During your recovery from a yeast infection, take some time off work in order to rejuvenate. If there is lingering tiredness after your illness, try to sleep in late when you can, and be especially conscious of eating high quality foods, and in particular avoid sweet foods, breads, alcohol, and follow the dietary as well as lifestyle recommendations as outlined in the Candida Crusher Program.

Will My Candida Come Back?

It shouldn't happen if you are sensible about your diet and lifestyle! As long as you limit your intake of the foods and drinks which launched you into this state in the first place. I have often found that a patient will consume one or more of a favourite whether it be chocolate, beer, bread, wine, junk food, cola drinks, etc. Yes – you have a high probability of getting the candida back if you go back to your old ways of eating too many refined and highly processed foods and drinks containing white sugar and flour. If you overindulge in alcohol, cigarettes and take pharmaceutical drugs like the oral contraceptive pill, steroids or antibiotics. If you over-extend yourself at work, play or exercise you will lower your immune system functionality and predispose yourself to the candida infection all over again as well. Consider candida as your teacher, did you learn any lessons? If you did and you were paying attention to the teacher you will find that your bad symptoms of candida should never come back again.

Do Heavy Metals Cause Candida?

No, not directly. Heavy metal toxicity, like many other toxins, can, over time, depress the immune system. Once the immune system is depressed, the candida can further affect immune function, leading to repeated opportunistic infections and greater fatigue. Mercury has ben implicated in the progression of a yeast infection, and you can read more about methyl mercury and candida in the section on detox in chapter 7.

Can Candida Damage My Thyroid Gland?

There is no evidence that candida can adversely affect the thyroid gland. That having been said keep in mind that the longer you have systemic candida, the more it can affect many bodily functions. If these problems are caused by candida, they will right themselves as the yeast organisms are eliminated.

Can You Die From Candida Overgrowth?

There is no known record of anyone actually dying from candida, however many long-term sufferers often wish they might! A serious candida yeast infection will not however disappear by itself without intervention. It will linger on and on, most often increasing the severity of symptoms over the years to the point of near incapacitation. This is why the problem should be addressed and eliminated as soon as possible. Don't be complacent; a minor yeast infection will become a major one in time so the sooner you identify whether you have a problem or not the better. Take the yeast infection survey now to determine if your yeast infection is mild, moderate or severe. Go to yesstinfection.org

Is There A Genetic Predisposition Towards A Yeast Infection?

It is not known if there is an actual genetic predisposition for a yeast infection. However, if one or both parents suffer from a candida yeast infection, either chronically or during the time of conception, and if the mother has a yeast infection during gestation, there is a greater than 50% chance that their children will also suffer from a yeast infection. This may be seen as a child with a weak constitution, early allergies, a propensity towards diaper rash, and longer recovery times after illnesses.

Is A Yeast Infection Related To Other Health Conditions?

Yeast infections can be linked with many different types of health complaints and can be a causative factor or may be found in conjunction (opportunistic) with other health complaints.

Can Yeast Infection Be Spread In Tanning Beds?

A yeast infection cannot be spread in a tanning bed, I have never heard of this before. A yeast infection can be passed however from one person to another by way of sexual contact or occasionally by wearing foot ware of a person who has athlete's foot.

Can A Tanning Bed Help Treat A Yeast Infection?

No, you will not cure a yeast infection by using a tanning bed. Yeast infections need lifestyle and dietary intervention and you will find a quicker resolution by using the right dietary supplements.

Can Ingrown Hairs Be Caused From A Yeast Infection?

Many yeast infections in the groin area are caused by ingrown hair that has become infected. The use of antibiotics to treat ingrown hair infection can also be a major contributing factor to yeast infections. One of the best ways to help prevent yeast infection causing ingrown hairs is to take steps to prevent ingrown hair when shaving or waxing.

Can Waxing Cause Yeast Infections?

No, I have not found that waxing of the vaginal area to be a cause of a yeast infection. In fact, regular waxing can help prevent a yeast infection in the groin area by allowing you to keep the area more clean and dry than you normally could.

Can A Yeast Infection Go Away By Itself?

No, a yeast infection generally will not go away by itself unless you take action and modify your diet and lifestyle. It may stay mild for years or become moderate or severe depending on your diet and lifestyle. Be sure to follow my Candida Crusher Program so that you will be able to permanently beat a yeast infection.

If A Doctor Says There Is No Such Illness As A Yeast Infection, What Options Do Patients Have?

Unfortunately, this is the view of many conventional doctors, but they are not as well informed as they believe. Yeast infections have been around for many years, doctors have been aware of yeast infections for over fifty years but some still believe that yeast infections only occur in women, and many believe that yeast infections do not even exist at all. The best thing to do is learn and do as much as possible to alleviate yeast infections by reading Candida Crushe. It may also help to switch to a doctor who is familiar with yeast infections or give the uninformed doctor a copy of the Candida Crusher. Hopefully in the years to come, many more physicians will know how to recognise and treat yeast infections.

Are Americans More Prone To Yeast Infection Than People From Other Nations?

Despite a relative abundance of resources, Americans have increased their likelihood of suffering from yeast infections because of their hectic lifestyle, poor food choices, lack of exercise, and drug, alcohol and caffeine consumption. People of less wealthy nations may be subject to other factors that are individually worse than Americans experience, but their overall lifestyle, less processed and nutrient rich diets and better family or social structures (thereby reducing stress) help counter-balance these.

Does Anyone Get Through Life Without A Yeast Infection?

Many people go through life with only a mild case of a yeast infection; others experience a major episode or recurring bouts of yeast infections that can dramatically compromise the quality of their life. Many others remain in outstanding health for most of their lives. However, these are usually people who are born with good constitutions and who look after their health as well.

Can Healthy People Get A Yeast Infection?

Not really, they may get a mild form but this will quickly disappear because their resistance is strong and their susceptibility low.

Can Someone Have Yeast Infections With No Symptoms?

Yes, but it is highly unlikely. What I do commonly find is that if somebody has been experiencing a yeast infection for a long period of time is that they become used to the symptoms. All persons with a yeast infection will experience signs and symptoms of varying degrees, and at times it may even be a relative or friend who will notice these signs and symptoms rather than the person experiencing the complaints.

Can Shaving Cause Yeast Infection?

No, but shaving the skin on the face or in the genital area can aggravate the sensitive skin and this can make the skin more prone to a yeast or bacterial infection, although this is highly unlikely to occur.

Can Tight Jeans Cause A Yeast Infection?

Yes they can, especially if a person wears nylon undergarments instead of cotton undergarments and there is an existing yeast infection no matter how small. If a yeast infection is noticed, it is best for the person to wear loose clothing and to ensure they wear 100% cotton undergarments.

Can Untreated Yeast Infections Cause Cramps?

Yes, I have certainly seen many patients with yeast infections over the years that have developed all manner of digestive pains and discomforts. The sensations can range from dull aches, cramps and pains right through to sharp and even debilitating stabbing pains.

Is Candida Albicans The Only Candida Species To Cause A Yeast Infection?

There are more than 20 different species of candida yeasts that are part of our normal daily lives; it is when there becomes an overgrowth of the yeast that a problem arises.

There are several other species of Candida becoming increasingly prevalent as the cause of vaginal yeast infection; they are *Candida tropicalis* and *Candida glabrata*. Only specific testing can determine which species is actually causing the infection. *Candida tropicalis* and *Candida glabrata* are becoming more resistant to the commonly available over the counter anti-fungal medications.

Under What Conditions Do Yeast Infections Thrive?

There has to be certain conditions present to provide an environment in which the yeast will grow out of control. Yeast thrives in a warm, dark and moist environment. Other common yeast infections we are familiar with are in the skin folds (this often happens in overweight people) and thrush in the mouth, which is common in infants.

Can Yeast Infections Occur Naturally?

Absolutely, yeast infections can and do appear naturally, but they are kept in balance by the beneficial bacteria (lactobacillus sp.) which are present in a person's digestive tract. It is when this delicate balance becomes completely imbalanced that a yeast overgrowth will occur.

Does Lack Of Sleep Cause Yeast Infections?

Insomnia or a lack of sleep does not directly cause a yeast infection, but it certainly can cause adrenal fatigue that can lower a person's immune system capabilities. Lack of sleep weakens the body and will increase a person's susceptibility to getting many different types of infections, including a yeast infection.

Is Yeast Infection Common In Someone With Cancer Who Is Going Through Chemotherapy?

Chronic illness and toxic treatments like chemotherapy are major stressors that the immune and digestive systems must respond to. In addition, because of the side effects of chemotherapy, and sometimes the cancer itself, nutrient consumption and absorption is often decreased, further increasing the body's susceptibility to a yeast infection. It is very important to provide proper yeast infection support during this time.

Does A Yeast Infection Increase Susceptibility To Infections?

Yeast infection often goes hand in hand with decreased immune function that makes someone more prone to acute and recurrent illness. There is an especially strong association between yeast infection and digestive infections, such as diarrhoea, dysbiosis and parasitic infections.

Is Yeast Infection Related To Depression?

It can be; a mild depression is sometimes one of the symptoms of a yeast infection, especially if the person has had a chronic yeast infection for many years with no resolution or recognition of their yeast related problems by their doctor. I have seen patients with anxiety and depression that had a bad yeast infection, and the depression and anxiety disappeared once the yeast infection was fully resolved.

Is A Yeast Infection Related To Chronic Fatigue Syndrome?

Yeast infections are a common component of chronic fatigue syndrome (CFS); many people with chronic conditions such as CFS have digestive issues including candida yeast infections. As the person's health becomes increasingly compromised, candida yeast infections become much more easily established and can contribute significantly to that person's poor quality of life.

Is Yeast Infection A Factor In People With HIV?

Yeast infections are a very common factor in people who are HIV positive. Unfortunately one of the treatments for Hepatitis C is the administration of immune suppressive drugs that contribute significantly to the proliferation of candida yeast infections.

This suppresses both the adrenal glands and the immune system, thus speeding the patient's decline. A relationship has been demonstrated between survival of HIV infected patients and the ability of their immune system to suppress pathogens such as candida yeast infections. In HIV, immune treatment and the eradication of yeast infections can be of significant benefit.

Does A Yeast Infection Cause Or Increase Allergies?

It has been long observed that people suffering from yeast infections definitely have greater allergic responses or become allergic to things that previously did not bother them. This is because yeast infections can contribute significantly to poor immune function and a condition known as leaky gut syndrome. Once the yeast infection has been brought back into a healthy balance and the bowel re-populated with beneficial bacteria, the allergic response decreases.

Are There Any Pre-Surgery Precautions That Will Protect From A Yeast Infection?

The likelihood of a yeast infection post-surgery is certainly there, with increasing amounts of people who just don't seem to come right after surgery due to intravenous antibiotics. Eat only high quality foods, especially good quality proteins and lots of dark green vegetables. Also use visualisation and/or relaxation methods to remain mentally and emotionally calm and positive throughout the procedure, and to heal more quickly afterwards. As far in advance of the surgery as possible, begin taking our recommended yeast infection products to ensure your immune system is boosted significantly.

Yeast Infection Treatment FAQs

I Have Been On Your Candida Crusher Program For One Week And Feel Really Terrible, Why? You Told Me I Was Going To Feel Better!

There are a few likely reasons for this to occur. Most likely you are having a reaction called "die off" which can occur as toxins flood your system due to yeast dying. You can read a lot more about the Herxheimer reaction in chapter 7, stage 3 of the Candida Crusher Program. There are several hints and tips in stage 3 of the program that will help you to alleviate any untoward reactions you may experience on the program.

Why Do I Still Feel So Bad After Being On The Candida Crusher Program For Three Months?

There are many potential scenarios here. One of the most important obstacles to cure is that the Candida Crusher Program is not followed carefully and diligently, and if it is and you STILL are not feeling well then you need to look a bit deeper at the hidden causes.

Please go to the trouble-shooting section – "What to do if you don't seem to come right" because this part of the Candida Crusher book was written to clarify poor recovery and what steps to take to set things right, you will find this near the end of chapter 7, in section 5.

How Do I Know The Candida Crusher Program Is Going To Work, Or Is Any Better Than Others I Have Tried?

Only you can be the judge of that by trying the Candida Crusher program for yourself. I have certainly experienced fantastic patient outcomes with this program, it has not let me down over the past twenty years that I have used it in my clinical practice. I have found that some patients don't recover, and these are generally the patients who for one of several reasons don't really engage in the program. How my program differs from others for example is that I believe in "test and measure", I recommend eight different home tests and like people to do two-weekly assessments. You can read more about these tests in Chapter 3 – Identifying and Testing for Candida Albicans. You will also find that I explain a lot more about the importance of your lifestyle in terms of your recovery than most books do. I have several real case studies throughout the book that illustrate the various points I am trying to make as well.

How Can I Measure The Effectiveness Of The Candida Crusher Program?

How the Candida Crusher program differs from any other yeast infection treatment plan for example is that I believe in test and measure, I recommend many different home tests and like people who undertake my program to do two-weekly assessments. You will find the Candida Test Tracker in the book. You can also track your symptoms with the Candida Symptom Tracker. You can read a lot more about these tests in Chapter 3 – Identifying and Testing for Candida Albicans.

Are There Any Effective Home Remedies For Yeast Infections?

There are several effective home remedies to use for yeast infections; one effective home remedy involves mixing one teaspoon of ordinary hydrogen peroxide with one cup of water. Use as douche once a day until the symptoms disappear. You may also want to consider colloidal silver, another most effective home treatment for a vaginal yeast infection. Try one teaspoon per cup of tepid water. While holistic practitioners often recommend these types of treatments, medical doctors sometimes frown on the use of home remedies for yeast infections.

Another way to use hydrogen peroxide or colloidal silver to cure yeast infections involves taking a bath with one pint of hydrogen peroxide (or a small glass of colloidal silver) mixed in a tub of water. When doing the hydrogen peroxide bath, take care if you do this at night because this can put so much oxygen in your system that you may have trouble sleeping.

Is Hydrogen Peroxide Effective In Yeast Infections?

Hydrogen peroxide occurs naturally in the vagina and helps prevent yeast infections in most cases. However, when the body produces too much yeast the naturally occurring hydrogen peroxide is overwhelmed and a yeast infection occurs.
Try to use hydrogen peroxide (obtainable from your drug store) by mixing it with water at the rate of one teaspoon per cup of water.

Can You Take Peroxide And Cranberry Juice Together To Treat A Yeast Infection?

Yes you could, this could be a successful combination of ingredients for yeast infections.

How Will A Doctor Treat My Yeast Infection Fast?

You doctor will use an antibiotic if he or she wants to treat a yeast infection quickly. In most cases, the yeast infection will recur because the primary cause was not addressed. I never recommend an antibiotic to treat a yeast infection; there are several excellent natural products you can use.

Is A Prescription Drug Necessary To Treat A Yeast Infection?

No, most cases of yeast infection can be remedied without prescription drugs. The treatments described in Candida Crusher by my, combined with the dietary supplements recommended are natural, relatively inexpensive and very effective.

Diagnosing Yeast Infection FAQs

How Do Doctors Diagnose Yeast Infections?

Most medical doctors are not aware of yeast infections in their patients. They only recognise major systemic candidiasis, which is the most extreme and life threatening form of having a yeast infection. Astute medical doctors who practice integrative medicine (a combination of natural medicine and conventional medicine) who are familiar with candida yeast infections can test the blood levels for candida antibodies or perform a stool test which will reveal the presence of candida. There are many other common tests that can be used more indirectly to detect the presence of a yeast infection, but the majority of medical doctors are not familiar with and do not know how to interpret these tests for indications of a yeast infection.

Are There Any Laboratory Tests That Detect A Yeast Infection?

The most simple and relatively inexpensive test that has recently become available for the home user is a simple blood test to determine if you have a yeast infection (CanDia5 test) and another test which will determine if you have a vaginal yeast infection, VagiCheck. These kits can be obtained and your test can be completed simply at home giving you a result within minutes.

One of the most accurate and valuable tests for detecting a yeast infection in my opinion is the stool analysis (CDSA x3), but it is best that you seek special interpretation by a trained practitioner to recognize and treat yeast infections based on these results.
Is there any Questionnaire or Survey I can complete myself to see if I have a Yeast Infection?

Absolutely, you can complete the yeast infection survey on www.yeastinfection.org is the internet's most comprehensive and widely used yeast infection survey to help those who in doubt of potentially having a yeast infection to make their own accurate diagnosis. In addition, there are many different home tests you can perform on yourself which are free and are available in the book the Candida Crusher. The survey is also in the Candida Crusher book.

Food And Nutrition Yeast Infection FAQs

Be sure to read section 1 of chapter 7, it contains much information relating to eating and candida. Also, check out the special food recommendations in section 4 of chapter 7.

Does Diet Have Anything To Do With Yeast Infections?

Yes, diet plays a critical role in a yeast infection. The phrase "garbage in, garbage out" aptly describes the relationship between poor diet and a yeast infection. A nutritionally inadequate diet that is high in sugar, caffeine and junk food places daily stress on the body that the digestive system has to respond to and, at the same time, deprives the body of the nutrients it needs to adequately function. This alone can lead to a yeast infection or make the body more vulnerable to a yeast infection when any additional stress such as an antibiotic is added. Similarly, good nutrition helps protect and sustain the digestive system, helping to protect against the development of yeast infections. When a yeast infection is already present, a healthy diet that supports the digestive system (especially when eating fermented and cultured foods) combined with the yeast infection supplements recommended can lead to recovery.

Do I Have To Follow A Specific Diet When Doing Your Program?

Yes you do. In fact you don't eat candida and what you avoid, while perhaps making you feel better, will not eliminate systemic candida. Many people contact our clinic after having been on the so-called 'yeast diets' for years and every time they go off for even a weekend, their symptoms come back, often stronger than before. We suggest avoiding concentrated sugars and refined white flour carbohydrate foods, as this will make you feel better while going through our program.

How Long Do I Need To Stay On The Candida Crusher Diet?

A very common question many ask me "How long do I have to stay on this diet?" Chances are that you will be staying on this diet in some form or another until you feel 100%, and then some more. Dr. William Crook, author of "The Yeast Connection" used to say "You stay on the diet as long as it takes and then some." You will probably avoid they key trigger foods which kept you in the candida yeast infection zone for several years, because after the yeast infection is gone you are going to feel so good you simply won't want to go back to feeling how you did. Most candida sufferers have one or two key foods that they love to consume regularly which will keep the condition going, sometimes for a dozen years or more. They partially eliminate foods like sugars, alcohol, and breads but consume that one key trigger food happening on a regular basis. Consequently, they partially recover only to slip back again and again.

The sooner you identify YOUR key food/s and or beverage/s and eliminate them once and for all, the sooner you will be able to rid yourself of the beast called yeast. I always recommend that you keep a record of how foods make you feel, and only you can decide if it is worth keeping that food or drink going for some time.

This question of "How long on the diet?" is a bit similar to the "Will my candida come back?" question. You stay on the diet long enough to get well, and then stay well permanently. I have found some patients stay on the candida diet for three months, which is probably the minimum time, some for six months and others for a year. I also know of several who just continue on with this diet approach indefinitely because they feel so good on it after experiencing a major reduction in weight, better sleep, more energy, improved moods and cognitive function.

Once a sense of balance comes back into your life, and by balance I mean dietary balance, lifestyle balance, etc.; then you will find that your yeast infection won't hang around because these infections thrive on an imbalance. It always pays to remain vigilant for at least one to one and a half years after your recovery. Be ready to slip back into the two-week induction phase of the candida diet anytime your feel those symptoms coming back. The more intuitive you become, the less the chances of any major aggravations or yeast related health hiccups in the future.

Should I Avoid ALL Fruits?

Many candida dietary experts go on to maintain that all fruits, except berries (blue berries are fine), lemons and limes, grapefruits, avocados and green apples (Granny Smith) are OK to consume. Some say that you should not eat any fruit until you have virtually eliminated all candida from your system. I would disagree here, as I have seen many patients who CAN eat fruits (within reason) quite OK whilst eliminating candida from their bodies. Whilst it is true that fruits in general are very high in sugar (fructose), it is a natural sugar that seems to be tolerated by many candida patients. I do believe however, that it makes sense to avoid all fruits (except the berries, lemons and limes, grapefruits, avocados and green apples) for at least the first two weeks.

When Can I Eat Bread Again?

I hear this question a lot! If you really want to know the answer to this question then you most probably haven't overcome one of the big (and probable) reasons for developing your yeast overgrowth in the first place, a craving and possible addiction to breads and the more refined carbohydrate foods. I have always found that the stronger the desire to want to start eating or drinking a particular food or beverage after beginning the Candida Crusher Program, the more likely this was one of the big problems to begin with. Some of the biggest dietary addictions are to the sweeter foods like chocolate, candies, alcohol and breads, but they can be to one of many other foods including peanut butter, soft creamy cheeses, crackers, donuts and all manner of take-out foods like pizza, hot dogs, Pepsi or Coke. The more you want it – the more you need to put your foot down and say…NO!

Focus on home cooked meals and get into the habit of eating meals based around meats and vegetables, just like your grandmother used to eat. Rely less on bread, because there is a habit to have a quick spread like honey of jam on bread and we want to keep away from sweet foods sufficiently long enough to restore the balance of the digestive system. You absolutely can't do without bread? Then try some flat bread, bread made without yeasts or sugar. This is bread made with plain flour, salt and water.

I Hate The Candida Crusher Diet And Want Something Sweet, What Can I Eat For A Treat?

You need to understand that it may have been you cravings and strong desires for "something sweet" which got you partly into this mess in the first place! A good trick to break your sweet cravings is to take 500mcg of Chromium picolinate twice daily with meals; this helps most people cope substantially with strong sugar cravings. As the candida population diminishes, so too will your cravings for sweet foods and drinks, because the bugs are no longer "calling your name" as I put it. Trust me, it gets easier and easier to say no to that coke, cheesecake or donut, you will get to the point where you can walk right past that triple chocolate cake and not even blink an eyelid, I have seen this happen with even the most hardened sugar addict many times over. Just hang in there; it gets a lot better after a few months. As you improve over several weeks, you can generally have fresh fruits again, but not to excess. Sweet fruits will often quell that strong craving for something sweet, but if you have a chronic case of yeast infection then please realise that the first several weeks you are best to avoid ALL sugars and yeasty foods as much as is possible. How bad do you want to beat this thing called yeast?

I Really Crave Bread (Or Wine, Sugar, Etc.) What Can I Do To Quell These Cravings?

If you follow the Candida Crusher Program carefully, these cravings will diminish within three weeks, I guarantee it. Just take chromium picolinate two to three times daily with meals (500mcg is a good dose) and be sure to eat plenty of protein. Have eggs with breakfast, fish like salmon or tuna or sardines for lunch (along with salads, vegetables, etc., and a good home cooked meal each evening.

Snack on health foods as suggested in my program. Eating smaller snack like meals more frequently helps tremendously with sweet cravings, and what you will find in particular is that as your yeast infection levels reduce, your strong and even killer desire for sweets will diminish in almost direct proportion to how your digestive function improves. At least that's what I have discovered in the clinic with countless women, and I've seen them all – the chocoholics, the biscuit (cookie) cravers, the donut lovers, the ice cream fanatics (some eat 2-3 litres every day), the Coca Cola drinkers (some drink up to 3 litres every day) and many more. Every person with an insatiable sweet craving will have his or her favourite food or drink or confectionary, what is yours? If you know exactly what it is then please become aware of your cravings for this food, and also become more aware when you buy it and if your levels of desire diminish over time. As your desire decreases for your "favourite", notice how your symptoms improve!

If A Piece Of Cake Accidentally Slips And Falls Into My Mouth, Do I Need To Go Right Back To The Beginning Of Your Program?

This is a good question, while accidents happen, they shouldn't happen to careful people! If you slip and fall, make the resolution to be stronger in the future. I explain this in detail in Candida Crusher. Everybody will fall sooner or later, and these slips may happen at birthday parties, weddings, BBQs, eating out with friends or family or at social functions generally. As you improve and the yeast bugs no longer "call your name" (your cravings will improve over time) you will find it easier to avoid such accidents. And going back to the beginning? No, you don't, but be careful because if you are very accident prone you may well have to start right from the beginning again.

Are There Any Benefits Of Drinking Buttermilk With A Yeast Infection?

Yes there are. Adding lactic acid bacteria to milk produces buttermilk and it is the good bacteria in the buttermilk that helps the body maintain a healthy balance of good and bad bacteria, thereby preventing yeast infections. The body reacts to the good bacteria and produces toxins that destroy bad bacteria and yeast cells.

Can A Poor Diet Cause Yeast Infection?

Absolutely, a poor diet is one of the main causative factors. Diets high in sugar containing foods, yeast or mold containing foods, refined foods, take-out foods and convenience foods in general are a recipe for developing a yeast infection. Be sure to read the Candida Crusher Program to learn the best foods to eat to avoid the possibility of developing a yeast infection.

Does Carrot Juice Help Yeast Infections?

Carrot juice can tend to be very high in sugars, it is surprisingly sweet! I do not recommend such juices for several months after beginning any kill or inhibition programs. You can have fresh carrot Juice after several months being in a spotless diet. Be careful!

Does Chlorophyll Cure Yeast Infections?

No, I do not recommend such drinks as "cures" for yeast infections. Chlorophyll drinks are certainly beneficial in that they help to balance the body's pH levels, but they do not cure a yeast infection as such.

Can Yeast Infections Raise Fasting Food Sugar?

Yeast infections do not raise fasting sugar levels, but they can be prone to lowering it. Sugar is the favourite food of yeast, and if a person has an invasive form of a yeast infection in the bloodstream, candida will feed on any sugar it can find including glucose or sugars in the bloodstream. Those with poorly controlled diabetes get frequent yeast infections because of sugar in the urine.

Dietary Supplement Yeast Infection FAQs

Be sure to read section 4 of chapter 7, it contains much useful information regarding to dietary supplements and candida.

Do I Need Dietary Supplements, I thought The Diet Was Sufficient Alone?

In section 1 of this chapter 7, the diet and nutrition section, you will have read about the supplementation recommendations. As I have mentioned earlier, while nutritional supplementation is not absolutely necessary at all, it does play a crucial role in fully recovering from a yeast infection. They will not only speed-up your recovery, but in many cases they will be found necessary for a complete and deep-seated recovery from the dysbiosis (bowel overgrowth of yeasts, poor bacteria, and parasites), leaky gut, fatigue and brain fog, food allergies and many other chronic health problems associated with a chronic yeast infection.

The CanXida supplements I have chosen and personally developed have been specifically selected based on my extensive experiences in working with many patients with chronic yeast infections for their cleansing, healing and deeply restorative effects. I will explain the significance of these formulations in section 4 of chapter 7 more fully, because it is important for you to understand why these supplements have been included as part of your Candida Crusher Program, and the necessity of taking them regularly.

I Have Been Told That Vitamins Can Cause A Yeast Infection

Perhaps some can, some vitamin C products I've seen contain up to 50 percent sugar! Yeast infection is generally caused by yeast overgrowth due to an imbalance in the flora of a person's digestive system, and not by dietary supplements. For example, excess sugars in a person's diet or refined carbohydrate foods will cause candida, or because the person took an antibiotic that destroyed his or her health intestinal bacteria allowing yeasts to thrive, but vitamins and minerals will not be a cause. Vitamins don't have anything to do with yeast infections.

What Are the Five Supplements You Recommend To Take On The Candida Crusher Program, And Why Do You Recommend These Particular Ones?

These are the five most important dietary supplements to use with a yeast infection in my experience:

1. CanXida Remove - Broad-spectrum Antifungal Formula

2. CanXida Restore - Probiotic Enzyme Formula

3. CanXida Rebuild - Natural Advanced Candida Multi-Vitamin

4. Good high quality Omega 3

5. Good high quality systemic renewal formula for Inflammation, Gut, Liver, Brain & Immune Support

To learn more about each product visit CanXida.com

I'm Taking Another Brand Of Dietary Supplements, Why Would Your Products Be Any Better?

Are you taking other supplement brands currently? They may be fine, and if you are having a good result then you may see no need to switch brands. My Candida Crusher supplements are different in that have been designed specifically by me, and based on more than two decades of yeast infection research, in addition to treating patients who have come to me with this complaint for the same period of time. I have worked out what works and what doesn't, and after having tried literally hundreds of products I have settled on a small core range that has proven to be effective time and again.

Each one of the five supplements I recommend has been based on the best quality raw materials I could find, and carefully selected based on several factors including compatibility with other nutrients, potency, effectiveness, shelf-life, as well as their specificity and sensitivity to not only yeast infections, but to bad bacteria, parasites and the various yeasts strains that candida patients present with. But the main choice was primarily because each specific ingredient in formulations has proven itself time and again to be the best when it comes to helping a person fully recover from their yeast infection.

You may want to think about switching to the Candida Crusher formulations which I recommend for a three to four month period and see the difference they make, I'm certain that you will notice the difference, and if you are improving with the Candida Crusher supplements then don't be in a hurry to stop. If money is an issue, just reduce you dosage and continue. You will save money in the long run with the most effective candida protocol by improving the quality of your life in a shorter period of time. And isn't that why you bought the Candida Crusher book, looking for the best possible solution to an annoying health problem that has been plaguing you for ages? What price do you put on your health?

If you are not taking the Candida Crusher formulations, and not improving on your current candida supplements that you are taking, then you will need to re-assess whether your current yeast infection program and products are having the desired effect. Many patients I see are wasting their hard-earned money by taking the wrong or ineffective supplements for their yeast infection. Please go to section 4 of chapter 7 and read about what I consider to be the best specialized nutrients and herbal medicines to take if you have a yeast infection, and see if your current products match the specifications of my targeted formulations.

But Can I Take My Usual Dietary Supplements and Drugs While Doing The Candida Crusher Program ?

Yes, you can continue taking your supplements and all prescribed medication as directed. In most cases I prefer the patient to only take what is absolutely essential, like prescribed pharmaceutical medications, and to discontinue any dietary supplements unless they are deemed absolutely necessary. Never discontinue any prescribed pharmaceutical medications without consulting your doctor, that is not a good idea.

It is best not to complicate your program, I have seen some patients take up to and over twenty or more nutritional and herbal supplements over the course of a day. It is best to stay with the recommendations I make in chapter 7, section 4 under "The Right Supplements and Herbal Medicines to Take". If you have any questions then ask your health-care professional who can best guide you.

Keep it simple is the best way to go, that way it will not only work out more cost effective, but you will also be in a much better position to be able to work out what supplement is working the best for you and when to increase, decrease or even stop taking certain products. Please be sure to read section 4 for much more information regarding what to take and when. I have tried just about every yeast infection dietary supplement on the market and now only recommend a few which work consistently, time and again.

Why Have You Recommended 5 Different Products?

The 5-product Candida Crusher supplementation protocol has been recommended after many years of trial and error. Initially I recommended an antifungal product and a probiotic alone, but then started to realize that better results were being achieved when I recommended digestive enzymes as patients reported less bloating, gas and increased digestive comfort. The multivitamin came into the protocol because I started to notice how much better people felt when they took the multi along with the digestive enzymes, they had more energy, slept better and suffered a lot less from any potential aggravations on the program. The omega 3 supplement was added a few years ago because I started to notice that those taking a daily omega experienced significantly less digestive discomfort, better bowel function and less aggravation from their diet, especially when they brought the potentially allergic foods back into their diet. This is why I have remained with this protocol that I now recommend. How can you just give one pill to accomplish all the above? It is pretty hard to expect to get the results I currently get with one or two tablets; there is only a limit as to how much you can cram into one tablet or capsule.

Those who take just an antifungal and probiotic will feel improvement, that I have no doubt, but when they follow my recommendations as far as supplementation is concerned and take the specialized enzyme formula and multi vitamin they will be amazed at the difference it makes. It is something you need to try for yourself before you declare that it's too much, because the only way you will experience the difference is by trying the protocol for yourself.

How Long Do I Need To Take
The Candida Crusher Supplements For?

It depends on which Candida Crusher dietary supplements you take and whether you have mild, moderate or a severe yeast infection. After having used countless different kinds of dietary supplements and herbal medicines from many different companies over the past twenty plus years, there is now a small core range five different specialized dietary supplements I recommend my patients to take when they have a yeast infection. I believe that the Candida Crusher 5-supplement combination works exceptionally well in those with candida especially over a 3 – 4 month period, but improvements keep on occurring even after 6 months or more and I have verified this clinically in many cases. I have personally developed this product range after much trial and error.

The duration of supplementation depends on the severity of your yeast infection, and it makes sense to take my yeast infection survey (see Yeastinfection.org) to determine whether you have a mild, moderate or severe yeast infection. I like patients to stay on the supplements for as long as it takes to get well, and then they no longer need supplements. In my experience, this is where many practitioners let their patients down – the patient will be placed on a candida kill product or probiotic for a few weeks or month or two, and then they stop. This could be due to either an improvement (and then the patient feels that there is no need for the supplement as they are "better" again), it may be a cost issue or a lack of follow-up or one of several other factors, but the important thing to remember is that it takes time to get well, ranging from weeks to several months. I typically have found that just as the patient is beginning to derive benefit from a dietary supplement it is discontinued! Is it a cost issue? Then simply reduce the dosage and take over a prolonged period of time, a lesser dosage is better than no dosage.

How Much Is This Going To Cost Me? I Have Spent A Small Fortune On Dietary Supplements And Practitioners Over The Years.

The Candida Crusher Program shouldn't cost much money, I generally tell people to expect to pay between three to seven dollars a day on average for dietary supplements, but this will lessen a great deal as time goes by, particularly after the first two to three months. The thing to bear in mind is that you will actually be saving money by making dietary changes; you will be eating in more and out less. This is a significant cost saving for many people. Just work out how much you will save if you stop buying take-out foods for a few months, stop buying alcohol, deserts, ice cream, and any sweet treats like chocolate. It is amazing how people view a health program designed to optimize their health and well-being as being costly, when in fact it is the lifestyle contributing to their health challenges which is actually the costly factor, a bottle of wine, a six-pack of beer or a take-out meal. And more so, it is more likely that the continuation of these poor health habits that may one day prove to be partly responsible for the development of a disease of such as diabetes, heart disease or cancer.

Did you know that most people spend more money in the last three months of their life actually trying to prolong their life, than they do in their entire life on health-care?

Please don't view a few dollars a day spent right now on preventive health-care as being "wasteful". See it rather as in investment in your healthy future, an insurance policy against premature chronic disease.

You take nothing with you after all, so do enjoy every moment you are alive and view money as a tool that can always be replaced. Time can never be replaced, and all we really have when you think about it is time, time to spend with those we love and care about, and isn't it worth feeling at your best in your allotted time? Of course it is, so I'm not really that interested in hearing your "small fortune" spending pennies today on restoring your health and preventing serious disease it will be the wisest money you will have spent, trust me on this one.

Can A Probiotic Cure My Yeast Infection?

Although a good probiotic can be very effective in preventing a candida overgrowth in the first place, and also in helping the digestive system restore function once a yeast infection is brought under control, there is certainly no evidence I have found to suggest that any probiotic can actually entirely cure candida, regardless of the strain involved. High-end quality probiotic strains can be most effective rather than most retail purchased products, which I have found to be therapeutically of little value. A survey conducted in America on the actual viability of probiotics, once GMP was enforced (Good Manufacturing Procedures) amongst probiotic manufacturers in 2010, revealed that over half were pretty much useless and contained mainly dead "beneficial" bacteria. You therefore need to be careful what you buy.

Once the candida becomes more widespread in the body you will find that probiotics have little effect unless you use a good eradication product and work hard out on diet modification, as I have outlined in section 1 (nutrition) in chapter 7. It is the combined and *consistent effort* placed on diet, supplements and lifestyle that will give you the results you are looking for in more than 90% of the most difficult cases of yeast infection I have seen.

What About Product X? I Read On The Internet It Is The Best
As you can well imagine, I have tried just about every single dietary supplement for candida yeast infections over the past two decades and found that there are only few which are a cut above the rest. In section 4, chapter 7 you can read all about "The Right Supplements and Herbal Medicines to Take".

Children And Baby Yeast Infection FAQs

Can You Use Diaper Rash Cream For Yeast Infection?

I have found in most cases of diaper rash that a high-quality Calendula officinalis cream works best. Always use a 100% natural diaper rash cream that does not contain any chemicals or irritants. A high quality cream or ointment can stop yeast infection rashes of many kinds, not just diaper rashes, but for optimal results use a cream which contains tea tree oil. Chapter 4 – the QUICK Start guide contains a lot more information about the best natural diaper rash solutions.

Can I Treat My Toddler's Yeast Infection With An Adult's Cream?

I would recommend that you use a gentle cream with an infant, preferably one containing aloe vera gel, tea tree oil, calendula and perhaps some eucalyptus oil.

Is Breast Feeding Possible When I Have A Yeast Infection?

Yes, absolutely, you can have a yeast infection and still breast feed at the same time. It shouldn't be a reason to stop you breast feeding, but do follow my Candida Crusher Diet for optimal results even if you are breast feeding. Be sure to eat plenty of garlic, include coconut products and follow my dietary advice. Be sure not to take an pharmaceutical antibiotic if you are pregnant, have a yeast infection and are breastfeeding however – you could make your yeast infection a lot worse and potentially seriously aggravate your baby, I have seen this all too many times.

Is Yeast Infection Common In Toddlers?

Infants and toddlers can easily get yeast infections when they are in diapers or just starting to toilet train because yeast can grow especially well in wet skin folds. The yeast infections that affect toddlers are caused by candida albicans, which is the most common cause of all types of yeast infections. Paediatricians can determine whether a rash on the groin or a thrush in the mouth of toddlers is yeast infection. To get a definite diagnosis a doctor may examine the scrapings of a yeast infection under the microscope.

Can Children have a Yeast Infection?

Yes, children are susceptible to the same causative factors for a yeast infection as adults. Children whose mothers had a candida yeast infection during their gestation and/or birth are especially vulnerable to developing a yeast infection. These children are often more sickly, are more likely to be prescribed antibiotics (which worsen yeast infections), are more prone to food allergies and take longer to recover from illnesses. However, they too can greatly benefit from proper yeast infection treatment and healthy lifestyle choices. We often see adolescents and young adults in our clinic with yeast infections, who benefit tremendously from the Candida Crusher Program.

Can a Yeast Infection be dangerous in Toddlers?

No, it is not a dangerous condition as such, just extremely annoying to both the child as well as the parents. It is best treated as early as possible otherwise it will eventually become a chronic condition.

Can Toddlers get Yeast infections from Antibiotics?

They most certainly can, and this is a common problem I see time and again in my clinic. Antibiotics destroy both the "good" and "bad" bacteria and the first organisms that tend to grow back are the yeasts. It is most important to give a toddler a probiotic after any antibiotic treatment, and better still to avoid giving antibiotics in the first place.

Male Yeast Infection FAQs

Can A Prostate Infection Be Transmitted?

Yes, a female partner can contract a urinary tract infection and worse (actual kidney infections) from a male partner who has prostatitis. I have seen this in several cases over the years and it usually starts after the couple began to have sex when the male had a history of a prostate infection. The male should be treated and the couple are best to observe good hygeine after sexual relations to reduce the chances of a cross-infection occuring. Better to be safe than sorry.

Can A Male's PSA Level Become Elevated Due To A Prostate Yeast Infection?

Yes, it most certainly can. The prostate serum antigen (PSA) level will only reveal an elevation if a man has an enlarged prostate, whether it be from an infection or from cancer. A Urologist will generally tell you that an elevated PSA reading cannot be due to a yeast infection, but I have seen this to be the case in many males over the years, and once their yeast infection was successfully treated their PSA reading went back to normal.

Can I Have Sex During A Prostate Infection?

You can but please bear in mind that you are at a high risk of potentially infecting your partner with a yeast infection.

Can Shaving Cause Yeast Infection?

No, but shaving the skin on the face or in the genital area can aggravate the sensitive skin and this can make the skin more prone to a yeast or bacterial infection, although this is highly unlikely to occur.

Can There Be A Yeast Infection In The Male Urethra?

Yes there can be, a yeast infection can commonly affect the male genital region including the skin in and around the penis and scrotom, the prostate and the urethra, although it is more common for the prostate to be affected (prostatitis) than the urethra.

Can Tight Jeans Cause A Yeast Infection?

Yes they can, especially if a person wears nylon undergarments instead of cotton undergarments and there is an existing yeast infection no matter how small. If a yeast infection is noticed, it is best for the person to wear loose clothing and to ensure they wear 100% cotton undergarments.

Female Yeast Infection FAQs

Be sure to read chapter 5, which has been devoted entirely to effectively treating a women's yeast infection.

Is Yeast Infection Possible While Breast Feeding?

Yes, you can have a yeast infection and still breast feed at the same time. It shouldn't be a reason to stop you breast feeding, but do follow my Candida Crusher Diet for optimal results even if you are breast feeding. Be sure to eat plenty of garlic, include coconut products and follow my dietary advice. Be sure not to take an antibiotic if you are pregnant, have a yeast infection and are breastfeeding however – you will make the yeast infection much worse and aggravate your baby.

Can A Vaginal Yeast Infection Be Passed To A Man And Cause A Prostate Infection?

Yes it can, just like a male can pass a yeast infection to a female, an infected female can pass a yeast infection to a male. Both male and female need to be cautious if they have a yeast infection because it is easily transmittable sexually. Take precautions, either avoid intimate contact until you are well or use protection.

Can Yeast Infection Spread To Your Bikini Line?

A yeast infection can affect any part of your skin, but favours the more moist, dark and warm areas of your body. You can have a yeast infection spread from your vaginal area to your bikini line, it is possible but with proper hygiene is much less likely to occur.

Can Untreated Yeast Infections Cause Health Problems During Pregnancy?

Yeast infections are extremely common during pregnancy because of the hormonal changes occurring within your body during this time. Before you have it treated with over the counter medications, do the vaginal home yeast test to first determine if you have a vaginal yeast infection or if in doubt check with your doctor. While a yeast infection does not harm the pregnancy or the baby, it may increase your baby's chance of having a yeast infection when he or she is born. If you are concerned then do see your doctor, and how it is treated will depend on where you are in your pregnancy.

An untreated yeast infection can worsen, causing further symptoms and potentially spread into the uterus. You will benefit significantly from the Candida Crusher Program if you do have a yeast infection.

Can Untreated Yeast Infection Lead To PID? (Pelvic Inflammatory Disease)

In general, bacteria that are transmitted through sexual contact and other bodily secretions most frequently can cause pelvic inflammatory disease. Bacteria that cause gonorrhoea and chlamydia cause more than half of all PID cases. Many studies suggest that a number of patients with PID and other sexually transmitted diseases are often infected with two or more infectious agents, and commonly these are Chlamydia trachomatis and Neisseria gonorrhoeae. Other organisms can also cause PID but are much less common.

Can A Yeast Infection Cause Spotting In A Woman?

Yes, vaginal yeast infections can cause spotting in women. Vaginal yeast infections occur when a fungus rapidly spreads throughout a woman's vagina and the vagina opening. Vaginal yeast infections consist of vaginal irritation, intense itchiness and even vaginal spotting, which may occur when a woman scratches her vaginal area in an effort to relieve the intense bouts of itchiness.

Can A Change Of Hormones Cause A Yeast Infection?

Absolutely, elevated levels of the hormone oestrogen are frequently found to be one of the major causes of yeast infections in women, and this can occur during pregnancy, whilst taking the oral contraceptive pill, before a menstrual period and hormone fluctuations around the menopause can also be a causative actor.

Can Codeine Cause A Yeast Infection In Women?

No, codeine will not cause a yeast infection. Codeine is a drug that reduces pain, calms coughs and helps you relax and sleep. Doctors will generally recommend this drug for pain but may also recommend it for a bad cough. Only use codeine for pain when milder pain medicines don't work. The side effects of codeine include constipation and temporary difficulties in passing urine. You may also experience nausea, vomiting, headaches and skin itching, and it may be the skin itching side effect that those who take codeine regularly may mistake for a yeast infection.

Can The Oestrogen Pill Cause A Yeast Infection?

Oestrogen is a prescribed pharmaceutical drug that contains oestrogens similar to those produced in people's bodies. People may use topical (on the skin, a cream) or oral (tablet) forms to treat some symptoms associated with a loss of oestrogens around menopause, which includes symptoms like hot flashes, or inflammation of the vagina that can result in pain during intercourse. There are many potential oestradiol side effects including dizziness, breast pain, increased risk for yeast infections, redness or irritation when the medication is used topically, and flu-like symptoms or arthritic pain.

Can High Doses Of The Birth Control Cause Yeast Infections?

Yes, high doses or the prolonged use of hormones (low grade) are implicated in vaginal yeast infections in particular.

Can Hormonal Imbalances Cause Yeast Infections?

Yes they can, increased levels of oestrogen before the menstrual period can be a causative factor in increasing the likelihood of developing vaginal thrush.

Can I Get Diarrhea From Monistat?

All pharmaceutical drugs may cause side effects, and Monistat has many side-effects including mild vaginal burning, irritation, or itching, constipation or diarrhoea, stomach pains, vomiting, severe allergic reactions (rash; hives; itching; difficulty breathing; tightness in the chest; swelling of the mouth, face, lips, or tongue); fever or chills; foul-smelling vaginal discharge; nausea; and even severe or prolonged vaginal burning, irritation, or itching.

Can Low Estrogen Cause A Yeast Infection?

Yes, having a low or high (or imbalanced) level of estrogen can make you more prone to a yeast infection. Low estrogen frequently leads to vaginal dryness and frequent urinary tract infections. Yeast infections are commonly due to changes in the genital area because of diminished secretions and changes in the pH balance of the vaginal tissues, this will be noticed in particular before periods or around menopause. It is the loss of natural lubrication that causes vaginal dryness and these changes in the vaginal tissue can lead to increased yeast as well as bacterial infections.

Can A Yeast Infection Affect My Sex Life?

Yes, very much so. A common complaint from both men and women suffering from a yeast infection is a decreased sex drive. This is because of several reasons, one reason is the both men and women can have genital yeast infections which dramatically increases their level of sexual discomfort, and secondarily because yeast infections can cause fatigue and a poor state of health and well being overall, thereby reducing a person's ability to enjoy a healthy sex life.

Does A Yeast Infection Affect A Woman's Menstrual Cycles?

A yeast infection can negatively affect many aspects of a woman's hormone cycles, including menstrual flow, PMS, peri-menopause and menopause.

Can Wearing Jeans Without Panties Cause Yeast Infections?

Not really, it is much more likely to occur if one wears panties, and then nylon panties instead of cotton ones. Wear cotton panties preferably rather than nylon.

Can Yeast Infections Be More Before The Periods?

Yes, they are more likely before the menstrual period because circulating oestrogen levels are likely to be higher at this stage of the menstrual cycle instead of being low.

Can You Experience Nipple Bleeding From An Untreated Yeast Infection?

A yeast infection of the nipple can most certainly be a causative factor in the nipple's ability to bleed, and this would most likely happen due to an increased level of itching, which would make a person want to rub or scratch the nipple.

Vaginal Yeast Infection FAQs

What Is A Vaginal Yeast Infection?

The vagina is the perfect environment for a candida yeast infection to thrive. Yeast is a fungus that normally lives in the vagina in small numbers, and a vaginal yeast infection means that way too many yeast cells are growing inside the vagina. Vaginal yeast infections are very common, and many women experience a vaginal yeast infection at some stage of their life. Although a yeast infection in the vagina can cause discomfort, these types of infections are not generally serious unless a woman has had a recurring vaginal yeast infection for a long period of time. Treatment is simple, just follow the instructions in chapter 5.

What Causes A Vaginal Yeast Infection?

A healthy vagina has many types of bacteria and a generally only a small number of yeast cells. The most common vaginal bacteria are beneficial bacteria called Lactobacilli acidophilus, which help keep the balance of the "good and bad": bacteria under control. Most yeast infections are caused by yeast called Candida albicans. When an event occurs which happens to change the balance of these organisms, the yeast can rapidly proliferate and cause various symptoms. One of the main ways to cause a vaginal yeast infection is by taking an antibiotic. Taking the oral contraceptive pill, hormone replacement therapies as well as being pregnant are all ways of assuring you have high levels of oestrogens in your body that can cause an elevation of yeast in the body as well. Chronic health problems such as diabetes or HIV may also be implicated in yeast infections.

What Are The Symptoms Of A Vaginal Yeast Infection?

There are many different symptoms that you may experience if you have a vaginal yeast infection, but the most common symptoms are itching, or soreness in the vagina and sometimes an uncomfortable pain or burning when you urinate or have sex. Occasionally a woman will in addition have a thick white discharge that can have a texture like curd or cottage cheese. The most likely time for an aggravation to occur is during the week before a woman's menstrual period.

Why Is My Vagina So Itchy? What Can I Do?

There are many reasons why your vagina is itchy; here are some of the best solutions. It the itching is recurrent, especially if you have recently engaged in sexual relations then it is best that you see your doctor and get checked out.

1. Avoid sexual relations with a person you think has a genital infection; even if in doubt avoid relations until you can be certain. This goes for guys too, men can be carriers of various common infections, and guys should not have sex with any woman who has an abnormal discharge.

2. If you have repeated issues with vaginal itching don't wear any tight clothing in that area.

3. Always wear 100% cotton undergarments, try to avoid nylon pantyhose and if you do wish to wear pantyhose then be sure that the crotch area of the pantyhose is made of cotton.

4. Use a non-perfumed soap when washing the vaginal area (a good quality tea tree oil soap is best) Rinse and dry the area very well, pat dry and try not to rub (skin irritation) the area. I recommend that you use a hair dryer to get the area very dry.

5. Try to avoid douches, unless you follow the instruction in Candida Crusher. You can douche but must follow a careful protocol or you will only potentially worsen the problem.

6. When at home and as often as you can, leave your undergarments off. Let fresh air circulate around the area.

7. AVOID sexual relations if you have an infection, wait until you have solved the problem or you will only worsen it and potentially spread the problem to your partner.

8. Be particularly careful if using toys during sex, you must very carefully wash and disinfect such items or you will only increase your risk of transmission back to yourself or another person.

9. It is best that you try to avoid scratching or rubbing the affected area. Keep your fingernails short if you just can't help yourself or you will worsen the problem. Patting the area will temporarily

lessen the itch; you may also like to try a warm or cold application to the area. I know some women who use ice cubes, whereas others will use a hot cloth.

10. If the itching does not resolve in a reasonable time frame you really do need to see your doctor and get professional assessment and treatment, you may have an STD or a bacterial vaginal infection. Try the vaginal yeast infection home test.

11. Are you menopausal and post-menopausal? You may be suffering from low oestrogen and have thinning of the skin in your vaginal area. Go and see your doctor, but if you have a discharge or want to know if you do have a yeast infection before you see your doctor, then try the vaginal yeast infection home test first. You should use a lubricant of their choice, as long as no infection is present. Sitz baths, cool or warm baths, cotton underwear, and a soothing vaginal cream will all help at night. Follow the Candida Crusher Program at the same time for best results if test results reveal that you do in fact have a yeast infection.

How Is A Vaginal Yeast Infection Treated?

The best way to treat a vaginal yeast infection is to follow the QUICK START Candida Crusher Guide (chapter 4) in the Candida Crusher book. If you have a chronic yeast infection condition then please read chapter 5 (Crushing Chronic Vaginal Yeast Infections) from my Candida Crusher book. You may like to treat a vaginal yeast infection at home yourself with a most effective vaginal antifungal cream you can buy without a prescription, and be sure to take recommended anti candida dietary supplements at the same time. It is best that you follow the Candida Crusher Program if you want the best possible outcome and a permanent resolution of your yeast infection. Are you pregnant and have a yeast infection? If you are pregnant, don't use any medicine for a yeast infection without talking to your doctor first. You will need to be very careful if you are using a cream or a suppository to treat any vaginal yeast infections if you depend on condoms or a diaphragm for birth control, because any chemicals in these products may weaken the latex.

My Vaginal Yeast Infection Keeps Recurring, What Is Wrong?

I my experience, many women will have a recurring vaginal yeast infection. If you keep getting your yeast infection back and rely on pharmaceutical creams and applicators you are wasting your time. It would pay to get checked out by your doctor in case you have an underlying chronic health complaint such as diabetes. The only way to make sure that you get a complete and permanent resolution is to follow my Candida Crusher Program.

Can Vaginal Yeast Infections Be Prevented?

In most cases a vaginal yeast infection can be prevented, here are several ways:

- Wear 100% cotton underwear or undergarments (avoid nylon).

- Avoid tight-fitting pants and panty hose.

- Change out of a wet swimsuit as soon as possible and keep the genital area dry.

- Allow your vagina to breath; sit back on your chair.

- Avoid douches and feminine sprays.

- Avoid scented toilet paper and deodorant tampons.

Is A Yeast Infection Swab Test Accurate?

It depends on the quality of the test and how it is performed. Home test kits are available through this website very soon.

Can Yeast From Vagina Be Spread To Nipples?

Yes it can, especially during sexual acts. It is important to maintain a high level of hygiene to avoid the cross contamination of a yeast infection from one part of the body to another.

Can Yeast In The Stool Cause Vaginal Yeast Infections?

Absolutely, and this is one of the most common ways for a woman to develop a vaginal yeast infection. During wiping, it is very important to wipe from front to back to avoid the contamination of any faecal matter from the anus to the vaginal region. Women have a much shorter uethra than men and are more prone to cross contamination this way.

For Those Who <u>Only Want the Best</u>, We Offer...

The World's Most Premium Herbal Based Gut Cleansing Formula For Candida & Gut Disorders

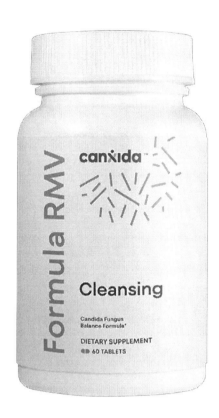

CanXida Remove (RMV) is:

- Clinician formulated based on +30 years of experience treating Candida, IBS, SIBO, Leaky Gut, IBD & more.

- Uses standardized ingredients in a **sustain release** form (targets all parts of GI tract).

- Gentle on the digestive sytem. Suitable for **seniors** & people with poor gut function.

- Designed to work even for **severe cases** where the patient has been sick for YEARS.

- Comes with 28 page User Guide booklet & YouTube channel with +2,000 gut health related videos to help patients get well.

Click Here or Visit <u>www.canxida.com</u> Today to Learn More

CanXida Products

The unique CanXida products can be found on CanXida.com.

This is a substantial website containing much information about yeast infection. You will find extracts from the Candida Crusher book on this website.

CanXida YouTube Channel

Access to 3000+ educational videos on topic of candida can be found at https://www.youtube.com/@canxida

Candida Overgrowth Quiz & Survey

You can take our candida overgrowth quiz here: https://quiz.yeastinfection.org/

Facebook: https://www.facebook.com/people/CanXida/100085663200612/

Instagram: https://www.instagram.com/canxidaguthealth/

Email: support@canxida.com

Phone: +1 (888) 508-3171

Laboratories

For Comprehensive Digestive Stool Analysis testing please contact Doctor's Data. Be sure to mention Dr. Eric Bakker, Candida Crusher. You can read all about this test in Chapter 3 - Diagnosing, Identifying & Testing for Candida Yeast Infections

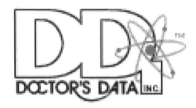

Doctor's Data, Inc.
3755 Illinois Avenue
St. Charles, IL 60174-2420
U.S.A

Customer Service
E-mail: inquiries@doctorsdata.com
Phone: 800.323.2784 (USA & Canada)
0871.218.0052 (United Kingdom)
630.377.8139 (Elsewhere)
Fax: 630.587.7860

For Food Allergy Testing please contact US Biotek. Be sure to mention Dr. Eric Bakker, Candida Crusher. You can read all about the Food Allergy Test in Chapter 3 - Diagnosing, Identifying & Testing for Candida Yeast Infections

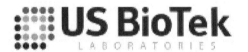

US BioTek Laboratories
13500 Linden Ave North
Seattle, WA 98133
USA
E-mail: http://www.usbiotek.com/Contact_Info.php
Phone: 206.365.1256
Fa: 206.363.8790

Appendix A:

There are many excellent books and research papers on yeast infection and natural health available, here are some of my favorites, if you want to learn more then you may wish to read them yourself. You may think that these books are old, but some of the best books on candida were written in the 1980's.

Adrenal Fatigue, The 21ˢᵗ Century Stress Syndrome By Dr. James L. Wilson D.C, N.D., PhD. 2001. Paperback 362 pages. Publisher: Smart Publications, CA, USA.

Allergies and Candida, with the 21st Century Solution, by S. Rochlitz, Human Ecology Balancing Sciences Inc., New York, 1988.

An Update On The Yeast Syndrome by Trowbridge, JP, Health News & Review,1992; 2: 10.

Candida - A Twentieth Century Disease by S. Lorenzani, Keats Publishing Inc., Connecticut, 1986.

Candida and Candidiasis by Richard A. Calderone (Editor) January 2002. Hardcover: 472 pages Publisher: American Soc. for Microbiology. USA.

Candida, The Symptoms, The Causes, The Cure by Dr. Luc De Shepper. Full of Life Publishers, 1986. Paperback, 176 pages.

Candida Albicans: Could Yeast Be Your Problem?
By Leon Chaitow September 1998. Paperback: 150 pages
Publisher: Inner Traditions Int. Ltd. USA.

Candida Can Be Beaten By Richard Turner and Elizabeth Simonsen, 1985. Paperback: 94 pages. Publisher Oidium Books, Australia.

Candida-Related Complex: What Your Doctor Might Be Missing
By Authors: Christine Winderlin, With Keith Sehnert
October 1996. Paperback, 303 pages. Publisher: Taylor Publishing Company. USA.

Chronic Candidiasis: Your Natural Guide to Healing with Diet, Vitamins, Minerals, Herbs, Exercise, and Other Natural Methods
By Michael T. Murray, Jennifer Basye Sander
2000. Paperback, 192 pages. Publisher: Crown Publishing Group. USA.

Chronic Fatigue Syndrome and The Yeast Connection by William G. Crook, MD, June 1992. Publisher Professional Books. USA.

Complete Candida Yeast Guidebook: Everything You Need to Know about Prevention, Treatment and Diet. By Jeanne Marie Martin. 2000 REVISED
Paperback, 528 pages. Publisher: Crown Publishing Group. USA.

Dr. James Wilson D.C, N.D, PhD. – Personal correspondence

Fatigue by L. Chaitow, Thorsons, London, 1988.

Feast Without Yeast: 4 Stages to Better Health.
By Bruce Sermon M.D., Ph.D. and Lori Kornblum. 1999. Paperback: 386 pages. Publisher: Wisconsin Institute of Nutrition, LLP. USA.

Hard To Stomach By Dr. John McKenna, 2002.
Paperback: 164 pages. Publisher Gill & Macmillan Ltd. Ireland.

Learning About Chronic Fatigue Syndrome Jesop C: Bolles EB, editor. NewYork, NY: Dell Medical, 1990. USA

Metabolic Abnormalities in Patients with Chronic Candidiasis: The Acetaldehyde Hypothesis. Orion Truss. J Orthomolecular Psych. 1984;13(2):66-93.

Natural Alternatives To Antibiotics By Dr. John McKenna, 1998. Paperback: 178 pages. Publisher Gill & Macmillan Ltd. Ireland.

Relief From Candida By Greta Sichel ND DO and Michael Sichel ND DO, 1990. Paperback: 131 pages. Publisher Sally Milner Publishing Pty. Ltd. Australia.

Relief Without Drugs By Dr. Ainslie Meares, M.D., D.P.M., 1974 Paperback: 191 pages. Publisher Fontana Books. Great Britain.

Nutrition and Candida Albicans By Dr. Leo Galland 1986 ed. J. Bland. New Canaan. Keats Pub.

Nutritional Factors In The Etiology Of The Premenstrual Tension Syndromes, by Abraham, GE, Journal of Reproductive Medicine, 1983; 28: 447-464.

Nutritional Medicine by Davies, S, Stewart, A, Pan Books, London, 1987.

Probiotics by Chaitow, L, Trenev, N, Thorsons, London , 1990.

Textbook of Medical Physiology by Guyton, AC, W.B. Saunders Co., Philadelphia , 1981.

The Candida Cure: Yeast, Fungus & Your Health by Ann Boroch, CNC. 2009. Softcover. 178 pages. Quintessential Healing Publishing, Los Angeles. USA.

Trace Elements, Hair Analysis and Nutrition by Passwater, RA, Cranton, EM, Keats Publishing Inc., Connecticut, 1983.

The Health Forum: Yeast, Parasites and Bacteria by Polly Hattemer November 2002. Paperback: 179 pages Publisher: Health Reflections Book Corp. USA.

The Lactic Acid Bacteria - Their Role in Human Health, by Plummer, N, BioMed Publications, West Midlands , 1992.

The Official Patient's Sourcebook on Oropharyngeal Candidiasis: A Revised and Updated Directory for the Internet Age By James N. Parker, M.D. (Editor), and Phillip M. Parker, Ph.D.(Editor)
August 2002. Paperback, 156 pages. Publisher: ICON Health Publications Series: Official Patient Guides. USA.

The Super Supplements Bible, by Rosenbaum ME, Bosco, D, Thorsons, London 1987.

The Yeast Connection Handbook: How Yeasts Can Make You Feel Sick All Over and the Steps You Need to Take to Regain Your Health By William G. Crook, MD Re-issue edition January 1999.
Paperback: 276 pages Publisher: Professional Books, Tn., USA.

The Yeast Connection: A Medical Breakthrough by William G. Crook, MD, James H. Brodsky October 1986. Publisher: Vintage Books

The Yeast Syndrome: How To Help Your Doctor Identify and Treat the Real Cause of Your Yeast-Related Illness   by John Parks Trowbridge, MD
November 1986. Softcover. Publisher: Bantam Books. USA.

The Missing Diagnosis By Orion C. Truss, 1983
Paperback: 175 pages. Publisher: The Missing Diagnosis . USA.

Victims of Thrush and Cystitis By Angela Kilmartin 1986.
Paperback: 198 pages. Publisher: Arrow Books Ltd. England.

Yeast Free And Healthy By Richard Turner and Elizabeth Simonsen, 1987. Paperback: 132 pages. Publisher Penguin Books. Australia.

Zinc and other Micro-Nutrients by Pfeiffer, CC Keats Publishing Inc., Connecticut , 1978.

REFERENCES

Made in the USA
Coppell, TX
12 June 2025

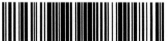

50590891R00393